Contraceptive Technology

16th Revised Edition

Robert A. Hatcher, MD, MPH
James Trussell, PhD
Felicia Stewart, MD
Gary K. Stewart, MD, MPH
Deborah Kowal, MA, PA
Felicia Guest, MPH, CHES
Willard Cates, Jr., MD, MPH
Michael S. Policar, MD, MPH

IRVINGTON PUBLISHERS, INC.
NEW YORK

Irvington Publishers, Inc.
Executive Offices: 522 E. 82nd St., Suite 1, New York, NY 10028
Customer service and warehouse in care of: Integrated Distribution Services
195 McGregor St., Manchester, NH 03102
(603) 669-5933

Editing and manuscript preparation: Deborah Kowal, MA

Proofreading and indexing: Marella Synovec, BA

Cover illustration: Digital Impact Design

Design and production: Octal Publishing, Inc.
                           8E Industrial Way
                           Salem, NH 03079

Library of Congress Catalogue Card Number: 78-641585

ISSN 0091-9721

ISBN 0-8290-3171-5 (Paperback)
ISBN 0-8290-3173-1 (Cloth)

1 3 5 7 9 10 6 4 2

Printed in the United States of America.

The paper used in this publication meets the minimum requirements of American National Standard for Information Sciences — Permanence of Paper for Printed Library Materials, ANSI Z39.48-1984.

Preface

> It seems inartistic and sordid to insert a pessary or a suppository in anticipation of the sexual act. But it is far more sordid to find yourself several years later burdened down with half a dozen unwanted children, helpless, starved, shoddily clothed, dragging at your skirt, yourself a dragged out shadow of the woman you once were.
>
> Margaret Sanger
> *Family Limitation*
> *11th Ed.,* undated

How quaint! we think. How outmoded in prose style, in politics, and in science! For family planners in the 1990s, Margaret Sanger's pioneering work in the early part of this century evokes our gratitude and admiration, but do we really place ourselves along a continuum with her? After all, look at what has happened since her day:

- For the couple with no STD concerns, contraception (and pregnancy anxiety) need no longer be linked in time and place with lovemaking. Oral contraceptives, implants, injectables, IUDs, and sterilization allow Margaret Sanger's "inartistic and sordid" disruptions to be avoided.

- The status of women has improved in this culture, and reproductive autonomy has become an even more politicized issue. The actions of lawmakers, lobbyists, and scientists keep these issues in flux: Just how much reproductive autonomy do we as a society want a woman to have? Many of us in reproductive health care have spent our entire professional lives with safe, legal abortion as a given. Others of us will never forget what it was like, before 1973, to tell a woman she was pregnant when she did not want to be.

- Human sexuality has become medicalized in the wake of the work by Masters and Johnson. More than any other health care professionals, family planners are likely to feel at home in helping patients connect the feelings and practices of their sexual lives with their health and well-being. Even personal sexuality is politicized in the 1990s, and we are asked to examine our sensitivity to personal and cultural variations in sexual expression and to find ways to be helpful to our patients without "my way is the right way" overtones.

- Our reproductive health care system designed for adults has struggled to meet the needs of adolescents as well. All methods of family planning require some degree of planning and communication skill, and teens often begin their sexual explorations long before these developmental skills are in place. We have begun to ask ourselves how we may help our patients who are too young to plan ahead effectively.
- The impact of personal reproductive decision making on global population growth is well understood. Thoughtful policy makers struggle to understand the consequences of population size and growth and the implications of reproductive freedom. A few leaders espouse a strength-in-numbers policy; a few promote family size limitation. Many link family planning not with population growth but instead with better health of women and children.

It is sometimes hard to sense the continuum that links us with our foremother and her co-workers in Brooklyn 75 years ago. In one sense, however, we meet each other across the years in absolute accord:

> The waste of life seemed utterly senseless. One by one worried, sad, pensive, and aging faces marshaled themselves before me in my dreams, sometimes appealingly, sometimes accusingly.

Margaret Sanger
An Autobiography
W.W. Norton, New York
1938, p. 89

We must first and foremost be about the business of helping our patients stay alive. As Margaret Sanger knew, the most adverse consequence of sexual intimacy is not pregnancy, it is death. In her day the villains were hemorrhage, puerperal fever, and syphilis. While unwanted pregnancy remains with us, our villains today are the viral pathogens, not only HIV but also HBV, HPV, HSV, and whatever new viruses find us next week or next year. With every patient, every visit, we must explore the viral STD issues, raising awareness, teaching appropriate risk-reduction skills, easing access to testing and diagnosis, arranging treatment of the highest quality for our infected patients, and modeling compassion and respect. Reproductive health is our chosen turf, and this sad, hard part of it is ours as well. Margaret Sanger would do no less.

The Authors
Atlanta, Georgia
Sacramento, California
Princeton, New Jersey

Dedication

Twelve years. That's a long time to withstand the squeeze on family planning funding, staff size, legislation, and political support. Thus, we welcome the new leadership to Washington, one that infuses new hope and new promise for our field of family planning and reproductive health care. For this, we are grateful.

However, we would not be able to respond to such rebounding optimism were it not for those individuals and organizations that held the field together over those difficult dozen years. It is to these wonderfully stubborn, never-say-die people that we dedicate this 16th edition:

- To our readers who provided the best of care despite a political climate hostile to family planning and STD management.
- To the bold souls in government who fought to protect a politically unpopular stance in favor of birth control, condoms, and abortion. We think in particular of courageous Title X family planning regional program consultants.

A few service-delivery organizations deserve special notice:

- State health departments. Often relegated to crowded, unrenovated buildings, professional staff continued to reach out to the women and men who had little access to other forms of reproductive health care.
- Feminist Women's Health Centers. Withstanding some of the most aggressive "rightist" campaigns, the physicians, nurses, and support staff endured and held their ground.
- Planned Parenthood. PPFA and its affiliates have been the voice and the symbol for our profession: taking the blows, acting as the diplomat, delivering desperately needed services.

You have our deepest gratitude. Onward.

The Authors

Robert A. Hatcher, MD, MPH
Director, Family Planning Program, Grady Memorial Hospital
Professor of Gynecology and Obstetrics
Emory University School of Medicine

James Trussell, PhD
Professor of Economics and Public Affairs
Director, Office of Population Research
Associate Dean, Woodrow Wilson School of Public Health and International Affairs
Princeton University

Felicia H. Stewart, MD
Gynecologist, Sutter Medical Group
Director of Research, Sutter Medical Foundation
Staff Physician, Planned Parenthood of Sacramento Valley
Sacramento, California

Gary K. Stewart, MD, MPH
Medical Director, Planned Parenthood of Sacramento Valley
Clinical Associate Professor Obstetrics and Gynecology
University of California Davis School of Medicine
Instructor, School of Public Health
University of California Berkeley

Deborah Kowal, MA, PA
Consultant, Reproductive Health Communications
Adjunct Assistant Professor of International Health
Emory University School of Public Health

Felicia Guest, MPH, CHES
Deputy Director for Training
Emory AIDS Training Network
Emory University School of Medicine

Willard Cates, Jr., MD, MPH
Director, Division of Training
Centers for Disease Control and Prevention
Adjunct Professor of Epidemiology and Biostatistics
Emory University School of Public Health
Adjunct Professor of Community Health and Preventive Medicine
Morehouse School of Medicine

Michael S. Policar, MD, MPH
Vice President for Medical Affairs
Planned Parenthood Federation of America, Inc.

Table of Contents

List of Tables

List of Figures

Sexuality and Reproductive Health

- Sexual feelings and sexual practices are inseparable aspects of reproductive health.
- Most patients appreciate having a safe forum for discussing, learning, and problem solving about sex.
- Understanding sexual behavior is critical for designing interventions that will reduce unintended pregnancy and STD risk taking.

- Few solid and generalizable data on sexual practices exist on which to base health interventions. Virtually no generalizable information is available on same-gender sexual practices.
- Safer sex guidance and help with a contraceptive choice can be conveyed only with good history-taking skills and comfort with explicit sexual information.

Sexuality and family planning are interdependent. Sexuality has to do with identity, roles, relationships, perceptions, and expectations, as well as biologic functions. The choice of a contraceptive, the actual use of the chosen method, the planning of a family, and the use of appropriate safer sex practices are more than pragmatic intellectual decisions and are deeply affected by the individual's feelings about sexuality and sense of self. Family planning is a very small aspect of sexuality. The technology of contraception is a significant part, but only a part, of family planning (see Figure 1-1). Family planning practitioners have a unique opportunity to supply sexual counseling services to patients who might otherwise have no readily available resource for help.

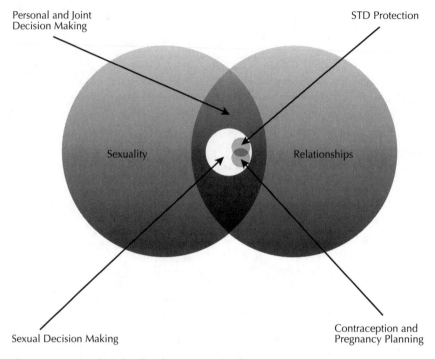

Personal and Joint
Decision Making

STD Protection

Sexuality

Relationships

Sexual Decision Making

Contraception and
Pregnancy Planning

Figure 1-1 Sexuality, family planning, and safer sex

Sexual Behavior Patterns in the United States

Human sexual interaction is surely the least understood, least investigated behavior in daily life, so family planning practitioners are thus placed at a serious disadvantage. Solid information on contraceptive use during vaginal heterosexual intercourse yields knowledge about contraceptive failure and pregnancy risk taking. Solid information on heterosexual and same-gender sexual practices (anal, vaginal, and oral intercourse) and partner networks (who does what with whom and when) yields knowledge about the transmission of STDs, including HIV. Understanding the psychological and social reasons for sexual behaviors is necessary for designing effective interventions for reducing risk taking with respect to pregnancy and infection. Understanding and combatting STD transmission can be even more difficult than understanding and combatting unintended pregnancy—the sexual behaviors that result in an STD are more varied and the sexual networks extend beyond the present into the past.

MYTHS, NONFACTS, AND FAKE KNOWLEDGE ABOUT ADULT SEXUAL BEHAVIORS

Our understanding of sexual behavior patterns in the United States is not likely to improve in the near future. Two nationally representative surveys of sexual behaviors—one of adults and the other of adolescents—were quashed by Secretary of Health and Human Services Louis Sullivan in 1991, despite the fact that research proposals were given very high priority by peer review panels at the National Institutes of Health.

In the absence of nationally representative surveys, research quackery abounds. So-called "surveys" have been conducted by women's and men's magazines and by others using invalid and unreliable survey instruments; results cannot be generalized to any defined population. Those who respond to such surveys constitute self-selected samples whose behaviors almost certainly differ substantially from behaviors of typical persons. For example, in a chapter on high-risk sexual practices in a standard reference volume on AIDS, these flawed statistics are cited as facts that pertain to Americans:[15]

1. Fifty-nine percent of males have experienced fellatio and 58% of females have experienced cunnilingus.[21,22]

2. Forty-three percent of married females have experienced anal intercourse, and 21% have anal intercourse occasionally or often.[41]

3. Among gay males, 80% and 69% (incorrectly cited as 71% and 54%) experienced insertive and receptive anal intercourse, respectively, in the past year.[5]

4. Thirty-six percent of males and 39% of females have engaged in anilingus.[26]

In addition, the latest Hite report claims that 70% of women married more than 5 years are having sex outside their marriages.[18] Another study claims that 26% of husbands and 21% of wives have had at least one outside sexual partner; 8% of husbands and 4% of wives have had six or more outside sexual partners.[7] The deficiencies of these and other studies that have produced "the penumbra of nonfacts and fake knowledge that informs the media and the public" were recently addressed in a report issued by the National Academy of Sciences,[44] especially the appendix to that volume by Smith.

WHAT (LITTLE) IS KNOWN ABOUT SEXUAL BEHAVIORS

With few exceptions, solid information about sexual behavior that does exist is limited to results of questions included in surveys primarily devoted to other topics, such as general social, family, or fertility surveys.

Premarital Heterosexual Intercourse

Heterosexual intercourse among teenagers has become common. As shown in Figure 1-2, the proportion of females having had premarital intercourse has risen dramatically over time: by age 15, from 4% of those born in the mid-1940s to 14% of those born in the early 1970s; by age 17, from 13% of those born in the mid-1940s to 40% of those born in the early 1970s. The number of premarital sexual partners has also increased over time, and less and less of the premarital experience is confined to the person who will become the spouse.

Because age at marriage has risen over the same period, one might speculate that the timing of first intercourse has remained constant, with intercourse that would formerly have occurred within marriage being replaced by premarital intercourse. However, as also demonstrated in Figure 1-2, the proportion of *all* females (regardless of marital status) having had intercourse at each age has also risen over time: by age 15, from 5% of those born in the mid-1940s to 14% of those born in the early 1970s; by age 17, from 20% of those born in the mid-1940s to 41% of those born in the early 1970s.[43]

Percentages of never-married adolescents having had sexual intercourse by age, race, and gender, derived from the 1988 National Survey of Adolescent Males (NSAM) and the 1988 National Survey of Family Growth (NSFG), are shown in Figure 24-3 in the chapter on Adolescent Sexual Behavior, Pregnancy, and Childbearing.

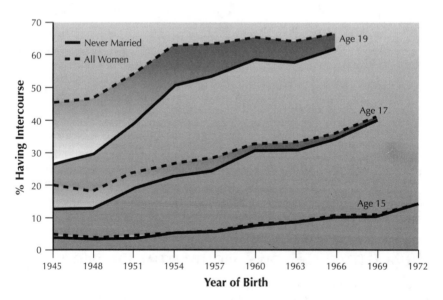

Source: Trussell and Vaughan (1991).

Figure 1-2 Percentage of women having intercourse by their 15th, 17th, and 19th birthday, obtained from retrospective reports in the 1988 NSFG

Lifetime Number of Partners and Number of Partners in the Past Year

One of the public health messages concerning STD and HIV risk reduction is to limit the number of sexual partners. As shown in Table 1-1, the majority of women reported having had more than one male sexual partner during their lifetime. Of particular interest in Table 1-2 are the percentages of married as well as unmarried persons having had more than one partner during the past year and the percentage of married persons who reported having no sexual partners in the past year.

Female respondents in the 1988 National Survey of Family Growth were asked whether they had changed their sexual behavior in seven specific ways (stopped having sex altogether, sex as often, sex other than heterosexual intercourse, sex with more than one man, sex with men not known well, sex with bisexual men, or sex with men who use needles to take drugs) since hearing about AIDS. Overall, 3% of married and 31% of unmarried women reported at least one change in their behavior.[a, 31]

Project Hope conducted a survey of 1,939 persons aged 16-50 in 1988.[46] Among males surveyed, 21.3% reported that they had reduced their number of sexual partners during the 5 years prior to the survey. Also among males, 5.9% reported having one or more partners who were commercial sex workers during the 5 years preceding the survey; of this group 7.7% reported that they had changed their behavior by no longer having intercourse with commercial sex workers.

Anal Intercourse

Unprotected anal intercourse is associated with an increased risk of STD and HIV infection. Results are available from only two nationally representative studies to estimate the prevalence of this behavior. In the Project Hope survey, 6.8% of females reported having unprotected anal intercourse in the 5 years preceding the survey, as did 16.3% of males (with females or males).[46] In the 1991 National Survey of Men (NSM), only 20% of men aged 20-39 reported having ever engaged in anal intercourse; of these, almost 50% had anal sex with only one partner in their lifetime.[6]

---

[a] Unfortunately, due to the wording of the questions, it is difficult to interpret the responses with any degree of precision. For example, the answers at best indicate the number of women who have changed their behaviors. Because one cannot assess the number who were at risk, one cannot determine what fraction of women at risk changed their behaviors. Moreover, it is not possible to know exactly what behaviors were changed. For example, when a woman responds to the question of whether she has limited sexual intercourse to one partner since hearing about AIDS, does she have in mind more than one partner in the same instant, more than one partner since approximately 1980, or alternating partners during some particular period of time?

Table 1-1 Lifetime number of male sexual partners of women, by current marital status, age, and race reported in the 1988 National Survey of Family Growth

		% **Reporting Number of Male Partners**									
	n	0	1	2	3	4	5	6	7–10	11+	mean
White											
Age 20–24	743	14	27	14	13	6	8	3	10	6	3.6
Single	406	24	20	13	10	5	7	3	12	7	3.7
Married	284	0	41	18	16	7	7	2	5	4	3.2
Post-Married	53	0	18	6	22	8	16	8	18	5	4.9
Age 25–29	960	5	28	12	13	9	9	4	11	9	5.1
Single	214	18	8	9	14	10	8	2	18	13	6.9
Married	622	0	39	13	13	9	9	4	6	7	3.9
Post-Married	124	0	12	10	14	12	11	9	18	16	7.3
Age 30–34	1,049	2	30	12	11	8	10	5	10	12	5.8
Single	111	13	15	9	7	9	6	4	17	20	9.3
Married	788	0	37	14	12	7	9	5	8	9	4.6
Post-Married	150	0	7	8	13	12	18	7	14	20	8.5
Black											
Age 20–24	479	7	20	13	18	11	10	5	9	7	4.7
Single	375	9	17	12	19	12	9	4	10	8	5.0
Married	80	0	33	19	15	7	14	7	5	0	3.0
Post-Married	24	0	6	10	24	8	14	14	10	14	6.8
Age 25–29	544	3	14	12	15	13	17	6	13	8	5.0
Single	312	6	5	10	13	12	21	7	16	8	5.7
Married	163	0	32	14	19	11	9	4	6	8	3.9
Post-Married	69	0	5	11	12	23	19	6	20	5	5.3
Age 30–34	531	2	11	12	16	16	15	8	13	8	5.5
Single	169	6	6	9	11	17	19	8	17	8	5.8
Married	216	0	22	20	18	13	12	6	7	3	3.8
Post-Married	146	0	2	5	19	18	15	12	16	14	7.7

Source: Trussell and Vaughan (1991).

Notes: (1) Row percentages may not add to 100 due to rounding.

(2) Percentages are computed with weighted observations; *n* is the number of unweighted observations.

Table 1-2 Number of sexual partners in the past year by gender, marital status, and age reported in the 1987 Telephone Survey conducted by the *Los Angeles Times* and the 1988 Personal Interview Survey conducted by the National Opinion Research Center

	% Reporting Number of Partners in Past Year			
	None	**1**	**2**	**3+**
Unmarried Men				
18–24	16.5	32.3	10.5	40.7
25–34	12.4	52.9	7.9	26.9
35–49	13.5	39.7	18.2	28.5
50–64	22.3	41.3	7.5	29.0
65+	74.0	17.2	4.6	4.2
Unmarried Women				
18–24	19.0	52.8	12.7	15.5
25–34	13.2	65.3	13.6	7.9
35–49	25.5	54.9	12.1	7.5
50–64	60.2	29.9	8.8	1.2
65+	93.7	6.3	0.0	0.0
Married Men				
18–24	0.0	83.6	2.5	13.9
25–34	1.0	92.7	2.3	4.0
35–49	4.6	90.7	1.7	3.1
50–64	5.9	91.7	0.9	1.6
65+	17.3	78.4	2.3	1.9
Married Men				
18–24	1.7	93.6	3.7	1.0
25–34	0.5	97.8	1.2	0.5
35–49	3.5	94.2	0.4	1.9
50–64	16.3	83.0	0.2	0.5
65+	21.7	77.5	0.1	0.7

Source: Turner et al. (1989), Table 2–3.

Notes: (1) Row percentages may not add to 100 due to rounding.

(2) Entries in the table were estimated by fitting a log-linear model to the pooled data from both surveys. Observed discrepancies between surveys are attributable to minor differences in the fractions of persons with no or one sexual partner.

In 1989, a representative sample of the population aged 18-54 years in Dallas County, TX, completed an anonymous questionnaire containing questions on selected sexual behaviors. In that survey, 4.5% of males and 19.9% of females reported receptive anal intercourse since January 1978 and 2.0% of males and 12.2% of females reported receptive anal intercourse during the year preceding the survey.[38]

A survey of first-year college students in Canada revealed that among women who had ever had intercourse, 18.6% had experienced anal intercourse.[27] Dramatic decreases in the frequency of unprotected receptive anal intercourse have been recorded among participants in several gay male cohort studies in large cities; however, relapses are common. Little information exists about younger gay men.[11,14,23,30,44]

Same-gender Sexual Behavior

Family planning practitioners have long understood that presuming heterosexuality in the reproductive health care setting can compromise care. However, we have little reliable data on same-gender practices and almost none on women. This section describes essentially all the generalizable studies.

- An analysis of five probability surveys of American men between 1970 and 1990 revealed that a minimum of 5%-7% of men have had some same-gender sexual contact during adulthood and that most of these contacts were infrequent.[37] Only one-quarter to one-half of those who reported same-gender contact during adulthood also reported having a male sexual partner during the year preceding the survey. A majority of men who reported same-gender contacts in adulthood also reported female sexual contacts contemporaneous with or subsequent to male contacts.

- In the Project Hope survey, 4.4% of males aged 16-24, 5.9% of males aged 25-34, and 3.5% of males aged 35-50 reported that they had sex with one or more men during the 5-year period preceding the survey.[46]

- Data from the General Social Survey (1988-1991) indicate that between 4% and 6% of adults have had same-gender sex. *Males:* 94.0% have had exclusively female partners, 4.8% have had both male and female partners, and 1.1% have had exclusively male partners. In the year before the survey, 97.5% had exclusively female partners, 0.5% had both male and female partners, and 2.0% had exclusively male partners. *Females:* 95.9% have had exclusively male partners, 3.5% have had both male and female partners, and 0.6% have had exclusively female partners. In the year before the survey, 99.2% had exclusively male partners, 0.1% had both male and female partners, and 0.7% had exclusively female partners.[32]

- A 1988 Harris poll found that among respondents aged 16–50, 4.4% of men reported having had a male sex partner and 3.6% of women reported having a female sex partner in the previous 5 years.[42]
- The 1991 National Survey of Men (NSM) found that only 2.3% of males aged 20-39 reported having had any same-gender sexual contact during the preceding 10 years and that only 1.1% reported exclusively same-gender sexual activity during that time.[6] It is possible that lower proportions were found in the NSM because the personal interviews with male respondents were conducted by female interviewers.

Before the time of the studies described here, health care providers could turn only to suspect data from the 1940s, because no other U.S. data existed. In 1948, the Kinsey report stated that 37% of the total male population had an overt homosexual experience to the point of orgasm between adolescence and old age, that 10% of males are more or less exclusively homosexual for at least 3 years between the ages of 16 and 65, and that 4% of white males are exclusively homosexual throughout their lives.[21] There are many reasons to doubt these figures, not the least of which is that the sample contained a disproportionate fraction of men who were or had been in prisons or jails.

Use of Male Condoms

One of the most important public health messages concerning STD and HIV risk reduction is to use condoms. Data on adolescent males indicate that condom use is much more widespread than do the data on adolescent females. In the 1988 NSAM, 57% of sexually active teenage males aged 15-19 reported use of a condom at last intercourse.[39] In contrast, only 31% of teenage females reported condom use at last intercourse in the 1988 NSFG.[43] Either males overreport use of condoms because they know that it is the socially responsible answer or females underreport condom use when a condom is used as an adjunct to another method.

Women may be slightly more likely to view condoms as birth control than as STD protection. In the 1988 NSFG, 4.07 million women reported currently using the condom as a contraceptive only. An additional 4.24 million women reported use of the condom as an STD prophylaxis but did not report use of the condom as a contraceptive, and 2.08 million used the condom for both purposes. Altogether 10.4 million women (of a total of 57.9 million women aged 15-44) reported use of condoms.[25]

The fractions of women using condoms as a contraceptive among those at risk of pregnancy were 30.6% among women aged 15-19 and 16.6% among women aged 20-24. The proportions of women using condoms as a contraceptive among those at risk of pregnancy increased between 1982

Sexual Behavior Patterns in the United States

and 1988 by 13.2 percentage points among women aged 15-19 and by 5.2 percentage points among women aged 20-24.[43] In the Project Hope survey, 21.1% of males and 22.1% of females reported that they had started to use condoms during the 5 years before the survey.[46]

In the 1991 NSM, 23.1% of married males and 44.9% of single males aged less than 30 reported using a condom at least once during the 4 weeks preceding the interview; the corresponding figures among males aged 30-39 were 16.2% and 27.6%, respectively.[40] In the 4 weeks preceding the interview, 10% of males had engaged in sexual activity that entailed risk of HIV infection; of these only 45% had used a condom during that period.

It would appear that in the U.S. culture, neither pregnancy risk nor STD risk compels couples to use condoms consistently. Lack of normative cultural modeling, personal denial of risk, fear of sexual awkwardness, fear of diminished pleasure, and fear of displeasing a partner may all contribute to these disheartening numbers.

Nonvoluntary Sexual Activity

Data from the 1987 National Survey of Children reveal that 12.7% of white females, 8.0% of black females, 1.9% of white males and 6.1% of black males had experienced nonvoluntary sexual intercourse by age 20.[33] One of every eight adult women surveyed in the National Women's Study reported that she had been the victim of at least one forcible rape sometime in her lifetime. Four in 10 rape victims have been raped more than once. At least 1.4 million women are raped each year.[34] Comparable data for adult males do not exist.

Lying to Obtain Sex

Public health practitioners routinely advise clients to avoid partners with a high risk of having an STD or HIV and to do so by questioning potential partners about their sexual histories. Unfortunately, these questions may not be met by truthful answers. A survey of 18-to 25-year-old students attending college in Southern California revealed that 47% of males and 42% of females would understate their number of previous sexual partners in order to have intercourse, 43% of men and 34% of women would not disclose a single episode of sexual infidelity in order to maintain a sexual relationship, and 20% of males and 4% of females would lie about having a negative HIV test in order to have sex.[9]

In the face of data such as these, it seems especially important to teach patients that not all sexual risks are ascertainable, and that abstinence, male and female condoms, and other safer sex practices can protect even from hidden risks.

Additional Information Needed: AIDS Modeling

Just how far our knowledge of sexual behavior falls short of what we need to know is best illustrated by a simple model of HIV (or any STD) transmission. Although simple, the model is a powerful tool for understanding whether a sexually transmitted infection will become epidemic or instead die out: $R = D \times I \times M$.[1]

R = Reproduction rate of the disease. The number of additional infections that will result from a single new infection. If R<1, the disease will eventually die out because each new infection fails to replace itself. If R>1, the disease will grow.

D = Number of years that an infected person remains infectious.

I = Probability that an infected partner will transmit the infection to an uninfected partner, depending on the specific sexual behaviors practiced, precautions taken to reduce risk, duration of the partnership, and other cofactors.

M = Effective average rate of acquiring new uninfected partners per year.[b]

One of the most powerful results of this model highlights the key role that those who have a comparatively large number of partners play in the initial spread of infection. Those few with many new partners ensure that infections will spread more rapidly. This simple model assumes that every uninfected person in the population has an equal probability of being selected as a sexual partner of an infected person. More realistic models must account for sexual networks. For example, if a population has two groups of persons and no person in group one has sexual intercourse with any person in group two, then regardless of the sexual behaviors *within* the two groups, no infection could be transmitted *between* the two groups. This distinction explains why infection can spread very rapidly in some groups while hardly affecting others.

While our knowledge of what U.S. couples actually do together is limited, we can use what data we do have about premarital heterosexual intercourse, numbers of partners, anal intercourse, same-gender sex, and use of male condoms to focus and enhance family planning and safer sex services. Our understanding of human sexual physiology on the individual level—arousal, response, and dysfunction—derives from pioneering research in the 1960s and 1970s. Reproductive health care providers are often very effective counselors on sexual issues for patients.

---

[b] M is not the average number of new sexual partners per person μ but instead is $\mu + \sigma^2/\mu$, where σ^2 is the variance of the number of new sexual partners per year. M is the number of partners associated with the average new partnership, which exceeds the average number of new partners per person, just as the size of the city in which the average person resides exceeds the average size of cities. The lesson is that both mean and variance matter. For example, among unmarried males aged 18–24, $\mu = 2.7$, but M = 8.4 ($\sigma^2 = 15.5$).

HUMAN SEXUAL PHYSIOLOGY

Sexual arousal may be caused by a dream, a fantasy, a memory, or any of the five senses: taste, smell, sight, hearing, or touch. Preferred forms of sexual expression may differ for each individual, for the same individual with different partners, or at different times with the same partner. Couples can enjoy a wide range of intimate sexual expressions—from holding hands, hugging, kissing, massage and dancing, to mutual masturbation, petting, anal stimulation, oral-genital sex, and the use of mechanical devices such as vibrators. One common factor can be found in all these expressions and that is *touching*. People need touching for nurture, for solace, for expressing simple affection, for communicating, and for sexual gratification. Penile-vaginal intercourse is only one way to touch and to make love, and it is not necessarily the most important way unless pregnancy is desired.

Two physiologic characteristics of sexual excitement are common to all mammals, including humans.

- Engorgement and dilatation of genital and pelvic blood vessels (also sometimes breasts) by means of increased arterial blood supply. This reaction has the secondary effects of penile erection (as cavernous penile bodies become congested with blood) and vaginal lubrication in females (as perivaginal vasculature becomes engorged and vaginal epithelial transudation occurs). Penile erection in men and vaginal lubrication in women are the major indicators of sexual excitement.

- Increased myotonia, or increased voluntary muscle tension. Individuals who undergo sexual excitation tend to display muscle tension, restlessness, voluntary and involuntary movements, thrusting, clasping, and/or grimacing.

Researchers describe four stages of sexual response: excitement, plateau, orgasm, and resolution. Sexual response is quite similar for both sexes (with a few very important differences):[28]

Stage	Sexual Response
Excitement	Pelvic engorgement, erection in males. Lubrication and dilatation of the upper vaginal canal in females. Both men and women have increased muscle tension, increased heart and respiratory rate, and increased blood pressure. Focus of attention is more and more centered on sexual matters.
Plateau	Sustained engorgement, muscle tension, elevated heart and respiratory rates, and elevated blood pressure for a period that may vary from minutes to hours.

Orgasm	Rhythmic contractions of pelvic voluntary and involuntary musculature in both sexes. In men, this action can result in ejaculation of semen. Men and women often experience a transitory change in sensorium (which the French have called "the little death") and a variety of somatic sensations sometimes described as a feeling of warmth arising from the pelvis.[4,16,17] Orgasm is a beginning of relief from tension.
Resolution	Gradual loss of muscle tension, progressive relaxation, and often a sense of drowsiness and contentment. Blood vessels open to drain pelvic and genital engorgement, and gradually (usually over a period of minutes) the individual returns to a nonexcited state.

One significant difference between men and women has to do with the ease of attaining multiple orgasms during a single sexual episode. Women are physiologically capable of moving from plateau to orgasm, back to plateau, and then back to orgasm one or several times.

Men have what is called a refractory period that follows ejaculation. During the refractory period, they have difficulty achieving a second erection, and, after they attain an erection, it may be difficult to have orgasm and ejaculate. The length of the refractory period gradually increases as men grow older. It may be only 5–15 minutes in an 18-year-old; by the age of 60, the refractory period may be 18–24 hours. The length of the refractory period varies widely from one man to another, and it may vary in a single individual according to how erotic the situation seems to be and according to his usual frequency of sexual experiences (the more often the man ejaculates as a usual habit, the shorter the refractory period).

FEMALE RESPONSE AND SENSITIVITY

Virtually any portion of a woman's skin may give pleasurable and exciting sensations when caressed, providing she is willing and not distracted by extraneous thoughts or events. Women tend to be whole-body oriented for sexual touching rather than genitally oriented as men are trained to be. Breast and nipple sensitivity tends to be high in most women, but some women do not find breast caressing particularly arousing.

For most women, the glans and shaft of the clitoris, the inner surfaces of the labia minora, and the first inch and a half of the vagina are the most sexually sensitive areas of all. Indeed, the clitoral head (glans) may be so exceedingly sensitive that direct touch is sometimes or always uncomfortable. Many women enjoy indirect clitoral touch by caressing the clitoral shaft rather than the glans. Women, as men, have (or may acquire) high levels of sexual responsiveness to anal penetration.

The old Freudian argument about clitoral versus vaginal orgasm is essentially dead. Neither is more mature than the other. Orgasms that arise primarily from clitoral stimulation may be perceived as different from orgasms that primarily arise from penile-vaginal thrusting. In fact, many women describe striking differences in their perception in sensation, intensity, and duration of orgasm depending upon how it is achieved (dream, fantasy, kissing, caressing, masturbation, partner manual stimulation, stream of water, oral stimulation, penile-vaginal thrusting, vibrator, anal intercourse, pelvic muscle contractions, etc.). Women vary greatly in what sort of stimulus produces orgasm. It is common to find healthy normal women who are orgasmic by some means, but not orgasmic with penile-vaginal thrusting alone.

Some women have an area of sexual sensitivity felt through the anterior wall of the vagina about halfway between the back of the pubic bone and the cervix. Fairly vigorous intravaginal massage in this area may lead to high levels of sexual excitement. This area has been called the Grafenberg or G spot. Orgasms from G spot stimulation or types of sexual stimulation may result in the rhythmic expulsion of fluid from the urethral meatus at orgasm in some women.[10] The nature of the ejaculate is the subject of some debate. It has been described as being a prostatic-like fluid that differs from urine in color, clarity, and odor and that does not stain.[45] Expulsion of fluid from the urethra at orgasm should be regarded as a normal variant female sexual response and not as an example of urinary incontinence. Usually a folded bath towel under the woman's hips is sufficient to keep sheets and bedclothes from becoming dampened. The source and function of these sexual events remain poorly understood in the mid-1990s.

MALE RESPONSE AND SENSITIVITY

Men tend to be conditioned to focus on genital sexual stimulation rather than whole-body touch arousal. Retraining to be comfortable and to accept and enjoy whole-body stimulation may be a desirable sexual goal for some men. In general, nipple stimulation may be as arousing for men as it is for women. Except for those men who do not respond to nipple caresses and those who deny their sensitivity because of the fear of being unmasculine, the remainder of men are likely to be pleased and excited by nipple stimulation. The sexual sensitivity of male genitalia varies strikingly according to anatomic area and the male's personal perceptions. The sites of highly pleasurable sensitivity (in order of decreasing response to touch) are as follows:

- Area of frenular attachment on ventral surface of penis, just behind the glans
- Coronal ridge of glans
- Urethral meatus
- Shaft of the penis
- Penile base located within the perineal area between the area of scrotal attachment and the anus
- Scrotum and testicles (gentle manipulation only)
- Perianal skin

CONTRACEPTION, SAFER SEX, AND SEXUAL FUNCTION

Fear of Infection

Worry about HIV, herpes, genital warts, and other incurable viral STDs often clouds the sexual experience for couples. It can be discouraging to realize that assuring protection from unwanted pregnancy is only half the battle for couples with any possible STD risk. Some people give up on sex altogether, some manage excellent safer sex techniques, but many more give up on safety. The clinician's task is to help at-risk patients to remain unflagging in their efforts to keep sex pleasurable and infection free, tailoring the advice to the sexual patterns of each individual patient.

Fear of Pregnancy and Infertility

Fear or hope for pregnancy may powerfully affect sexual desire and performance. For men, the subject of pregnancy may cause concerns, but their level of concern tends to be lower than for women. Even among premenarchal, postmenopausal, contracepting, or sterilized women, the fantasy, memory, hope, fear, anticipation, dread, joy, or desperation and despondency of pregnancy have an impact on identity that men generally do not feel. A woman who has more children than she wants may feel that she literally risks the further destruction of her life every time she has penile-vaginal intercourse. An infertile woman may put her feminine identity on the line every month she tries to conceive, and is likely to feel emotionally intimidated by the typical infertility workup.

Instructions to time intercourse around ovulation prove particularly stressful for both partners. Such instructions are likely to precipitate a crisis in performance anxiety as well as power and control conflicts in even well-adjusted couples. After couples begin timed intercourse, the man may experience an inability to achieve or maintain erections and the couple may have major battles. The spontaneity and romantic parts of lovemaking disappear, and couples often panic. Couples trying timed intercourse often need counseling and vacations from performance.

Lactation

In Western civilization, female breasts have four functions:

- Sexual enticement (both visually and tactilely attractive);
- Sexual excitement for the female—tactile stimulation of the breast by hand, mouth, clothing, etc., initiates physiologic sexual responses in most but not all women;
- Female identity for women—size, shape, prominence, and change in breast structure often have powerful and immediate impact on a woman's self-image; and
- Nutrition for infants.

Not surprisingly, these four functions occasionally get intermingled and lead to confusion among men and women. When mammary hypertrophy, nipple enlargement, and areolar darkening take place during pregnancy, men are often simultaneously excited and confused about whether it is all right to be excited by these changes. Some couples may have confusion about the woman as sexual/erotic partner versus the woman as nurturing mother. Women are confused by feelings of sexual excitement and orgasm that sometimes occur during infant nursing and many experience conflict between nurturing and erotic roles. Men who make love to lactating women are confused about whether they may enjoy breasts as erotic objects while milk flows from them and whether they can enjoy breasts as nurturing objects (*i.e.*, to be nursed) as part of erotic play.

Reassure patients about the naturalness of sexual feelings associated with breast appearance and usage. Remind women that if they choose to rely on the lactational amenorrhea method (LAM) as a temporary method of contraception, they must feed their baby on demand, avoid any bottle feedings, and provide minimal supplements by cup or spoon. To avoid pregnancy, they must begin using another method of contraception when they resume menstruation, when they reduce the frequency or duration of breastfeedings, when they introduce bottle feeds, or when their baby turns 6 months old. If they are breastfeeding and providing bottle supplements, remind women to begin using a birth control method no later than the time of their first postpartum exam (which would ideally occur 3 weeks rather than 6 weeks after delivery). See Chapter 17.

Birth Control Pills

Couples who value the fact that pills do not interrupt lovemaking may find it difficult to add condoms or other latex barriers for STD protection.

One of the occasional side effects of oral contraceptives is decreased sex drive (diminished libido) or, more properly, diminution or loss of sexual desire. A woman whose usual sexual response pattern is well established over time (*i.e.*, one who knows herself) is likely to recognize immediately any loss of desire that closely follows the initiation of a new birth control pill as an undesirable effect of the pill. Such patients will usually report their symptom.

From time to time, clinicians are asked to begin young women on birth control pills in anticipation of their first intercourse. Often these young women have very limited or no previous sexual experience but plan to begin intercourse soon and wish to prepare for that time with contraception. A small percentage of these women may have diminished desire as a result of the pill, but in the absence of prior sexual experience they have no basis for comparison. When, after the initiation of regular sexual intercourse, they find themselves less excited, less interested, and less pleased than they had imagined they would be, they often begin to define themselves as sexually neutral rather than blame the lack of desire on birth control pills.

Diaphragms and Other Vaginal Barriers

Many women who request diaphragms are initially uncomfortable with and lack the agility to insert the device covered by slippery contraceptive cream or gel. During attempts to insert it, the diaphragm sometimes takes flight like a pliable Frisbee. A poorly fitted diaphragm may cause discomfort, and certainly distrust, thus inhibiting sexual enjoyment.

Inserting the diaphragm, sponge, or cap before the beginning of a sexual interaction may seem to imply anticipation and expectation of intercourse. On the other hand, carrying the equipment when going out for a date feels uncomfortable for some women, and can certainly alter the negotiation between partners. Inserting the method during precoital play, although still carrying some flavor of deliberate planning and experience, also carries the risk of interrupting a tender and romantic interlude with a purely mechanical task. Some authorities suggest that both partners participate in insertion, but this interaction rarely seems opportune with a new lover. The extra lubrication these products supply is pleasant for some couples and a messy interference for others.

Anxiety about STDs can diminish sexual pleasure with vaginal barrier methods.

Condoms

Some men leak seminal fluid from the urethral meatus when their penis is fully erect. This so-called pre-ejaculatory fluid or lubricating fluid is believed to be largely a secretion of Cowper's glands, small glands that drain into the urethra beneath the prostate. Each drop of this pre-ejaculatory fluid may contain HIV and/or other pathogens (although not motile sperm capable of causing pregnancy).[19,36] For this reason, for couples with any STD risk, a male condom should be put on or a female condom inserted before any vaginal, anal, or oral contact, not just when ejaculation seems imminent. To put on or insert the condom early also makes it easier to include this activity as part of genital foreplay, and couples are less likely to consider it as an interruption of lovemaking.

Some men lose their erection rapidly after ejaculation whereas others maintain a relatively erect penis for some time, perhaps as long as 15–20 minutes. Because even a few minutes of rest and relaxation while the penis is still inside the partner may mean a small flaccid penis for some, all men are encouraged to hold the rim of the male condom at the base of the penis as they withdraw. Doing so tends to prevent the condom from slipping off.

Coitus Interruptus

Although coitus interruptus or withdrawal has definite value as a method of birth control, its utility as a safer sex technique is unknown. It has rather major disadvantages for relational and recreational intercourse. It encourages attention on performance rather than pleasure and encourages spectatoring. Withdrawal requires the man to do the opposite from his usual desire (*i.e.*, pull out and move away from his partner when his desire is to push deeper, clasp, and hold more firmly). For some heterosexual couples, this contraceptive method may leave the woman in a state of high excitement without orgasmic relief. Having separated the partners, withdrawal may not encourage leisurely afterplay. If withdrawal is a couple's usual method of contraception, they should make a special effort to reinstitute sexual play after withdrawal to make sure both partners have achieved gratification and relief of sexual tension.

In adult or X-rated movies the man often withdraws, ejaculates after a few moments of manual stroking, and then rapidly reinserts. It should be noted that this withdrawal is for the purpose of showing the viewer his ejaculation and is not for contraception. Rapid reinsertion when seminal fluid is still in the urethra as well as on the glans and shaft is not a satisfactory technique for contraception. Reinsertion should probably not take place without mechanical cleansing of the male genitalia (washcloth and warm water with or without soap) and urination to flush the urethra.

Abstinence

Couples may achieve satisfaction with sexual abstinence providing both select this alternative as the one that most closely meets their individual needs. A relationship can be almost anything so long as both partners agree on what it is to be. When one partner does not agree to abstinence but does not wish to give up the relationship, then a continuing conflict arises that will have emotional consequences for each individual and for the couple. One or both partner(s) may choose abstinence for contraception, for protection from an STD, as part of sexual aversion, or as a symptom of alcoholism or other addiction, depression, or distraction. The person who feels abandoned because of his/her partner's decision for abstinence may use masturbation as an alternative, may reluctantly accept abstinence also, or may sometimes choose to seek another partner outside of the primary relationship.

The couple practicing sexual abstinence may lose a major method of non-verbal communication in their relationship and may find it difficult to compensate by communicating in less intimate ways. They must make special efforts to maintain or strengthen other forms of communication.

FEMALE AND MALE SEXUAL DYSFUNCTIONS

When anything occurs to distract a person from excitement, then erection (in men), lubrication (in women), and orgasm/ejaculation (in both sexes) may be impeded. Pharmacologic agents that affect the autonomic nervous system or have a potentially sedative effect may cause a change in sexual function. History-taking, laboratory tests, and physical exams are aimed at defining the condition and establishing a differential diagnosis.

LOSS OF DESIRE – MEN AND WOMEN

Problems of sexual desire may be expressed as diminished desire, absent desire with sexual response when stimulated, absent desire with little or no response when stimulated, or aversion. Aversion implies the creation of negative feelings to the point of causing withdrawal from sexual interaction. Aversion may be general or expressed only for some specific ideas, beliefs, or practices. Among people who have diminished desire, inhibiting childhood training and *anticipation* of failure, embarrassment, pain, or inadequacy are as important as actual inhibiting or painful experiences.

In contrast to loss of desire, discrepancies in levels of desire between sexual partners are extremely common. When a relationship has become dysfunctional, one partner often wants sexual intimacy far more often than the other. These exaggerated discrepancies tend to disappear as the partners solve other problems and restore their ability to communicate and negotiate.

Organic disease may negatively affect female sexual responsiveness just as it may interfere with male responsiveness. Estrogen deficiency with secondary vaginal atrophy (whether postsurgical or postmenopausal) may lead to dyspareunia. This condition can often be treated successfully with topical or systemic estrogen therapy if atrophy is not of such excessive duration as to be irreversible. Organic pelvic or genital disease may lead to dyspareunia and eventual secondary loss of desire.

Birth control pills may diminish desire in some women, but diminished desire is more often associated with psychological factors (depression, grief, suppressed anger, histrionic personality, etc.).

Chronic fatigue affects both male and female sexual responsiveness. Any time a primary care-giver parent has a child who is not yet in kindergarten or cares for an elderly parent, then chronic fatigue should be considered as an important factor in her or his problem.

Generally debilitating diseases and conditions such as childbirth, surgery, cancer, chronic dieting, or excessive weight loss may temporarily or permanently diminish desire and responsiveness.

FEMALE SEXUAL DYSFUNCTIONS

Anorgasmia

Anorgasmia may be the result of not yet learning how to have an orgasm (preorgasmia or primary anorgasmia) or of having lost the ability to have an orgasm (secondary anorgasmia). Perhaps 10% of women over age 25 have not yet learned how to have an orgasm.

Primary anorgasmia (preorgasmia). Failing to be orgasmic may be a complication of the sexually inhibiting cultures that are common in Western civilization. Some women are orgasmic during their first sexually exciting experience, and others never learn to have an orgasm. Learning to be orgasmic may occur in preschool female children who learn to masturbate by themselves or are taught by peers, or it may occur in 70- to 80-year-old women who take part in preorgasmic support groups. Sex therapists in general do not believe that women physiologically lack the capacity to learn to be orgasmic. Learning to have a first orgasm is relatively easy; learning to have an orgasm in every desired situation or with high frequency may be less easy for many women.

Women who have primary anorgasmia sometimes have achieved a relatively low level of sexual excitement and may think of intercourse and/or other sexual activities as pleasant. They may get most of their reward from touching, holding, kissing, caressing, attention, and approval. Women who regularly achieve high levels of sexual response without orgasmic release of tension may find the experience frustrating. Emotional irritability, restlessness, and pelvic pain or a heavy pelvic sensation may occur because of vascular engorgement.[29]

In taking a history for the presence or absence of orgasm in women, the fundamental issue is whether the patient has felt high levels of sexual tension or excitement followed by relief of tension and relaxation. Individual descriptions of orgasm are highly variable, and many women may not be able to find words to describe the experience. The characteristic high tension followed by relief and relaxation is an essentially universal indicator of orgasm.

Women who have not yet had an orgasm usually have some combination of the following:

- Sociocultural inhibitions that interfere with normal masturbation experimentation as well as other sorts of sexual experimentation that would otherwise lead to learning.
- Lack of factual knowledge about sex and sexuality that interferes with normal sexual development to a major degree.
- Absence of an adequate role model for a warm, sensuous, emotionally responsive, earthy, knowledgeable woman.
- Extreme religious orthodoxy. Religious devotion, *per se*, is not related to inhibited sexual function, but extreme or neurotic religious belief may well be.
- Lack of opportunity to practice in a safe, secure, socially acceptable, private atmosphere (alone or in a relationship) in a situation that offers approval and support for self-experimentation.
- A partner who cannot or will not provide sexual stimulation.
- A partner who has rapid ejaculation.
- A partner who has primary or secondary erective difficulty.

Of these eight factors the first and second appear to be most important in clinical practice. Learning to become orgasmic may be accomplished alone, with a partner, as a member of a group training class, in couples counseling, or in individual counseling. Excellent guides exist for counselors and patients to use in achieving comfort with their sensuous selves and their sexual selves.[4,16] The opportunity to practice self-stimulation alone and without the distraction of a partner's presence greatly facilitates the learning process for those who can accept self-stimulation. For those who cannot accept self-stimulation, use of a steady or pulsating stream of water (as in a tub or shower-spray attachment) is sometimes acceptable. Vibrators offer powerful stimulation and a ready means of learning to be orgasmic for some women, although it may be difficult for vibrator users to move successfully to less intense forms of stimulation.

Secondary anorgasmia. Secondary anorgasmia is the loss of ability to become orgasmic after some history of orgasmic function in the past. Women who have lost the capacity to have orgasms usually have a causal event close to the time when this capacity was lost. The causal event may be alcoholism, depression, grief, medication, illness, or estrogen deprivation associated with menopause. The causal event may also be something that has violated the patient's sexual value system.[29]

Almost every woman is able to list the things she needs in order to feel all right about herself, her partner, the relationship, and the sexual interaction. These things are roughly divided into biophysical and psychosocial needs. Unless these needs are fulfilled, she is likely to be sexually unresponsive. When an unmet need is recognized and corrected, her responsiveness usually returns. Needs may be as simple as a warm, private, and comfortable place or as complex as trust, love, respect, and warmth.[29]

Situational anorgasmia. Women who are orgasmic in some situations and not in others are situationally anorgasmic. Many women reach orgasm through self-stimulation, a partner's manual or oral stimulation, or using a vibrator, but not from penile-vaginal intercourse. Or a woman may be orgasmic with one partner but not another, or only on vacation, or only with a certain type or amount of foreplay. These common variations should not be thought of as illness or abnormality; they are within the range of normal sexual expression. The patient, however, may wish for a change in her sexual expression and should be offered help and advice to do so.

Encourage a woman with these complaints to explore alone and with her partner those factors that may affect whether or not she is orgasmic, such as fatigue, emotional concerns, feeling pressured to have sex when she is not interested, or her partner's sexual dysfunction. Advice may be offered about (1) improving communication with her partner regarding her needs, (2) avoiding performance anxiety by being aware of this problem, (3) focusing on sensations rather than cerebration, and (4) using voluntary muscle contractions to increase levels of sexual tension.

The female-above position may be recommended for penile-vaginal intercourse, as it may allow for greater stimulation of the clitoris by the penis or symphysis pubis or both, and it allows the woman to control movement better. Aside from this advice, the most helpful technique involves *bridging*.

Bridging is the use of a successful sexual stimulation in conjunction with the desired technique so that the body learns to associate orgasm with the desired technique. If, for example, the woman is readily orgasmic with manual stimulation but not with penile-vaginal thrusting, then she is encouraged to combine the two regularly until her body has learned to associate high levels of excitement and orgasm with thrusting.

Random anorgasmia. Some women are orgasmic, but not in enough instances to satisfy their sense of what is appropriate or desirable. Women who wish for a higher frequency of orgasm may be anxious about performance, distracted, or not using muscle tension to enhance their responsiveness. Often such women seem to have trouble giving up control and allowing themselves to be fully responsive. Therapy can be aimed at helping them give up the need to keep their sexual feelings under control at all times. In other cases, a partner's lack of skill may be a cause.

Dyspareunia

Dyspareunia is penis-in-vagina intercourse that is painful. Clinicians should consider dyspareunia primarily a physical problem rather than an emotional problem until proven otherwise. In most instances, when dyspareunia began, a physical cause was present. When pain from whatever cause occurs, the woman may be distracted from pleasure and excitement, and both vaginal lubrication and vaginal dilatation diminish or disappear.

When the vagina is dry and undilated, penile thrusting is painful, and this pain leads to further loss of pleasure and to distraction. Instead of a self-perpetuating cycle of pleasure, a self-perpetuating cycle of pain is established. The pain that comes from anticipation and expectation of more pain may persist even after the original source of pain (a healing episiotomy, for example) has disappeared.

When taking a history of dyspareunia, therefore, one may identify two different types of problems:

- Dyspareunia *during* the first 2 weeks or so of its manifestation, either as pain on penile insertion or movement of the penis in the vagina (often due to local conditions of vulva or vagina), or as pain on deep penetration of the penis into the vagina, often due to deep pelvic pathology.
- Dyspareunia *after* the first 2 weeks or so of its manifestation, often strongly influenced by a self-perpetuating cycle. The original cause of pain may still exist or may have disappeared, leaving the woman with anticipatory pain associated with a dry, tight vagina and sometimes with vaginismus as well.

Dyspareunia is treated by the following steps:

- Carefully taking a history.
- Carefully examining the pelvis to duplicate as closely as possible the discomfort and to identify a site or source of the pelvic pain.
- Clearly explaining to the patient what has happened, including sites and causes of pain.
- Removing the source of pain when it is possible to do so.
- Prescribing very large amounts of water-soluble sexual or surgical lubricant during intercourse. Discourage petroleum jelly. Moisturizing skin lotion (Lubriderm, Keri-Lotion) may be recommended as an alternative lubricant unless the patient is using a condom or other latex product for contraception and/or safer sex. Lubricant should be liberally applied (two tablespoons full) to both the penis and vulva/introitus. A folded bath towel under the woman's hips helps prevent spillage on bedclothes.
- Instructing the woman to take the penis in her hand and control insertion herself rather than letting the man do it.
- Encouraging the couple to add pleasant, sexually exciting experiences to their regular interactions, such as showering together (in which the primary goal is not cleanliness), mutual caressing without intercourse, or use of sexual books and pictures. Such activities tend to increase both natural lubrication and vaginal dilatation, both of which decrease friction and pain.

- Recommending a change in coital position to one admitting less penetration for women who have pain on deep penetration due to pelvic pathology (endometriosis, pelvic inflammatory disease, etc.) but whose pathology is not sufficient to justify pelvic surgery.

Maximum penile penetration is achieved when the woman is on her back with her pelvis rolled up off the bed and her thighs tightly compressed against her chest with her calves over the man's shoulders. If she changes to a posture in which her hips are flat on the bed and her thighs are away from her chest, penile penetration will be reduced. The further her thighs are away from the chest, the more penile penetration will be reduced. Minimal penetration occurs when the woman is on her back with her legs extended flat on the bed and close together while her partner's legs straddle hers. In this position vaginal penetration is shallow, but her thighs tend to press her labia together to give good penile clasping and increased vulvar contact.

If no vaginal penetration is tolerable, the couple may substitute interfemoral intercourse. In interfemoral intercourse the woman lies either prone or supine with her ankles locked (crossed). A triangular space between the upper thighs and vulva in most women makes a satisfactory alternative to vaginal penetration and permits both vulvar and penile shaft stimulation. In slender women the space is larger and the woman may need to use her hands with fingers hooked to hold the thrusting penis against her vulva.

The prognosis for resolution of dyspareunia is excellent, even when long-standing, self-perpetuating pain is a factor.

Vaginismus

Vaginismus is a painful or spastic contraction of a woman's pelvic floor muscles that occurs with attempted penetration of the vagina. Young women may be painfully unable to begin having intercourse. Vaginismus is commonly seen in the gynecologic examining room among young women who appear afraid of their first pelvic examination. Rather than being uncooperative patients, such young women are suffering from a reflex phenomenon that they have as yet not learned to control. In both of those situations vaginismus is a primary process.

Vaginismus is also sometimes seen as a secondary process. A woman who has had severe dyspareunia from some physical cause may develop secondary vaginismus as a reflex. Women who have been traumatized genitally (rape, child abuse, examination by a callous clinician) may also develop secondary vaginismus.

In general, women who have vaginismus are strongly motivated to change. Women who have been traumatized often have the most problems with a pelvic exam. Many of these patients can learn to break their cycle of spastic contractions with one limited pelvic exam done with extreme gentleness (including a one-fingered vaginal exam and omission of the rectal exam). Tell women that they are in charge, that nothing will be done without their knowledge and permission, and that all parts of the examination will be explained in detail in advance. As the exam progresses, reassure the woman that her pelvic findings are normal (if indeed they are normal).

Some women may require vaginal dilatation as part of the treatment of vaginismus. The best vaginal dilator is the woman's own finger which she can insert with the aid of a little lubricant. Occasionally, it may be necessary to use mechanical dilators. For this purpose, the most useful objects are the tapered disposable plastic containers in which plastic syringes are supplied. By using containers of graduated sizes, the clinician has a good idea what progress is being made. The average volume of an erect penis is about 57 cc. By the time most patients can accommodate a 35 cc or 50 cc syringe carrier, they can usually discard dilators and have intercourse. Relaxation techniques are also useful in resolving vaginismus.

MALE SEXUAL DYSFUNCTIONS

Male sexual dysfunctions are often strongly affected by male cultural imperatives. Our culture stresses unfortunate facets of sexuality for the "masculine ideal," such as numbers of partners, numbers of acts, ejaculations, impregnation, and duration of intromission, instead of sensuous interaction. Many men come to think of sexual interactions in terms of performance or accomplishment instead of pleasure, and often have performance anxiety as a result.

Rapid Ejaculation (Premature Ejaculation)

When ejaculation occurs without any sense of voluntary control, and within a minute or so of insertion of the penis into the partner, it may be called rapid in the sense that time available for sexual pleasure is quite limited for both people. No accurate data on the frequency of rapid ejaculation exist, but perhaps a third of men under age 25 and 10% of men over age 40 ejaculate quickly. Although a few men tend to ejaculate more rapidly in response to anxiety or stress, the majority of men who ejaculate rapidly do so from their earliest partner experiences. Over time, many men learn ejaculatory control.

When rapid ejaculation represents a sexual concern for either or both partners, it can be treated by behavioral retraining. Treatment involves various techniques, such as the use of squeeze or stop-start as defined by Masters and Johnson and others.[29,35]

Erective Difficulty (Impotence)

Erective difficulty in men may be primary or secondary. Primary erective difficulty (inability to sustain an erection sufficiently for insertion) is not common and usually has to do with high levels of anxiety about sexual performance. The treatment is psychotherapy for anxiety.

Secondary erective difficulty is quite common. Researchers have suggested that secondary erective difficulty exists when an individual is unable to maintain an erection in 25% of his coital opportunities.[29] Nothing is magical about 25%, and when a patient expresses concern about losing or maintaining an erection on more than an occasional basis, an evaluation is appropriate.

Secondary erective loss may be psychogenic, but more likely is secondary to organic disease or pharmacologic substances. Psychogenic erective loss is most commonly associated with a history of rapid ejaculation or following an episode of acute alcohol or drug intoxication, but it may be related to extreme religious orthodoxy, domineering parents, anxiety about sexual orientation, or chronic intellectual or emotional stress. Performance anxiety is most often the common denominator.

In general, men with erective loss caused by organic disease have an insidious onset with no specific history of a precipitating event. Their loss is persistent and progressively worsens, and they may have loss of erections under other circumstances as well (nighttime, masturbation, erotic situations). They may or may not lose sexual desire.

In contrast, men whose erective loss is primarily psychogenic sometimes have a history of acute onset with a specific precipitating event. Thereafter, the erective loss is selective, intermittent, and transient. It does not occur on all occasions or with all partners. A history of good to fair erections during foreplay that disappear on attempted insertion is particularly common. Men with psychogenic erective loss usually maintain their ability to masturbate and respond to erotic situations. Nighttime erections usually continue.

Organic erective loss.   Organic erective loss is associated with four types of organic disease.

1. Endocrine disease. In rare cases, sexual dysfunction is secondary to testicular failure with low serum testosterone. Determining the serum testosterone can help establish this diagnosis. Elevated prolactin levels associated with erective loss suggest a prolactin-secreting pituitary tumor that can be treated with good result. Diabetes mellitus is commonly associated with sexual dysfunction in three different circumstances:

   • Diabetic men have the same sorts of psychogenic erective loss as other men.

- Previously undiagnosed diabetics who are not in good metabolic control may experience dysfunction, but this condition is usually reversible with good metabolic control.
- Men with long-standing diabetes and diabetic neuropathy may develop erective loss or loss of sexual responsiveness over time. This loss is usually not reversible, and men with this loss may be candidates for a penile prosthesis, or other approaches to restore erection.

2. Vascular disease. Any disease that obstructs arterial blood supply to the genitalia may impede erection. Examples include penile small vessel disease (demonstrable with Doppler studies of penile blood flow), generalized obliterative arterial disease, thrombosis of the aortic bifurcation, or aortic aneurysm.

3. Neurologic disease. Any lesion from the spinal cord to the genital innervation may interfere with erection, ejaculation, or both. Included are such widely varying problems as cord trauma, cord tumors, multiple sclerosis, diabetic neuropathy, and surgical ablation of autonomic pathways.

4. Generally debilitating disease. Debilitating diseases that affect a man's sexual function include cancer, late HIV, chronic malnutrition, and starvation, among others.

Men who have sexual dysfunction and organic disease require careful medical evaluation and consultation. Although patients with organic disease sometimes first complain of sexual dysfunction, it is far more common to see sexual dysfunction in men whose organic disease is well known and long established. In either case, a qualified clinician should reevaluate the patient's physical health.

Pharmacologic erective loss. Besides alcohol (both acute intoxication and physical damage from chronic usage) and habituating drugs, three major categories of pharmacologic agents are commonly associated with loss of desire, erection, ejaculation, or orgasm in men (and women):

- Antihypertensive therapy (including diuretics)
- Antidepressants and antipsychotic agents
- Antiulcer therapeutic agents (except simple antacids)

Any pharmacologic agent that affects the autonomic nervous system or has a potentially sedative effect may in some people cause change in sexual function. The change in function is often dose-related and idiosyncratic, so a change in type of medication or dosage level may relieve the sexual loss. Remember that alcohol and/or drug usage is a common cause of sexual dysfunction and relationship dysfunction as well.

Psychogenic erective loss.   Virtually every man by the age of 40 has had one or more instances in which he wished to have an erection and was not able to do so. A man tends to react to this experience in one of two ways. Either he feels some mild concern, or he views the situation with alarm and anxiety and suggests to himself that something in the apparatus is broken and perhaps will never work properly again. On subsequent occasions the man with the first reaction has little thought of the previous incapacity, whereas the man with the second reaction evaluates his performance repeatedly and begins a continuing internal dialogue with himself about his performance. This process is called *spectatoring*. Most sexually dysfunctional men and women begin spectatoring and, by so doing, rapidly distract themselves from sexual excitement and pleasure.

Psychogenic erective loss is reversed by treating the performance anxiety and spectatoring that caused the loss. Spectatoring is thwarted by describing the process and its harmful effects to both sexual partners and encouraging each to control it. Awareness is necessary before self-control can be instituted. Self-control will decrease spectatoring as patients are encouraged to focus on pleasure and enjoyment rather than performance. Encourage both partners to focus on sight, sound, smell, touch, and taste and to fill their minds with sensation rather than allowing themselves to become distracted by thinking. Performance anxiety can also be relieved by temporarily forbidding the couple to have any kind of insertive sex, but instead encouraging them to practice touching, caressing, and kissing, and to share other sensuous and erotic experiences. Forbidding insertive sex relieves the anxiety about the presence or absence of erection. Under such circumstances, erection usually returns rapidly.

Ejaculatory Delay

Sometimes ejaculatory delay is called retarded ejaculation, inhibited ejaculation, or ejaculatory incompetence. Ejaculatory delay is a much less judgmental title. Delayed ejaculation almost always occurs with oral, vaginal, or anal intercourse rather than with masturbation, unless it is related to medication or disease. It is often secondary to performance anxiety, but may also be a learned behavior (anger at partner, unilateral contraception decision, etc.) or may occur in a man who has a usual masturbatory pattern to which he is accustomed and which he cannot duplicate with his partner. As a consequence, he may find sexual activities with his partner insufficiently stimulating to produce orgasm.

Men who have acquired a pattern of withholding ejaculations can often be retrained by having them masturbate to orgasm on successive days in closer and closer proximity to the partner's genitals. For example, for a heterosexual man, masturbatory ejaculation takes place on the vulva, and then in the vagina. This experience often breaks the pattern of withholding.

Men who have become accustomed to a particular way of masturbating that they cannot duplicate with a partner can be encouraged to learn to masturbate to orgasm and ejaculation in a variety of alternative ways and thus retrain themselves to respond.

Men who withhold ejaculation as a part of passive-aggressive behavior patterns will require psychotherapy to overcome their passive-aggressive style, rather than sexual therapy *per se*. They need to understand the relation between withheld ejaculation and passive-aggressive behavior.

BRIEF SEXUAL HISTORY AND COUNSELING TECHNIQUES

Originally the sex history was a sometime component of the menstrual and gynecologic history of women patients, where age at first (heterosexual) intercourse, frequency of intercourse, and inquiry about pain or discomfort with intercourse were couched in a strictly medical context. Clinicians attuned to STD issues may also have asked about number of sexual partners, especially in public health settings. Men may have been asked about genitourinary symptoms or discomfort, but rarely were invited to discuss sexual issues.

Masters and Johnson and other sex researchers medicalized human sexuality in the 1960s and 1970s, and clinicians sometimes expanded sex history-taking to include questions for men and women about presence or absence of desire, satisfaction with sexual experiences, and sexual dysfunction. Referral to sex therapists became a fairly common occurrence in urban areas.

The 1980s and 1990s brought a different focus to the sex history. The primary goals today are to look for behaviors that put the male or female patient at risk for chronic or even lethal viral STDs, and to assist the patient with risk-reduction skills.

CURRENT HISTORY-TAKING PRACTICE

A sex history is by no means a standard practice in all health care settings. For example:

- A 1986 telephone survey of 1,000 primary care physicians in California found that only 10% asked new patients questions that would pick up HIV risk behaviors. Less than 4% ask patients to fill out a history form that asks about sexual orientation and practices.[24]
- A 1991 study of 768 faculty, fellows, and residents at a teaching hospital in a low-HIV-prevalence area found that only 11% routinely asked patients about HIV risk behaviors.[13]

- A 1991 telephone survey of 1,350 U.S. adults found that only 19% had ever discussed AIDS with a physician, and more than half of those initiated the conversation themselves.[3]

When physicians at an HMO in California were asked in 1992 why they were reluctant to discuss HIV risks with patients, they mentioned lack of time, perceiving the patient to be not at risk, giving priority to other health issues, believing the patient would ask if he or she wanted information, and feeling discomfort with discussion of sex and drug use behaviors.[3] Patients, however, may be more comfortable discussing these issues. Some 91% of 228 patients in a Boston university-based general medical practice felt that a discussion of sex with a physician is appropriate.[12] Only 7% of respondents in the national telephone survey cited above said they would be reluctant to discuss sex with a physician.[3] This level of comfort is impressive, given that most sexual histories are done on the very first visit.

A FRAMEWORK FOR SEXUAL HISTORY-TAKING IN THE 1990s

If you only have time to ask one question of each patient, a reasonable choice might be this:[8]

What do you do to protect yourself from AIDS?

No matter what your patient answers, you can always take her or him one step further along in skill development. The patient who responds, "Who, me?" can be encouraged to look closely at whether there is any chance of STD risk in her or his present or past life. The patient who says, "I use condoms every time I have sex" can be praised, reinforced on correct condom use, advised about where to get free or inexpensive condoms, reminded that condoms sometimes slip off or break, and then praised some more!

If you have 2-5 minutes, you can ask these 10 questions to get a basic history. You can ask oral questions or give patients a questionnaire to complete, guided primarily by your understanding of literacy skills and cultural feelings in your patient population about open sexual discussion. Always provide a private setting, assure the confidentiality of the recorded information, and tell patients you ask these questions of all patients because sexual issues contribute greatly to overall physical and emotional health and well-being.

1. Have you had a sexual experience with another person in the past year?

2. (If yes,) With how many different people in this year? One? Two or three? Four to 10? More than 10?

3. (If yes,) In this year, have you had sex with men, with women, or with both?

4. What can you tell me about your sexual life before this last year?
5. Have you ever had a sexually transmitted disease of any kind?
6. Have you ever shared needles or injection equipment with another person for any reason?
7. Have you ever felt that a sex partner put you at risk for any reason?
8. What do you do to protect yourself from AIDS?
9. What do you do to protect yourself from unplanned pregnancy?
10. Is there anything else about your sexual lifestyle that I need to know to ensure good medical care?

Questions 1 and 2 ask about the most recent 12 months because accurate recall of sexual practices may deteriorate after that time.[20] A "yes" response leads to questions 2 and 3. A "no" leads to question 4. If question 4 reveals no previous sexual experiences with another person, the history is complete. If question 4 reveals previous sexual experiences, inquire further about numbers and genders of partners.

Question 2 is asked so that the patient can feel safe giving any answer, responding to the multiple choice cue. This technique can minimize the tendency to guess—and give—the "right" answers.

Question 3 cues the clinician to inquire about any risk behaviors specific to same-gender and opposite-gender practices, and also helps the clinician know what specific body areas should be examined for sexually related disease or injury and/or tested for STD. Perhaps most importantly, this question guards against making unfounded assumptions about sexual orientation.

Question 4 is an open-ended question to help ascertain the degree to which the most recent 12 months have been typical in the patient's sexual life. Have there been more or fewer sexual encounters in the past? More or fewer partners? More or less STD and pregnancy risk taking?

Question 5 elucidates perhaps the clearest "red flag" issue in sexual risk taking. Behavior that puts a person at risk for one STD can put a person at risk for any and all STDs.

Question 6 must include inquiry not only into the shared use of uncleaned needles and injection equipment for street drugs, but also for tattooing, skin piercing, and for steroid use to promote muscle development.

Question 7 seeks to uncover partners who are obviously physically sick, have genital sores, use needle drugs, or for other reasons cause the patient to worry about HIV and other STDs. Unfortunately, behaviors that may be associated with high STD risk, such as use of injection drugs and male bisexuality, are some of the most secret, carefully hidden behaviors in the U.S. culture. In settings where the patient feels high levels of trust for the clinician, this question can also uncover abuse, rape, battering, and other coercive sexual situations.

Question 8 permits an assessment of current safer sex practices. The clinician can always take the patient one step further in skill development.

Question 9 permits an assessment of current contraceptive practice, the patient's perception of personal child-bearing potential, and her/his plans for future childbearing. Skill-building can begin where the patient is, and move forward.

Question 10 is a mop-up question. In a trusting relationship, the clinician may be able to pick up loneliness, depression, abuse, addiction, self-destructive sexual practices that may or may not trouble the patient, relationship issues, or sexual dysfunction. Much of the time, this question will yield little or nothing.

If you have longer than 5 minutes, add questions about transfusions before April 1985, workplace exposure to blood, specific sexual practices, gynecologic problems related to sexual function, relationships, alcohol and drug use, and sexual dysfunction.

Ask questions about specific sexual practices to learn what parts of the body might be affected by trauma or infection, such as these for a woman who has sex with men:

- Does your partner ever put his penis in your mouth?
- Does your partner ever put his penis in your rectum (butt, anus)?
- Does your partner ever put his mouth on your sex organs (genitals, vulva)?
- About how often do you have sex with your partner?

Ask questions about gynecological problems:

- Does intercourse or other sexual activity ever cause you physical pain or discomfort?
- How many times have you used an over-the-counter treatment for a vaginal infection in the past year?

Ask questions about relationships:

- Do you have a steady sex partner?
- (If yes,) How would you describe that relationship?
- Has anyone ever asked you to do something sexual against your will? (These issues may not be held as a "sexual" memory for some patients, but rather as a violent memory.)

Ask questions about substance use:

- How many drinks of beer, wine, and hard liquor did you consume in the last 7 days?
- What prescription medicines do you take?
- Do you take any medicines or drugs from a nonmedical source?
- Have you ever traded sex for things you wanted or needed?

- In the past year when you've been sexual with a partner, were you more likely to be totally sober, using some form of alcohol, some form of drugs, or both?

Ask questions about sexual dysfunction:

- Some of our patients have concerns about their sexual lives. What about you? Is there anything about your sexual life that you would like to be different?

Certainly no set of questions will be ideal for all patients in all settings, and these questions are offered solely as a point of departure, ready to be adapted to the care setting and to the communication style of the clinician. A few final comments on implementing the sexual history:

- It is appropriate to allow patients to defer the history until a later visit, or to decline to discuss sexual issues altogether. Once you have expressed your conviction that the sexual history is a normal and valuable part of the health history for all people, the patient will decide whether to risk the loss of privacy and face possible embarrassment, anxiety, or rejection.
- Document only what is critical to good patient care, and rigorously protect the written record under lock and key. Some health care providers return the sex history questionnaire to the patient once it has been discussed, assuring that only minimal information will be recorded.
- Avoid taking an "ophthalmic" sex history, that is, deciding from across the room what kind of sex life a patient has based on appearances, such as:
  - single people have active sex lives;
  - older people do not have active sex lives;
  - sexually experienced people know how to use birth control and safer sex techniques; and
  - married people are heterosexual.
- Remember that terminology can sometimes get in the way of clarity with sexual history-taking. For example, teens may not know the word "monogamous." Lay people may think "sexually active" means vigorous sex, or lots of partners. Many people who engage in same-gender sexual practices do not think of themselves as "homosexual."

THE PLISSIT COUNSELING MODEL

The PLISSIT counseling model was developed for health care workers who are not psychiatrists, psychologists, or sexual therapists but who wish to address the sexual needs and concerns of their patients and make appropriate referrals when necessary.[2] Few patients who have a sexual problem or dysfunction are beyond help, if they want to change and if the clinician is willing to help. By simply allowing them a place to ventilate or by providing basic information, the clinician can often help patients solve their problems. The PLISSIT model consists of four stages: **P**ermission giving, **L**imited **I**nformation giving, **S**pecific **S**uggestions, and **I**ntensive **T**herapy.

Permission giving is not the same as telling the patient what to do. Permission is usually for thoughts, feelings, or behaviors and may be expressed as permission to do or not to do. Permission giving from a knowledgeable professional figure is quite powerful. Bringing up the topic of sex with a patient is part of permission giving.

Limitation must be imposed on permission giving. The health care worker is not required to give permission for thoughts, feelings, or behaviors that violate his or her own professional value system, but the clinician is required by professional honesty to indicate to the patient that such is the case and to be frank about differing beliefs and values among professionals. For example, no qualified professionals approve of rape or child sexual abuse. The law requires that any individual who suspects or has knowledge of child abuse report that information immediately to the police. This duty supersedes medical confidentiality. Professionals ought not approve of behaviors that threaten the physical or psychological health of patients and their partners.

Limited information usually involves discussing anatomy and physiology as well as dispelling myths about sex. This task is often fairly easy for health care workers to do since we know a lot of anatomy and physiology and patients often know little or none. Because sexual myths are common, trained health workers can usually dispel them if given a chance to discuss sex.

Specific suggestions involve skill-building such as changing position for intercourse and other activities, using lubricants (for dyspareunia), or using a squeeze or stop-start technique (for rapid ejaculation).

Intensive therapy will almost certainly prove too time-consuming and involved for all but those who are specially trained and wish to devote considerable time to such work. Intensive therapy may be necessary for body image problems, relationship problems, identity issues, depression, personality disorders, or psychoses.

Patients are rarely hesitant to provide sexual information if the examiner seems professional, concerned, self-confident, and nonjudgmental. Even though the patient may offer no data on the first visit, the experience demonstrates the history-taker's willingness to deal with these special subjects, and, often on subsequent visits, patients will offer additional significant and useful data.

If the patient has beliefs or practices that may be harmful or dysfunctional (not merely different from those of the health care worker), then talking about the consequences of those beliefs and practices and discussing alternatives is appropriate. Refusing to offer care for ethical reasons and then failing to recommend an alternative source of reputable help is not appropriate.

Health care workers need to be honest with themselves about what problems they have the knowledge, skills, and time to handle. Patients who will require more therapy than is available immediately will need appropriate referral to another source of counseling or sexual therapy. A well-trained reproductive health practitioner can probably handle most of his or her patients' sexual questions and concerns without referral. Only a small minority of patients will need referral to a sexual therapist.

REFERENCES

1. Anderson RM, May RM. Epidemiological parameters of HIV transmission. Nature 1988;333(6173):514-519.
2. Annon JS. The behavioral treatment of sexual problems. Vol. 1, Brief therapy. Honolulu HI: Mercantile Printing, 1974:100-105.
3. Anonymous. Are physicians prepared to answer questions about HIV? AIDS Alert 1992;7(2):23-26.
4. Barbach LG. For yourself: the fulfillment of female sexuality. Garden City NY: Anchor Press, 1976.
5. Bell AP, Weinberg MS. Homosexualities: a study of diversity among men and women. New York NY: Simon and Schuster, 1978.
6. Billy JOG, Tanfer K, Grady WR, Klepinger DH. The sexual behavior of men in the United States. Fam Plann Perspect 1993;25(2):52-60.
7. Blumstein P, Schwartz P. American couples: money, work and sex. New York NY: Morrow, 1983.
8. Bush DM. Personal communication, November 10, 1991.
9. Cochran SD, Mays VM. Sex, lies, and HIV. N Engl J Med 1990;322(11):774-775.
10. Darling CA, Davidson JK, Conway-Welch C. Female ejaculation: perceived origins, the Grafenberg spot/area, and sexual responsiveness. Arch Sex Behav 1990;19(1):29-47.
11. Ekstrand ML, Coates TJ. Maintenance of safer sexual behaviors and predictors of risky sex: the San Francisco Men's Health Study. Am J Public Health 1990;80(8):973-977.
12. Ende J, Rockwell S, Glasgow M. The sexual history in general medicine practice. Arch Intern Med 1984;144(3):558-561.
13. Ferguson KJ, Stapleton JT, Helms CM. Physicians' effectiveness in assessing risk for human immunodeficiency virus infection. Arch Intern Med 1991;151(3): 561-564.
14. Freeman A, Cohn D, Corby N, Wood R. Patterns of sexual behavior change among homosexual/bisexual men—selected U.S. sites, 1987-1990. MMWR 1991;40(46):792-794.

15. Glasel M. High-risk sexual practices in the transmission of AIDS. In: DeVita VT, Hellman S, Rosenberg SA (eds). AIDS: etiology, diagnosis, treatment, and prevention. Philadelphia PA: JB Lippincott, 1988:355-367.

16. Heiman J, Lo Piccolo J, Lo Piccolo L. Becoming orgasmic: a sexual growth program for women. New York NY: Prentice-Hall, 1976.

17. Hite S. The Hite report. New York NY: MacMillan, 1976.

18. Hite S. Women and love: a cultural revolution in progress. New York NY: Alfred A. Knopf, 1987.

19. Ilaria G, Jacobs JL, Polsky B, Koll B, Baron P, MacLow C, Armstrong D, Schlegel PN. Detection of HIV-1 DNA sequences in pre-ejaculatory fluid. Lancet 1992;340(8833):1469.

20. Kauth MR, St. Lawrence JS, Kelly JA. Reliability of retrospective assessments of sexual HIV risk behavior: a comparison of biweekly, three-month, and twelve-month self-reports. AIDS Educ Prev 1991;3(3):207-214.

21. Kinsey AC, Pomeroy WB, Martin CE. Sexual behavior in the human male. Philadelphia PA: WB Saunders, 1948.

22. Kinsey AC, Pomeroy WB, Martin CE, Gebhard PH. Sexual behavior in the human female. Philadelphia PA: WB Saunders, 1953.

23. Lambert B. Relapses into risky sex found in AIDS studies. New York Times, June 22, 1990:A18.

24. Lewis CE, Freeman HE. The sexual history-taking and counseling practices of primary care physicians. West J Med 1987;147(2):165-167.

25. London KA, Mosher WD. What is current use of a contraceptive method? Hyattsville MD: National Center for Health Statistics, 1990.

26. Lowe W, Kretchmer A, Petersen JR, Nellis B, Lever J, Hertz R. The Playboy readers' sex survey: part four. Playboy 1983;30(7):130,132,192,194,196-198,200,203.

27. MacDonald NE, Wells GA, Fisher WA, Warren WK, King MA, Doherty JA, Bowie WR. High-risk STD/HIV behavior among college students. JAMA 1990;263(23):3155-3159.

28. Masters WH, Johnson VE. Human sexual response. Boston MA: Little, Brown & Co., 1966.

29. Masters WH, Johnson VE. Human sexual inadequacy. Boston MA: Little, Brown & Co., 1970.

30. McKusick L, Coates TJ, Morin SF, Pollack L, Hoff C. Longitudinal predictors of reductions in unprotected anal intercourse among gay men in San Francisco: the AIDS behavioral research project. Am J Public Health 1990;80(8):978-983.

31. McNally JW, Mosher WD. AIDS-related knowledge and behavior among women 15-44 years of age: United States, 1988. Adv Data, Number 200. Hyattsville MD: National Center for Health Statistics, 1991.

32. Michael RT, Laumann EO, Gagnon JH. The number of sexual partners of adults in the U.S. Hyde Park IL: National Opinion Research Center, University of Chicago, 1992.

33. Moore KA, Nord CW, Peterson JL. Nonvoluntary sexual activity among adolescents. Fam Plann Perspect 1989;21(3):110-114.

34. National Victim Center and Crime Victims Research and Treatment Center. Rape in America. Arlington VA: National Victim Center, April 23, 1992.

35. Perelman MA. Treatment of premature ejaculation. In: Lieblum ST and Pervin L (eds). Principles and practice of sex therapy. New York NY: Guilford Press, 1980:204-205.

36. Pudney J, Oneta M, Mayer K, Seage G, Anderson D. Pre-ejaculatory fluid as potential vector for sexual transmission of HIV-1. Lancet 1992;340(8833):1470.
37. Rogers SM, Turner CF. Male-male sexual contact in the U.S.A.: findings from five sample surveys, 1970-1990. J Sex Res 1991;28(4):491-519.
38. RTI. Report on the Dallas County household HIV survey. Research Triangle NC: Research Triangle Institute, 1990
39. Sonenstein FL, Pleck JH, Ku LC. Sexual activity, condom use and AIDS awareness among adolescent males. Fam Plann Perspect 1989;21(4):152-158.
40. Tanfer K, Grady WR, Klepinger DH, Billy JOG. Condom use among U.S. men, 1991. Fam Plann Perspect 1993;25(2):61-66.
41. Tavris C, Sadd S. The Redbook report on female sexuality. New York NY: Delacorte, 1977.
42. Taylor H. Number of gay men more than 4 times higher than the 1 percent reported in a recent survey. New York NY: Louis Harris & Associates, April 26, 1993.
43. Trussell J, Vaughan B. Selected results concerning sexual behavior and contraceptive use from the 1988 National Survey of Family Growth and the 1988 National Survey of Adolescent Males. Working Paper #91-12. Princeton NJ: Office of Population Research, Princeton University, 1991.
44. Turner CF, Miller HG, Moses LE (eds). AIDS: sexual behavior and intravenous drug use. Washington DC: National Academy Press, 1989.
45. Weisberg M. Physiology of female sexual function. Clin Obstet Gynecol 1984;27(3):697-705.
46. Wells JA, Sell RL. Project Hope's international survey of AIDS educational messages and behavior change: France, the United Kingdom, and the United States. Chevy Chase MD: Project Hope, 1990.

The Menstrual Cycle

- Understanding how menstrual cycle hormone patterns affect the maturation and release of an egg from the ovary, and uterine preparation for implantation, is fundamental to understanding how many methods of contraception work.

- Learning to identify cyclic fertility signs can empower women and their partners when they want to maximize fertility, or when they want to avoid pregnancy.

Female fertility is cyclic, unlike male fertility, which is relatively constant. Ovulation occurs only once a month and is regulated by a hormone system that involves the hypothalamus, pituitary gland, and ovaries. Figures 2-1 and 2-2 summarize events in this system, as well as hormone effects on the uterine lining (endometrium), body temperature, and cervical mucus. Facts for the brief synopsis in this chapter are drawn from *Clinical Gynecologic Endocrinology and Infertility* by Speroff, Glass, and Kase[2] and from *Infertility, Contraception and Reproductive Endocrinology* by Mishell and Davajan.[1] Both of these excellent texts provide more extensive descriptions of menstrual cycle physiology and clinical management of problems that may be associated with cyclic hormone patterns.

MENSTRUAL CYCLE LENGTH

For simplicity, all events presented in this chapter have been adjusted to a 28-day cycle, the average menstrual cycle length. Traditionally the cycle is divided into two parts—the follicular phase and the luteal phase—

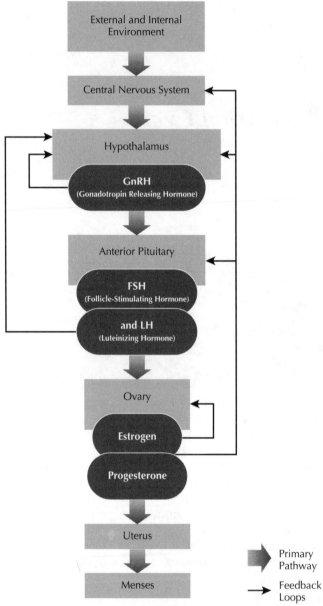

Primary hormone pathways (➡) in the reproductive system are modulated by both negative and positive feedback loops (→). Prostaglandins, secreted by the ovary and by uterine endometrial cells, also play a role in ovulation, and may modulate hypothalamic function as well.

Figure 2-1 Regulation of the menstrual cycle

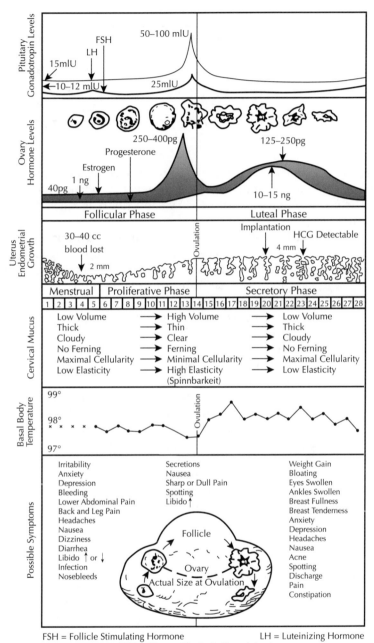

FSH = Follicle Stimulating Hormone   LH = Luteinizing Hormone
HCG = Human Chorionic Gonadotropin

Figure 2-2 Menstrual cycle events: hormone levels, ovarian, and endometrial patterns, and cyclic temperature and cervical mucus changes

Table 2-1 Menstrual cycle phases

Cycle Days	Ovarian Phase	Endometrial Phase
1–5	Follicular Phase	Menstrual Phase
6–14	Follicular Phase	Proliferative Phase
15–28	Luteal Phase	Secretory Phase

named by the changes that occur in the ovary. Cyclic patterns of hormone release by the ovary also induce cyclic changes in the endometrium (see Table 2-1). The first day of menstrual flow, by convention, is called day 1 of the menstrual cycle.

The time interval between ovulation and the onset of menstruation, the luteal phase, is consistently close to 14 days for all women (normal range 12–17 days). The length of the follicular phase is not as consistent. Differences in normal ovulatory cycle length (25–35 days) are primarily accounted for by variation in the time required for follicle development.

A woman is most likely to conceive if fresh sperm are present in the reproductive tract when ovulation occurs. The woman's oocyte (egg) retains maximal potential for fertilization for 12–24 hours. Sperm retain potential for fertility for a significantly longer interval; precisely how much longer is not known, but is estimated to be about 3 days.

Cycle days of maximal fertility are the 3 days before ovulation: intercourse on any one of these days results in a 20% probability of pregnancy (approximately). The next most fertile is the day of ovulation, when the probability of pregnancy is approximately 15% (see Tables 2-2 and 22-5). The likelihood of pregnancy is much lower on other cycle days (0%–10%). In practice, however, this information is usually difficult to apply to patient care because the precise day of ovulation is not known with certainty unless the woman has been carefully monitored to detect ovulation.

Table 2-2 Cycle length and maximal fertility

Cycle Length	Day of Ovulation (Cycle Day)	Maximal Fertility Interval (Cycle Days)
25 Days	11	8–10
28 Days	14	11–13
32 Days	18	15–17

THE FOLLICULAR PHASE

Cycle day 1 is the first day of menstrual bleeding. The endometrial lining begins to shed because levels of estrogen and progesterone in the bloodstream decline during the last few days of the preceding cycle. The endometrium loses its estrogen and progesterone support. If estrogen and progesterone patterns during the previous cycle were normal, the matured endometrial lining is ready for an orderly separation between the innermost basal layer and the two outer layers. When the endometrial lining is hormonally mature, shedding can occur at about the same time throughout the lining and can be completed within a few days, so the woman's menstrual period seems "normal."

If hormone events in the preceding weeks have not been normal, shedding patterns are less predictable. A woman who has had an anovulatory cycle or has developed a persisting functional cyst (see Chapter 20) may fail to bleed, or her bleeding may not follow the usual pattern. Prolonged bleeding, for example, may occur if development of the uterine lining is incomplete or is not uniform throughout the uterus.

OVARY FOLLICLE DEVELOPMENT

In the ovary, cycle day 1 marks the beginning of the follicular phase. Initial follicle development begins independent of hypothalamic and pituitary hormones. During the first few days of the cycle, numerous ovarian follicles begin growing. Most of these are destined to grow briefly, then recede (become atretic). Meanwhile, the pituitary increases its release of follicle stimulating hormone (FSH). The hypothalamus has sensed low estrogen and progesterone levels at the end of the preceding cycle, and has responded by secreting pulses of gonadotropin-releasing hormone (GnRH). GnRH pulses stimulate FSH release from the nearby pituitary gland. As FSH rises, one group of newly developing follicles is at just the right stage to be able to respond to FSH. This follicle cohort accelerates in growth and secretes increasing quantities of estrogen.

DOMINANT FOLLICLE SELECTION

In the cohort, one follicle will be the leader in estrogen secretion. Since estrogen induces an increase in follicle FSH *receptor* content, the estrogen leader soon also has more FSH receptors. With more FSH receptors, its growth response to FSH is amplified. This follicle is able to outperform the other follicles in its cohort, and by cycle day 5–7 has become the dominant follicle. The dominant follicle is indirectly responsible for the demise of the others in the cohort. Increasing estrogen production by this follicle and the other follicles in the cohort causes a decrease in pituitary FSH release, so the follicles that are less responsive to FSH are no longer able to continue growth. Because it has more FSH receptors, the dominant follicle continues to grow. It produces rapidly increasing estrogen and also the single, mature oocyte for that cycle.

The endometrium responds to ovarian production of estrogen by initiating renewal of the uterine lining, beginning the proliferative phase of the endometrial cycle. Regeneration begins from the basal (innermost) layer as early as cycle day 2, and rising estrogen levels stimulate proliferation of endometrial cells (multiplication), so that the lining becomes thicker. Glycogen storage also occurs during the proliferative phase of endometrial development.

Increasing estrogen also causes increased cervical mucus production. As ovulation approaches, the woman may notice copious, clear secretions in the vagina that look like egg white and feel wet. The mucus can be stretched into a strand several inches long (spinnbarkeit) and forms a fern pattern when dried on a microscope slide.

OVULATION

As midcycle approaches, and the oocyte and follicle near maturity, the sustained, rising level of estrogen stimulates increases in luteinizing hormone (LH) release by the pituitary gland. LH, in turn, stimulates production of progesterone and androgen by the ovary beginning a day or two before ovulation. The mature follicle itself provides the final ovulation signal: its increasing estrogen production reaches the threshold required to trigger a sudden and spectacular increase in LH. Ovulation will occur 34–36 hours after the LH surge begins, 10–12 hours after its peak.

The LH surge is an important temporal reference point for the cycle. Subsequent cycle hormone events, ovulation, and the onset of menstrual shedding 13, 14, or 15 days after the LH peak occur at uniformly predictable times for all women. The LH surge initiates the final steps in oocyte maturation: completion of the first meiotic division, preparing the chromosomes to split into two separate sets. The LH surge also stimulates synthesis of prostaglandins and proteolytic enzymes (enzymes that can break down protein molecules) in the follicle that are essential for rupture of the follicle and extrusion of the oocyte. Rising progesterone production at midcycle also activates proteolytic enzymes and stimulates the rise and peak in FSH secretion that occurs just prior to ovulation. FSH allows the oocyte, with its accompanying clump of cumulus cells, to become free-floating inside the follicle.

As LH reaches it peak, ovarian estrogen production is temporarily inhibited, so estrogen levels dip temporarily just before ovulation. A brief interval of midcycle endometrial bleeding is a fairly common result. The LH surge also causes a midcycle increase in androgen hormone production by the ovary. The ovary normally secretes androgens ("male" hormones, including testosterone) in small amounts. The rise in androgens just before and during ovulation may explain the midcycle peak in sexual activity that occurs among normally cycling women.

The mature follicle is a spectacular sight, a bulge 2 cm in diameter on the surface of the ovary. Its *rupture* releases 5 cc–10 cc *of follicular fluid* containing the barely visible, pinhead-sized, oocyte mass, *and may be accompanied by bleeding. So it is not surprising that lower abdominal pain is often associated with ovulation.* Diurnal timing of ovulation is surprisingly consistent. Ovulation occurs for 90% of women between 4 p.m. and 7 p.m. except during the spring months (March through June), when timing is more evenly distributed around the clock.

THE LUTEAL PHASE

After the follicle ruptures, the follicle walls collapse in a convoluted shape. The cells in the wall take up lipids and lutein pigment, which give them a yellow appearance. With this transformation the follicle earns a new name, corpus luteum, and is easily visible to the naked eye on the surface of the postovulatory ovary. This change begins the luteal phase in the ovary cycle; the corpus luteum secretes estrogens, progestins, and androgens. Normal follicle development before ovulation is a prerequisite for normal corpus luteum function. After ovulation, maintenance of corpus luteum function also requires sustained LH secretion from the pituitary.

Progesterone production and renewed estrogen production increase during the first half of the luteal phase. During this interval, the single corpus luteum secretes 80% of all the progesterone produced during the cycle. A serum progesterone level of more than 3 ng/ml is good evidence that ovulation has occurred. The peak should reach 8–10 ng/ml about 8 days after ovulation. A lower peak level may indicate inadequate corpus luteum function.

Rising progesterone causes a change in cervical mucus: it becomes scant, thick, and sticky. So the wet, abundant mucus present at the time of ovulation subsides quickly within a day or so after ovulation.

In response to rising levels of estrogen and progesterone, the endometrial lining changes in character. Glycogen storage is greatly increased, and the vascular and glandular structure of the lining assumes its mature form, ready to supply glucose to a free-floating embryo and an environment hospitable to implantation. This phase of endometrial development is called the secretory phase.

Progesterone and estrogen levels reach their peak in the middle of the luteal phase. Pituitary secretion of FSH and LH decreases in response to the increasing progesterone and estrogen levels. The corpus luteum then begins a process of regression and involution unless "rescued" by human chorionic gonadotropin (HCG) produced in detectable amounts by a newly beginning pregnancy as soon as 7 days after fertilization. *If pregnancy occurs, HCG supports continued corpus luteum function and thus maintains estrogen and progestin levels sufficient to prevent endometrial shedding* until the placenta is able to provide these hormones. Continued corpus luteum function is necessary for the first 7–9 weeks of pregnancy. If pregnancy does not occur, then corpus luteum function declines, estrogen and progesterone levels fall, and the stage is set for endometrial shedding and the beginning of a new cycle.

Occasionally, an especially exuberant corpus luteum fails to degenerate on schedule. This results in the most common type of functional ovarian cyst. A cyst may continue to produce estrogen and progesterone for several weeks or even months, sometimes causing a delayed or abnormal menstrual period.

FERTILIZATION AND EARLY PREGNANCY EVENTS

Fertilization involves a complex series of events that occur over a period of many hours. The sperm attaches to a receptor on the egg cell's protein halo, called the zona pellucida. The zona responds by becoming impervious to other sperm, and the sperm releases enzymes that allow it to penetrate the zona and also induces final maturation of the egg chromosomes. Next the sperm contacts the egg cell membrane, and the egg responds by surrounding the sperm head and fusing its membrane with the sperm membrane. Chromosomes in the sperm head decondense and both male and female chromosome pronuclei migrate within the cell to meet, fuse membranes, form a chromosome spindle, and prepare for cell division.

Fertilization usually occurs in the fallopian tube lumen; tubal fluid and cumulus cells from the ovary that accompany the egg at ovulation provide nutrition for early cell division. Cell division continues for the first 2 days or so in the tube lumen resulting in a ball of cells called a morula. By the third day, the morula reaches the uterine cavity where it continues early embryo development for another 2 to 3 days before beginning the process of implantation.

Approximately 6 days after ovulation, the embryo, now at the blastocyst stage, is ready to begin implantation. The blastocyst sheds the zona pellucida, and rests on the endometrial surface. At the point of contact, microvilli on the embryo's surface flatten and form close junctions with adjacent endometrial cell membranes. The endometrial cells respond by reorganizing underneath the blastocyst to allow blastocyst cells to grow into and underneath the endometrial surface. By day 12, the embryo implants just under the endometrial surface, nourished by maternal blood pools in embryonic tissue destined to form the placenta.

Fertilization, early embryonic development, and implantation are complex and delicate processes. Many eggs and sperm are abnormal and incapable of fertilization; some carry chromosome abnormalities incompatible with embryonic survival. Once fertilization occurs, many precisely coordinated biochemical events must occur for development and implantation to be successful. As a result, *spontaneous loss is very common: approximately 50% of embryos do not survive*. Because most of these losses occur during the first 2 weeks after ovulation, the woman is not likely to recognize the spontaneous pregnancy loss. Spontaneous loss is less common after the first 2 weeks; approximately 15% of pregnancies that are clinically evident (an expected menstrual period is late) subsequently end in spontaneous abortion.

M ENSTRUAL CYCLE REGULATION

Regulation of the menstrual cycle begins in the hypothalamus. Cells in the hypothalamus integrate information from the external and internal environment relayed to them by other parts of the central nervous system. *It is through the hypothalamus that factors such as stress or starvation affect menstrual patterns.* Hypothalamic cells also respond to a variety of circulating hormone levels that create feedback loops. These allow the hypothalamus to alter its messages in response to hormone effects it has induced.

HYPOTHALAMUS HORMONE RELEASE

GnRH, the hypothalamic messenger to the pituitary gland, is released in a pulsatile pattern and travels directly to the anterior pituitary through the hypothalamic pituitary portal vessels, a network of blood vessels that links the hypothalamus directly to the pituitary gland. Subtle changes in the amplitude and frequency of GnRH pulses determine what response (if any) occurs in the pituitary. The normal frequency of GnRH pulses is approximately one pulse every 70–90 minutes during the follicular phase of the cycle, and one pulse every 100–200 minutes during the luteal phase. For normal pituitary patterns, GnRH pulses must remain within a fairly critical range in frequency and amplitude. In response to GnRH pulses during the follicular phase, the pituitary releases FSH; pulse patterns during the luteal phase trigger release of both FSH and LH.

PITUITARY HORMONES

FSH and LH from the pituitary travel in the bloodstream to their target organs, the ovaries. In response, the ovaries produce estrogen, progesterone, androgens including testosterone, and precursor hormones including androstenedione. Ovarian estrogen plays a crucial role in menstrual cycle regulation. Through feedback loops, estrogen influences the hypothalamus, the pituitary, and also the ovaries' own sensitivity to FSH and LH. *Anything that prevents estrogen secretion, blocks its actions, or alters its normal fluctuations during the cycle, can disrupt reproductive function.*

GnRH pulse activity is affected by neurotransmitters such as dopamine and norepinephrine, and by beta endorphins, all of which can be influenced by circulating estrogen and progesterone levels. Endorphin production is directly increased by estrogen and by progesterone. The endorphin level, in turn, modulates GnRH pulse frequency to complete a feedback loop. Maximal endorphin stimulation occurs with both estrogen and progesterone together, so endorphin levels are highest during the luteal phase; lowest at the beginning of menses. Endorphins influence hypothalamic regulation of sexual behavior, body temperature, and food and water intake. They also influence functions outside the hypothalamus including pain perception, mood, memory, and respiratory function.

Drugs that alter neurotransmitter metabolism can affect hypothalamic secretion of GnRH and prolactin-releasing hormone (PRL). This is the reason that excessive prolactin hormone production (hyperprolactinemia) and disturbed menstrual cycle patterns often occur among women who are taking medications such as methyldopa, reserpine, chlorpromazine, propranolol, phentolamine, haloperidol, cyproheptadine, and tricyclic antidepressants such as imipramine. Marijuana also causes a decrease in GnRH pulse activity and can impair reproductive function.

FEEDBACK AND REGULATION

Feedback loops and fine tuning in the menstrual cycle exploit several different physiologic mechanisms. Hormone receptors and hormone binding to proteins in the bloodstream, for example, both play roles in these processes. Hormones act on their target cells by way of receptors: specific sites on or inside the cell bond with the incoming hormone and initiate the cell's response to the hormone. Feedback loops often involve changes in the receptor content of target cells; an increased or decreased receptor content results in increased or decreased responsiveness of the cell to any given level of incoming hormone.

Anti-hormones such as 486 RU, the synthetic anti-progestin, exert their effect by binding with receptor sites in the target cells, but in a form that does not initiate the cell's normal hormone response. Effective anti-hormones form bonds that are tighter and more enduring than those formed by the active hormone. Thus the anti-hormone is able to monopolize receptor sites, depriving active hormone of its chance to act.

The therapeutic effects of synthetic GnRH agonist drugs such as nafarelin acetate (Synarel) and leuprolide acetate (Lupron) also occur because of receptor alteration. These drugs, similar in structure to natural GnRH, cause an initial stimulation of pituitary hormone release. Repeated administration of the synthetic agonist, however, causes a decrease in pituitary gland GnRH receptors. Pituitary responsiveness to GnRH decreases, and in turn, so do levels of FSH and LH. With very low FSH, estrogen secretion by the ovary falls drastically.

HORMONE BINDING

Sex hormone binding globulin (SHBG) plays an important role in determining the activity of ovarian steroid hormones. Produced in the liver, it binds to estradiol and testosterone molecules circulating in the bloodstream, leaving only 1% of these hormones in the free, fully active state. The blood SHBG level modulates the impact of estrogen or testosterone produced in the ovary or absorbed from hormone medication. Many factors, including hormone medications, influence the SHBG level. It is increased during pregnancy, with hyperthyroidism, and with elevated estrogen or estrogenic medication. SHBG levels are decreased by androgens, corticoids, and growth hormone. One of the reasons that oral contraceptives containing new progestins such as norgestimate or gestodene have less androgenic effects than their predecessors is that they cause a very significant increase in blood SHBG.

OTHER HORMONE ROLES

Many other hormones are involved in menstrual cycle physiology. Some of these hormones such as prostaglandins and beta endorphins also have important roles outside the reproductive system. Some are specialized reproductive system hormones just now being identified and characterized, such as inhibin (sometimes called folliculostatin) and OMI (oocyte maturation inhibitor). These are particularly interesting because of the possibility that their characteristics could be exploited for contraceptive purposes.

Inhibin, a peptide hormone secreted by ovarian follicle granulosa cells, *suppresses FSH release*. By secreting inhibin, the leading ovarian follicle secures its dominance by suppressing FSH stimulation available to other follicles. Ovarian follicles also contain activin, closely related in molecular structure to inhibin, but with an opposite action. Activin directly stimulates FSH release.

The factor present in follicular fluid that prevents the oocyte from resuming meiosis is called OMI (oocyte maturation inhibitor). Because of

OMI, which is secreted by follicle granulosa cells, the oocyte remains dormant from the time that oocytes are established during fetal life, until the precise moment years later when that specific follicle reaches dominance and maturity. OMI suppression ends within hours following the LH surge.

REFERENCES

1. Mishell DR Jr, Davajan V. Infertility, contraception and reproductive endocrinology. 3rd ed. Oradell, NJ: Medical Economics Co., 1991.
2. Speroff L, Glass RH, Kase NG. Clinical gynecologic endocrinology and infertility. 4th ed. Baltimore: Williams & Wilkins Co., 1989.

HIV and AIDS

- Many of our reproductive health care patients are infected with HIV, and half of them are not aware of their infection.
- AIDS cases, and presumably HIV infections, in U.S. women aged 15-44 are increasing rapidly.
- Every patient merits some attention to HIV prevention skill building. Ask each patient, "What do you do to protect yourself from AIDS?"
- Reproductive health care settings are a critical conduit to HIV testing and diagnosis, especially in high-prevalence areas.
- Ensure that infected patients have access to primary and reproductive health care, either by direct treatment or careful referral.

The epidemiologic trends in the global and U.S. HIV pandemic offer little cause for optimism. Numbers grow, the ratio of infected men and women approaches 1:1, and women aged 15-44 constitute one of the fastest-growing segments of the U.S. epidemic.

HIV is first and foremost a global issue, with 80% of reported AIDS cases in developing countries, where only 6% of the world's HIV prevention resources are spent. Between 38 and 108 million people will be infected by the year 2000. Perhaps 4.7 million women are already infected, and on almost every continent AIDS is a leading cause of death among young women. Most of these women have been infected via sexual exposure to infected men.[44]

U .S. TRENDS

Overall, 11.4% of United States adult and adolescent cases have been among women (see Table 3-1). This female portion has increased from 3% of reported AIDS cases in 1981 to 13% in 1992-1993.[31,14] In nine U.S. cities,

Table 3-1 AIDS in adults and adolescents, United States, cumulative through March 1993

	Male %	Female %
Exposure Category		
Men/sex/men (MSM)	58	—
Injecting drug (ID)	21	49
MSM/ID	6	—
Hemophilia	1	0
Heterosexual	4	36
Blood, tissue	1	6
Other/risk not identified	8	9
Racial/Ethnic Group		
White, not Hispanic	56	25
Black, not Hispanic	27	53
Hispanic	16	20
Asian/Pacific Islander	<1	<1
American Indian/Alaska Native	<1	<1
Age		
<13	1	6
13–19	<1	1
20–24	3	6
25–44	75	73
≥45	20	14

Source: Centers for Disease Control and Prevention (1993a).

AIDS is the leading cause of death among women aged 25-44 years.[18] Each year, AIDS deaths among men and women account for more than 750,000 years of life lost before age 65.[19] About a quarter of women with AIDS are 20-29 years old, suggesting that many were infected in their teen years.

Injecting-drug use has played a huge role in the first decade of AIDS in U.S. women. About 49% of AIDS cases have been among women who injected drugs with shared and uncleaned injection equipment. Thousands more women have been infected by male sex partners who were injecting-drug users.[14] In 1992-1993, injecting drugs directly and indirectly accounted for almost two-thirds of reported cases in adult and adolescent U.S. women.[14] Among AIDS cases, about 93% of the 164 U.S. women who report sex only with other women have been injecting-drug users.[20,21] Risk behavior surveys conducted in STD, abortion, family planning, and pre-natal clinics in 1989-1991 revealed a 2.8% positivity rate among 470 women who reported sex with both men and women. Their infection was associated with personal use of injected drugs and with sex with high-risk or infected men.[45]

Heterosexually acquired AIDS in U.S. women is increasing rapidly. Sex with an HIV-infected male accounted for 36% of all AIDS cases in U.S. adult and adolescent women since 1981, and for 50% of cases reported in 1992. Heterosexual exposure is a major risk factor in younger women, accounting for 49% of cumulative cases among women aged 20-24 years and 50% among women aged 13-19 years[14] (see Table 3-2).

African-American and Hispanic women are disproportionately represented in reported AIDS cases, due in part to injecting-drug use in urban segments of these ethnic groups, especially in Atlantic Coast cities. About 84% of children with perinatally acquired AIDS are African American or Hispanic.

Another persistent and disturbing trend is that younger U.S. groups of infected people have higher proportions of females than do older groups. Among AIDS cases reported in 1992-1993, 14% of those aged 25 and older were female, compared with 26% aged 20-24 and 33% of those aged 13-19.[14]

Estimates of HIV seroprevalence provide important information for planning the medical care of infected women and their children (See Table 3-3). The 1.5/1000 rate of infection among all childbearing women in 38 states underscores the magnitude of woman-to-offspring transmissions. AIDS deaths are projected to orphan 80,000 U.S. children and adolescents by the year 2000.[47]

The U.S. women already infected with HIV are demographically similar to people who seek reproductive health care in many publicly funded family planning, prenatal, abortion, and STD service sites. Thus, our patients fit the profile for women at risk for HIV infection, and we have an urgent responsibility to teach them skills to reduce their HIV risk.

Table 3-2 AIDS in persons younger than 25, United States, cumulative through March 1993

	Male 20–24 %	Female 20–24 %	Male 13–19 %	Female 13–19 %	Male and Female <13 %
Exposure Category					
Men/sex/men (MSM)	65	—	33	—	—
Injecting drug (ID)	12	36	7	23	—
MSM/ID	10	—	5	—	—
Hemophilia	4	0	43	1	4
Heterosexual	3	49	3	50	—
Blood, tissue	1	3	4	9	7
Mother at risk, infected	—	—	—	—	87
Risk not identified	4	11	5	17	2

Source: Centers for Disease Control and Prevention (1993a).

Table 3-3 Selected seroprevalence rates among U.S. women

Group	Time Period	Seroprevalence (%)
Childbearing women[1]	1988–1990	0.15
Job Corps entrants[2]	1987–1992	0.4
Publically funded HIV test recipients[3]	1989–1990	3.0 HIV test site 2.2 STD clinic 3.7 drug treatment 0.5 family planning clinic 0.9 prenatal/obstetric clinic 6.3 prison
Military applicants[4]	1985–1990	0.06

Sources: 1. Gwinn et al. 1991.
2. Conway 1993.
3. Centers for Disease Control and Prevention 1991.
4. Division of HIV/AIDS 1991.

HIV PREVENTION IN THE REPRODUCTIVE HEALTH CARE SETTING

It would be hard to imagine a reproductive health care patient who *does not* merit some sort of HIV prevention intervention. Even the patient in a long-term monogamous relationship is theoretically one partner away from HIV. Many patients are not in long-term monogamous relationships at all. Many patients need new skills in order to be effective HIV prevention educators for their own children.

The care provider has several key tasks in HIV prevention:

- **Ask each and every patient, "What do you do to protect yourself from AIDS?"**[4] You can always take him or her one step further in skill mastery, even in a brief discussion. You may be able to determine the patient's readiness for behavior change by assessing the answer given to your question, using a theoretical framework for personal behavior change that has been used and studied extensively in U.S. HIV prevention programs. See Chapter 23, Table 23-1 for details.

- **Assess substance use for each patient and for his or her sex partner(s)** with direct behavior-based questions such as those described in the section on "A Brief Sexual History and Counseling Techniques" in Chapter 1. The riskiest behavior of all is personal injecting-drug use with shared, uncleaned injection equipment. Having sex with a infected drug user is also extremely risky, and because injecting-drug use in the present or past is often a carefully hidden practice, some patients will be exposed to this sexual risk without being aware of it. Addiction to non-injected drugs or alcohol also increases HIV risk because of potentially self-destructive risk taking to obtain drugs, money, food, and/or shelter.

- **Teach explicit safer sex skills,** including correct use of male and female condoms and other latex and synthetic barriers, to all at-risk patients (see Table 3-4). Use audiovisual, print, and electronic teaching aids appropriate to the patient's skill, culture, language, and age.
- **Teach skills, not just facts.** Most Americans know what AIDS is, know it is lethal, and know it is transmitted through sex and shared uncleaned injecting-drug equipment. Sexual decisions may not be based on reason, however, and human beings may act not out of what they *know*, but out of what they *feel* and *see*.[40] Patients need our help,

Table 3-4 Safer sex options for physical intimacy

Safe
> Massage
> Hugging
> Body rubbing
> Dry kissing
> Masturbation
> Hand-to-genital touching (hand job) or mutual masturbation
> Erotic books and movies
> All sexual activities, when both partners are monogamous, trustworthy, and known
> by testing to be free of HIV

Possibly Safe
> Wet kissing with no broken skin, cracked lips, or damaged mouth tissue
> Vaginal or rectal intercourse using latex or synthetic condom correctly
> Oral sex on a man using a latex or synthetic condom
> Oral sex on a woman using a latex or synthetic barrier such as a female condom,
> dental dam, or modified male condom, especially if she does not have her period
> or a vaginal infection with discharge
> All sexual activities, when both partners are in a long-term monogamous relationship
> and trust each other

Unsafe in the absence of HIV testing and trust and monogamy
> Any vaginal or rectal intercourse without a latex or synthetic condom
> Oral sex on a man without a latex or synthetic condom
> Oral sex on a woman without a latex or synthetic barrier such as a female condom,
> dental dam, or modified male condom, especially if she is having her period or has
> a vaginal infection with discharge
> Semen in the mouth
> Oral-anal contact
> Sharing sex toys or douching equipment
> Blood contact of any kind, including menstrual blood, or any sex that causes tissue
> damage or bleeding

Source: Adapted from Planned Parenthood (1987).

therefore, with skills for forging relationships with low-risk people, skills for sexual negotiating in relationships, and skills for operating from an internal value system rather than from external pressure.

CONTRACEPTIVE CHOICE AND HIV PREVENTION

Male condom efficacy. Latex and synthetic condoms are the best way to reduce STD/HIV risk during intercourse and fellatio. Numerous studies have shown that male condoms help prevent the transmission of HIV,[7] but it remains difficult to give patients precise answers about *how much* protection they can count on. One problem is that we do not know how to factor in slippage and breakage effects (see Chapter 7 on Condoms). Studies of women at high risk for HIV, including commercial sex workers and women who are partners of infected men, have shown protective effects with male condoms, but it is not clear what other behavioral and biological factors play a role in HIV transmission. For example, a study of 256 sexually active serodiscordant heterosexual couples who were followed for a median of 22 months found no seroconversions in the 123 couples who always used condoms and 12 seroconversions in the 122 couples who used condoms intermittently. Additional factors that may have played a role in transmission were advanced disease in the HIV-infected partner, genital infection, and ejaculation (rather than withdrawal).[29] Care providers must assure patients that male condoms clearly help in HIV prevention, but more precise quantifying of condom efficacy depends on personal circumstances.

Timing when to put on a male condom is a practical issue. Some men leak seminal fluid from the urethral meatus once the penis is fully erect, and this clear pre-ejaculatory fluid can contain HIV and other pathogens (although not motile sperm capable of causing pregnancy).[36,52] When a condom is used for safer sex, it must be rolled on the penis well before the penis has any contact with the partner's mouth, vagina, anus, or any broken skin.

The take-home message for all patients: Always using male condoms and always using them correctly *works*. Halfway measures do not work.[54]

Spermicide benefits and risks. For two decades, nonoxynol-9-based spermicide products have been the "chicken soup" of reproductive health care, as we have generally advised users of other contraceptive methods to add a spermicide for improved contraceptive efficacy and for protection against STDs. In 1993, this advice was being questioned in the context of HIV risk, in part because spermicide-mediated vulvovaginal microabrasions could theoretically increase susceptibility to HIV. Data to help us solve this dilemma are limited and sometimes flawed,[7,41,53] but clearly, women who have compromised vulvar and vaginal tissue—especially with few or no symptoms to alert them—could have some measure of increased susceptibility to HIV. It is unclear how their male partners might be affected by vulvovaginal microabrasions in an HIV-infected woman.

Other contraceptive use.   One powerful reason women of all ages like oral contraceptives, other hormonal methods, IUDs, and surgical sterilization for birth control is that nothing mechanical or intrusive gets in the way of sex. Therefore, special effort may be needed to encourage these patients to add male or female condoms for STD/HIV protection. Data show an inverse relationship between the use of more effective methods and concurrent condom use. In Baltimore, for example, more than three-quarters of sterilized women never used a condom, compared with 46% of non-sterilized women.[12] Among 12,000 U.S. high school students, 19% of pill users used condoms at last intercourse, compared with 54% of other sexually active students; pill use was the single strongest predictor of failure to use condoms, even stronger than alcohol or drug use or multiple partners.[24] We are a long way from pills-plus-condoms as the cultural norm for protected sex. Unfortunately this behavior is rarely modelled in the media, and pregnancy often feels more like a genuine personal threat than HIV does. Almost everybody knows someone who has been involved in an unplanned pregnancy, while many people have never (to their knowledge) known anyone with HIV.

Oral contraceptives increase the vascularity of the cervical epithelium and alter certain immune parameters.[8] Whether pill use increases susceptibility to HIV in any way, for women or for their male partners, remains unknown. This issue is currently undergoing investigation. Meanwhile, advise all pill users to use male or female latex or synthetic condoms as well, unless they are certain that both partners are free of HIV and other STDs.

Advice for contraceptive patients.   Until further data are available, it seems prudent to advise all patients as follows:

- If at all possible, use male or female latex or synthetic condoms each and every time you suspect any risk of HIV transmission but choose to have intercourse anyway.

- If you cannot use condoms, vaginal spermicides are a second-best option to prevent bacterial infections such as gonorrhea and chlamydia.

- Any tissue damage on the vulva or vagina could increase susceptibility to HIV and other STDs. Avoid intercourse until you are healed. See your clinician for help with healing.

- If you use contraceptive sponges or other spermicide products, be alert for tender, red, or raw tissue. Avoid intercourse and avoid spermicides (including spermicide-coated condoms) until you are healed. Ask your clinician to check you carefully for signs of irritation any time you have routine exams, because vaginal irritation may not cause any symptoms.

These directions can be modified for gay male, lesbian, and bisexual patients.

SPECIAL CONSIDERATION IN HIV PREVENTION

Romance. It is difficult to hold simultaneously the two thoughts, "I'm in love with you," and "You might pose an infection risk to me." Romantic (germ-free) fantasy is a hallmark of midadolescence,[39] and many people never manage to be clear-eyed about romance even when realism pervades all other aspects of the adult worldview. Therefore, the reproductive health care provider is frequently in the unenviable position of bubble-burster, attempting to foster self-protective health behavior where there is only desire, emotional neediness, and single-minded devotion to the idealized love relationship.

Effective HIV prevention counseling with patients who are in love does not set up the beloved as a bad person, but stresses that all people can and do harm other people even when they do not mean to, and that people who love each other would certainly try to help each other maintain good health!

Power imbalance. Sometimes women patients express interest in and even personal commitment to HIV prevention steps but have little hope of enlisting the cooperation of their male partners. They say, for example, "You might as well not give me any condoms, because I know he won't use them." In all U.S. cultural groups, women typically lack economic, social, and personal power equal to that of men. Even when couples negotiate and achieve a relationship with equal decision-making power, they are likely to have begun the relationship with a power imbalance.

Perhaps the most direct way for women's care providers to address this issue is to urge women to bring in their partners and to offer prevention skill-building for these men, either together with the female partner or alone. When men cannot or will not come in, telephone counseling with a male counselor can be offered instead. When no way exists to speak directly with the patient's partner, give patients specially targeted audiotape or print messages to give to men. Remember that cultural norms vary substantially in how sexual decisions get made and by whom, so be sure counseling is grounded in the cultural reality of your patient population.

A woman-controlled vaginal microbicide is a high research priority for HIV prevention, but it is at least a decade away. Meanwhile, women at risk must be encouraged to use male and female latex or synthetic condoms and other safer sex techniques consistently, even when they are unaccustomed to such expressions of personal power.

Special needs of adolescents. The critical challenge for reproductive health care providers in this decade is to implement effective HIV prevention strategies for adolescents who are entering into sexual and drug-use experimentation. Interventions in the 1980s and early 1990s have increased knowledge and sometimes led to modest behavior change, but in general, adolescents still take many risks. Among urban adolescents moving into young adulthood, risk-taking behaviors remained about the same from 1985 to 1990,[58] regardless of their knowledge about HIV, number of sources of information, acquaintance with infected people, perception of personal risk, or experience with HIV test counseling. Most young people disliked condoms, did not use them on a regular basis, and did not trust condoms to be protective.[58]

A bold six-step plan for improving HIV prevention strategies with adolescents is essential:[35]

- Use teenagers as spokespersons, and not irresponsible stereotypes, in prevention campaigns.
- Replace abstinence-only campaigns with a more balanced approach aimed at delaying first intercourse and other sexual experimentation.
- Saturate the adolescent environment with appropriate and explicit risk-reduction messages.
- Link prevention programs with easy access to testing and medical services.
- Help adults learn to deal with sexuality and HIV, including parents, teachers, youth workers, and health care workers.
- Link on-site condom availability with HIV prevention programs in schools and youth agencies.

Reproductive health care providers must be in the forefront to adapt these suggestions to our own communities, fighting for the lives of our young patients.

HIV TESTING AND COUNSELING

No more important conduit to HIV testing services exists than the reproductive health care provider. Almost 300,000 HIV antibody tests were conducted on blood from women in family planning, prenatal, and abortion clinics through 1990, as part of national seroprevalence surveys,[30] and more than 200,000 tests (with a 0.6% seropositivity rate) were performed in 1991 in family planning clinics.[11]

WHEN TO OFFER TESTING

Reproductive health care providers are almost certainly going to increase HIV testing activity in this decade, both on-site and by referral. Testing should be offered liberally:

- Any time the patient *requests* testing, even if your own assessment of his or her HIV risk would not indicate testing.
- To all patients routinely, if you provide care in an area where HIV seroprevalence is high. (Discussion of a threshold seroprevalence for routine prenatal HIV testing, for example, has fallen in the 1 in 100 to 1 in 1,000 range.[25])
- Any time history reveals a present or past sex or drug use risk behavior. (See Chapter 1 for a sample brief history format.)
- Any time the patient is pregnant or planning a pregnancy.
- Any time you diagnose recurrent vulvovaginal candida or other sexually transmitted infection (see Chapter 4).
- Any time you diagnose infections or constitutional signs consistent with HIV infection (see next section).
- Any time history reveals consensual or coerced sex with a stranger whose health history and status remain unknown.
- Any time the patient had a blood transfusion between 1977 and April 1985 or has received multiple transfusions or blood products for any reason.
- Any time the patient has lived in an area of the world where HIV is endemic.
- Any time the patient has history of a workplace or other injury or accident that might result in HIV exposure.

Test Counseling

The decision to be tested for HIV belongs to the patient. The provider's role is to explain how the test is done, what the routine screening procedure will and will not reveal, characteristics of anonymous and confidential testing, and instructions on learning test results. Some patients do not return for test results, so use the pre-test session to teach personalized and explicit risk-reduction skills. Table 3-5 presents a counselor's checklist for the pre-test session, and Table 3-6 presents a checklist for giving positive test results to patients. Upon their return visit, patients with negative test results should receive guidance as follows:

- Explicit and personalized sex and drug risk-reduction guidance
- Discussion of the possibility of a false negative result from infection less than 6 months in duration
- Guidance for next test interval, if appropriate

Counselors who do test counseling full-time generally allow 15-30 minutes for a pre-test, 10-15 for a negative post-test, and 30-45 for a positive post-test session.

Table 3-5 Counseling checklist for pre-test counseling

Understand why patient desires testing
Positive result means infected and able to infect others; not necessarily AIDS
Negative result means probably not infected; can become infected later if risk continues
Test can be falsely positive, falsely negative, indeterminant
Personalized and explicit risk reduction skills, including referral if needed
Anonymous vs. confidential testing
State requirements for reporting test results
Possible benefits of testing
- provides peace of mind
- helps diagnose symptoms
- allows early care if infected
- provides opportunity to inform and protect partner(s) if infected
- adds information for childbearing decisions
- allows access to disability programs if infected

Possible drawbacks of testing
- anxiety waiting for results
- positive result causes extreme emotional stress
- possible distancing from some loved ones if infected
- possible loss of job, housing if infected
- probable loss or other difficulty with health insurance if infected
- awkwardness, risk of telling sex or needle-sharing partners

Evaluate coping skills and personal support network
Allow patient to make uncoerced decision
Informed consent
Appointment and instructions for return visit

Sources: American Medical Association (1993) and Centers for Disease Control and Prevention (1993d).

SPECIAL ISSUES IN COUNSELING AND TESTING

Resistance.   Reproductive health care providers dread telling a young woman she has a lethal, incurable illness. Test counseling is time-consuming; it also requires specialized training and mastery of new referral resources. Be careful to provide sensitive staff training and support both before and after your work setting initiates testing and counseling.

Anonymous vs. confidential testing.   *Anonymous* testing never links a name to the serum sample presented for evaluation (although age, county of residence, sex, and other general demographic characteristics are often recorded). The anonymous patient is given a number code to bring back after a specific interval for getting test results. *Confidential* testing is name-linked, and information is protected to a degree determined by state

Table 3-6 Counseling checklist for positive test results

Give result and assess understanding of result, face to face

Attend to and comfort patient as long as needed

Assess emotional state, with referral to psychological support services if needed

Assist with referral for primary health care

Assist with plan for informing loved ones, sex or needle-sharing partners; encourage testing as appropriate

Assist with plan to avoid transmission
- abstinence as option
- easy access to free condoms
- option counseling for pregnant women
- contraception as appropriate; 20%-30% transmission rate to offspring
- personalized, explicit safer-sex guidance as needed
- personalized, explicit instructions on safer injecting-drug use and treatment, as needed
- no donation of blood, semen, tissue, organs
- no sharing of toothbrushes, razors
- no breastfeeding

Assist with health maintenance
- stress hope, optimism
- refer to support group
- advise on nutrition, rest, exercise
- reduce/eliminate tobacco, alcohol, other drugs
- avoid new STDs
- refer to 24-hour talk lines
- refer to HIV service organizations
- inform dentist, other caregivers

Assure emotional stability before terminating session; schedule a second post-test visit or refer as needed

Sources: American Medical Association (1993) and Centers for Disease Control and Prevention (1993d).

law and the formal policies and staff commitment to confidentiality at the particular testing site.

Allow patients to choose the method they prefer, and be prepared to make a careful referral for anonymous testing if you do not provide it on-site. Most labs are willing to work out a coding system for anonymous serum samples. Patients not offered anonymous testing and reluctant to have an HIV test on record are likely to go to a test site where they are not known and to use a false name.

Discourage patients from donating blood as a way to get HIV testing, because of the possibility they will donate falsely negative blood early in HIV infection.

Test accuracy. Both the serum ELISA test and the Western blot confirmatory test are very sensitive and specific,[54] but neither test is perfect, so an HIV antibody test is reported as positive on a given serum sample *only after* at least two ELISA tests and one Western blot or other confirmatory test are all positive. Known causes of false ELISA test results are given in Table 3-7. As with any laboratory screening test, population seroprevalence is the single biggest factor in determining a test's predictive value; the higher the seroprevalence, the greater the likelihood that a positive test result means that the person is really infected.[55]

Always regard laboratory test results in the context of the total patient history and clinical picture, and re-evaluate when the two are not in accord. The 23-year-old needle-drug-using woman with thrush who tests negative merits further evaluation, as does the healthy 30-year-old lesbian woman with no drug use or transfusion history who tests positive.

Pregnancy. Many U.S. women learn they have HIV when testing is done as part of routine prenatal care. Frequently these women are not aware of any personal HIV risk factors. Pregnancy option counseling then becomes an important component of post-test counseling (see Table 3-6), and the patient has an enormous amount of highly emotional information to absorb at once. Pregnant infected women make the same sorts of reproductive decisions as do uninfected women, with similar percentages of pregnancies and live births. Knowledge of HIV infection may increase the likelihood that a woman would seek pregnancy termination if her infection is diagnosed during early pregnancy.[60]

Charting. Charting of HIV test results is clearly important for ongoing medical care. On the other hand, some insurance companies have denied health insurance coverage on the basis of even a *negative* test result in the chart, reasoning that some risk behavior must be present in the

Table 3-7 False results with HIV antibody ELISA testing

False Negatives
Test performed too early, <3–6 months after infection
History of replacement transfusion
Bone marrow transplant
Use of test kit for antibody only to p24 antigen
Tester error

False Positives
Cross-reacting antibodies such as those against class II human leukocyte antigens, most often seen in multiparous women, persons with multiple transfusions
Cross-reacting autoantibodies against smooth muscle or parietal cells, anti-mitochondrial antibodies, antinuclear antibodies, anti-T-cell antibodies
Tester error

Source: Adapted from Saag (1992).

patient's life. This dilemma can be addressed by maintaining HIV-related information in a separate chart, by using a code for HIV test results, or by removing HIV-related information before releasing the chart. This latter practice is required by law in some states. State and local professional associations may offer helpful guidance for appropriate charting that does not compromise patient or care provider.

M EDICAL CARE AND PSYCHOSOCIAL SUPPORT FOR INFECTED PATIENTS

CHARACTERISTICS OF HIV IN WOMEN

The course of HIV in women appears to be similar to the illness in men. In limited studies of women, laboratory findings, early symptoms, late illnesses, treatment responses, and duration of illness are fairly consistent with findings in men.[3] Women also have a whole constellation of gynecologic problems.

Adults with HIV typically feel well for months or years, then progress from minor skin and constitutional symptoms, to discrete opportunistic illness, to a cascade of illnesses, to end-stage disease. Whether all people with HIV ultimately progress to illness and death is not yet clear. In a cohort of men infected for 11 years, 19% remained symptom-free while 54% progressed to AIDS.[22] Table 3-8 reviews the typical characteristics, duration, CD4 cell count, and reproductive health concerns of each stage of HIV infection.

Most HIV specialists recommend that infected patients receive their primary health care from a clinician experienced with and comfortable with HIV care. Reproductive health care will ideally be managed in the primary health care setting also, but often the primary care provider and reproductive health care provider are in different sites, so careful attention to shared information, shared decision making, and collaboration is essential.

A natural role for the reproductive health care provider is to assist patients with health promotion strategies, low-risk activities that engender optimism and may contribute to slowing HIV progression. Provide guidance on nutrition, stress management, exercise, rest, and reduction or elimination of tobacco, alcohol, or drugs.[38]

PSYCHOSOCIAL CARE AND SUPPORT

Women with HIV are likely to be caregivers themselves, accustomed to attending to the needs of children, spouse, parents, and others, and they may resist moving into a self-care mode. Women may make sure their children's clinic appointments are kept, for example, but be less diligent about keeping their own appointments. Gently remind the patient that she deserves care as well.

Table 3-8 Stages of HIV infection

	Infection → Seroconversion	Symptom-Free	Early Symptoms	Discrete Illness → Cascade of Illness → Endstage
Characteristics	Some notice a flu-like illness that resolves in ± 2 weeks Would test negative for HIV antibody in "window period" that typically lasts 6–12 weeks after infection	Likely to test positive 6–12 weeks after infection Without test, may have no reason to suspect infection With test, difficult to resolve feeling well with ominous diagnosis With test, loss of sense of health, and loss of uncomplicated sex Not yet clear whether some people have HIV and do not progress to illness	Fevers, night sweats, zoster, candida, hairy leukoplakia, skin problems, weight loss, fatigue, loss of appetite Symptoms often prompt testing and diagnosis Offer antiretroviral drugs (AZT, DDI, etc.) Evaluate for TB Loss of strength, looks, stamina, long-range planning	Average interval from infection to AIDS is 11 years Opportunistic infections: bacterial, viral, fungal, parasitic; mild or severe Neoplastic: Kaposi's sarcoma, lymphoma, cervical cancer Neurologic: dementia, memory, affect, gait, peripheral neuropathy Evaluate for TB Many medications daily, side effects common Loss of job, ability to care for self, ability to interact with others Saying goodbye
Duration	Average 6–12 weeks	Few months to many years	Few months to several years	Few months to several years, and lengthening
CD4 Cell Count/µL	Normal or high Normal = 400–1200	Typically > 500	Typically < 500	AIDS diagnosis automatic at ≤ 200
Reproductive Health Concerns	No test available for early diagnosis and so sex partner(s) and offspring may be placed at risk	No reason to suspect risk to sex partner(s) and offspring without testing May be tested as part of routine prenatal screening Offer anticipatory guidance on future pregnancy planning Pap every 6 months, aggressive management of abnormal findings Offer personalized, explicit safer-sex skill building Pregnancy likely to be uncomplicated by HIV	Aggressive, recurrent vulvovaginal candida; other aggressive STDs should prompt HIV evaluation Pregnancy likely to be uncomplicated by HIV Pap every 6 months, aggressive management of abnormal findings Aggressive management of gynecologic infections Assess contraception, safer sex status	Assist with arranging child care Pregnancy may result in prematurity, low birth weight, premature rupture of membranes, other complications Pap every 6 months, aggressive management of abnormal findings Aggressive management of gynecologic infections Assess contraception, safer sex status
Risk of Transmission to Offspring	20%–30% each pregnancy	20%–30% each pregnancy	20%–30% each pregnancy	20%–30% each pregnancy. Unclear whether risk increases as illness progresses

Source: Adapted from McKusick (1992).

Sometimes the infected woman is not the only infected person in her household; her spouse or partner and one or more children may also have HIV, so the disruption of daily life may be profound.

When infected women discuss their biggest worries and concerns, several fundamental needs are often mentioned:

- Housing
- Income
- A good caregiver for children when mother/patient is not feeling well
- Worry about health of children
- Dread about disclosing illness to a particular loved one, especially a child
- Fear of losing ability to care for oneself
- Relationship with spouse/partner
- Coping with addiction

Any guidance, support, and referral you can offer to assist with these fundamental concerns is likely to be welcome and helpful. Remember that for a women in poverty, HIV may not be at the top of her list of things to worry about.

CONTRACEPTIVE MANAGEMENT

HIV-infected women, like all women, are more likely to succeed with a contraceptive they have chosen for themselves and feel comfortable using, so the whole range of methods can be offered, with the probable exception of the IUD. (Many care providers are reluctant to expose the patient to the risk of pelvic infection secondary to IUD insertion.) The goal is high contraceptive efficacy, low risk of woman-to-partner HIV transmission, and low risk of partner-to-woman STD transmission. This goal is met by options such as oral contraceptives plus male latex or synthetic condoms. In reality, infected women often choose a method of birth control without regard to disease transmission factors, just as uninfected women often do. Table 3-9 describes characteristics of contraceptives specific to HIV issues.

GYNECOLOGIC MANAGEMENT

The keys to successful management of gynecologic infections in HIV-infected women are prompt diagnosis, aggressive treatment, and secondary prophylaxis when appropriate.

Candida. Vulvovaginal candidiasis is typically an early manifestations of HIV,[37] and recurrent candida is common, occurring up to 45% of the time.[5] First-line treatment is one of the over-the-counter topical antifungals

Table 3-9 Contraception and the HIV-infected woman

Method	Possible Benefits	Possible Drawbacks
Oral Contraceptives	Good efficacy with consistent use	Unclear interaction of steroids and immune function
	Scanty blood loss to avoid anemia	Interaction with certain antibiotics and other drugs
		Possible increased shedding of virus from cervix
		No STD protection
		May increase anergy
IUD		Risk of uterine infection secondary to insertion
		No STD protection
		Increased days of bleeding, possible anemia, partner transmission
Norplant Depo-Provera	Good low-maintenance efficacy	Unclear interaction of steroids and immune function
		No STD protection
		May increase anergy
Diaphragm, Cap, Sponge, Other Vaginal Barriers	Limited STD protection	
Male and Female Condom	Good STD protection	Male condom requires partner cooperation
Surgical Sterilization	Good low-maintenance efficacy for women ready to terminate childbearing	No STD protection

Sources: Denenberg (1993a) and (1993b), Clemetson (1993).

(See Chapter 4, candidiasis). If topical treatment proves unsatisfactory, use oral Ketoconazole, 200–400 mg/day for 14 days, then a 5-day course each month for 6 months. Liver function should be monitored before and throughout treatment.[48]

Cervical disease. Human papillomavirus-mediated cervical disease may progress more rapidly in HIV-infected women. Consider 6-month Pap smear intervals and colposcopy/biopsy of any abnormal Pap findings. Treatment of abnormal or neoplastic cervical disease should be prompt and aggressive. HIV-infected women with preinvasive and invasive cervical cancer may have more rapid recurrence and die sooner than uninfected women. Of 10 infected women in one series who died, nine died of cervical disease and one died of AIDS, underscoring the need for aggressive treatment in infected women.[42,43,48]

Pelvic inflammatory disease (PID).   Most HIV specialists recommend inpatient management of PID using standard treatment regimens for all women[16] (see Chapter 4, pelvic inflammatory disease). With proper treatment, the course of PID in HIV-infected women is similar to PID in other women.[48,61]

Herpes.   Herpes lesions may be more extensive, more painful, and slower to heal in the presence of HIV infection. Suppressive doses of acyclovir are often prescribed.

Menstrual problems.   Women with HIV may report new problems with heavy bleeding, irregular periods, and premenstrual syndrome. HIV, medications, emotional stress, or all three may contribute to the problem.[27] Infected women, like other women, cope with menopause. Oral contraceptives may be helpful for menstrual regulation and hormonal replacement therapy for menopause.[28] Hormonal intervention also may be offered for heavy bleeding and anemia and to ease discomfort. All menstrual irregularities merit a full evaluation. Do not assume HIV is always the culprit.[28]

Pregnancy and HIV.   Thousands of U.S. women with HIV give birth each year.[34,57] Generally, HIV-infected women who are not late in the course of illness have uneventful pregnancies with normal labor and delivery. Just as with any woman with serious systemic illness, women very late in HIV illness may have complicated pregnancies, including prematurity, low birth weight, and premature rupture of membranes. However, the effects of HIV on pregnancy are hard to differentiate from the effects of poverty, poor health care, or addiction.[48]

HIV medications are often continued in pregnancy for women with late-stage illness, namely ≤200 CD4 cells. When the woman is moderately immunocompromised, from 200-500 CD4 cells, her own judgment is crucial as she evaluates the benefit of treatment for herself versus any possible adverse effects of medication on the developing fetus.[48] Women with normal immune function, with 400-500 or more CD4 cells, will often choose to be medication-free during pregnancy.

Each offspring of an infected woman faces a 20%-30% (range 13%-45%) risk of being infected *in utero,* during birth, or while breastfeeding.[33] Infants will all test positive for HIV antibody at birth because of the presence of maternal antibodies in infant blood. The HIV test becomes accurate for the infant's true status at 15-18 months. Many infected infants become ill before the first birthday.[33] Negative HIV serology in a totally healthy 18-month-old is proof that the child had been spared infection.[33]

Reproductive decision making for the infected woman is similar to uninfected women, and desire for a child is often profound. Infected women have freedom to make reproductive choices for themselves just as other U.S. women do. Counseling for the infected woman who is pregnant or contemplating pregnancy includes the following:[2]

- Impact of HIV on pregnancy
- Impact of pregnancy on HIV
- Effect of treatment on patient and fetus
- Risk of woman-to-offspring transmission
- Risk of breastfeeding for HIV transmission
- Course of HIV in perinatally infected infants

Unfortunately for counselor and patient alike, relatively little is known about most of these issues.

Counseling for pregnancy optimally includes a full understanding of the patient's personal support network, a full understanding of stressors in her life, and her overall physical and psychosocial status. Once all this groundwork is in place, consider walking the patient through these five scenarios, helping her predict how she will feel, how others will feel, and what will happen:[2]

- She becomes sick in pregnancy and has to decide whether or not to take medication that could harm the fetus.
- She will not know the child's HIV status for 18 months.
- After birth, she feels well, but her baby gets sick and possibly dies.
- After birth, she gets sick and possibly dies, but her baby stays healthy.
- Both she and her baby get sick and possibly die.

Clearly, this is difficult counseling work, best carried out by counselors with experience, compassion, and ability to help with the feelings of grief and loss that these scenarios will likely generate. The goal is to guide each patient to an uncoerced, thoughtful decision.

WORKPLACE SAFETY

An intense and persistent concern with personal safety is normal and common when health care workers take care of HIV-infected patients, even in an ambulatory setting. When agency policies and procedures and staff training are managed appropriately, worker safety can be maintained at high levels. Workplace safety with regard to HIV and other blood-borne pathogens has several essential components:

- Universal Precautions or another infection control system for protecting the worker (and patient) from body fluid exposure

- Hepatitis B vaccination for all workers with any risk of exposure to blood or bloody body fluid
- A post-exposure plan for appropriate management of needlesticks and other accidental exposures
- Appropriate procedures for respiratory isolation for tuberculosis.

INFECTION CONTROL

In the ambulatory reproductive health care setting, most care providers use Universal Precautions (UP). This means they treat all blood, bloody body fluids, semen, vaginal secretions, amniotic fluid, cerebrospinal fluid, serosal transudates and exudates, and inflammatory exudates as potentially infectious.[9,32] Basic instructions are as follows:

- Wash hands before and after every patient contact.
- Dispose of needles and sharps in puncture-resistant containers, and *never recap needles.*
- Wear gloves when likely to touch body fluids, mucous membranes, or broken skin.
- Wear protective eyewear and mask when eyes and mucous membranes may be splashed.
- Wear a water-repellent gown when clothing could be soiled with body substances.

Body substance precautions (BSP) or body substance isolation (BSI) is another good infection control system. This approach follows a single standard of precaution in anticipating exposure to all body fluids. UP takes into account the type of infection expected, and BSP is based on how much body fluid contact is expected. Both systems emphasize use of barriers, exposure prevention, and no special labeling so that all patients and laboratory specimens receive the same highly protective infection control procedures.[32]

OCCUPATIONALLY ACQUIRED HIV

Between three and five cases of occupationally acquired HIV continue to be reported annually to the CDC.[15] These workers had no known personal risk behaviors, a negative HIV antibody test at the time of exposure, and a subsequently positive test.[13] Most exposures were among laboratory workers and nurses. A larger number of workers have been reported to CDC with possible occupationally acquired HIV, with no known personal risk factors but without documented seroconversion. Nurses, laboratory workers, physicians, and health aides predominate in this group.

Needlesticks and other percutaneous exposures have accounted for 84% of cases, with some mucocutaneous exposures and one both percutaneous and mucocutaneous exposure.[13] Almost all exposures have been to blood. No infections have been observed from blood exposure to intact skin, from airborne droplets, or from environmental surfaces.[32] The exact proportion of occupationally acquired infections reported to the CDC is unknown.

The rate of occupational HIV infection following a single needlestick or other percutaneous exposure is about 0.3%, in more than 2,000 reported accidental exposures in the U.S. and other countries. The risk of infection from mucocutaneous exposure is too low to quantify.[32]

Of course, many thousands of health care workers have acquired HIV through sex and the other typical transmission routes. Whether HIV-infected health care workers pose any risk to their patients is not well understood. We will not likely ever know precisely what happened in the Florida dental practice that led to six patient infections. Other retrospective studies—voluntary HIV testing of patients cared for by infected physicians, surgeons, and dentists—have found no evidence of infection in any of 19,000 patients evaluated.[49] Infected dentists, physicians, and other care providers are usually advised to make practice decisions in consultation with the personal physician, supervisor, and other professional groups as appropriate.

PERSONAL PERSPECTIVE ON WORKPLACE SAFETY

To work in health care in the 1990s, each of us must accept the fact that the workplace is not, and has never been, 100% safe. Ultimately we are each responsible for our own safety and must insist on sound workplace policies and procedures, high-quality barriers and other equipment, and adequate staff training. In emergency situations, we must take the extra seconds to protect ourselves and our coworkers with barriers and careful sharps disposal. Most important, we must find a way to maintain compassionate touching, even when a latex barrier must sometimes come between provider and patient.

REFERENCES

1. American Medical Association. HIV blood test counseling: physician guidelines, 2nd edition. Chicago IL: American Medical Association, 1993.
2. Bermon N. Family and reproductive issues: reproductive counseling. AIDS Clinical Care 1993;5(3):45-47.
3. Brettle RP, Leen CLS. The natural history of HIV and AIDS in women. AIDS 1991;5(11):1283-1292.

4. Bush DM. Personal communication to F. Guest, November 10, 1991.
5. Carpenter CCJ, Mayer KH, Stein MD, Liebman BD, Fisher A, Fiore TC. Human immunodeficiency virus infection in North American women: experience with 200 cases and a review of the literature. Medicine 1991;70(5):307-325.
6. Cates W Jr., Stewart FH, Trussell J. Commentary: the quest for women's prophylactic methods—hope vs science. Am J Public Health 1992;82(11):1479-1482.
7. Cates W Jr., Stone KM. Family planning, sexually transmitted diseases and contraceptive choice: a literature update—part I. Fam Plann Perspect 1992; 24(2):75-84.
8. Cates W Jr., Stone KM. Family planning, sexually transmitted diseases and contraceptive choice: a literature update—part II. Fam Plann Perspect 1992;24(3):122-128.
9. Centers for Disease Control and Prevention. Guidelines for prevention of transmission of human immunodeficiency virus and hepatitis B virus to health-care and public-safety workers. MMWR 1989;38(S-6):1-37.
10. Centers for Disease Control and Prevention. Characteristics of, and HIV infection among, women served by publicly funded HIV counseling and testing services. MMWR 1991;40(12)195-197;203-204.
11. Centers for Disease Control and Prevention. Publicly funded HIV counseling and testing—United States, 1991. MMWR 1992;41(34):613-617.
12. Centers for Disease Control and Prevention. Surgical sterilization among women and use of condoms—Baltimore, 1989-1990. MMWR 1992;41(31):568-569; 575.
13. Centers for Disease Control and Prevention. Surveillance for occupationally acquired HIV infection—United States, 1981-1992. MMWR 1992;41(43):823-825.
14. Centers for Disease Control and Prevention. HIV/AIDS surveillance report 1993(a);5(1):1-10.
15. Centers for Disease Control and Prevention. HIV/AIDS surveillance report 1993(b);5(3):13-17.
16. Centers for Disease Control and Prevention. 1993 sexually transmitted diseases treatment guidelines. MMWR 1993(c);42(RR-14):1-73.
17. Centers for Disease Control and Prevention. Technical guidance on HIV counseling. MMWR 1993(d);42(RR-2):11-17.
18. Centers for Disease Control and Prevention. Update: mortality attributable to HIV infection/AIDS among persons age 25-44 years—United States 1990 and 1991. MMWR 1993(e);42(25):481-486.
19. Centers for Disease Control and Prevention. Years of potential life lost before age 65—United States, 1990 and 1991. MMWR 1993(f);42(13):251-253.
20. Chu SY, Buehler JW, Fleming PL, Berkelman RL. Epidemiology of reported cases of AIDS in lesbians, United States 1980-89. Am J Public Health 1990;80(11):1380-1381.
21. Chu SY, Hammett TA, Buehler JW. Update: epidemiology of reported cases of AIDS in women who report sex only with other women, United States, 1980-1991. AIDS 1992;6(5):518-519.
22. Clement M, Hollander H. Natural history and management of the seropositive patient, In: Sande MA, Volberding PA (eds). The medical management of AIDS, 3rd ed. Philadelphia PA: W.B. Saunders, 1992.

23. Clemetson DBA, Moss GB, Willerford DM, Hensel M, Emonyi W, Holmes KK, Plummer F, Ndinya-Achola J, Roberts PL, Hillier S, Kreiss J. Detection of HIV DNA in cervical and vaginal secretions: prevalence and correlates among women in Nairobi, Kenya. JAMA 1993;269(22):2860-2864.
24. Collins J, Holtzman D, Kann L, Kolbe L. Predictors of condom use among U.S. high school students, 1991. Abstract # WSC134. Presented at the Ninth International Conference on AIDS, June 6-11, 1993, Berlin, Germany.
25. Committee on Prenatal and Newborn Screening for HIV Infection, Institute of Medicine, Hardy LM (ed). HIV screening of pregnant women and newborns. Washington DC: National Academy Press, 1991.
26. Conway GA, Epstein MR, Hayman CR, Miller CA, Wendell DA, Gwinn M, Karon JM, Peterson LR. Trends in HIV prevalence among disadvantaged youth. JAMA 1993;269(22):2887-2889.
27. Denenberg R. Female sex hormones and HIV. AIDS Clinical Care 1993(a);5(9): 69-71;76.
28. Denenberg R. Gynecological care manual for HIV positive women. Durant OK: Essential Medical Information Systems, 1993(b).
29. DeVincenzi I, for the European Communities Study Group on heterosexual transmission of HIV, European Centre for the Epidemiological Monitoring of AIDS, Paris, France. Heterosexual transmission of HIV in a European cohort of couples. Abstract # WSC021. Presented at the Ninth International Conference on AIDS, June 6-11, 1993, Berlin, Germany.
30. Division of HIV/AIDS, National Center for Infectious Diseases. National HIV seroprevalence summary: results through 1990. Atlanta GA: Centers for Disease Control and Prevention, 1991.
31. Ellerbrock TV, Bush TJ, Chamberland ME, Oxtoby MJ. Epidemiology of women with AIDS in the United States, 1981 through 1990. JAMA 1991;265(22):2971-2975.
32. Gerberding JL. HIV transmission to providers and their patients, In: Sande MA, Volberding PA (eds). The medical management of AIDS, 3rd ed. Philadelphia PA: W.B. Saunders, 1992.
33. Grossman M. Pediatric AIDS, In: Sande MA, Volberding PA (eds). Medical Management of AIDS, 3rd ed. Philadelphia PA: W.B. Saunders, 1992.
34. Gwinn M, Pappaioanou M, George JR, Hannon WH, Wasser SC, Redus MA, Hoff R, Grady GF, Willoughby A, Novello AC, Petersen LR, Dondero TJ, Curran JW. Prevalence of HIV infection in childbearing women in the United States. JAMA 1991;265(13):1704-1708.
35. Hein K. "Getting real" about HIV in adolescents. Am J Public Health 1993;83(4):492-494.
36. Ilaria G, Jacobs JL, Polsky B, Koll B, Baron P, MacLow C, Armstrong D, Schlegel PN. Detection of HIV-1 DNA sequences in pre-ejaculatory fluid. Lancet 1992;340(8833):1469.
37. Imam N, Carpenter CCJ, Mayer KH, Fisher A, Stein M, Danforth SB. Hierarchical pattern of mucosal candida infections in HIV-seropositive women. Am J Medicine 1990;89(2):142-146.
38. Jewett JF, Hecht FM. Preventive health care for adults with HIV infection. JAMA 1993;269(9):1144-1153.
39. Johnson R. Adolescent growth and development In: Hofmann A, Greydanus D (eds). Adolescent medicine, 2nd ed. Norwalk CT: Appleton & Lange, 1989.
40. Keeling R. Personal communication, May 20, 1993.

41. Kreiss J, Ngugi E, Holmes K, Ndinya-Achola J, Waiyaki P, Roberts PL, Ruminjo I, Sajabi R, Kimata J, Fleming TR, Anzala A, Holton D, Plummer F. Efficacy of nonoxynol-9 contraceptive sponge use in preventing heterosexual acquisition of HIV in Nairobi prostitutes. JAMA 1992;268(4):477-482.

42. Maiman M, Fruchter RG, Guy L, Cuthill S, Levine P, Serur E. Human immunodeficiency virus infection and invasive cervical carcinoma. Cancer 1993;71(2):402-406.

43. Maiman M, Fruchter RG, Serur E, Remy JC, Feuer G, Boyce J. Human immunodeficiency virus infection and cervical neoplasia. Gynecol Oncol 1990; 38(3):377-382.

44. Mann JM, Tarantola DJM, Netter TW (eds). AIDS in the world. Cambridge MA: Harvard University Press, 1992.

45. McCombs SB, McCray E, Wendell DA, Sweeney PA, Onarato IM. Epidemiology of HIV-1 infection in bisexual women. J Acquir Immune Defic Syndr 1992; 5(8):850-852.

46. McKusick L, Counseling across the HIV spectrum. HIV Frontline 1992;No. 8, June 1992:1-8.

47. Michaels D, Levine C. Estimates of the number of motherless youth orphaned by AIDS in the United States. JAMA 1992;268(24):3456-3461.

48. Minkoff HL, DeHovitz JA. Care of women infected with the human immunodeficiency virus. JAMA 1991;266(16):2253-2258.

49. Mishu B. HIV-infected surgeons and dentists: looking back and looking forward. JAMA 1993;269(14):1843-1844.

50. Nanda D, Minkoff H. HIV in pregnancy—transmission and immune effects. Clin Obstet Gynecol 1989;32(3):456-466.

51. Planned Parenthood Federation of America. New medical standards for HIV testing and counseling. Memorandum dated August 13, 1987.

52. Pudney J, Oneta M, Mayer K, Seage G, Anderson D. Pre-ejaculatory fluid as potential vector for sexual transmission of HIV-1. Lancet 1992;340(8833):1470.

53. Rekart ML, Barnett JA, Manzon LM, Wittenberg L, McNabb A. Nonoxynol-9: its adverse effects. Abstract # SC36. Presented at the Sixth International Conference on AIDS, June 23, 1990, San Francisco, California.

54. Roper WL, Peterson HB, Curran JW. Commentary: condoms and HIV/STD prevention—clarifying the message. Am J Public Health 1993;83(4):501-503.

55. Saag MS. AIDS testing: now and in the future. In: Sande MA, Volberding PA (eds). The medical management of AIDS, 3rd ed. Philadelphia PA: W.B. Saunders, 1992.

56. Sloand EM, Pitt E, Chiarello RJ, Nemo GJ. HIV testing: state of the art. JAMA 1991;266(20):2861-2866.

57. Sperling RS, Stratton P, and members of Obstetric-Gynecologic Working Group of AIDS Clinical Trials Group of National Institute of Allergy and Infectious Diseases. Obstet Gynecol 1992;79(3):443-448.

58. Stiffman AR, Earls F, Dore P, Cunningham R. Changes in acquired immunodeficiency syndrome-related risk behavior after adolescence: relationships to knowledge and experience concerning human immunodeficiency virus infection. Pediatrics 1992;89(5):950-956.

59. Stone KM, Peterson HB. Spermicides, HIV, and the vaginal sponge [editorial]. JAMA 1992;268(4):521-523.

60. Sunderland A, Minkoff HL, Handte J, Moroso G, Landesman S. The impact of human immunodeficiency virus serostatus on reproductive decisions of women. Obstet Gynecol 1992;79(6):1027-1031.

61. Wofsy CB. Therapeutic issues in women with HIV disease. In: Sande MA, Volberding PA (eds). The medical management of AIDS, 3rd ed. Philadelphia PA: W.B. Saunders, 1992.

Sexually Transmitted Diseases

- Sexually transmitted diseases (STDs) are the most frequent infections encountered by reproductive health professionals.
- STD prevention depends on both individual behavior (*e.g.*, contraceptive choice) and effective diagnosis/ treatment.
- STDs have four crucial long-term sequelae:
  1) tubal occlusion leading to infertility and ectopic pregnancy
  2) neonatal morbidity and mortality caused by transmission during pregnancy and childbirth
  3) genital cancers
  4) epidemiologic synergy with HIV transmission

In the 1990s, clinicians in family planning must also master the field of sexually transmitted diseases (STDs). The STD problem is steadily growing; increased numbers of people are becoming infected with more severe infections.[4] Persistent viral infections, including the human immunodeficiency virus (HIV), herpes simplex virus (HSV), hepatitis B virus (HBV), and human papillomavirus (HPV), have afflicted millions of people with incurable illness; syphilis and resistant strains of once easily cured gonorrhea are at high levels; long-term consequences of pelvic inflammatory disease (PID) such as infertility, ectopic pregnancy, and chronic pain have all increased in number of women affected and in importance;[58] and neoplastic sequelae such as cervical cancer and hepatocellular carcinoma have been closely linked to STDs.

Preventing the acquisition of infection is the most effective way to reduce the adverse consequences of STDs. However, diagnosing and treating current infection can also prevent personal complications and interrupt community transmission. This chapter provides general background about STD management in the family planning setting and current approaches to diagnosing and treating the most common STDs.

MAGNITUDE AND RISKS OF STDs

The number of people infected with sexually transmitted diseases or affected by the consequences of STDs is a major problem for our society.[11] The estimated total number of people newly infected with symptomatic STDs is approximately 13 million.[45] In the 1990s, the annual cost of PID and its consequences was estimated to be $4.2 billion for the United States.[55] Infertility consequent to PID alone accounts for over $1 billion of health care costs, to say nothing of the human misery. Although deaths due to STDs (primarily syphilis and PID) have declined over the past four decades, STDs still cause almost one-third of reproductive mortality in the United States.[28]

Individuals under age 25 account for a majority of STD cases. Two-thirds of reported cases of gonorrhea and chlamydia occur in persons 24 years of age or younger.[12] Rates of chlamydia, gonorrhea, vaginitis, and pelvic inflammatory disease are all highest in adolescents and decline exponentially with increasing age. STD cases are concentrated in socio-geographic clusters, the so-called "core-populations."[43] For example, low-income people in urban areas are more likely to have an STD than people of higher socioeconomic status or those who live in suburban or rural areas.

Most STDs show a biological sexism. Women suffer more severe long-term consequences including PID, infertility, ectopic pregnancy, chronic pelvic pain, and cervical cancer. Women are less likely to seek health care if infected because a greater percentage of their STDs is asymptomatic. Moreover, most STDs are more difficult to diagnose in women than in men. Additionally, due to the fluid dynamics of intercourse, women are more likely than men to acquire a sexually transmitted infection from any single sexual encounter.

The probability of unprotected sexual intercourse leading to an STD or its consequences differs from the risk of unintended pregnancy (Table 4-1). The likelihood of pregnancy changes during the menstrual cycle. The risk of acquiring an STD depends on (1) having intercourse with an infected person, (2) the transmissibility of the particular STD, and (3) the gender of the infected person. For example, the risk of acquiring gonorrhea from a single coital event (where one partner is infectious) is approximately 25% for men and 50% for women. The probability of suffering consequences from an STD depends on whether or not the person received proper diagnosis and treatment (Table 4-1).

Table 4-1 Comparative risk of adverse consequences from coitus—STD and unintended pregnancy

Unintended pregnancy/coital action[53]	
	17%–30% midcycle
	<1% during menses
Gonococcal transmission/coital act[33]	
	50% infected male, uninfected female
	25% infected female, uninfected male
PID per woman infected with cervical gonorrhea[42]	
	40% if not treated
	0% if promptly and adequately treated
Tubal infertility per PID episode[60]	
	8% after 1st episode
	20% after 2nd episode
	40% after 3rd or more episodes

One of the fundamental concepts affecting the field of STD is the "epidemiological synergy" between HIV and other STDs.[57] The best evidence supports the interrelationship between those organisms causing genital ulcers (HSV, syphilis, chancroid) and the transmission or acquisition of HIV. Moreover, because the immune dysfunction caused by HIV disease makes the ulcerative symptoms persist, the infections have a potentiating influence on each other. Additionally, those STD-producing symptoms of vaginal and/or urethral discharge (gonorrhea, chlamydia, trichomoniasis) have also been associated with higher levels of HIV infection. Thus, family planning clinicians must always suspect HIV in persons diagnosed with another STD.

STD PREVENTION AND PERSONAL BEHAVIORS

Different individuals accept different levels of risk to satisfy personal needs. Not everyone will follow every recommendation but, with the proper knowledge, each person can make his or her own informed choices. Just as with eating properly, exercising, using seat belts, and many other daily health decisions, everyone will weigh differently the factors affecting sexual choices. Thus, simplistic messages urging absolutist policies are ineffective.[14]

Preventive measures for avoiding transmission of all STDs are generally consistent with guidelines for reducing the risk of HIV infection (See Chapter 3). Risk-free options include completely abstaining from sexual activities that involve semen, blood, or other body fluids, or that allow for skin-to-skin contact.[54] Alternatively, having a mutually faithful relationship with an uninfected partner eliminates any STD risk. Examining a partner for lesions, discussing each new partner's previous sexual history, and avoiding partners who have had many previous sexual partners can augment other measures to prevent the transmission of STDs.

Good health habits also require a regular assessment of one's body. Like breast self-examination, a genital self-examination (GSE) is a simple exercise that should be performed by sexually active persons. GSE helps patients become educated about the symptoms and signs of STDs and how to look for them. Those who suspect abnormalities can have their conditions diagnosed and treated earlier than those who wait for an annual check-up or for severe symptoms to occur. Early treatment is more effective than later treatment, decreases the risk of serious consequences, and can prevent the patient from transmitting the disease to new partners. Educating patients about their bodies and teaching them to be active participants in their health care gives them more control over their reproductive destiny.

OVERLAP OF STD AND FAMILY PLANNING FIELDS

Professionals in the fields of family planning and STD control are increasingly working together for common reproductive health goals.[15,25] Family planners can assist STD control in several ways:

- Educating all patients about the realities of STDs
- Extending their diagnostic services to include risk assessment, STD screening and voluntary HIV testing
- Ensuring that all persons diagnosed with an STD get appropriate treatment, preferably before leaving the family planning facility
- Counseling individuals about the need for simultaneous treatment for their sex partner(s)
- Assisting patients in choosing a contraceptive that will reduce their risk of acquiring an STD[37]

The emergence of HIV infection/AIDS has emphasized the importance of educating all family planning clients about using condoms for infection prevention, even in conjunction with other contraceptive methods for pregnancy prevention. Recent data indicate that as many as 10% of selected populations use supplementary condoms in high-risk settings to prevent STDs, in addition to another contraceptive method.[41]

STD services have already been integrated into family planning clinics to varying degrees.[24] Laboratory methods for the diagnosis of most STDs can be performed in nearly all family planning settings.[59] For example, routine chlamydia screening in Region X family planning clinics has been associated with measurable declines in this STD over the past 4 years.[9] In addition, some family planning clinics have extended their range of services to male clients, including STD diagnosis, treatment, and counseling. Finally, family planners have become familiar with their local STD programs in order to provide appropriate referrals.

The sensitive area of STD partner notification is not part of the usual family planning menu of services. However, stimulated in part by HIV prevention resources, an increasing number of family planning counselors are being trained in this essential public health process. Partner notification requiring field outreach is probably most easily handled by the STD program.[48] Client confidentiality is a crucial foundation for partner notification activities,[8] just as it is in all aspects of family planning and STD care.

STD AND CONTRACEPTION

Choice of contraception has a direct impact on STD risk (Table 4-2). Condoms protect against both bacterial and viral STDs. Spermicides prevent infection with chlamydia and gonorrhea, but their role in preventing viral infections (including HIV) has not been scientifically established.[17] Diaphragms (usually used with spermicides) provide a mechanical barrier against cervical infection, but they have been associated with vaginal and

Table 4-2 Effects of contraceptives on bacterial and viral STD

Contraceptive Methods	Bacterial STD	Viral STD
Condoms	Protective	Protective
Spermicides	Protective against cervical gonorrhea and chlamydia	Undetermined *in vivo*
Diaphragms	Protective against cervical infection; associated with vaginal anaerobic overgrowth	Protective against cervical infection
Hormonal	Associated with increased cervical chlamydia; protective against symptomatic PID	Not protective
IUD	Associated with PID in first month after insertion	Not protective
Natural Family Planning	Not protective	Not protective

Source: Cates and Stone (1992).

bladder infections. Oral contraceptives are associated with an increase in chlamydia detected in the cervix, but protect against symptomatic PID. IUDs are associated with PID, especially in the first month after insertion.[26]

STD AND OTHER RISK BEHAVIORS

In addition to sexual practices, other behaviors have been linked to STDs. Douching has been associated with an increased risk of PID and ectopic pregnancy.[27] Postcoital washing or urination have been poorly studied, but have little impact, if any, on reducing the risk of acquiring an STD. Postcoital urination can, however, wash away bacteria that could cause cystitis and is generally recommended for women susceptible to cystitis.

Drug use is playing an increasingly important role in transmission of STDs. Besides the risks associated with needle-sharing (hepatitis B, HIV infection), using drugs such as crack cocaine has been associated with sexual behaviors which increase a person's risk of acquiring and transmitting many STDs.[39] Specific outbreaks of syphilis and antibiotic-resistant gonorrhea have been linked to crack-related behaviors. Also, use of other drugs, especially alcohol, have been associated with high-risk sexual practices.

STD DIAGNOSIS AND TREATMENT IN THE FAMILY PLANNING SETTING

Managing STD in family planning clinics requires that the clinician have a high index of suspicion. Often a patient will have two or more concurrent STDs. Clinicians should be alert for symptoms different from those normally associated with the primary STD infection. All STDs presumed to be present must be treated. For example, whenever gonorrhea is diagnosed, providing dual therapy for both gonorrhea and chlamydia is epidemiologically indicated, cost-effective, and safe for the patient.

All states require that the five traditional "venereal diseases" (syphilis, gonorrhea, chancroid, LGV, granuloma inguinale) be reported to public health officials; many other states have instituted reporting systems for STDs such as chlamydial infections, genital herpes, and genital warts. In addition, AIDS and HIV reporting is a definite public health priority. Accurate reporting of STDs helps (1) identify trends in disease, (2) gain resources for high prevalence communities, and (3) evaluate STD intervention efforts. Family planning officials should confer with STD control officials to ensure prompt and accurate reporting of the notifiable STDs.

Counseling patients with STD requires a different approach than generally used in family planning settings. With couples trying to prevent unplanned pregnancies, non-directive counseling allows maximum opportunity to choose the best contraceptive method for them. However, for patients who have STDs, *directive counseling* is important to (1) prevent new infections; (2) increase compliance with treatment and follow-up; and (3) offer patients guidance for subsequent discussion with their partner(s). Patients must be made aware of both the serious potential consequences of STDs and the behaviors that increase the likelihood of reinfection. Thus, with STD, in addition to the importance of counseling to the individual, it plays a complementary role of reducing infection in the community.

1. Make sure that the patient understands what disease she/he has, how it is transmitted, why it must be treated, and exactly when and how to take prescribed medication. Such education can improve the patient's compliance with the treatment. Unpleasant side effects from many medications may discourage the patient from continuing treatment. For example, doxycycline taken on an empty stomach may cause nausea that prompts the patient to stop medication early.

2. Strongly urge patients to finish their entire supply of medication even though their symptoms may diminish or disappear in a few days. Discontinuing antibiotics before the infection is completely cured can not only lead to recurrent infection, but also increases the likelihood that hard-to-cure strains of the pathogen may flourish.

3. Enhance the patient's somatic and emotional comfort to enhance compliance with the treatment. Nausea, pain, itching, or other physiologic discomforts should be symptomatically treated, if possible. The psychosocial component of genital discomfort can be exceedingly important in STD treatment and must be sensitively addressed. Remember, patients may be afraid or ashamed to ask a partner to seek treatment, may be embarrassed to admit their sexual practices, and may be concerned about confidentiality. Physicians frequently have the same difficulty. Telling patients that they have a sexually transmissible infection rather than disease may prevent some people from feeling stigmatized.

4. Notify and treat sexual partner(s) to prevent both reinfection of the patient and spread of disease through the community. Systems for assisting patients in notifying their partners include coaching them in partner notification techniques (patient referral) and tracing partners using STD caseworkers (provider referral). As indicated earlier, an increasing number of family planning professionals are being trained in partner notification skills.

5. Advise all patients to avoid intercourse while they complete the full course of therapy. After the infection is cured, urge the patient to continue using condoms to prevent repeated infection, especially if a woman wishes to have children in the future or continues to have intercourse with new partners.

S TD AND PREGNANCY

Pregnant women and their sexual partners should be questioned about risk of STDs and counseled about possible neonatal infections.[10] Because of the severe effects that STDs may have on a fetus, routine prenatal care should include testing for infections with syphilis, hepatitis B, chlamydia, and gonorrhea (Table 4-3). While some authorities recommend routine screening for HIV as well, others recommend screening only those with acknowledged risk factors. Routine screening for HPV and HSV is *not* recommended.

Table 4-3 Risks of sexually transmitted organisms in pregnancy and childhood

Organism	Maternal Infection Rate (%)[1]	Infant Effects	Risk From Infected Mother	Prevention	Treatment of Neonate
Neisseria gonorrhoeae	1–30	Conjunctivitis, sepsis, meningitis	Approximately 30%	Screening– culture mother; apply ocular prophylaxis	Ceftriaxone
Chlamydia trachomatis	2–25	Conjunctivitis, pneumonia, bronchiolitis, otitis media	25%–50% conjunctivitis 5%–15% pneumonia	Screening in third trimester– culture mother; apply ocular prophylaxis	Erythromycin
Treponema pallidum	0.01–15	Congenital syphilis, neonatal death	50%	Serologic screening in early and late pregnancy	Penicillin
Hepatitis B virus	1–10	Hepatitis, cirrhosis	10%–90%	Active HBV immunization	Post-exposure passive HBV immunization
Herpes simplex virus	1–30	Disseminated, central nervous system, localized lesions	3% recurrent at delivery, 30% primary at delivery	Cesarean delivery if lesions present at delivery	Vidarabine, Acyclovir
Human papilloma–virus	10–35	Laryngeal papillomatosis	rare	None	Surgical
Human immuno– deficiency virus	0.01–20	Pediatric AIDS	22%–39%	Pregnancy prevention	Zidovudine

Source: Cates (in press).

[1] Percent of pregnant women with evidence of infection.

Management of the specific STDs is discussed in the sections pertaining to each disease. HIV and pregnancy is discussed in Chapter 3. For more complete information on STDs in pregnant women, refer to "Guidelines for Perinatal Care,"[3] jointly published by the American Academy of Pediatrics and the American College of Obstetrics and Gynecology.

STD AND SEXUAL ASSAULT

In cases of sexual assault and abuse, clinicians must address not only the physical and psychological trauma, but also the possibility of pregnancy and the risk of STDs. Any of the sexually transmissible agents, including HIV, can be acquired during a sexual assault.[23,31] Some STDs, such as gonorrhea or syphilis, are almost exclusively sexually transmitted and are therefore useful markers of assault. Because of their high incidence and the possibility of non-sexual transmission, STDs such as trichomoniasis, HPV, and bacterial vaginosis are less conclusive evidence of assault. In general, cultures provide higher sensitivity and specificity than non-culture tests.

CDC recommends the following approach to dealing with STD risks after sexual assault or sexual abuse:

ADULT

Evaluation If possible, the initial evaluation should be performed within 24 hours of the assault and should include cultures for *N. gonorrhoeae* and *C. trachomatis*; a vaginal specimen examination for *T. vaginalis* and bacterial vaginosis (BV); a pregnancy test; and a frozen serum sample kept for possible future testing. Repeat evaluations should be scheduled for 2 weeks later unless treatment has already been administered.

Treatment Presumptive treatment remains controversial. While no regimen provides coverage against all potential pathogens, the following should be effective against gonorrhea, chlamydia, and syphilis:

Empiric Regimen for Victims of Sexual Assault

- Hepatitis B vaccination—first dose
- Ceftriaxone 125 mg given IM
- Metronidazole 2 g given orally
- Doxycycline 100 mg orally 2 times a day for 7 days

and

Condoms should be used until test results are reported.

CHILDREN

In general, identification of a sexually transmissible agent in a child beyond the neonatal period suggests sexual abuse. However, unlike gonorrhea or syphilis, specific infections such as BV, genital mycoplasmas, and genital warts are not conclusive evidence of sexual abuse. Evaluation is essentially the same as described for adult victims, except that culture specimens should be collected from the pharynx and rectum as well as from the vagina or urethra because the child's report of assault may not be complete. Presumptive treatment may be given at the family's request.

For more complete information regarding laboratory procedures, diagnosis and treatment for sexual assault and abuse victims, refer to the *1993 Sexually Transmitted Diseases Treatment Guidelines.*

S TD RESOURCES

The diagnosis and treatment recommendations that follow are based on Centers for Disease Control and Prevention's (CDC) *1993 STD Treatment Guidelines.*[19] For further information on STDs, or copies of the most recent guidelines, contact Technical Information Services, National Center for Prevention Services, CDC, Atlanta, GA 30333, 404/639-1819.

An excellent comprehensive textbook, covering the entire field of STDs, is *Sexually Transmitted Diseases* available from McGraw-Hill.[30] A more practical clinical handbook for STD diagnosis and treatment was developed by the University of Washington. This publication, *The Practitioner's Handbook for the Management of STDs,*[50] which contains useful diagrams and algorithms to facilitate management of STDs, should be part of every family planning clinic's library and can be obtained by writing:

Health Sciences Center for Educational Resources
Distribution, SB-56
University of Washington
Seattle, Washington 98195

The American Social Health Association maintains a hotline for people to call for recent information about STDs. Patients may appreciate having this toll-free number: (800) 227-8922.

A LPHABETICAL CATALOG OF SEXUALLY TRANSMITTED DISEASES

Acquired immunodeficiency syndrome (AIDS) and **HIV** (human immunodeficiency virus) **infections** are covered in Chapter 3.

Acute urethral syndrome (dysuria-pyuria syndrome) can be caused by *E. coli, C. trachomatis, N. gonorrhoeae,* or other gram-negative bacteria.[51]

Bacterial cystitis itself is not sexually transmitted. "Honeymoon" cystitis is believed to be caused by friction against the urethra during sexual intercourse. Thus the etiology is traumatic rather than infectious, and the trauma allows vaginal organisms to ascend into the bladder.

Prevalence. Depending on the population studied, as many as 10%-25% of reproductive-aged women report dysuria during the previous year.

Symptoms. Painful, urgent, and frequent urination, as well as dyspareunia, characterizes this syndrome. Occasionally hematuria is the precipitating event for seeking clinical evaluation. If a patient's temperature exceeds 101° F or if costovertebral angle pain or tenderness are present, pyelonephritis is a possible cause.

Diagnosis. Women with $\geq 10^5$ organisms per ml of urine of coliform bacteria or *Staphylococcus saprophyticus* have bacterial cystitis; however, smaller number of organisms may also cause symptoms. Women with dysuria, frequency, pyuria (10 WBCs per 400x field on microscopic examination of urinary sediment), and a negative Gram stain of unspun urine have the acute urethral syndrome. A definitive diagnosis of the etiologic organism requires cultures of the urethra or urine. Dysuria may also be caused by vaginitis or genital herpes simplex virus infection.

Treatment. Acute urethral syndrome can be treated with doxycycline 100 mg two times a day. The length of therapy is dictated by clinical response, but 1-2 weeks is the usual course. Initial episodes of bacterial cystitis can be treated with appropriate single-dose therapy such as sulfamethoxazole 1.6 g plus trimethoprim (Bactrim or Septra) 320 mg.

Potential complications. Left untreated, infections of the lower genito-urinary tract can ascend to the upper tract, leading to acute pyelonephritis, chronic pyelonephritis, and eventual kidney failure.

Behavioral messages to emphasize. Understand how to take any prescribed oral medications. Drink copious fluids to flush the genitourinary system. If *C. trachomatis* or *N. gonorrhoeae* organisms are isolated, refer sexual partner(s) for examination. Return for evaluation 4–7 days after initiation of therapy.

Bacterial Vaginosis is a syndrome in which several species of vaginal bacteria (including *Gardnerella vaginalis, Mycoplasma hominis*, and various anaerobes) interact to produce vulvovaginitis symptoms. Bacterial vaginosis is a sexually associated condition, but is not usually considered a specific sexually transmitted infection.

Symptoms. Excessive or malodorous discharge is a common finding. Other signs or symptoms include erythema, edema, and pruritis of the external genitalia.

Diagnosis. The presumptive criteria are typical clinical symptoms of vulvovaginitis, elevated vaginal pH (greater than 4.7), and identification of clue cells (small coccobacillary organisms associated with epithelial cells) in a saline wet mount or gram stain of vaginal discharge. The diagnosis is further supported when a mixture of the vaginal discharge and 10% KOH liberates a fishy odor of volatile amines. Cultures for *G. vaginalis, M. hominis,* or *Mobiluncus* are not useful and are *not* recommended for diagnosing this syndrome.

Treatment. Only patients with symptomatic disease require treatment. Metronidazole, 500 mg taken orally, twice daily, for 7 days or metronidazole 2 g, orally, in a single dose.[38] Alternatives are:

(1) Clindamycin cream 2%, one applicatorful (5 g) intravaginally at bedtime for 7 days;

(2) Metronidazole gel 0.75%, an applicatorful (5 g) intravaginally, two times a day for 5 days; and

(3) Clindamycin 300 mg taken orally two times a day for 7 days.

Clindamycin vaginal cream is the preferred treatment in first trimester pregnancy. During second and third trimester, oral metronidazole is the preferred treatment. Treatment is not recommended for asymptomatic carriers of *G. vaginalis* or male partners of women with this syndrome.

Potential complications. Secondary excoriation may occur. Recurrent infections are common. Several studies have associated bacterial vaginosis with an increased risk of salpingitis.

Behavioral messages to emphasize. Understand how to take or use any prescribed medications. Return if the problem is not cured or recurs. Avoid drinking alcohol until 24 hours after completing metronidazole therapy.

Candidiasis is caused by *Candida albicans* (and other Candida species), dimorphic fungi that grow as oval, budding yeast cells and as chains of cells (hyphae). Candida are normal flora of the skin and vagina and are *not* considered to be sexually transmitted infections.

Symptoms. Clinical presentation varies from no signs or symptoms to erythema, edema, and pruritis of the external genitalia. The type of symptoms or signs alone does *not* distinguish the microbial etiology. Male sexual partners may develop urethritis, balanitis, or cutaneous lesions on the penis.

Diagnosis. The presumptive criteria are typical clinical symptoms of vulvovaginitis and microscopic identification of yeast forms (budding cells) or hyphae in Gram stain or KOH wet-mount preparations of vaginal discharge. Candidiasis is definitively diagnosed when a vaginal culture is positive for *C. albicans* or other *Candida* species in a symptomatic woman. However, cultures are not recommended. Yeasts are part of the resident microbiota of the vagina and anogenital skin. Cultures for *Candida* species may detect clinically insignificant infections, which should not be treated.

Treatment. Offer miconazole nitrate (vaginal suppository 200 mg) intravaginally at bedtime for 3 days; OR miconazole nitrate 2% vaginal cream, one full applicator (5 g) intravaginally at bedtime for 3 days (and applied externally for vulvitis); OR clotrimazole (vaginal tablets 200 mg), one vaginal suppository daily for 3 days; OR butoconazole nitrate cream 2% 5 g intravaginally for 3 days. Many effective treatment regimens exist, but 3- to 7-day regimens are preferred for severe or complicated infections. Note: Treatment with antibiotics predisposes women to develop vulvo-vaginal candidiasis.

Potential complications.   Secondary excoriation may occur. Recurrent infections are common. Persistent candidiasis may indicate HIV infection.

Behavioral messages to emphasize.   Understand how to take or use any prescribed medications. Return if the problem is not cured or recurs. Wear a sanitary pad to protect clothing. Change pads frequently. Avoid panty hose and non-cotton panties to reduce moisture. Store suppositories in a refrigerator. Continue taking medicine even during your menstrual period.

Chancroid is caused by *Hemophilus ducreyi*, a gram-negative bacillus with rounded ends commonly observed in small clusters along strands of mucus. On culture, the organism tends to form straight or tangled chains.

Prevalence.   Chancroid occurs more frequently in the developing than in the developed world. Specific chancroid outbreaks have occurred in high-risk settings, generally associated with prostitute contact.

Symptoms.   Women are frequently asymptomatic. Usually a single (but sometimes multiple) painful ulcer, surrounded by an erythematous halo, appears in men. Ulcers may be necrotic or severely erosive with a ragged serpiginous border. Painful inguinal lymphadenopathy presents in about half the cases and may rupture in 25%-60% of cases. Ulcers usually occur on the coronal sulcus, glans, or shaft of the penis.

Diagnosis.   A clinical presentation consistent with chancroid symptoms involving the genitalia, a unilateral bubo, or both, suggests chancroid. Because other STDs cause genital ulcers (principally syphilis and herpes), all lesions should be examined with darkfield microscopy when adequate facilities exist. Appropriate serologic tests should be performed. When the only organisms seen in a bubo aspirate or ulcer smear are arranged in chains or clumps along strands of mucus and they are morphologically similar to *H. ducreyi*, the diagnosis of chancroid is highly likely. The diagnosis is definitive when *H. ducreyi* is recovered by culture or appropriate selective media. Biopsy may be diagnostic but is not usually performed.

Treatment.   Prescribe azithromycin 1 g orally in a single dose; OR ceftriaxone 250 mg IM in a single dose; OR erythromycin base 500 mg taken orally four times a day for 7 days. Alternatives are amoxicillin 500 mg plus clavulanic acid 125 mg orally three times a day for 7 days; OR ciprofloxacin 500 mg orally twice a day for 3 days. Persons infected with HIV have higher rates of treatment failure with single-dose therapy. The susceptibility of *H. ducreyi* to this combination of antimicrobial agents varies throughout the world. Evaluate the results of therapy after a maximum of 7 days and continue therapy until ulcers or lymph nodes have healed. Fluctuant lymph nodes should be aspirated through healthy, adjacent, normal skin.

Incision and drainage or excision of nodes will delay healing and are contraindicated. Apply compresses to ulcers to remove necrotic material. All sexual partner(s) should be simultaneously treated.

Potential complications. Systemic spread is not known to occur. Lesions may become secondarily infected and necrotic. Buboes may rupture and suppurate, resulting in fistulae. Ulcers on the prepuce may cause phimosis or paraphimosis. Recalcitrant serpiginous ulcerations may take months or years to heal.

Behavioral messages to emphasize. Because genital ulcer disease can be a risk for HIV infection, get an HIV test. Refer sex partner(s) for examination as soon as possible. Return for evaluation 3–5 days after therapy begins and thereafter return weekly for evaluation until the infection is entirely healed. The prepuce should remain retracted during therapy, except in the presence of preputial edema. Clean the ulcerative lesions three times daily. Use condoms to prevent future infections.

Chlamydia is the common name for infections caused by *Chlamydia trachomatis*. Genital chlamydial infection, the most common bacterial STD in the United States, is the leading cause of preventable infertility and ectopic pregnancy.[18] An estimated 4 million new cases occur annually.[56] Like viruses, chlamydiae are obligate intracellular parasites and can be isolated in the laboratory only by cell culture. Unlike viruses, *C. trachomatis* is susceptible to inexpensive, readily available antibiotics. Because many chlamydial infections are asymptomatic and probably chronic, widespread screening is necessary to control this infection.[22] For further information about the syndromes caused by *C. trachomatis*, see Mucopurulent Cervicitis, Nongonococcal Urethritis, and PID in this chapter. Doxycycline 100 mg taken orally, twice a day for 7-10 days OR azithromycin 1 g orally, taken once, are the recommended regimens for all sites of chlamydial infection.[52] Alternatives are ofloxacin 300 mg orally two times a day for 7 days; OR erythromycin base 500 mg orally four times a day for 7 days; OR erythromycin ethyl succinate 800 mg orally four times a day for 7 days; OR and sulfisoxazole 500 mg orally four times a day for 10 days.

Genital Warts (Condyloma acuminata) are caused by human papillomavirus (HPV), a small, slowly growing DNA virus belonging to the papovavirus group.

Prevalence. Genital warts account for more than 1 million physician office visits, making condyloma the most common symptomatic viral STD in the United States.[35] Including Pap smears revealing cervical HPV infections, an estimated 3 million HPV cases are diagnosed yearly. More sensitive measures of HPV indicate up to half of all sexually active young women are infected with this virus.[7] Cases of condyloma have been correlated with earlier onset of sexual activity, and a higher frequency of multiple sexual partners than among controls.

Symptoms. Single or multiple soft, fleshy, papillary or sessile, painless keratinized growths appear around the vulvovaginal area, penis, anus, urethra, or perineum. Women infected with condyloma may exhibit typical growths on the walls of the vagina or cervix and may be unaware of their existence. Regular genital self-examinations are often helpful in detecting such growths on the external genitalia of both women and men. From 60% to 90% of male partners of women with condyloma have HPV infection on the penis, although infection may not be visible to the naked eye.

Diagnosis. A diagnosis may be made on the basis of typical clinical signs on the external genitalia or of koilocytosis on Pap smear specimens. Colposcopy is valuable for diagnosing flat warts, which are difficult to see. Tests for the detection of the virus' DNA are now widely available, although the clinical utility of these tests in managing individual patients is questionable. Therapeutic decisions should *not* be made on the basis of this test. Exclude the possible diagnosis of condylomata lata by obtaining a serologic test for syphilis. A biopsy is usually unnecessary clinically but would be required to make a definitive diagnosis. Some types of warts in the anogenital region are strongly associated with genital dysplasia and carcinoma. Where neoplasia is a possibility, take a biopsy of atypical lesions and pigmented or persistent warts before initiating therapy. Women infected with HIV have an increased risk of progressive HPV-cervical disease.[21]

Treatment. Several different treatment modalities can be used: (1) cryotherapy with liquid nitrogen or cryoprobe; (2) podofilox, 0.5% solution for self-treatment (genital warts only); and (3) podophyllin, 10%-25% in compound tincture of benzoin applied to wart (avoid normal tissue). When taking podophyllin, limit the total volume of solution applied to <0.5 ml per treatment session. Wash off thoroughly in 1-4 hours. Treat <10 cm^2 per session. If warts persist after four weekly applications, use alternative treatments. Podophyllin should not be used during pregnancy or with cervical, urethral, oral, or anorectal warts. Other alternative therapies: weekly applications of 80%-90% trichloroacetic acid, CO_2 laser surgery, electrosurgery, surgical removal (scissor or curette). Interferon therapy is not recommended.

HPV infection is a chronic condition even when asymptomatic. No therapy has been shown to eradicate the virus. In 80% of cases, HPV recurs after some length of time. HPV has been demonstrated in adjacent tissue even after attempts to eliminate subclinical HPV by extensive laser vaporization of the anogenital area. The effect of genital wart treatment on HPV transmission and the natural history of HPV is unknown. Therefore, the goal of treatment is the temporary removal of exophytic warts and the amelioration of symptoms and signs, not the eradication of HPV.

Potential complications. Lesions may enlarge and destroy tissue. Giant condyloma, while histologically benign, may simulate carcinoma. In pregnancy, warts enlarge, are extremely vascular, and may obstruct the birth canal to necessitate a cesarean delivery. Neither routine HPV screening tests nor cesarean delivery for prevention of the transmission of HPV to the newborn is indicated. The perinatal transmission rate is unknown, although it is thought to be low.

Behavioral messages to emphasize. Return for regular treatment until lesions have resolved. Once warts have responded to therapy, no special follow-up is necessary. Anogenital warts are contagious to uninfected sex partners. The majority of partners are probably already infected. Examination of sex partners is not necessary. Use of condoms may help reduce transmission to those who are uninfected. Annual Pap smears are crucial.

Gonorrhea is caused by *Neisseria gonorrhoeae*, a gram-negative diplococcus.

Prevalence. Approximately 700,000 cases of gonorrhea were reported in 1992, making it the most commonly reported communicable disease in the United States. When unreported cases are included, an estimated 1.5 million cases occur every year.

Symptoms. Symptomatic men usually have dysuria, increased frequency of urination, and purulent urethral discharge. An estimated one-quarter of infected men can be asymptomatic. Women may have abnormal vaginal discharge, abnormal menses, dysuria, or may be asymptomatic. Pharyngeal gonorrhea can produce symptoms of pharyngitis.

Diagnosis. Presumptive diagnosis relies on microscopically identifying typical gram-negative intracellular diplococci on smear of urethral exudate (men) or endocervical material (women). Diagnosis, especially in women, also relies on microscopic visualization of bacteria with typical colonial morphology, positive oxidase reaction, and typical Gram-stain morphology, grown in a selective culture medium. Ideally, all gonorrhea cases should be diagnosed by culture to facilitate antimicrobial susceptibility testing, but use of nonculture tests may increase the number of women tested. A definitive diagnosis is required if the specimen is extragenital, from a child, or medicolegally important.

Treatment. Because of the high percentage of penicillin-resistant *N. gonorrhoeae* in most areas of the United States, an alternative antibiotic is recommended for treating gonorrhea.[61] In addition, in many areas about one-fourth of men and two-fifths of women with gonococcal infections also have a coexisting chlamydial infection. For this reason, using *both* a single-dose anti-gonococcal drug and 1 week of doxycycline for chlamydia is epidemiologically indicated.[49] The recommended therapies for gonorrhea include ceftriaxone, 125 mg IM, once; ciprofloxacin 500 mg take PO once; cefixime 400 mg taken orally once; or ofloxacin 400 mg taken orally once. For chlamydia, use doxycycline, 100 mg taken orally, two times a day for 7 days. Patients with a history of oral-genital sex should be treated with a regimen effective against pharyngeal gonorrhea.

Potential complications. Up to 40% of untreated women with cervical gonorrhea develop PID and are at risk for its sequelae (see PID section), including involuntary sterility and pelvic abscesses. Men are at risk for epididymitis, urethral stricture, and sterility. Newborns are at risk for ophthalmia neonatorum, scalp abscess at the site of fetal monitors, rhinitis, or anorectal infection. All infected untreated persons are at risk for disseminated gonococcal infection.

Behavioral messages to emphasize. Understand how to take any prescribed oral medications. Return for a checkup 4–7 days after completing therapy. Refer sexual partner(s) for examination and treatment. Avoid sex until patient and partner(s) are cured. Use condoms to prevent future infections. Women should insist on condom use during pregnancy if partner(s) may have gonococcal infection.

Granuloma Inguinale (Donovanosis) is caused by *Calymmatobacterium granulomatis* (formerly known as *Donovania granulomatis*), a bipolar, gram-negative bacterium (Donovan body) that, in a crush preparation, appears in vacuolar compartments within histiocytes, white blood cells, or plasma cells.

Prevalence. Although one of the traditional venereal diseases, granuloma inguinale is rare in the United States.

Symptoms. Initially, single or multiple subcutaneous nodules appear at the site of inoculation. Nodules erode to form granulomatous, heaped ulcers that are painless, bleed on contact, and enlarge slowly. Spread by autoinoculation is common.

Diagnosis. The typical clinical presentation is sufficient to suggest the diagnosis. Resolution of the lesions following specific antibiotic therapy supports the diagnosis. The patient's or partner's history of travel to the tropics (particularly India or Papua New Guinea) helps to substantiate the clinical impression. A microscopic examination of scrapings of biopsy specimens from the ulcer margin reveals the pathognomonic Donovan bodies. Tissue culture of *C. granulomatis* is not feasible.

Treatment. The following regimens are listed in order of preference: tetracycline hydrochloride 0.5 g taken orally four times a day for 21 days or until the lesion completely heals; OR streptomycin 0.5 g IM four times a day for at least 21 days; OR chloramphenicol 0.5 g taken orally three times a day for at least 21 days; OR gentamicin 40 mg IM twice daily for at least 21 days. Erythromycin and trimethoprim/sulfamethoxazole regimens have also been reported to be effective. Penicillins are not effective.

Potential complications. Lesions may become secondarily infected. Fibrous, keloid-like formations may deform the genitalia. Pseudoelephantoid enlargement of the labia, penis, or scrotum occurs. Necrosis and destruction of the genitalia may result. Toxic manifestations include fever, malaise, secondary anemia, cachexia, and death.

Behavioral messages to emphasize. Understand how to take any prescribed oral medication. Return for evaluation 3–5 days after therapy begins. Assure examination of sexual partner(s) as soon as possible. Return weekly or biweekly for evaluation until the infection is entirely healed.

Hepatitis B is caused by hepatitis B virus (HBV), a DNA virus with multiple antigenic components.

Prevalence. In the United States, approximately 5%–20% of segments of the general population show evidence of past HBV infections. An estimated 150,000 new cases of HBV infection are transmitted sexually each year. Heterosexual intercourse is now the predominant mode of HBV transmission.[1] In developing countries and in homosexual male populations, the overall prevalence of HBV markers may be more than 80%.

Symptoms. Most HBV infections are clinically inapparent. When present, symptoms include serum sickness-like prodrome (skin eruptions, urticaria, arthralgias, arthritis), lassitude, anorexia, nausea, vomiting, headache, fever, dark urine, jaundice, and moderate liver enlargement with tenderness.

Diagnosis. HBV infection is clinically indistinguishable from other forms of viral and other hepatitis. A patient with the typical clinical symptoms and exposure to the serum of a patient with definitive or presumed HBV infection may be presumed to have HBV infection. Serodiagnosis of HBV infection is the best method for clinicians to reach a definitive diagnosis. Positive results of the following tests are reliable:

1. Hepatitis B surface antigen (HBsAg): Acute HBV infection or, with no acute disease exposure, the chronic carrier state, the person is infectious.

2. HBe antigen: More infectious than if just HBsAg-positive, because indicates active viral replication

3. Anti-HBsAg: Past infection with present immunity.

4. Anti-HB core antigen: Past or current infection.

Treatment. No specific therapy exists. Supportive and symptomatic care should be provided. HBV is the only STD for which we have a vaccine. Two vaccines made from recombinant genetic material are currently available. Specific vaccination and post-exposure prophylaxis strategies are of proven efficacy in preventing hepatitis B. Vaccinating all newborn infants and adolescents against hepatitis B is currently recommended.[3,6] In addition, the Advisory Committee on Immunization Practices recommends vaccinating all persons with recent STD and those who have a history of sexual activity with more than one partner in the previous 6 months.

Potential complications. Long-term sequelae include chronic, persistent, active hepatitis; cirrhosis; hepatocellular carcinoma; hepatic failure; and death. Rarely, the course may be fulminant with hepatic failure.

Behavioral messages to emphasize. Clinical follow-up intervals are determined by symptoms and the results of liver function tests. Persons at risk for sexual transmission of HBV are also at risk for HIV and other STDs. Reducing the number of sexual contacts and avoiding contact with HBV carriers are ways to avoid contracting the disease.

Herpes Genitalis is caused by herpes simplex virus (HSV) types 1 and 2 DNA viruses that cannot be distinguished clinically. HSV type 2 (HSV-2) is much more common in genital disease.

Prevalence. Symptomatic primary (or initial) HSV infections affect an estimated 200,000 persons each year. Recurrent HSV infections are much more common. An estimated 30 million Americans are infected with genital HSV, though most infections are asymptomatic.[32] Persons without symptoms probably transmit most HSV infections.[36,40]

Symptoms. Single or multiple vesicles, which are usually pruritic, appear anywhere on the genitalia. Vesicles spontaneously rupture to form shallow ulcers that may be very painful. Lesions resolve spontaneously with minimal scarring. The first clinical occurrence is termed first episode infection (mean duration 12 days). Subsequent, usually milder, occurrences are termed recurrent infections (mean duration 4.5 days). The interval between clinical episodes is termed latency. Viral shedding occurs intermittently without clinical symptoms during latency. Genital sites of HSV infection have six times the rate of clinical recurrence as oral sites, and HSV-2 genital infections are five times more likely to recur than is HSV type 1 (HSV-1).

Diagnosis. When typical genital lesions are present or a pattern of recurrence has developed, herpes infection should be suspected. A presumptive diagnosis is further supported by direct identification of multinucleated giant cells with intranuclear inclusions in a clinical specimen prepared by Papanicolaou or other histochemical stain OR by an increased CF or other serologic titer in convalescent serum. An HSV virus tissue culture demonstrates the characteristic cytopathogenic effect following inoculation of a specimen from the cervix, the urethra, or the base of a genital lesion. Nonculture tests, although not as sensitive as culture, may be used.

Treatment. No cure for HSV has been found; however, the antiviral drug acyclovir has been helpful in reducing or suppressing symptoms. Oral acyclovir is the most clinically useful form of the drug, both in treating clinically symptomatic episodes and in suppressing or reducing recurrent outbreaks. For clinical illness, oral acyclovir is given in 200 mg capsules five times a day for 7-10 days or until clinical resolution occurs. To prevent recurrences, the same dosage two to five times a day has been used as daily suppressive therapy. Topical therapy with acyclovir is substantially less effective than therapy with the oral drug. Intravenous acyclovir is used to treat uncommon disseminated forms of herpes infection requiring hospitalization.

The safety of systemic acyclovir in pregnant women has not been established. In pregnant women without life-threatening disease, systemic treatment should not be used to treat recurrent genital herpes episodes or, as suppressive therapy, to prevent reactivation near term.

Potential complications. *Male and female patients:* HSV infection can cause neuralgia, meningitis, ascending myelitis, urethral strictures, and lymphatic suppuration. *Female patients:* HSV infections have been associated with fetal wastage. *Neonates:* Virus from an active genital infection may be transmitted during vaginal delivery causing neonatal herpes. Neonatal herpes ranges in severity from clinically inapparent infections to local infections of the eyes, skin, or mucous membranes, to severely disseminated infection that may involve the central nervous system. The full-blown infection has a high fatality rate, and survivors often have ocular or neurologic sequelae.

Behavioral messages to emphasize. Keep involved area clean and dry. Because both initial and recurrent lesions shed high concentrations of the virus, abstain from sexual contact lesions while you are symptomatic. The risk of HSV transmission also exists during asymptomatic intervals. Because of the large number of persons with asymptomatic HSV infections, most HSV is transmitted by this group. Condoms offer some protection.

The risk of transmission to the neonate from an infected mother is highest among women with primary herpes infection (the first time they have been infected with either type-1 or type-2 HSV) at the time of delivery, less with women with nonprimary first episode disease, and low among women with recurrent herpes.[2] At the onset of labor, all women should be carefully questioned about symptoms and examined. Women without signs or symptoms may be delivered vaginally.[44] Infants delivered through an infected birth canal should be cultured and followed carefully.

Genital herpes (and other diseases causing genital ulcers) has been associated with an increased risk of acquiring HIV infections.[29] Evaluating asymptomatic partners has little value for preventing transmission of HSV.

Human Papillomavirus (HPV) See Genital Warts.

Lymphogranuloma Venereum (LGV) is caused by immunotypes L1, L2, or L3 of *C. trachomatis*.

Prevalence. LGV infections are more common than ordinarily believed. They are endemic in Asia and Africa but are rare in the United States.

Symptoms. The primary lesion of LGV is a 2mm–3 mm painless vesicle or nonindurated ulcer at the site of inoculation. Patients commonly fail to notice this primary lesion. Regional adenopathy follows a week to a month later and is the most common clinical symptom. A sensation of stiffness and aching in the groin, followed by swelling of the inguinal region, may be the first indications of infections for most patients. Adenopathy may subside spontaneously or proceed to the formation of abscesses that rupture to produce draining sinuses or fistulae.

Diagnosis. LGV is often diagnosed clinically and may be confused with chancroid. The LGV complement fixation test is sensitive; 80% of patients have a titer of 1:16 or higher. Levels of 1:64 are considered diagnostic. Because the sequelae of LGV are serious and preventable, treatment should not be withheld pending laboratory confirmation. A definitive diagnosis requires isolating *C. trachomatis* from an appropriate specimen and confirming the isolate as an LGV immunotype. However, these laboratory diagnostic capabilities are not widely available.

Treatment. Prescribe doxycycline 100 mg taken orally two times a day for 21 days. Tetracycline 500 mg taken orally four times a day for 21 days is an alternative. Other alternative therapies include: erythromycin 500 mg orally four times a day for 21 days; OR sulfisoxazole 500 mg orally four times a day for 21 days. Fluctuant lymph nodes should be aspirated as needed. Incision and drainage or excision of nodes will delay healing and are contraindicated.

Potential complications. Dissemination may occur with nephropathy, hepatomegaly, or phlebitis. Large polypoid swelling of the vulva (esthiomene), anal margin, or rectal mucosa may occur. The most common severe morbidity results from rectal involvement: perianal abscess and rectovaginal or other fistulae are early consequences, and rectal stricture may develop 1–10 years after infection.

Behavioral messages to emphasize. Understand how to take any prescribed oral medications. Return for evaluation 3–5 days after therapy begins. Assure examination of sexual partner(s) as soon as possible.

Molluscum Contagiosum is caused by molluscum contagiosum virus, the largest DNA virus of the poxvirus group.

Prevalence. As an STD, molluscum contagiosum occurs infrequently, about 1 case for every 100 cases of gonorrhea. Outbreaks have been reported among groups at high risk for other STDs.

Symptoms. Lesions are 1mm–5 mm, smooth, rounded, firm, shiny flesh-colored to pearly-white papules with characteristically umbilicated centers. They are most commonly seen on the trunk and anogenital region and are generally asymptomatic.

Diagnosis. Infection is usually diagnosed on the basis of the typical clinical presentation. Microscopic examination of lesions or lesion material reveals the pathognomonic molluscum inclusion bodies.

Treatment. Lesions may resolve spontaneously without scarring. However, they may be removed by curettage after cryoanesthesia. Treatment with caustic chemicals (podophyllin, trichloroacetic acid, silver nitrate) and cryotherapy (liquid nitrogen) have been successful. If every lesion is not extirpated, the condition may recur.

Potential complications. Secondary infection, usually with staphylococcus, may occur. Lesions rarely attain a size greater than 10 mm in diameter.

Behavioral messages to emphasize. Return for reexamination 1 month after treatment so that any new lesions can be removed. Partner(s) should be examined.

Mucopurulent cervicitis (MPC) can be caused by *C. trachomatis, N. gonorrhoeae* (rarely), or possibly mycoplasmas.

Prevalence. Based on extrapolation from local studies, mucopurulent cervicitis probably occurs more frequently than male urethritis. Up to 3 million cases per year may occur annually.

Symptoms. The mucopurulent discharge is exuded from the cervix. Often the patient does not recognize the discharge or may perceive it as normal vaginal discharge.

Diagnosis. A presumptive diagnosis is made by finding mucopus on a swab of the endocervical secretions or filiability (bleeding) on the first endocervical swab. Some clinicians diagnose MPC by finding 30 or more polymorphonuclear leukocytes per microscopic field at a magnification of 1000X. A definitive etiologic diagnosis is made when either gonorrhea is diagnosed by Gram stain or culture, or when *C. trachomatis* is detected by one of the following techniques: culture, monoclonal antibody immunofluorescence, or enzyme immunoassay.

Treatment. Chlamydia is treated with doxycycline, 100 mg taken orally, twice a day for 7-10 days. See specific treatments for gonorrhea, listed previously.

Potential complications. PID, infertility, and pelvic abscesses may complicate infection. In addition, neonatal chlamydial infections, such as ophthalmia or pneumonia, may be acquired during delivery if the mother has an infected endocervix. If a pregnant woman is infected, she may be at risk for spontaneous abortion, stillbirth, and postpartum endometritis.

Behavioral messages to emphasize. Understand how to take any prescribed oral medication. Refer sexual partner(s) for examination and treatment if infected with *C. trachomatis* or *N. gonorrhea.* Avoid sex until patient and your partner(s) are cured. Return early if symptoms persist or recur. Use condoms to prevent future infections.

Nongonococcal Urethritis (NGU) is caused by *Chlamydia trachomatis*
about 50% of the time. Other sexually transmissible agents causing 10%–15% of NGU include *Ureaplasma urealyticum, Trichomonas vaginalis,* and herpes simplex virus. The etiology of the remaining cases is unknown.

Prevalence. NGU appears more frequently than gonorrhea in both public STD clinics and private practices. More than 2 million cases annually are estimated to occur in men.

Symptoms.   Men usually have dysuria, urinary frequency, and mucoid to purulent urethral discharge. Many men have asymptomatic infections.

Diagnosis.   Men with typical clinical symptoms are presumed to have NGU when their gonorrhea tests are negative and they have either white blood cells (WBCs) on gram stain of urethral discharge or sexual exposure to an agent known to cause NGU. Asymptomatic men with negative gonorrhea tests are also presumed to have NGU if they ≥5 WBCs per oil immersion field on an intraurethral smear. Gonococcal and nongonococcal urethritis may coexist in the same patient.

Treatment.   When the etiology is *C. trachomatis, U. urealyticum,* or unknown, the following treatment is recommended: doxycycline, 100 mg taken orally, twice daily for at least 7 days. An alternative for patients in whom tetracyclines are contraindicated or not tolerated, or who fail their first trial of doxycycline, is erythromycin, 500 mg taken orally, four times a day for at least 7 days. For *T. vaginalis* or herpes simplex infections, see the sections of this chapter that deal specifically with these agents.

Potential complications.   Urethral strictures or epididymitis may occur. If transmitted to female sexual partners, the condition may result in mucopurulent cervicitis and PID. If *C. trachomatis* is transmitted to a pregnant woman, complications may include neonatal infections such as ophthalmia or pneumonia.

Behavioral messages to emphasize.   Understand how to take any prescribed oral medications. Refer sexual partner(s) for examination and treatment. Avoid sex until you and your partner(s) are cured. Use condoms to prevent future infections.

Pelvic Inflammatory Disease (PID)   can be caused by varying combinations of *N. gonorrhoeae, C. trachomatis,* anaerobic bacteria, facultative gram-negative rods (such as *E. coli*), *Mycoplasma hominis,* and a variety of other microbial agents. Clinical PID is usually of polymicrobial etiology. *N. gonorrhoeae* and *C. trachomatis* may cause antecedent inflammation, which makes the tubes susceptible to invasion by anaerobic organisms.[16]

Prevalence.   PID accounts for nearly 180,000 hospitalizations every year in the United States. More than 1 million episodes occur annually. Among American women of reproductive age, one in seven reports having received treatment for PID.[5]

Symptoms.   Based on retrospective reports, many women with PID have atypical or no symptoms. Women may have pain and tenderness involving the lower abdomen, cervix, uterus, and adnexae, possibly combined with fever, chills, and elevated white blood cell (WBC) count and erythrocyte sedimentation rate (ESR). The condition is more likely if the patient has multiple sexual partners, a history of PID, has recently had an intrauterine device (IUD) inserted, or is in the first 5–10 days of her menstrual cycle.

Diagnosis.　Women who have the typical clinical symptoms are presumed to have PID if other serious conditions, such as acute appendicitis or ectopic pregnancy, can be excluded. The diagnosis of PID is often based on imprecise clinical findings.[34] Clinicians should use objective criteria to monitor response to antibiotics, especially if ambulatory treatment is given. Direct visualization of inflamed (edema, hyperemia, or tubal exudate) fallopian tube(s) during laparoscopy or laparotomy makes the diagnosis of PID definitive. Cultures of tubal exudate may help establish the microbiologic etiology.

Treatment.　Because the causative organism is usually unknown at the time of the initial therapy, clinicians should use treatment regimens that are active against the broadest possible range of pathogens.

Hospitalization and inpatient care: Strongly consider hospitalizing patients with acute PID when (1) the diagnosis is uncertain; (2) surgical emergencies, such as appendicitis and ectopic pregnancy, are not definitely excluded; (3) a pelvic abscess is suspected; (4) severe illness precludes outpatient management; (5) the woman is pregnant; (6) the woman is unable to follow or tolerate an outpatient regimen; (7) the woman has failed to respond to outpatient therapy; (8) clinical outpatient follow-up after 48–72 hours of antibiotic treatment cannot be arranged; (9) the patient is a prepubertal child; or (10) the woman is infected with HIV. Some experts recommend that all patients with PID be hospitalized for treatment, with special consideration given to adolescents both to preserve their fertility and improve their compliance.

Combined drug therapy is recommended in all cases since the full bacterial etiology of PID is not clear and is generally polymicrobial. Treat inpatients with doxycycline, 100 mg IV twice daily, PLUS cefoxitin, 2.0 g IV four times a day OR cefotetan, 2.0 g IV twice daily at least 2 days after the patient clinically improves. Continue doxycycline 100 mg taken orally, twice daily after discharge to complete at least 14 days of therapy. This regimen provides optimal coverage for all strains of *N. gonorrhoeae* and *C. trachomatis*. It may not provide optimal treatment for anaerobes, pelvic mass, or an IUD-associated PID. An alternative inpatient regimen is the combination of clindamycin 900 mg IV three times a day, PLUS gentamicin 2 mg/kg IV loading dose and maintenance 1.5 mg/kg IV three times daily.

Ambulatory treatment: Prescribe ofloxacin 400 mg twice daily PLUS either clindamycin 450 mg four times a day OR metronidazole 500 mg two times a day for 14 days. Accepted regimens also include cefoxitin 2 g, IM along with probenecid, 1 g taken orally; OR ceftriaxone 250 mg IM, followed by doxycycline 100 mg taken orally twice daily for 14 days.

Potential complications.　Potentially life-threatening complications include ectopic pregnancy and pelvic abscess. Other sequelae are involuntary infertility, recurrent or chronic PID, chronic abdominal pain, pelvic adhesions, premature hysterectomy, and depression.

Behavioral messages to emphasize. For outpatient therapy, return for evaluation 2–3 days after initiation of therapy. Return for further evaluation 4–7 days after completing therapy. Refer sexual partner(s) for evaluation and treatment (up to half of sexual partners of women with PID are infected but asymptomatic). Avoid sexual activity until you and your partner(s) are cured. If you used an IUD, consult with a family planning physician. Use condoms to prevent future infections. Understand how to take any prescribed oral medications.

Syphilis is caused by *Treponema pallidum,* a spirochete with 6–14 regular spirals and characteristic motility.

Prevalence. Primary/secondary syphilis currently affects approximately 40,000 persons each year in the United States, occurring more frequently in low-income minority heterosexual populations.[47] Congenital syphilis occurs in about 1 in 10,000 pregnancies.[20] Recent syphilis outbreaks have been associated with the exchange of sex for drugs, especially crack cocaine. Over the past decade, syphilis reached its highest level in the past 40 years.[46]

Symptoms.

Primary: The classical chancre is a painless, indurated ulcer, located at the site of exposure. The differential diagnosis for all genital lesions should include syphilis.

Secondary: Patients may have a highly variable skin rash, mucous patches, condylomata lata, lymphadenopathy, alopecia, or other signs.

Latent: Patients are without clinical signs of infection.

Diagnosis.

Primary: Patients have typical lesion(s) and either a positive darkfield exam; or a fluorescent antibody techniques in material from a chancre, regional lymph node, or other lesion; or their present serologic test for syphilis (STS) titer is at least fourfold greater than the last; or they have been exposed to syphilis within 90 days of lesion onset.

Secondary: Patients have the typical clinical presentation and a strongly reactive STS; condyloma lata will be darkfield positive.

Latent: Patients have serologic evidence of untreated syphilis without clinical signs.

Primary and secondary syphilis are definitively diagnosed by demonstrating *T. pallidum* with darkfield microscopy or fluorescent antibody technique. A definitive diagnosis of latent syphilis cannot be made under usual circumstances.

Treatment.

Primary, secondary, or early syphilis of less than 1 year's duration: benzathine penicillin G, 2.4 million units IM.

Syphilis of indeterminate length or of more than 1 year's duration: benzathine penicillin G, 7.2 million units total; 2.4 million units IM weekly for 3 successive weeks.

Patients allergic to penicillin: doxycycline 100 mg taken orally two times a day. Note: Duration of therapy depends upon estimated duration of infection. If less than 1 year, treat for 14 days; otherwise, treat for 28 days.

For penicillin-allergic pregnant women or for doxycycline-intolerant patients only: erythromycin (stearate, ethyl succinate or base) 500 mg taken orally, four times a day for 2 weeks.

For congenital syphilis or if the patient is simultaneously infected with syphilis and HIV, refer to *1993 STD Treatment Guidelines.*

Potential complications. Both late syphilis and congenital syphilis, complications of early syphilis, are preventable with prompt diagnosis and treatment. Sequelae of late syphilis include neurosyphilis (general paresis, tabes dorsalis, and focal neurologic signs), cardiovascular syphilis (thoracic aortic aneurism, aortic insufficiency), and localized gumma formation.

Behavioral messages to emphasize. Because genital ulcers may be associated with HIV infection, get an HIV test. Return for follow-up serologies 3 and 6 months for early syphilis, and 6 and 12 months for late latent disease. HIV-positive patients should return 1, 2, 3, 6, 9, and 12 months after therapy; pregnant partners should be followed monthly. Understand how to take any prescribed oral medications. Refer sexual partner(s) for evaluation and treatment. Avoid sexual activity until you and your partner(s) are cured. Use condoms to prevent future infections.

Trichomoniasis is caused by *Trichomonas vaginalis,* a motile protozoan with an undulating membrane and four flagella.

Symptoms. Excessive, frothy vaginal discharge is common, although clinical presentation varies from no signs or symptoms to erythema, edema, and pruritis of the external genitalia. Dysuria and dyspareunia are also frequent. The type of symptoms or signs alone does NOT distinguish the microbial etiology. Male sexual partners may develop urethritis, balanitis, or cutaneous lesions on the penis. Males rarely display symptoms.

Diagnosis. Trichomoniasis is diagnosed when a vaginal culture or fluorescent antibody is positive for *T. vaginalis* OR typical motile trichomonads are identified in a saline wet mount of vaginal discharge. Trichomonads found by Pap smear are not diagnostic of active infection.

Treatment. Prescribe metronidazole, 2.0 g taken orally, at one time, OR metronidazole, 500 mg taken orally, twice daily for 7 days. Metronidazole-resistant *T. vaginalis,* although uncommon, has been reported from most states.

Potential complications. Secondary excoriation may occur. Recurrent infections are common. Several studies have associated trichomoniasis with an increased risk of salpingitis, low birth weight, and prematurity.

Behavioral messages to emphasize. Understand how to take or use any prescribed medications. Return if the problem is not cured or recurs. Use condoms to prevent future infections. Avoid drinking alcohol until 24 hours after completing metronidazole therapy.

REFERENCES

1. Alter MJ, Hadler SC, Margolis HS, Alexander WJ, Hu PY, Judson FN, Mares A, Miller JK, Moyer LA. The changing epidemiology of hepatitis B in the United States. JAMA 1990;263(9):1218-1222.
2. American College of Obstetrics and Gynecology. Technical Bulletin No. 122. Perinatal herpes simplex virus infections. ACOG Technical Bulletin 1988;102:1-5.
3. American College of Obstetrics and Gynecology and American Academy of Pediatrics. Guidelines for Perinatal Care, 3rd edition. Washington DC: American College of Obstetrics and Gynecology, and American Academy of Pediatrics, 1992.
4. Aral SO, Holmes KK. Sexually transmitted diseases in the AIDS era. Scientific American 1991;264(2):62-9.
5. Aral SO, Mosher WD, Cates W Jr. Self-reported pelvic inflammatory disease in the United States, 1988. JAMA 1991;266(18):2570-2573.
6. Arevalo JA, Washington AE. Cost-effectiveness of prenatal screening and immunization for hepatitis B virus. JAMA 1988;259(3):365-369.
7. Bauer HM, Ting Y, Greer CE, Chambers JC, Tashiro CJ, Chimera J, Reingold A, Manos MM. Genital human papillomavirus infection in female university students as determined by a PCR-based method. JAMA 1991;265(4):472-477.
8. Bayer R, Toomey KE. HIV prevention and the two faces of partner notification. Am J Public Health 1992;82(8):1158-1164.
9. Britton TF, DeLisle S, Fine D. STDs and family planning clinics: a regional program for chlamydia control that works. Am J Gynecol Health 1992;6:80-87.
10. Brunham RC, Holmes KK, Embree JE. Sexually transmitted diseases in pregnancy. In: Holmes KK, Mårdh P-A, Sparling PF, Wiesner PJ, Cates W Jr, Lemon SM, and Stamm WE (eds). Sexually transmitted diseases, 2nd edition. New York NY: McGraw-Hill, 1990:771-802.
11. Cates W Jr. Sexually transmitted diseases: the scale of the problem in the developed and developing world. In: Job-Spira N, Spencer B, Moatti JP, and Bouvet E (eds). Public health and sexual transmission of diseases: directions for future research and health policy. Paris: John Libbey Company, 1990:26-32.
12. Cates W Jr. Teenagers and sexual risk taking: The best of times and the worst of times. J Adolesc Health Care 1991;12:84-94.
13. Cates W Jr. Sexually transmitted diseases. In: Sachs BP, Beard R, Papiernik E (eds). Health care for women and babies: analysis of medical, economic, ethical and political issues. Oxford: Oxford University Press (in press).
14. Cates W Jr, Hinman AR. AIDS and absolutism: the demand for perfection in prevention. N Engl J Med 1992;327(7):492-494.
15. Cates W Jr, Stone KM. Family planning, sexually transmitted diseases, and contraceptive choice: a literature update—part I. Fam Plann Perspect 1992;24(2):75-84.
16. Cates W Jr, Rolfs RT Jr, Aral SO. Sexually transmitted diseases, pelvic inflammatory disease, and infertility: an epidemiologic update. Epidemiol Rev 1990;12:199-220.
17. Cates W Jr, Stewart FH, Trussell J. The quest for women's prophylactic methods: hopes vs. science. Am J Public Health 1992;82(11):1479-1482.

18. Cates W Jr, Wasserheit JN. Genital chlamydial infection: epidemiology and reproductive sequelae. Am Journal Obstet Gynecol 1991;164(6 Pt 2):1771-1781.
19. Centers for Disease Control and Prevention. 1993 sexually transmitted diseases treatment guidelines. MMWR 1993;42(RR-14):1-73.
20. Centers for Disease Control. Policy guidelines for the prevention and control of congenital syphilis. MMWR 1988;37(suppl no. S-1):1-13.
21. Centers for Disease Control and Prevention. Risk for cervical disease in HIV-infected women—New York City. MMWR 1990;39:846-849.
22. Centers for Disease Control and Prevention. Recommendations for the prevention and control of *Chlamydia trachomatis* infections. MMWR 1993;42(RR-12):1-36.
23. Davies AG, Clay JC. Prevalence of sexually transmitted disease infection in women alleging rape. Sex Transm Dis 1992;19(5):298-300.
24. Donovan P. Family planning clinics: facing higher costs and sicker patients. Fam Plann Perspect 1991;23(5):198-203.
25. Donovan P. Testing positive: sexually transmitted diseases and the public health response. New York NY: Alan Guttmacher Institute, 1993.
26. Farley TMM, Rosenberg MJ, Rowe PJ, Chen J-H, Meirik O. Intrauterine devices and pelvic inflammatory disease: an international perspective. Lancet 1992;339(8796):785-788.
27. Forrest KA, Washington AE, Daling JR, and Sweet RL. Vaginal douching as a possible risk factor for pelvic inflammatory disease. J Natl Med Assoc 1989;81(2):159-165.
28. Grimes DA. Deaths due to sexually transmitted diseases: the forgotten component of reproductive mortality. JAMA 1986;255(13):1727-1729.
29. Holmberg SD, Stewart JA, Gerber AR, Byers RH, Lee FK, O'Malley PM, Nahmias AJ. Prior herpes simplex virus type 2 infection as a risk factor for HIV infection. JAMA 1988;259(7):1048-1050.
30. Holmes KK, Mårdh PA, Sparling PF, Wiesner PJ, Cates W Jr, Lemon SM, Stamm WE (eds). Sexually transmitted diseases, 2nd edition. New York NY: McGraw-Hill, 1990.
31. Jenny C, Hooton TM, Bowers A, Copass MK, Krieger JN, Hillier SL, Kiviat N, Corey L, Stamm WE, Holmes KK. Sexually transmitted diseases in victims of rape. N Engl J Med 1990;322(11):713-716.
32. Johnson RE, Nahmias AJ, Magder LS, Lee FK, Brooks CA, Snowden CB. A seroepidemiological survey of the prevalence of herpes simplex virus type 2 in the United States. N Engl J Med 1989;321(1):7-12.
33. Judson FN. Gonorrhea. Med Clin N Amer 1990;74(6):1353-1366.
34. Kahn JG, Walker CK, Washington AE, Landers DV, Sweet RL. Diagnosing pelvic inflammatory disease. JAMA 1991;266(18):2594-2604.
35. Koutsky LA, Galloway DA, Holmes KK. Epidemiology of genital human papillomavirus infection. Epidemiol Rev 1988;10:122-163.
36. Koutsky LA, Stevens CE, Holmes KK, Ashley RL, Kiviat NB, Critchlow CW, Corey L. Underdiagnoses of genital herpes by current clinical and viral-isolation procedures. N Engl J Med 1992;326(23):1533-1539.
37. Lande RE. Controlling sexually transmitted diseases. Popul Rep Series L (9);1993.
38. Lugo-Miro VI, Green M, Mazur L. Comparison of different metronidazole therapeutic regimens for bacterial vaginosis. A meta-analysis. JAMA 1992;268(1):92-95.
39. Marx R, Aral SO, Rolfs RT, Sterk CE, Kahn JG. Crack, sex, and STD. Sex Transm Dis 1991;18(2):92-101.

40. Mertz GJ, Benedetti J, Ashley R, Selke SA, Corey L. Risk factors for the sexual transmission of genital herpes. Ann Intern Med 1992;116(3):197-202.
41. Mosher WD. AIDS-related behavior and condom use in the United States: an evaluation of the data. Presented at the annual meeting of the Population Association of America, Denver, Colorado, April 30, 1992.
42. Platt R, Rice PA, McCormack WM. Risk of acquiring gonorrhea and prevalence of abnormal adnexal findings among women recently exposed to gonorrhea. JAMA 1983;250(23):3205-3209.
43. Potterat JJ. 'Socio-geographic space' and sexually transmissible diseases in the 1990s. Today's Life Science 1992;December:16-31.
44. Prober CG, Hensleigh PA, Boucher FD, Yasukawa LL, Au DS, Arvin AM. Use of routine viral cultures at delivery to identify neonates exposed to herpes simplex virus. N Engl J Med 1988;318(14):887-891.
45. Quinn TC, Cates W Jr. Epidemiology of sexually transmitted diseases in the 1990s. In: Quinn TC, Gallin JI, and Fauci AS (eds). Advances in host defense mechanisms: sexually transmitted diseases, Vol. 8. New York NY: Raven Press, 1992:1-37.
46. Rolfs RT, Cates W Jr. The perpetual lessons of syphilis. Arch Dermatol 1989;125(i):107-109.
47. Rolfs RT, Nakashima AK. Epidemiology of primary and secondary syphilis in the United States, 1981 through 1989. JAMA 1990;264(11):1432-1437.
48. Rothenberg RB, Potterat JJ. Strategies for management of sex partners. In: Holmes KK, Mårdh P-A, Sparling PF, Wiesner PJ, Cates W Jr, Lemon SM, Stamm WE (eds). Sexually transmitted diseases, 2nd edition. New York NY: McGraw-Hill, 1990:1081-1086.
49. Stamm WE, Guinan ME, Johnson C, Starcher T, Holmes KK, McCormack WM. Effect of treatment regimens for *Neisseria gonorrhoeae* on simultaneous infection with *Chlamydia trachomatis*. N Engl J Med 1984;310(9):545-549.
50. Stamm WE, Kaetz SM, Beirne MB, Ashman JA. The practitioner's handbook for the management of STDs. Seattle, Washington: Health Sciences Center for Educational Resources, 1988.
51. Stamm WE, Wagner KF, Amsel R, Alexander ER, Turck M, Counts GW, Holmes KK. Causes of the acute urethral syndrome in women. N Engl J Med 1980;303(8):409-415.
52. Toomey K, Barnes R. Treatment of *Chlamydia trachomatis* genital infection. Rev Infect Dis 1990;12 (Suppl 6):S645-655.
53. Trussell J, Kost K. Contraceptive failure in the United States: a critical review of the literature. Stud Fam Plann 1987;18(5):237-283.
54. Turner CF, Miller HG, Moses LE (eds). AIDS: sexual behavior and intravenous drug use. Washington DC: National Academy Press, 1989:166-167.
55. Washington AE, Katz P. Cost of and payment source for pelvic inflammatory disease. Trends and projections, 1985 through 2000. JAMA 1991;266(18): 2565-2569.
56. Washington AE, Johnson RE, Sanders LL, Barnes RC, Alexander ER. Incidence of *Chlamydia trachomatis* infections in the United States: using reported *Neisseria gonorrhoeae* as a surrogate. In: Oriel D, Ridgway G, Schachter J (eds). Chlamydial infections. Cambridge, England: Cambridge University Press, 1986:487.

57. Wasserheit JN. Epidemiological synergy. Interrelationships between human immunodeficiency virus infection and other sexually transmitted diseases. Sex Transm Dis 1992;19(2):61-77.

58. Wasserheit JN, Holmes KK. Reproductive tract infection: challenges for international health policy, programs, and research. In: Germain A, Holmes KK, Piot P, Wasserheit JN (eds). Reproductive tract infections: global impact and priorities for women's reproductive health. New York NY: Plenum Press, 1992:7-33.

59. Wentworth BB, Judson FN, Gilchrist MJR (eds). Laboratory methods for the diagnosis of sexually transmitted diseases, second edition. Washington DC: American Public Health Association, 1991.

60. Westrom L, Joesoef R, Reynolds G, Hadgu A, Thompson SE. Pelvic inflammatory disease and fertility: a cohort study of 1,844 women with laparoscopically verified and 657 control women with normal laparoscopic results. Sex Transm Dis 1992;19(4):185-192.

61. Zenilman JM. Gonorrhea: clinical and public health issues. Hosp Pract 1993;Feb:31-50.

The Essentials of Contraception: Effectiveness, Safety, & Personal Considerations

- Most methods have a low risk of failure if they are used correctly and consistently.
- Simultaneous use of two methods dramatically lowers the risk of failure.
- Even a low annual risk of contraceptive failure implies a high risk of failure during a lifetime of use.

- In general, contraceptives pose little risk to a user's health, although personal risk factors should influence personal choice.
- Preserving future fertility by lowering STD risk has become a critical issue in contraceptive decision making.

Choosing a contraceptive is an important decision. A method that is not effective for an individual can lead to the serious consequence of an unwanted pregnancy. A method that is not safe for the user can create unfortunate medical consequences. A method that does not fit the individual's personal lifestyle is not likely to be used correctly or consistently. Who makes the choice? Users themselves should make the decisions about the contraceptives they select, taking into consideration the feelings and attitudes of their partners.

Through counseling, patients can choose the most suitable contraceptives. Family planning providers can also influence the user's motivation and ability to use the method correctly.[12] Encourage clients to educate themselves about the various methods available. Simply stressing the "clinician's advice" makes women dependent upon a particular clinician's interpretation of current knowledge. Direct clients toward available literature (such as this book or the many resources listed in Chapter 28). Virtually everyone will use a variety of methods throughout a lifetime and should be knowledgeable enough to consider various contraceptive methods. The patient's choice of a contraceptive depends on several major factors: effectiveness, safety, noncontraceptive benefits, and personal considerations.

CONTRACEPTIVE USE: LEVELS AND TRENDS

Information on levels and trends in contraceptive use in the United States is particularly good because it is based on the National Surveys of Family Growth (NSFG). In these periodic surveys conducted by the National Center for Health Statistics, about 8,500 women aged 15-44 are interviewed about topics related to childbearing, family planning, and maternal and child health.

- Among the 58 million women of reproductive age (aged 15-44), about 60% (35 million) were using some method of contraception, according to the 1988 NSFG.
- Among the 40% (23 million) who were not currently using a method, only about one-sixth were at risk of pregnancy. The remaining five-sixths were not at risk because they had been noncontraceptively sterilized, were sterile, were trying to become pregnant, were pregnant, were interviewed within 2 months after the completion of a pregnancy, or were not having intercourse.

About 90% of the women at risk were using a contraceptive. Ten percent of all women at risk of unintended pregnancy did not use any contraceptive. Today, the most popular contraceptive methods are oral contraceptive pills (10.7 million), female sterilization (9.6 million), condoms (5.1 million), and male sterilization (4.1 million).[23] See Table 5-1 for information on contraceptive method use by age of woman. Between 1982 and 1988, contraceptive method choices changed somewhat:[44]

- Condom use increased from 15.1% to 26.4% among 15- to 19-year old women at risk of pregnancy, generally because of the concern over AIDS and sexually transmitted diseases. Condom use also increased among those at risk aged 20-24 (from 9.4% to 12.8%) and 25-29 (from 9.9% to 14.2%).
- Pill use among women at risk increased in the age groups 20-24 (from 48.3% to 59.8%), 25-29 (from 31.7% to 39.7%), and 30-34 (from 15.5% to 20.4%), possibly because information about noncontraceptive benefits offset some of the fears and misinformation about pills.
- Use of no method among teenagers dropped by 7.9 percentage points (from 27.7% to 19.8%) between 1982 and 1988 despite an increase of 6.0 percentage points (from 33.4% to 39.4%) in exposure to risk caused by a rise in the proportion sexually active.

Table 5-1 Percent of women at risk[†] of pregnancy and percent at risk[†] currently using various methods from the 1988 National Survey of Family Growth

Age	% at Risk[†]	% Using among Women at Risk [†]									Sterilization	
		Pill	Condom	Diaphragm	Periodic Abstinence	Withdrawal	IUD	Spermicide	Sponge	No Method	Female	Male
15–19	39.4	47.7	26.4	0.8	0.7	2.5	0.0	0.8	0.6	19.8	0.2	0.2
20–24	66.5	59.8	12.8	3.4	1.5	3.0	0.3	0.6	1.0	11.8	4.4	1.5
25–29	72.1	39.7	14.2	4.8	2.0	3.0	1.0	1.5	1.9	10.4	15.4	5.5
30–34	73.6	20.4	11.0	8.1	2.7	2.1	2.9	2.3	0.7	7.4	29.9	12.5
35–39	75.0	4.6	11.3	7.3	2.9	0.5	2.6	2.7	1.4	6.3	41.9	18.4
40–44	71.0	3.0	9.4	3.6	2.0	1.1	3.3	1.4	0.2	7.6	46.9	21.1
15–44	66.7	27.8	13.2	5.2	2.1	2.0	1.8	1.7	1.0	9.7	24.8	10.5

Source: Trussell and Vaughan (1991).

[†] At risk = those who have had intercourse more than once AND who EITHER are current contraceptive users OR are nonusers who have had sex in the past 3 months and are not trying to become pregnant, are not pregnant, or were not interviewed within 2 months after the completion of a pregnancy and are not sterile.

- Use of the IUD, diaphragm, and periodic abstinence among women under age 30 virtually disappeared.

- Among women over age 30, IUD use declined dramatically (from 8.7% to 2.9% among women aged 30-34 and from 7.0% to 2.6% among women aged 35-39).

- Use of sterilization among women at risk aged 15-44 increased from 28.9% to 35.3% between 1982 and 1988. All of this increase is attributable to female sterilization, since the prevalence of male sterilization actually dropped slightly. The prevalence of female sterilization increased among women at risk in every age group.

CONDOM USE

Actually, use of condoms has increased more than these figures on "current" method indicate. First, concomitant use of condoms and sterilization, oral contraception, IUD, or diaphragm is coded in the NSFG as use of that other method, while concomitant use of condoms and any contraceptive other than these four methods is recoded as use of the condom. When the data in Table 5-1 are retabulated to capture all condom use among women at risk of pregnancy, regardless of whatever other methods were used as well, the total number of condom users in 1988 rises by 19%, from 5.09 to 6.04 million. The fractions of women using condoms among those at risk of pregnancy rise from 26.4% to 30.6% among women aged 15-19 and from 12.8% to 16.6% among women aged 20-24. Retabulation of the 1982 data causes the proportions of women using condoms among those at risk of pregnancy to increase from 15.1% to 17.4% among women aged 15-19 and from 9.4% to 11.4% among women aged 20-24. Retabulation results in an increase between 1982 and 1988 in the proportions of women using condoms among those at risk of pregnancy of 13.2 percentage points among those aged 15-19 and of 5.2 percentage points among those aged 20-24.[44]

Moreover, women probably do not report occasional use of condoms as an adjunct method in the NSFG. The reason is that women are asked to report all methods they have "used for one month or more." To determine current use, women are asked whether they are still using the last method they reported. Episodic use of an adjunct method may not be perceived as use for 1 month or more. Evidence for this conclusion is provided by examining any use of a condom at last intercourse (a separate question in a different section of the questionnaire than the questions used to determine current use). Among women in 1988 who were exposed to the risk of pregnancy and who reported that they used a condom at last intercourse, 14.4% did not report the condom (either alone or as an adjunct method) as their current method. This percentage is even higher among women aged 15-19 (24.8%) and aged 20-24 (16.8%). Nevertheless, even condom use at last intercourse may be underreported in the NSFG if women fail to report condoms used as an adjunct to their regular method.[44]

In the 1988 NSFG, women were also asked which methods they use "to keep you or your partner from catching diseases." Responses to the question reveal that 4.24 million women reported use of the condom as an STD prophylaxis but did not report use of the condom as a contraceptive. Altogether 10.4 million women of a total of 57.9 million women aged 15-44 reported use of condoms for prevention of pregnancy or STDs or both.[19]

E FFECTIVENESS: "WILL IT WORK?"

"Is the condom really effective?"
"Which would be the most effective method for me?"
"Why did one magazine say diaphragms are 98% effective and another say they are 80% effective?"
"Can you still get pregnant if you take your pills every day on schedule?"

"Will it work?" is the question usually asked first and most frequently about any birth control method. Because this question cannot be answered with certainty for any particular couple, most clinicians and counselors try to help patients understand something of the difficulty of quantifying efficacy.

It is useful to distinguish between measures of *contraceptive effectiveness* and measures of *contraceptive failure*. If 18% of women using the diaphragm were to become accidentally pregnant in their first year of use, then the method would have a failure rate of 18%. However, it does not follow that the diaphragm is 82% *effective*, because it is not true that 100% of these women would have become pregnant if they had not been using the diaphragm but had instead relied on chance. It may have been that 90% of these diaphragm users would have become pregnant had they relied on chance. If that were true, then the use of the diaphragm reduced the number of accidental pregnancies from 90% to 18%—a reduction of 80%. In this sense, the diaphragm could be said to be 80% effective at reducing pregnancy in the first year. But if only 60% of these women would have become pregnant if they did not use contraception, then the diaphragm would be only 70% effective.[a] Because no study can ascertain the proportion of women who would have become pregnant had they not used the contraceptive under

---

[a] Strictly, effectiveness is the proportionate reduction in the monthly probability of conception c. If this monthly probability is constant across women and over time, then the proportion conceiving in one year with no contraceptive use is $1-(1-c)^{12}$. Therefore, in the first example above c=0.1746 and in the second example c=0.0735. Using a contraceptive with effectiveness e reduces the proportion becoming pregnant in one year to $1-\{1-c(1-e)\}^{12}$. Hence, in the first example, diaphragm effectiveness, strictly measured, is 90.6% and in the second example it is only 77.7%.

investigation, effectiveness cannot be measured directly. Therefore, we focus attention entirely on *failure rates* or probabilities, which are directly measurable. However, we continue to use the term *effectiveness* in its loose everyday sense throughout this book. We also provide estimates of the proportion of women who would become pregnant if they did not use contraception, so that the reader may calculate rough effectiveness rates if they are needed.

EFFICACY DURING TYPICAL AND PERFECT USE

Our current understanding of the results in the literature on contraceptive efficacy is summarized in Table 5-2. More complete explanations of the derivations of the statistics in Table 5-2 are provided in Chapter 27. In addition, tables summarizing the efficacy literature for each method are contained in that chapter.

Typical Use

In the second column of Table 5-2, we provide estimates of the probabilities of failure during the first year for the *typical* user of each method in the United States:

- For spermicides, periodic abstinence, the diaphragm, male condom and pill, estimates were derived from the experience of married women in the 1976 and 1982 National Surveys of Family Growth (NSFG), so that the information pertains to nationally representative samples of users regularly exposed to risk of pregnancy.[41]

- Probabilities of failure for the cervical cap and the sponge were based on results of two clinical trials in which women were randomly assigned to use the diaphragm or sponge or the diaphragm or cervical cap.

- Estimates for methods such as the IUD, sterilization, Depo-Provera, and Norplant were derived from large clinical investigations. The estimate for the female condom is based on the only clinical trial of this method.

- Estimates for withdrawal and chance were based on evidence from surveys and clinical investigations, respectively.

Perfect Use

In the third column, we provide our best guess of the probabilities of *method* failure during the first year among *perfect* users. A method is used perfectly when it is used consistently according to a specified set of rules. For many methods, perfect use requires use at every act of intercourse. Virtually all method failure rates reported in the literature have been calculated

Table 5-2 Percentage of women experiencing a contraceptive failure during the first year of typical use and the first year of perfect use and the percentage continuing use at the end of the first year, United States

Method (1)	% of Women Experiencing an Accidental Pregnancy within the First Year of Use		% of Women Continuing Use at One Year[3] (4)
	Typical Use[1] (2)	Perfect Use[2] (3)	
Chance[4]	85	85	
Spermicides[5]	21	6	43
Periodic Abstinence	20		67
Calendar		9	
Ovulation Method		3	
Sympto-Thermal[6]		2	
Post-Ovulation		1	
Withdrawal	19	4	
Cap[7]			
Parous Women	36	26	45
Nulliparous Women	18	9	58
Sponge			
Parous Women	36	20	45
Nulliparous Women	18	9	58
Diaphragm[7]	18	6	58
Condom[8]			
Female (Reality)	21	5	56
Male	12	3	63
Pill	3		72
Progestin Only		0.5	
Combined		0.1	
IUD			
Progesterone T	2.0	1.5	81
Copper T 380A	0.8	0.6	78
LNg 20	0.1	0.1	81
Depo-Provera	0.3	0.3	70
Norplant (6 Capsules)	0.09	0.09	85
Female Sterilization	0.4	0.4	100
Male Sterilization	0.15	0.10	100

Emergency Contraceptive Pills: Treatment initiated within 72 hours after unprotected intercourse reduces the risk of pregnancy by at least 75%.[9]

Lactational Amenorrhea Method: LAM is a highly effective, *temporary* method of contraception.[10]

Source: Updated from Trussell et al. (1990b). See Chapter 27.

incorrectly and are too low (see the discussion below). Hence, we cannot justify our estimates rigorously except those for the ovulation method of periodic abstinence;[38] the cervical cap;[30,42] the diaphragm;[42] the sponge;[42] and the female condom;[10] those for methods with little scope for user error (implants, injectables, and sterilization); and those for the pill and IUD, which are based on extensive clinical trials with very low failure rates. Even the estimates for the female condom, diaphragm, cervical cap, and sponge are based on only one or two studies. Our hope is that our understanding of efficacy during perfect use for these methods will be enhanced by additional studies, and that the total gap in our knowledge for methods such as spermicides, the male condom, withdrawal, and other variants of periodic abstinence will be closed by future research.

Continuation Rates

The fourth column displays the first-year probabilities of continuing use. They are based on the same sources used to derive the estimates in the first column (typical use).

Alternative Estimates of Failure During Typical Use

Alternative estimates of the probabilities of failure during the first year of typical use are provided in Table 5-3. These are based on the 1986 Australian

Table 5-3 Percentage of women experiencing a contraceptive failure in the first year of typical use. United States and Australia

Method	United States 1976 and 1982 NSFGs Shown in Table 5-2. Married Women, Standardized	Australia 1986 AFS. All Women, Not Standardized	United States 1988 NSFG Uncorrected for Abortion. All Women, Not Standardized	United States 1988 NSFG Corrected for Abortion. All Women, Not Standardized	United States 1988 NSFG Corrected for Abortion. All Women, Standardized
(1)	(2)	(3)	(4)	(5)	(6)
Pill	3	2	5	8	7
Male Condom	12	8	7	15	16
Diaphragm	18	21	10	16	22
Withdrawal	19	14			
Periodic Abstinence	20	18	21	26	31
Spermicides	21	22	13	25	30

Sources: 1976 and 1982 NSFGs, Trussell et al. (1990b); 1986 AFS, Bracher and Santow (1992); 1988 NSFG, Jones and Forrest (1992).

Family Survey[2] and on the 1988 NSFG.[15] The estimates in the second column are the same as those in the second column of Table 5-2. They are standardized probabilities of failure among married women based on the 1976 and 1982 NSFGs. They differ from the estimates in the other columns because they are based on the experience of married women only. Also, they are standardized to reflect the estimated probabilities of failure that would be observed if users of each method had the same characteristics (age distribution, fraction seeking to prevent rather than delay further childbearing, parity distribution, and fraction living in poverty). The estimates in the third column are based on Australian women (62% of whom were married or cohabiting, ranging from only 45% of those using the pill to 92% of those using periodic abstinence or withdrawal) who were using a method for the first time. The estimates in the fourth column are based on all women aged 15-44 in the 1988 NSFG regardless of marital or cohabitation status. Those in the fifth column are revised to reflect estimated underreporting of induced abortion in the 1988 NSFG. The estimates in the sixth column are corrected for estimated underreporting of abortion and standardized on a common distribution of age, poverty status, and marital status.

Our preferred estimates in Table 5-2 are very similar to those from the Australian Family Survey and are slightly lower than the unstandardized estimates based on the 1988 NSFG corrected for underreporting of abortion, even though the estimates pertain to different populations of users. We decided to retain our prior estimates based on the 1976 and 1982 NSFGs instead of updating these to reflect the 1988 NSFG for two reasons. First, we conclude that the correction for underreporting of abortion produces estimates that are too high, especially for the pill, the condom, periodic abstinence, and spermicides, probably because women in abortion clinics (surveys of whom provided the information for the correction) overreport use of a contraceptive at the time they became pregnant. Moreover, it seems likely that women in personal interviews for the NSFG also would tend to overreport use of a contraceptive at the time of a conception leading to a live birth. Evidence for this suspicion is provided by a 6% first-year failure rate for the IUD (a method with little scope for user error) among married women in the 1976 and 1982 NSFGs. This rate is much higher than rates observed in clinical trials of IUDs.[41] We would naturally expect overreporting of contraceptive use in both the NSFG and in surveys conducted in abortion clinics: responsibility for the pregnancy is shifted from the woman (or couple) to the method. Thus, we suspect that failure rates based on the NSFG would tend to be too low because induced abortions (and contraceptive failures leading to induced abortions) are underreported but would tend to be too high because contraceptive failures leading to live births are overreported. These two sources of bias would tend to cancel, whereas adjustment for underreporting of induced abortion would make the failure rates too high.

Second, we would prefer to present standardized estimates for married women only, or at least for women regularly cohabiting with a sexual partner, so that they reflect probabilities of failure for those having sexual intercourse regularly. Estimates standardized for user characteristics for married women uncorrected for estimated underreporting of abortion are not available for the 1988 NSFG.

EFFICACY OVER TIME

We confine attention to the first-year probabilities of failure solely because probabilities for longer durations are generally not available. Failure rates at these longer durations for most methods (but not Norplant) should be lower than failure rates during the first year, primarily because those users prone to fail do so early, leaving a pool of more successful contraceptive users (or those who are relatively infertile) as time passes. Nevertheless, probabilities of failure cumulate over time. Suppose that 15%, 12%, and 8% of women using a method experience a contraceptive failure during years 1, 2, and 3, respectively. The probability of not failing within 3 years is obtained by multiplying the probabilities of *not failing* for each of the three years: 0.85 times 0.88 times 0.92, which equals 0.69. Thus, the percentage failing within 3 years is 31% (=100%–69%).

The lesson here is that the differences among failure probabilities for various methods will increase over time. For example, suppose that each year the typical proportion failing for the pill is 3% and for the diaphragm is 18%. Within 5 years, 14% of pill users and 63% of diaphragm users will accidentally become pregnant.

CONTRACEPTIVE FAILURES IN A LIFETIME

Data from the National Survey of Family Growth (NSFG) conducted in 1982 indicate that during the 3-year period 1979-1982, about 1.61 million contraceptive failures occurred per year and the typical woman would experience 0.81 failures during her lifetime.[43] This statistic must be interpreted precisely. It is the average number of failures that a hypothetical woman would experience if during her life she faced at each age the risk of contraceptive failure actually observed in the period 1979-1981. These age-specific risks are governed by the proportions of women having intercourse, their frequency of intercourse, the mix of contraceptive methods, the consistency and correctness of contraceptive use, the outcomes of pregnancies (births or induced abortions), and the underlying fecundity of the woman and her partner(s). Therefore, the estimate is very unlikely to pertain to any individual woman or even a cohort of women, because all the proximate determinants listed above are likely to change over time.

Nevertheless, the estimate is a convenient summary statistic that pertains to a specific period of time.

Since the total fertility rate (TFR) during the period 1979-1981 averaged 1.82,[25] these results imply that the typical woman will experience one contraceptive failure for every 2.25 live births during her lifetime, so that contraceptive failures are not uncommon relative to live births. We suspect that many readers will be surprised that the average lifetime number of contraceptive failures is so low, but several factors operate to make it smaller than one might expect:

- First, the average annual risk of contraceptive failure (which includes women at all durations of use) is much smaller than the first-year rates published in the literature and summarized in Table 5-2, because failure rates decline with duration of use.[41,47,48,49]
- Second, substantial fractions of women are not exposed to the risk of contraceptive failure because they or their partners have been sterilized. In the preceding analysis, 38.8%, 53.7%, and 55.8% of the women aged 30-34, 35-39, and 40-44, respectively, were protected by sterilization. When intervals during which women were protected by sterilization are removed when calculating the age-specific contraceptive failure rates, one obtains an estimate of 0.97 lifetime contraceptive failures for the typical woman who relies solely on reversible methods when she does use contraception.
- Third, contraceptive failures cannot be experienced by women who do not use contraception. The annual numbers of contraceptive failures experienced by teenagers are particularly low for this reason. When intervals during which contraception was not used (except for the gestation period following a contraceptive failure) are also removed from the denominators of the age-specific failure rates, one obtains an estimate of 1.96 lifetime failures for the typical woman who seeks to avoid pregnancy throughout her lifetime by relying solely on reversible methods.[43]

FACTORS THAT INFLUENCE EFFICACY

Both contraceptive providers and their patients can better understand why contraceptive failure rates can vary so widely from study to study if we recall that many factors influence efficacy. Factors that affect contraceptive failure rates and probabilities reported in the literature can be usefully divided into three categories: (1) the inherent effectiveness of the method when used correctly and consistently (perfect use) and the technical attributes of the method that facilitate or interfere with proper use, (2) characteristics of the user, and (3) competence and honesty of the investigator in planning and executing the study and in analyzing and reporting the results.

Inherent Efficacy

For some methods, such as sterilization, implants, and injectables, the inherent efficacy is so high, and proper and consistent use is so nearly guaranteed, that extremely low failure rates are found in all studies, and the range of reported probabilities of failure is quite narrow. For other methods such as the pill and IUD, inherent efficacy is high but there is still room for potential misuse (forgetting to take pills or failure to check for the proper placement of IUD strings), so that the second factor can contribute to a wider range of reported probabilities of failure. In general, the studies of sterilization, injectable, implant, pill, and IUD failure have been very competently executed and analyzed. Studies of periodic abstinence, spermicides, and the barrier methods display a wide range of reported probabilities of failure because the potential for misuse is high, the inherent effectiveness is relatively low, and the competence of the investigators is mixed.

User Characteristics

Characteristics of the users can affect the failure rate for any method under investigation, but the impact will be greatest when the typical failure rates are highest, either because the method is inherently less effective or because it is hard to use consistently or correctly.

Imperfect use. The user characteristic that is probably most important is imperfect use of the method. Unfortunately, nearly all investigators who have attempted to calculate "method" and "user" failure rates have done so incorrectly. Investigators routinely separate the accidental pregnancies into two groups. By convention, pregnancies that occur during a month in which a method was used improperly are classified as user failures (even though, logically, a pregnancy might be due to failure of the method, if it was used correctly on some occasions and incorrectly on others), and all other pregnancies are classified as method failures. But investigators do not separate the exposure (the denominator in the calculation of failure rates) into these two groups.

For example, suppose that two method failures and eight user failures occur during 100 women-years of exposure to the risk of pregnancy. Then the common calculation is that the user failure rate is 8% and the method failure rate is 2%; the sum of the two is the overall failure rate of 10%. By definition, however, method failures can occur only during perfect use and user failures cannot occur during perfect use. If there were 50 years of perfect and 50 years of imperfect use in the total of 100 years of exposure, then the method failure rate would be 4% and the user failure rate would be 16%, and the difference between the two rates (here 12%) provides a measure of how forgiving of imperfect use the method is. However, since investigators do not generally inquire about perfect use except when a pregnancy occurs, the proper calculations cannot be performed. The importance of perfect use is demonstrated in the few studies where the requisite information on quality of use was collected. For example, in a WHO study of the ovulation method of periodic abstinence, the proportion of women becoming pregnant among those who used the method perfectly during the first year was 3.1%, whereas the corresponding proportion failing during a year of imperfect use was 86.4%.[38] In a large clinical trial of the cervical cap conducted in Los Angeles, among the 5% of the sample who used the method perfectly, the fraction failing during the first year was 6.1%. Among the remaining 95% of the sample who at least on one occasion used the cap imperfectly, the first-year probability of failure was nearly twice as high (11.9%).[30]

Frequency of intercourse. Among those who use a method consistently and correctly (perfect users), the most important user characteristic that determines contraceptive failure is frequency of intercourse. For example, among condom, diaphragm, and spermicide users and those who relied on "chance" in the 1982 National Survey of Family Growth, unmarried women had lower failure rates than did married women, almost certainly because the unmarried had intercourse less frequently.[13] In another study in which users were randomly assigned to either the diaphragm or the sponge, diaphragm users who had intercourse four or more times a week became pregnant in the first year twice as frequently as those who had intercourse less than four times a week.[20] In that clinical trial, among women who used the diaphragm at every act of intercourse, only 3.4% of those who had intercourse fewer than three times a week became pregnant in the first year, compared with 9.7% of those who had intercourse more than three times per week.[42]

Age. A woman's biological capacity to conceive and bear a child declines with age. This decline is likely to be pronounced among those who are routinely exposed to sexually transmitted infections such as chlamydia and gonorrhea. Among those not so exposed, the decline is likely to be moderate until a woman reaches her late 30s.[21] Although many investigators have found that contraceptive failure rates decline with age,[13,33,34,49] this effect almost surely overstates the pure age effect because age in many studies primarily captures the effect of coital frequency, which declines both with age and with marital duration.[45] User characteristics such as race and income seem to be less important determinants of contraceptive failure.

Influence of the Investigator

The competence and honesty of the investigator also affect the published results. The errors committed by investigators range from simple arithmetical mistakes to outright fraud.[41] One well-documented instance of fraud involved the Dalkon shield. In a two-page article published in the *American Journal of Obstetrics and Gynecology*, a first-year probability of failure of 1.1% was presented and the claim made that "only the combined type of oral contraceptive offers slightly greater protection."[8] It was not revealed by the researcher that some women had been instructed to use spermicides as an adjunctive method to reduce the risk of pregnancy, nor that he was part-owner of the Dalkon Corporation. Furthermore, he never subsequently revealed (except to the A.H. Robins Company, which bought the shield from the Dalkon Corporation but did not reveal this information either) that as the original trial matured, the first-year probability of pregnancy more than doubled.[22]

The United States' system of drug testing, which demands that the company wishing to market a drug be responsible for conducting studies to assess its efficacy and safety, provides incentives for the unscrupulous to present less-than-honest results. Some actions that are not deliberately dishonest are, nevertheless, not discouraged by the incentives in the present system. For example, a woman who becomes pregnant may be discarded from a clinical trial if the researcher decides that she did not fit the protocols after all. Or one can be less than vigilant in trying to contact patients lost to follow-up (LFU). The standard assumption made at the time of analysis is that women who are LFU experience accidental pregnancy at the same rate as those who are observed. This assumption is probably innocuous when the proportion LFU is small. But in many studies the proportion LFU may be 20% or higher, so that what really happens to these women could drastically affect the estimate of the proportion failing. Our strong suspicion is that women LFU are more likely to experience a contraceptive failure than are those still in the trial. For example, one study found that the failure rate for calendar rhythm rose from 9.4 to 14.4 per 100 women-years of exposure as a result of resolution of cases LFU.[35]

Methodological Pitfalls

Several methodological pitfalls can snare investigators. One of the most common is a misleading measure of failure called the Pearl index, which is obtained by dividing the number of accidental pregnancies by the number of years of exposure to the risk of unintended pregnancy contributed by all women in the study. This measure can be misleading when one wishes to compare failure rates obtained from studies with different average amounts of exposure. The likelihood of failure declines over time because the less effective users are removed as they become pregnant. Those still using after long durations are unlikely to fail, so that an investigator could (wittingly or unwittingly) drive the reported failure rate toward zero by running the trial "forever." As discussed in Chapter 25, life-table measures of failure are easy to interpret and control for the distorting effects of varying durations of use. Another problem occurs when deciding which pregnancies to count. Most studies count only the pregnancies observed and reported by the women.

If, on the other hand, a pregnancy test were administered every month, the number of pregnancies (and hence the failure rate) would increase because early fetal losses not observed by the woman would be added to the number of observed pregnancies. Such routine pregnancy testing in the more recent pill trials has resulted in higher failure rates than would otherwise have been obtained and makes the results not comparable to other pill trials or trials for other methods. Other, more technical, errors that have biased reported results are discussed elsewhere.[36,39,41]

The incentives to conduct research on contraceptive failure vary widely from method to method. Many studies of the pill and IUD exist because companies wishing to market them must conduct clinical trials to demonstrate their efficacy. In contrast, few studies of withdrawal exist because investigating this method leads to no financial reward. Moreover, researchers face differing incentives to report unfavorable results. The vasectomy literature is filled with short articles by clinicians who have performed 500 or 1,000 or 1,500 vasectomies. When they report accidental pregnancies (curiously, pregnancy is seldom mentioned in discussions of vasectomy "failures," which focus on the continued presence of sperm in the ejaculate), their pregnancy rates are invariably low. Surgeons with high pregnancy rates simply do not write articles calling attention to their poor surgical skills. Likewise, drug companies do not commonly publicize their failures. Even if investigators prepared reports describing failures, journal editors would not be likely to publish them.

GOALS FOR TEACHING EFFICACY

Keep these thoughts in mind when counseling about contraceptive effectiveness:

1. **Failure rate estimates apply to groups, not an individual user.** For example, a 3% probability of failure during the first year for the pill will not protect the careless user and may not apply to 14-year-old girls who are less likely to be compliant. The 18% probability of failure during the first year from a diaphragm study need not discourage a careful and disciplined woman who has infrequent intercourse from using a diaphragm. Help your patients understand that numbers are not what protect—correct and consistent use protects.

2. **Make sure your staff provides consistent information.** One study of the information provided by family planning staff indicated that providers tended to give the lowest reported probabilities of failure for pills and IUDs, probabilities of failure during typical use for diaphragms and foam, and higher-than-typical probabilities of failure for condoms.[37] Thus, family planning providers may extensively bias their patient education in favor of methods they provide most fre-

quently. In spite of their safety, condoms, withdrawal, and spermicides get an undeserved low efficacy score within many family planning clinics and offices. You can avoid unintentional bias by deciding carefully what failure rates your clinic or staff members are going to use.

3. **Technology fails people just as people fail technology.** In the past, patients were often told that accidental pregnancies were their own fault because they did not use their method correctly or carefully. Contraceptives are imperfect and can fail even the most diligent user.

4. **Using two methods at once dramatically lowers the risk of accidental pregnancy**, provided they are used consistently. If one of the methods is a condom or vaginal barrier, protection from disease transmission is an added benefit. For example, the probabilities of failure during the first year of perfect use of male condoms and spermicides are estimated to be 3% and 6%, respectively, in Table 5-2. During perfect use, the contraceptive mechanisms of condoms and spermicides operate independently, since lack of independence during typical use would most likely be due to imperfect use (either use both methods or not use either). The annual probability of failure during simultaneous perfect use of condoms and spermicides would be 0.1%, the same as that achieved by the combined pill (0.1%) and LNg20 IUD (0.1%) during perfect use. Even if the annual probabilities of failure during perfect use for the condom and spermicides were twice as high—6% and 12%, respectively—the annual probability of failure during simultaneous perfect use would be only 0.4%, comparable to that of the minipill (0.5%) and the Copper T 380A IUD (0.6%) during perfect use.[16]

5. **Methods that protect a person for a long time** (sterilization, implants, IUDs, and long-acting injections) **tend to be associated with higher contraceptive efficacy**, primarily because there is little scope for user error.

SAFETY: "WILL IT HURT ME?"

"I smoke. Won't the pill give me a heart attack?"
"Could the IUD puncture my womb?"
"Will I be able to get pregnant after stopping my method?"

In general, contraception poses few serious health risks to users. Moreover, the safety considerations of contraceptive methods are not as great as those of pregnancy-related complications. Unplanned and unwanted pregnancies place women at risk unnecessarily. Women in many other countries will experience an even greater advantage in using contraceptive methods, especially in comparison to pregnancy-related mortality. Nonetheless, some contraceptives pose potential risk to the user:

- First, the method itself may have inherent dangers: the method might be associated with death, hospitalization, surgery, medical side effects, infections, loss of reproductive capacity, or pain.
- Second, accidental pregnancy is associated with risk: a particular woman must assess both the likelihood of contraceptive failure and the dangers that a pregnancy would pose.
- Third, future fertility may be influenced by contraceptive choice.

These risks are briefly addressed here. More detailed discussion appears in the chapters devoted to each method.

MAJOR HEALTH RISKS

When it comes to the most serious outcome of all—death—the absolute level of risk is extraordinarily low for most women. Table 5-4 puts into perspective some of the risks of everyday life in the United States. Although the information in this table should not be used to deny the concerns of a woman who is worried about pills, abortion, or tampons, it may help her compare these risks with other risks she voluntarily faces in her life.

Other major health risks are not only uncommon, they are most likely to occur in women who may have underlying medical conditions that may be influenced by hormonal contraception:

- Cardiovascular disease: The pill has been associated with an increased risk of myocardial infarction and stroke. About one death in 100,000 users under the age of 45 has been attributable to use of the pill.[14] Risk increases with age because risk factors such as hypertension, thromboembolic disease, diabetes, and a sedentary lifestyle increase with age. Smoking is a definite risk factor.[50]
- Cancer: The association between cancer of the breast and cervix and the use of the pill remains under scrutiny.
  - It may be that specific subpopulations of users are at an increased risk for breast cancer.[32] Risk factors for breast cancer include having a family history of breast cancer and delayed or no childbearing.
  - Cervical cancer has been reported more often in pill users, although the correlation may be due to other, unidentified factors that place the OC user at a higher risk.[3] Risk factors for cervical cancer include having had multiple sexual partners and cigarette smoking.

Conversely, the pill appears to protect users against cancers of the endometrium[4] and ovary.[5] Barrier methods used in conjunction with spermicides decrease the user's risk of cervical cancer.[26,29]

Table 5-4 Voluntary risks in perspective

Activity	Chance of Death in a Year
Risks for Men and Women of All Ages Who Participate In:	
Motorcycling	1 in 1,000
Automobile Driving	1 in 6,000
Power Boating	1 in 6,000
Rock Climbing	1 in 7,500
Playing Football	1 in 25,000
Canoeing	1 in 100,000
Risks for Women Aged 15–44 Years:	
Using Tampons	1 in 350,000
Having Sexual Intercourse (PID)	1 in 50,000
Preventing Pregnancy:	
Using Birth Control Pills	
Nonsmoker	1 in 63,000
Smoker	1 in 16,000
Using IUDs	1 in 100,000
Using Diaphragm, Condom, or Spermicide	None
Using Fertility Awareness Methods	None
Undergoing Sterilization:	
Laparoscopic Tubal Ligation	1 in 67,000
Hysterectomy	1 in 1,600
Vasectomy	1 in 300,000
Continuing Pregnancy	1 in 11,000
Terminating Pregnancy:	
Legal Abortion	
Before 9 Weeks	1 in 260,000
Between 9 and 12 Weeks	1 in 100,000
Between 13 and 15 Weeks	1 in 34,000
After 15 Weeks	1 in 10,200

Sources: Atrash et al. (1990);
Cates (1980);
Dinman (1981);
Lawson et al. (1992);
Peterson et al. (1982);
National Center for Health Statistics (1986).

FUTURE FERTILITY

An important issue in helping a couple evaluate safety as they choose a contraceptive may be their future childbearing aspirations. There are several important considerations to keep in mind in order to protect the future fertility of contraceptive patients:

- **Abstinence** is the single most effective and risk-free means of protecting future fertility.
- **Pregnancy** and the outcomes of pregnancy carry substantial risks to future fertility.
- **The pill**, which has a protective effect against acute gonococcal pelvic inflammatory disease and decreases the risk of ovarian cyst surgery and fibromyomata, may be the ideal contraceptive option for the woman who wants to be sexually active for a number of years before bearing children.[14] On the other hand, oral contraceptives appear to increase a woman's risk of acquiring chlamydia infection.[51] Perhaps the *best contraceptive option for a young healthy woman who wishes to delay her childbearing is the pill/condom combination.*
- **Mechanical and chemical barriers** combined offer the greatest protection against tubal damage.[7]
- **The IUD**, which causes a 1.6-fold increase in the risk of pelvic inflammatory disease, is probably the least desirable option for women who want to preserve fertility.[28]
- **Sterilization** must be considered permanent.

SIDE EFFECTS

Often the minor side effects of contraceptives, in addition to the more serious complications, influence whether an individual selects a certain method. "What physical changes will I undergo?" "Will I be annoyed by spotting, weight gain, cramping, or the sensation of using a given method?" Clinicians cannot dismiss the important role that side effects play when an individual must repeatedly assess whether to continue using a method or whether to use it consistently.

Side effects can be hormonally or mechanically induced. Headaches, weight gain, and depression can be side effects of hormonal methods. Menstrual changes such as spotting and decreased or increased bleeding can be caused by hormonal or mechanical methods. Physical sensations such as decreased penile sensitivity or pressure on pelvic walls or uterine cramping are generally caused by mechanical methods. Other mechanically induced side effects include urinary tract infection due to diaphragm rim pressure or vaginal trauma from vaginal barrier methods.

With the great majority of these side effects, instruction and patient education can help users accept and understand what is happening. The appearance of side effects that are not serious is not a reason to avoid use of a method.

PRECAUTIONS

Some women are more likely than others to encounter problems with a specific method of birth control, so considering the precautions to the use of methods is important when a woman chooses her contraceptive. Most of the serious pill and IUD problems could be avoided by (1) eliminating the use of these methods among women who are medically at risk and (2) teaching the user to recognize the early danger signals for serious complications.

The authors prefer to avoid the concept of contraindications to any given method. Certain words trigger such vivid images in our minds that they virtually block out all rational communication about anything else. In family planning and reproductive health, phrases that may effectively stop the patient from absorbing any new information include the following: Your pregnancy test is positive. You have an abnormal pap smear. You have a small lump in your breast that we need to evaluate further. Your HIV test is positive.

Some conditions are not open to much qualification. To a certain extent, contraindication is such a word. Health educators, journalists, clinicians, and clients need only see the word *contraindication* linking a medical condition and a medication and all attempts to qualify the degree of contraindication are virtually futile. Hence, in the following chapters a table describing precautions replaces tables in previous editions describing contraindications to various methods.

- Precautions—Refrain from providing the method to women with medical conditions that may increase their risk of serious complications.
- Exercise caution—Carefully follow the woman's health situation and monitor her for adverse side effects.
- Provide with care—Provide follow-up care and instruct the woman about early danger signals.

GOALS FOR TEACHING SAFETY

1. **Try to educate the patient about misconceptions.** People who are afraid do not respond well to rational persuasions. Many patients hold certain opinions about contraceptives—that the pill is very dangerous even to healthy, nonsmoking young women or that injectables lead to permanent sterility. However, if you see that you are getting nowhere, stop. Help each client select a method that can be used without fear.

2. **Make sure that you and your staff know all about the major side effects** of contraceptives, such as the relationship between pill use and blood clots or reproductive cancers. Give accurate information.

3. **Tell patients what they need to know** even if they do not ask. Patients do not always ask the questions they need answered.

4. **Compare the contraceptive risks** with the risks a woman faces if she becomes pregnant. In general, the risks of pregnancy, abortion, and delivery are far greater than those for using a contraceptive.

5. **Help patients make a contraceptive choice that will protect them from both pregnancy and sexually transmitted infections**. Safety concerns often overlap with worries about infections.

6. **Teach patients the danger signals** of the methods they select. If a danger signal does appear, the informed user can quickly seek help.

N ONCONTRACEPTIVE BENEFITS

Although the noncontraceptive benefits provided by certain methods are not generally the major determinant for selecting a contraceptive method, they certainly can help patients decide between two or more suitable methods. (See Table 5-5.)

As the AIDS epidemic continues, methods that reduce the user's risk of acquiring HIV infection provide a noncontraceptive benefit that may weigh as heavily as the contraceptive benefit. Any sexually active person who may be at risk of acquiring infection with the human immunodeficiency virus (HIV), human papillomavirus (HPV), gonorrhea, syphilis, chlamydia, herpes, or other sexually transmitted diseases should consider barrier methods, especially condoms. More women are beginning to appreciate this noncontraceptive benefit of condoms: women seeking safer sex now buy 30% to 40% of condoms.[31]

Oral contraceptives offer several noncontraceptive benefits: protection against pelvic inflammatory disease (PID), cancers of the ovary and endometrium, recurrent ovarian cysts, and benign breast cysts and fibroadenomas.[14] As women who have suffered menstrual cramps and discomforts can attest, the pill eases these problems. Make it a practice to tell your patients about the noncontraceptive benefits of the various methods. If patients have additional reasons for using the contraceptives, their motivation to use the methods correctly and consistently will probably be improved.

Table 5-5 Major methods of contraception and some related safety concerns, side effects, and noncontraceptive benefits

Method	Dangers	Side Effects	Noncontraceptive Benefits
Pill	Cardiovascular complications (stroke, heart attack, blood clots, high blood pressure, hepatic adenomas)	Nausea, headaches, dizziness, spotting, weight gain, breast tenderness, chloasma	Protects against PID, some cancers (ovarian, endometrial) and some benign tumors (leiomyomata, benign breast masses) and ovarian cysts; decreases menstrual blood loss and pain
IUD	Pelvic inflammatory disease, uterine perforation, anemia	Menstrual cramping, spotting, increased bleeding	None known except progestin-releasing IUDs which may decrease menstrual blood loss and pain
Male Condom	None known	Decreased sensation, allergy to latex, loss of spontaneity	Protects against sexually transmitted diseases, including AIDS; delays premature ejaculation
Female Condom	None known	Aesthetically unappealing and awkward to use for some	Protects against sexually transmitted diseases, including on the vulva
Implant	Infection at implant site	Tenderness at site, menstrual changes	May protect against PID; lactation not disturbed; may decrease menstrual cramps, pains and blood loss
Injectable	None definitely proven	Menstrual changes, weight gain, headaches	May protect against PID; lactation not disturbed; may have protective effects against ovarian and endometrial cancers
Sterilization	Infection	Pain at surgical site, psychological reactions, subsequent regret that the procedure was performed	None known; may have beneficial effects *vis a vis* PID
Abstinence	None known	Psychological reactions	Prevents infections including AIDS
Abortion	Infection, pain, perforation, psychologic trauma	Cramping	None known
Barriers: Diaphragm, Cap, Sponge	Mechanical irritation, vaginal infections, toxic shock syndrome	Pelvic pressure, cervical erosion, vaginal discharges if left in too long	Protects somewhat against sexually transmitted diseases
Spermicides	None known	Tissue irritation	Protects against many sexually transmitted diseases
Lactational Amenorrhea Method (LAM)	None known	Mastitis from staphylococcal infection	Provides excellent nutrition for infants under 6 months old

PERSONAL CONSIDERATIONS

The best methods of birth control for patients are those that will be in harmony with their wishes, fears, preferences, and lifestyles. Table 5-6 lists questions designed to help patients determine whether or not a birth control method under consideration is a realistic choice. These questions may

Table 5-6 Contraceptive comfort and confidence scale

Method of birth control you are considering using: _____

Length of time you used this method in the past: _____

Answer **YES** or **NO** to the following questions:

	YES	NO
1. Have I had problems using this method before?		
2. Have I ever become pregnant while using this method?		
3. Am I afraid of using this method?		
4. Would I really rather not use this method?		
5. Will I have trouble remembering to use this method?		
6. Will I have trouble using this method correctly?		
7. Do I still have unanswered questions about this method?		
8. Does this method make menstrual periods longer or more painful?		
9. Does this method cost more than I can afford?		
10. Could this method cause me to have serious complications?		
11. Am I opposed to this method because of any religious or moral beliefs?		
12. Is my partner opposed to this method?		
13. Am I using this method without my partner's knowledge?		
14. Will using this method embarrass my partner?		
15. Will using this method embarrass me?		
16. Will I enjoy intercourse less because of this method?		
17. If this method interrupts lovemaking, will I avoid using it?		
18. Has a nurse or doctor ever told me NOT to use this method?		
19. Is there anything about my personality that could lead me to use this method incorrectly?		
20. Am I at any risk of being exposed to HIV (the AIDS virus) or other sexually transmitted infections if I use this method?		
Total Number of **YES** Answers:		

Most individuals will have a few "yes" answers. "Yes" answers mean that potential problems may arise. If you have more than a few "yes" responses, you may want to talk with your physician, counselor, partner, or friend to help you decide whether to use this method or how to use it so that it will really be effective for you. In general, the more "yes" answers you have, the less likely you are to use this method consistently and correctly at every act of intercourse.

be used exactly as is or they may be adapted for local use without permission. "Don't know" answers point to a need for more thinking, more introspection, or more information. "Yes" answers may mean the user might not like or be successful with the method. Most individuals will have a few "yes" answers. "Yes" answers mean that potential problems may lie in store. If clients have more than a few "yes" responses, they may want to talk to their physician, counselor, partner, or friend. Talking it over can help them to decide whether to use this method, or how to use it so it will really be effective for them. In general, the more "yes" answers they have, the less likely they are to use this method consistently and correctly.

Reproductive life span. The typical woman in the United States spends about 36 years—more than half of her life span of 79 years—at potential biological risk of pregnancy, during the time from menarche (at age 12.5) to natural menopause (at age 48.4).[11] What matters most to a woman when she considers a contraceptive will ordinarily change over the course of her reproductive life span. As is shown in Table 5-7, different reproductive stages are associated with distinct fertility goals and sexual behaviors. From menarche to first birth, the primary fertility goal is to postpone pregnancy and birth. Between the first and last births, the primary goal is to space pregnancies leading to births. Between the last birth and menopause, the goal is to cease childbearing altogether. The biggest demands on a contraceptive method are generated during the period between first intercourse and first birth, when the typical woman will have several sexual partners with high coital frequency; the typical woman will attach great importance to preventing pregnancy and STDs and to a method's reversibility and ease of use. In the last stage of her reproductive life span, from the last birth to menopause, the most important factor is a method's efficacy at preventing pregnancy.

Because the information is presented in tabular format, Table 5-7 gives the misleading impression that the stages of reproductive life are approximately equal in length. However, as is shown in Figure 5-1, more than half the entire reproductive life span—18.4 years or 51% of the reproductive span of 35.9 years—is spent trying to avoid further childbearing, in the stage from the last birth to menopause. The typical woman accomplishes this goal via female or male sterilization. A further 13.5 years or 38% of the reproductive span, from menarche to the first birth, is characterized by no desire to become pregnant. Thus, of a total reproductive span of 35.9 years during which a woman is potentially biologically at risk of conception, only 4.0 years (11% of the total), from the first to the last birth, are characterized by any desire to become pregnant. Even this figure is exaggerated since a great fraction of this stage is spent in the pregnant or lactating state or trying to postpone the next pregnancy.

Table 5-7 The stages of reproductive life

	Adolescents/Young Adults		Later Reproductive Years	
	Menarche to First Intercourse	**First Intercourse to First Birth**	**First Birth to Last Birth**	**Last Birth to Menopause**
Fertility Goals				
Births	Postpone	Postpone	Space	Stop
Ability to Have Children	Preserve	Preserve	Preserve	Irrelevant
Sexual Behavior				
# of Partners	None	Multiple?	One?	One?
Coital Frequency	Zero	Moderate to High	Moderate	Moderate to Low
Coital Predictability	Low	Moderate to High	High	High
Importance of Method Characteristics				
Pregnancy Prevention		High	Moderate	High
PID Prevention		High	Moderate	Low
Not Coitus-Linked		High	Low	Moderate
Reversibility		High	High	Low
Most Common Methods				
Most Common		Pill	Pill	Sterilization
Next Most Common		Condom	Condom	Pill, Condom

Source: Forrest (1993).

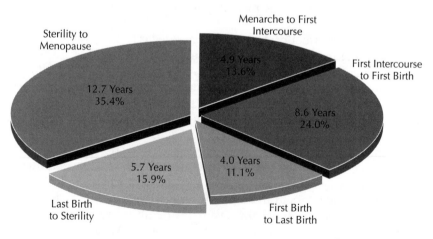

Figure 5-1 Time spent in the stages of reproductive life

Source: Forrest (1993).

Cost of contraceptives. We cannot provide contraceptives without considering the patient's financial circumstances.[18] A woman should be told in advance what her ongoing expenses will be. If cost will impose a major hardship, then offer an alternative contraceptive or a means of obtaining the desired contraceptive less expensively. The economic implications of using some forms of contraception have become significant (see Table 5-8).

Pattern of sexual activity. Regarding their contraceptive choices, women and men should be influenced by their number of partners and their frequency of intercourse.

The number of partners affects the risk of sexually transmitted diseases (STDs). In more obvious cases, the individual will have more than one partner at any given time. Less obvious are the individuals who practice serial monogamy. That is, they have only one partner at a time; however, the relationships are not permanent and so at the end of one relationship, the individual will move on to a new partner. Indeed, having more than one lifetime partner is the norm, and it is not uncommon for unmarried men and women to have more than one partner per year (see Chapter 1). The methods that would most protect individuals from STDs require commitment, understanding, and assertiveness by the client. The practitioner recommending the use of condoms (male or female) or other barrier protection must be prepared to take the time required to discuss risks, encourage behavioral change, and teach skills.

Table 5-8 Cost of contraceptive methods, based on assumption of 100 acts of intercourse annually

Method	Unit Cost ($)	Annual Cost ($)	Comments
Cervical Cap	20 plus 50-150 for fitting	Cost of spermicide: 85	
Male Condom	0.50	50	Add cost of spermicide if used
Female Condom	2.50	250	Add cost of spermicide if used
Diaphragm	20 plus 50–150 for fitting	Cost of spermicide: 85	
Depo-Provera	35/injection	140	
IUD	120 plus 40–50 for insertion/lab tests	160 for Progestasert; 20 for Cu T 380A if retained 8 years*	
Norplant	350/kit plus 150–250 for insertion/removal	130–170 if retained 5 years*	5-year cost: 650–850
Pill	10–20/cycle	130–260	
Spermicides	0.85/application	85	
Sponge	4/pack of 3	133	

* Norplant and Cu T 380A have considerably higher annual costs if devices are removed prior to expiration; however, Wyeth Laboratories will refund cost of implants if removed before 6 months.

The frequency of intercourse also has bearing on a person's contraceptive choice. For example, the woman who has infrequent intercourse may not wish to use a method that requires daily medication or continuous exposure to possible side effects posed by pills or IUDs. On the other hand, infrequent intercourse may also indicate that a client is at risk of unpredicted intercourse. These clients may need to develop skills in "expecting the unexpected."

Access to medical care. Certain subpopulations in our society have difficulty gaining access to the health care system; they do not understand the system or cannot afford it or find that it shuns them. Others may find their access hampered by too long a wait at the clinic. Studies in other nations have shown that access has great bearing on contraceptive compliance and choice.[46] Presumably, the degree of access can influence women in the United States. Access can be eased for all clients by providing a full year's supply of contraceptives. While many clinicians do provide 13 cycles of pills, for example, most do not offer sufficient quantities of condoms. If access (or motivation) may be a problem, then the client should have access to bags containing 20, 40, or more condoms.

GOALS FOR TEACHING ABOUT PERSONAL CONSIDERATIONS

Key concepts for discussing and teaching about contraceptive choice and personal considerations include these:

1. **The patient decides which personal considerations matter**. Only the potential user can weigh all the elements for personal choice, and the clinician will not be able to predict what matters. Privacy? Lubrication? Light periods? What big sister uses? Do not guess; ask.

2. **It is a long way from the exam room to the bedroom**. We offer methods as medicines in a clinical setting, and then our patients go home and use them in a sexual setting, be it a bedroom, motel room, car seat, or tent. Remember to help your patients think through the sexual aspects of contraception.

3. **Give patients permission to make a second (or third) contraceptive choice**. They may not like the first method at all and will need to know it is okay to come back and try something else. Besides, it is always good to know how to use several methods.

4. **Encourage your patients to talk about birth control issues with their partners**. How can one person decide if a method of birth control will be compatible with a couple's personal and sexual styles? Help your clients practice discussing birth control with their partners if this is new territory for them.

5. **Personal considerations are likely to change over time**. Teenagers and 35-year-olds will use very different criteria as they evaluate their contraceptive choices. Encourage patients to rethink their contraceptive needs as life and sex and bodies change over time.

6. **Teach patients a wise and cautious approach to sexual activity**. All sexually active people need to know the risk factors for STDs and HIV infection. They need to know how to avoid those risk factors.

REFERENCES

1. Atrash HK, Koonin L, Lawson H, Franks A, Smith J. Maternal mortality in the United States, 1979-1986. Obstet Gynecol 1990;76(6):1055-1060.
2. Bracher M, Santow G. Premature discontinuation of contraception in Australia. Fam Plann Perspect 1992;24(2):58-65.
3. Brinton LA, Reeves WC, Brenes MM, Herrero R, de Britton RC, Gaitan E, Tenorio F, Garcia M, Rawls WE. Oral contraceptive use and risk of invasive cervical cancer. Int J Epidemiol 1990;19(1):4-11.
4. CASH. Combination oral contraceptive use and the risk of endometrial cancer. The Cancer and Steroid Hormone Study of the Centers for Disease Control and the National Institute of Child Health and Human Development. JAMA 1987a;257(6):796-800.
5. CASH. Reduction in risk of ovarian cancer associated with oral contraceptive use. The Cancer and Steroid Hormone Study of the Centers for Disease Control and the National Institute of Child Health and Human Development. N Engl J Med 1987b;316(1):650-655.
6. Cates W. Putting the risks in perspective. Contraceptive Technology Update 1980;1(8):111.
7. Cramer DW, Goldman MB, Schiff I, Belisle S, Albreacht B, Stadel B, Gibson M, Wilson E, Stillman R, Thompson I. The relationship of tubal infertility to barrier method and oral contraceptive use. JAMA 1987;257(18):2446-2450.
8. Davis HJ. The shield intrauterine device: a superior modern contraceptive. Am J Obstet Gynecol 1970;106(3):455-456.
9. Dinman BD. The reality and acceptance of risk. JAMA 1980;244(11):1226-1128, and JAMA 1981;246(11):1196-1197.
10. Farr G, Gabelnick H, Sturgen K. The Reality® female condom: efficacy and clinical acceptability of a new barrier contraceptive. Durham NC: Family Health International, 1993.
11. Forrest JD. Timing of reproductive life stages. Obstet Gynecol 1993;82(1):105-110.
12. Gallen M, Lettenmaier C. Counseling makes a difference. Popul Rep 1987;15(3), Series J(35).
13. Grady WR, Hayward MD, Yagi J. Contraceptive failure in the United States: estimates from the 1982 National Survey of Family Growth. Fam Plann Perspect 1986;18(5):200-209.
14. Harlap S, Kost K, Forrest JD. Preventing pregnancy, protecting health: a new look at birth control choices in the United States. New York NY: The Alan Guttmacher Institute, 1991.
15. Jones EF, Forrest JD. Contraceptive failure rates based on the 1988 NSFG. Fam Plann Perspect 1992;24(1):12-19.

16. Kestelman P, Trussell J. Efficacy of the simultaneous use of condoms and spermicides. Fam Plann Perspect 1991;23(5):226-227, 232.
17. Lawson H, Frye A, Atrash HK, Ramick M, Smith J. Legal abortion mortality in the United States: 1972 to 1987. Atlanta GA: Division of Reproductive Health, Centers for Disease Control and Prevention, 1992.
18. Lewis MA. Do contraceptive prices affect demand? Stud Fam Plann 1986;17(3): 126-135.
19. London KA, Mosher WD. What is current use of a contraceptive method? Hyattsville MD: National Center for Health Statistics, 1990.
20. McIntyre SL, Higgins JE. Parity and use-effectiveness with the contraceptive sponge. Am J Obstet Gynecol 1986;155(4):796-801.
21. Menken J, Trussell J, Larsen U. Age and infertility. Science 1986;233(4771):1389-1394.
22. Mintz M. At any cost: corporate greed, women, and the Dalkon shield. New York NY: Pantheon Books, 1985.
23. Mosher WD, Pratt WF. Contraceptive use in the United States, 1973-88. Adv Data 1990; Number 182:1-10.
24. National Center for Health Statistics. Advance report of final mortality statistics, 1984. Mon Vital Stat Rep 1986;35(6):1-44.
25. National Center for Health Statistics. Advance report of final natality statistics, 1989. Mon Vital Stat Rep 1991;40(8-Suppl):1-55.
26. Parazzini F, Negri E, La Vecchia C, Fedele L. Barrier methods of contraception and the risk of cervical neoplasia. Contraception 1989;40(5):519-530.
27. Peterson HB, DeStefano F, Greenspan JR, Ory HW. Mortality risk associated with tubal sterilization in United States hospitals. Am J Obstet Gynecol 1982;143(2): 125-129.
28. Petitti DB. Reconsidering the IUD. Fam Plann Perspect 1992;24(1):33-35.
29. Richardson AC, Lyon JB. The effect of condom use on cervical intraepithelial neoplasia. Am J Obstet Gynecol 1981;140(8):909-913.
30. Richwald GA, Greenland S, Gerber MM, Potik R, Kersey L, Comas MA. Effectiveness of the cavity-rim cervical cap: results of a large clinical study. Obstet Gynecol 1989;74(2):143-148.
31. Rinzler CA. The return of the condom. Am Health 1987;6(6):97-107.
32. Romieu I, Berlin JA, Colditz G. Oral contraceptives and breast cancer: review and meta-analysis. Cancer 1990;66(11):2253-2263.
33. Schirm AL, Trussell J, Menken J, Grady WR. Contraceptive failure in the United States: the impact of social, economic, and demographic factors. Fam Plann Perspect 1982;14(2):68-75.
34. Sivin I, Schmidt F. Effectiveness of IUDs: a review. Contraception 1987;36(1): 55-84.
35. Tietze C, Poliakoff SR, Rock J. The clinical effectiveness of the rhythm method of contraception. Fertil Steril 1951;2(5):444-450.
36. Trussell J. Methodological pitfalls in the analysis of contraceptive failure. Stat Med 1991;10(2):201-220.
37. Trussell J, Faden R, Hatcher RA. Efficacy information in contraceptive counseling: those little white lies. Am J Public Health 1976;66(8):761-767.
38. Trussell J, Grummer-Strawn L. Contraceptive failure of the ovulation method of periodic abstinence. Fam Plann Perspect 1990;22(2):65-75.

39. Trussell J, Hatcher RA, Cates W, Stewart FH, Kost K. A guide to interpreting contraceptive efficacy studies. Obstet Gynecol 1990(a);76(3):558-567.

40. Trussell J, Hatcher RA, Cates W, Stewart FH, Kost K. Contraceptive failure in the United States: an update. Stud Fam Plann 1990(b);21(1):51-54.

41. Trussell J, Kost K. Contraceptive failure in the United States: a critical review of the literature. Stud Fam Plann 1987;18(5):237-283.

42. Trussell J, Strickler J, Vaughan B. Contraceptive efficacy of the diaphragm, sponge and cervical cap. Fam Plann Perspect 1993;25(3):100-105, 135.

43. Trussell J, Vaughan B. Aggregate and lifetime contraceptive failure in the United States. Fam Plann Perspect 1989;21(5):224-226.

44. Trussell J, Vaughan B. Selected results concerning sexual behavior and contraceptive use from the 1988 National Survey of Family Growth and the 1988 National Survey of Adolescent Males. Working Paper #91-12. Princeton NJ: Office of Population Research, Princeton University, 1991.

45. Trussell J, Westoff CF. Contraceptive practice and trends in coital frequency. Fam Plann Perspect 1980;12(5):246-249.

46. Tsui AO, Ochoa LH. Service proximity as a determinant of contraceptive behaviour: evidence from cross-national studies of survey data. In: Philips JF, Ross JA (eds). Family planning programmes and fertility. Oxford, England: Clarendon Press, 1992:222-256.

47. Vaughan B, Trussell J, Menken J, Jones EF. Contraceptive failure among married women in the United States, 1970-1973. Fam Plann Perspect 1977;9(6):251-258.

48. Vaughan B, Trussell J, Menken J, Jones EF, Grady W. Contraceptive efficacy among married women aged 15-44 years, United States. Vital Health Stat 1980;Series 23(5):1-62.

49. Vessey M, Lawless M, Yeates D. Efficacy of different contraceptive methods. Lancet 1982;1(8276):841-842.

50. Vessey MP, Villard-Mackintosh L, McPherson K, Yeates D. Mortality among oral contraceptive users: 20 year follow up of women in a cohort study. BMJ 1989;299:1487-1491.

51. Washington AE, Gove S, Schachter J, Sweet RL. Oral contraceptives, Chlamydia trachomatis infection and pelvic inflammatory disease: a word of caution about protection. JAMA 1985;253(15):2246-2250.

Abstinence and the Range of Sexual Expression

- Abstinence can be primary or secondary. Primary abstainers have not had a sexual experience with another person. Secondary abstainers are sexually experienced persons who have chosen to avoid some or all sexual activity with another person.

- Many abstainers choose to avoid intercourse but engage in other forms of sexual intimacy.

- Secondary abstinence, or celibacy, is the choice of many sexually experienced adolescents and adults. It is not an extremist position in the age of viral STDs.

- The care provider's role is to support the choice of abstinence and to teach negotiation and planning skills for using abstinence effectively and safely.

Abstinence, here defined as refraining from vaginal or anal insertive sex, is a common practice in the United States and in other areas of the world. Historically, sexual abstinence has probably been the single most important factor in curtailing human fertility.[1] Until age 17, abstainers in the United States outnumber persons who have had intercourse (see Chapter 2 on Adolescent Pregnancy).[3]

U.S. surveys from the late 1980s show that 12.4% of unmarried men and 13.2% of unmarried women aged 25-34 had no sex partners in the past 12 months; among married people, 4.5% of men and 3.5% of women aged 35-59 had no active sex partners in the past year.[5] Another study found that 13% of 30- to 34-year-old single white women in the U.S. have never had a sexual partner.[4]

People of all ages deliberately choose to abstain. It is important for family planning professionals to welcome abstinence as normal, common, and acceptable. It is also crucial to separate persons whose abstinence is freely and happily chosen from those whose chastity is dysfunctional or forced upon them. The latter may require help; the former deserve respect, encouragement, and support. All abstemious persons should be offered education about the other methods of birth control and safer sex available to them, including:

- Effective over-the-counter products
- Sources for prescription methods
- Postcoital options
- STD protection skills

THE RANGE OF SEXUAL EXPRESSION

Although abstinence has become associated with saying "no," viewed from another perspective, abstinence can mean saying "yes" to a number of other sexual activities. All human beings need touching—for nurture, for solace, for communication, for simple affection. Most human beings enjoy erotic touching as well, a specialized language of sexual gratification and more intimate forms of affection. Penis-in-vagina intercourse belongs somewhere along this touch continuum because it propagates the species and because many people find it immensely pleasurable.

For some people, erotic touching equals insertive intercourse, nothing more or less. Most people, however, have a more expansive view of sexual expression, and other activities give them pleasure and meaning. Holding hands, kissing, massage, solo masturbation, mutual masturbation, dancing, oral-genital sex, fantasy, and erotic books and movies all fit along the sexual continuum, as do many other activities. Taste, smell, vision, and hearing may matter as much as touch for erotic power.

INDICATIONS FOR ABSTINENCE OR OTHER FORMS OF SEXUAL EXPRESSION

When the only goal of abstinence is to avoid unwanted pregnancy, then all forms of sexual expression are available to a couple except for penis-in-vagina intercourse. When a goal of abstinence is to avoid STDs, then oral-genital sex, anal-genital sex, and other practices that expose the partner to pre-ejaculatory fluid, semen, cervical-vaginal secretions, or blood must be reconsidered. Some couples avoid these practices altogether, and others employ condoms, latex dams, or other barriers to inhibit body fluid transmission during these practices. The care provider's role is to offer factual, explicit guidance on safer-sex options (see Chapter 3 on HIV Infection).

Consider discussing abstinence even with adolescents who have experimented with intercourse and other sexual behaviors. Once young men and women have satisfied their initial curiosity about intercourse, and once they feel socially comfortable with their level of sexual sophistication, they may be willing to become experienced abstainers, removing themselves at least for a while from the health risks of intimate sex. Family planning care providers can help young people learn that the door between abstinence and sexual activity opens in both directions.

For times when vaginal or anal intercourse may be unwise from a medical standpoint for one or both partners, other forms of erotic touching may make more sense. Some situations where insertive sex may be advised against and where alternatives may be recommended include:

- Known or suspected sexually transmitted disease (also avoid other sexual practices that transmit pre-ejaculatory fluid, semen, cervical-vaginal secretions, and blood)
- Post-operative pain or tenderness, such as from episiotomy, hemorrhoidectomy, vasectomy, and other procedures
- Pelvic, vaginal, or urinary tract infection
- Gastrointestinal illness or infection
- Dyspareunia or other pelvic pain
- Undiagnosed postcoital bleeding
- Untreated postmenopausal atrophic vaginitis
- Late third trimester of pregnancy, postpartum, or postabortion
- Postmyocardial infarction
- Certain disabling physical conditions
- Known or suspected allergic sensitization to partner's semen
- Therapy for a variety of sexual problems may include exploration of avenues of sexual gratification other than intercourse. Temporarily forbidding intercourse takes performance pressure off couples struggling with erection difficulty, orgasm difficulty, or rapid ejaculation.

INSTRUCTIONS FOR USING ABSTINENCE

1. **Decide what you want to do about sex** at a time when you feel clearheaded, sober, and good about yourself. If you have a partner, decide together at a time when you feel close to each other but not sexual. For example, try talking while you take a walk and hold hands.
2. **Decide in advance** what sexual activities you will say "yes" to and discuss these with your partner.
3. **Tell your partner,** very clearly and in advance—not at the last minute—what activities you will not do.

4. **Avoid high-pressure sexual situations,** stay sober, and stay out of the empty house, or the back seat.

5. **If you say "no"** say it so it is clear that you mean it. Here are a few techniques for saying "no":[2]

Technique	Example
Simple "no"	"No, thanks." or "No."
Emphatic "no"	"No! I don't want to do that!"
Repetitive "no"	"No." "No." "No."
Turn the tables	"You say that if I love you I would. But if you really loved me, you wouldn't insist."
Give a reason	"I'm not ready." "We can't be too careful in this age of AIDS." "I have decided to abstain for a while."
Leave the scene	Walk out of there.
Steer clear	If you suspect you will be pressured, don't go out with the person.
Call in the cavalry	Threaten to tell someone with authority or power (counselors, relative, police, etc.)
Safety in numbers	Double date; keep trusted friends nearby.

6. **Learn more about your body** and how to keep it healthy. Appreciate the marvel of your body.

7. **Learn about birth control and safer sex,** so you will be ready if you change your mind. Always keep condoms around. Always.

8. **Learn about emergency birth control options** in case you have intercourse when you didn't expect it.

Emergency Contraceptive Pills: Treatment initiated within 72 hours of unprotected intercourse reduces the risk of pregnancy from unprotected intercourse by at least 75%. (See Chapter 16.)

REFERENCES

1. Hajnal J. European marriage patterns in perspective. In: Glass DV, Eversley DEC, (eds). Population in history: essays in historical demography. London: Aldine, 1986:101.
2. Grossman L, Kowal D. Kids, drugs, and sex. Preventing trouble. Brandon, VT: Clinical Psychology Publishing Co., 1987.
3. Jones EF, Forrest JD, Goldman N, Henshaw SK, Lincoln R, Rossoff JI, Westoff CF, Wulf D. Teenage pregnancy in developed countries: determinants and policy implications. Fam Plann Perspect 1985; 17(2): 53-63.

4. Trussell J, Vaughan B. Selected results concerning sexual behavior and contraceptive use from the 1988 National Survey of Family Growth and the 1988 National Survey of Adolescent Males. Princeton NJ: Princeton University, Office of Population Research, Working Paper #91-12, 1991.
5. Turner CF, Miller HG, Moses LE. AIDS: sexual behavior and intravenous drug use. Washington DC: National Academy Press, 1989.

Condoms

- Unlike other, more effective nonbarrier contraceptives, condoms, if used consistently and correctly, prevent both unintended pregnancy and sexually transmitted infection.
- When used consistently and correctly, condoms are the most effective method for preventing HIV infection.
- Condoms can be used with other contraceptives when STDs are a concern. Other more effective contraceptives—sterilization, oral contraceptives, Norplant implants, Depo-Provera, and intrauterine devices—do not prevent HIV infection or other STDs.

- Except for coitus interruptus, condoms are the only readily reversible method of birth control for men.
- Condoms rarely break during vaginal intercourse. Further, not every broken condom results in pregnancy or infection.
- The provision of condoms in large numbers at a low or at no cost and the promotion of positive images of condoms need to become major public health priorities.

The condom is one of the most popular contraceptive methods used in the United States. According to the 1988 National Survey of Family Growth, an estimated 5.1 million women (13.2% of women at risk for unintended pregnancy) reported using condoms as a contraceptive method (see Table 5-1 on page 109). Moreover, an additional 4.2 million women reported using condoms exclusively for protection from sexually transmitted infections.[30] From 1982-1988, a trend toward increasing use of condoms was observed among 15- to 29-year-old women at risk for pregnancy (see Chapter 5). From 1987 to 1989, condom sales in the United States rose more than 60%,[8] then increased only a few percentage points per year.[29]

For centuries, mechanical barriers covering the penis have been used for protection against pregnancy and infection, for decoration, and occasionally to produce penile or vaginal stimulation.[20] A sheath worn over the penis can be traced as far back as 1350 B.C., when Egyptian men wore decorative covers for their penises. In 1564 A.D., the great Italian anatomist Fallopius described the use of linen sheaths. Protective sheaths from animal intestines soon followed. It was not until the 18th century that penile sheaths made from animal intestines were given the name "condom" and popularized as a means of "protection from venereal disease and numerous bastard offspring."[4] With the advent of vulcanized rubber in the 1840s came the mass production of condoms (or "rubbers") from synthetic materials.

M ECHANISM OF ACTION

Placed over the erect penis, a condom acts as a mechanical barrier, preventing direct contact with semen, genital lesions and discharges, or infectious secretions. Most U.S. condoms available today are manufactured from latex (*i.e.,* "latex" or "rubber" condoms) while a small proportion (about 5%) are made of processed collagenous tissue from the intestinal caecum of lambs (*i.e.,* "skin" or "natural membrane" condoms).[8]

Both synthetic condoms and skin condoms prevent pregnancy by blocking the passage of sperm through their surfaces. Skin condoms are not recommended for protection against sexually transmitted diseases, however. The surface of the skin condom (unlike the synthetic condom) contains small pores that have been shown in laboratory tests to permit the passage of viruses including hepatitis B virus, herpes simplex virus, and HIV.[5]

An extended feature found in some prelubricated latex and skin condoms is the presence of a small volume of spermicide applied to the inside and/or outside of the condom. Spermicide is a surfactant that has been found to actively kill sperm. The main spermicide used in the United States is nonoxynol-9. (See Chapter 8 for further discussion on spermicides.) It is unknown whether the spermicidal condom is more effective in actual use than a regular lubricated condom.

CONDOM OPTIONS

Consumers can choose from a wide selection of condoms in the United States. The brand names and attributes of condoms currently available in the U.S. are presented in Table 7-1. The more than 100 brands of condoms (including four brands of skin condoms) represent different sizes, shapes, thicknesses, presence or absence of lubricants or spermicides, and presence

Table 7-1 A consumer's guide to condoms

Brand (Manufacturer)	Reservoir End	Lubri-cated	Sperm-icide	Pre-Shaped	Width (in.)	Length (in.)	Thickness (mm)	Color
Latex Condoms								
Beyond Seven (Okamoto, USA)	Y	Y	N	N	2.05	7.9	0.048	Blue
Beyond Seven Plus (Okamoto, USA)	Y	Y	Y	N	2.05	7.9	0.048	Blue
Birds 'N Bees (RFSU of Sweden)	Y	Y	N	Y	2.05	7.3	0.045–0.065	Green
Blue Circle Coin (Safetex)	Y	N	N	Y	2.05	7.2	0.069	Blue
Crown (Okamoto, USA)	Y	Y	N	N	2.09	7.9	0.048	Pink
Embrace (Safetex)	Y	Y	N	Y	2.05	7.2	0.069	Pink
Excita Extra (Schmid)	Y	Y	Y	N	2.05	7.5	0.07	Transparent
Excita Fiesta (Schmid)	Y	Y	N	N	2.05	7.5	0.07	Assorted
Gold Circle (Safetex)	Y	N	N	N	2.05	7.2	0.069	Transparent
Gold Circle Coin (Safetex)	Y	N	N	N	2.05	7.2	0.069	Transparent
Green Circle Coin (Safetex)	Y	N	N	Y	2.05	7.2	0.069	Green
Kilroy (RFSU of Sweden)	Y	Y	Y	Y	2.06	7.3	0.055–0.075	Transparent
Kimono (Mayer Labs)	Y	Y	N	Y	2.13	8.0	0.06	Transparent
Kimono PLUS (Mayer Labs)	Y	Y	Y	Y	2.13	8.0	0.06	Transparent
Kimono Microthin (Mayer Labs)	Y	Y	N	Y	2.13	8.0	0.05	Transparent
Kimono Microthin Plus (Mayer Labs)	Y	Y	Y	Y	2.13	8.0	0.05	Transparent
Kiss of Mint (Ansell)	Y	N	N	Y	2.05	7.0	0.03–0.09	Neutral
Lady Protex Lubricated (Schmid)	Y	Y	N	N	2.05	7.5	0.07	Neutral
Lady Protex Spermicidal (Schmid)	Y	Y	Y	N	2.05	7.5	0.07	Neutral
Lifestyles Assorted Colors (Ansell)	Y	Y	N	Y	2.05	7.0	0.03–0.09	Assorted

(continued)

Table 7-1 A consumer's guide to condoms *(cont.)*

Brand (Manufacturer)	Reservoir End	Lubri-cated	Sperm-icide	Pre-Shaped	Width (in.)	Length (in.)	Thickness (mm)	Color
Latex Condoms (Continued)								
Lifestyles Assorted Colors With Nonoxynol-9 (Ansell)	Y	Y	Y	Y	2.05	7.0	0.03–0.09	Assorted
Lifestyles Extra Strength (Ansell)	Y	Y	N	N	2.05	7.0	0.03–0.09	Neutral
Lifestyles Extra Strength With Nonoxynol-9 (Ansell)	Y	Y	Y	N	2.05	7.0	0.03–0.09	Neutral
Lifestyles Lubricated (Ansell)	Y	Y	N	Y	2.05	7.0	0.03–0.09	Neutral
Lifestyles Non-Lubricated (Ansell)	Y	N	N	Y	2.05	7.0	0.03–0.09	Neutral
Lifestyles Ribbed (Ansell)	Y	Y	N	Y	2.05	7.0	0.03–0.09	Neutral
Lifestyles Snugger Fit (Ansell)	Y	Y	N	Y	1.93	6.3	0.03–0.09	Neutral
Lifestyles Spermicidally Lubricated (Ansell)	Y	Y	Y	Y	2.05	7.0	0.03–0.09	Neutral
Lifestyles Tuxedo (Ansell)	Y	Y	N	Y	2.05	7.0	0.03–0.09	Black
Lifestyles Ultra Thin (Ansell)	Y	Y	N	Y	2.05	7.0	0.03–0.09	Neutral
Magnum (Carter-Wallace)	Y	Y	N	N	2.3	7.5	NA	Transparent
Magnum With Spermicidal Lubricant (Carter-Wallace)	Y	Y	N	N	2.3	7.5	NA	Transparent
Mamba (RFSU of Sweden)	Y	Y	N	Y	2.03	6.9	0.05–0.07	Yellow
MAXX (Mayer Labs)	Y	Y	N	Y	2.34	8.25	0.06	Transparent
MAXX Plus (Mayer Labs)	Y	Y	Y	Y	2.34	8.25	0.06	Transparent
Mentor (Carter-Wallace)	Y	Y	N	N	2.0	7.0	NA	Transparent
Mentor Plus (Carter-Wallace)	Y	Y	Y	N	2.0	7.0	NA	Transparent
Okeido (RFSU of Sweden)	Y	Y	N	N	2.13	7.6	0.05–0.06	Transparent

(continued)

Table 7-1 A consumer's guide to condoms *(cont.)*

Brand (Manufacturer)	Reservoir End	Lubri-cated	Sperm-icide	Pre-Shaped	Width (in.)	Length (in.)	Thickness (mm)	Color
Latex Condoms (Continued)								
Pleasure Plus (Reddy Health Care)	Y	Y	N	Y	2.0	7.3	0.08	Transparent
Prime Assorted Colors (Ansell)	Y	Y	N	Y	2.05	7.0	0.03–0.09	Neutral
Prime Lubricated (Ansell)	Y	Y	N	N	2.05	7.0	0.03–0.09	Neutral
Prime Non-Lubricated (Ansell)	Y	N	N	N	2.0	7.5	0.03–0.09	Neutral
Prime Snugger Fit (Ansell)	Y	Y	N	Y	1.93	7.0	0.03–0.09	Neutral
Prime Spermicidally Lubricated (Ansell)	Y	Y	Y	Y	2.05	7.0	0.03–0.09	Neutral
Prime Ultra Thin (Ansell)	Y	Y	N	N	2.05	7.0	0.03–0.07	Neutral
Prime Textured (Ansell)	Y	Y	N	N	2.05	7.0	0.07–0.09	Neutral
Profil (RFSU of Sweden)	Y	Y	N	Y	2.05	7.3	0.055–0.075	Transparent
Rainbow (Safetex)	Y	Y	N	Y	2.05	7.2	0.069	Assorted
Ramses Extra (Schmid)	Y	Y	Y	N	2.05	7.5	0.07	Transparent
Ramses Extra Ribbed (Schmid)	Y	Y	Y	N	2.05	7.5	0.07	Transparent
Ramses Extra Strength (Schmid)	Y	Y	Y	N	2.05	7.5	0.10	Neutral
Ramses Non-Lubricated Mint Scented (Schmid)	Y	N	N	N	2.05	7.5	0.07	Neutral
Ramses Safe Play Lubricated (Schmid)	Y	Y	N	N	2.05	7.5	0.07	Neutral
Ramses Safe Play Spermicidal (Schmid)	Y	Y	Y	N	2.05	7.5	0.07	Neutral
Ramses Sensitol (Schmid)	Y	Y	N	N	2.05	7.5	0.07	Transparent
Ramses Ultra Thin Lubricated (Schmid)	Y	Y	N	N	2.05	7.5	0.04	Neutral
Ramses Ultra Thin Spermicidal (Schmid)	Y	Y	Y	N	2.05	7.5	0.04	Neutral

(continued)

Table 7-1 A consumer's guide to condoms *(cont.)*

Brand (Manufacturer)	Reservoir End	Lubri- cated	Sperm- icide	Pre- Shaped	Width (in.)	Length (in.)	Thickness (mm)	Color
Latex Condoms (Continued)								
Red Circle Coin (Safetex)	Y	N	N	Y	2.05	7.2	0.069	Red
Rough-Rider (Ansell)	Y	Y	N	Y	2.05	7.0	0.10–0.17	Neutral
Saxon (Safetex)	Y	Y	N	Y	2.05	7.2	0.069	Transparent
Saxon Spermicidal (Safetex)	Y	Y	Y	N	2.05	7.2	0.069	Transparent
Saxon Ultra Thin (Safetex)	Y	Y	N	Y	2.05	7.2	0.069	Transparent
Saxon Wet Lube (Safetex)	Y	Y	N	N	2.05	7.2	0.069	Transparent
Saxon Gold Ultra Lube (Safetex)	Y	Y	N	N	2.05	7.2	0.069	Transparent
Saxon Gold Ultra Ribbed (Safetex)	Y	Y	N	Y	2.05	7.2	0.069	Transparent
Saxon Gold Ultra Sensitive (Safetex)	Y	Y	N	Y	2.05	7.2	0.069	Transparent
Saxon Gold Ultra Spermicidal (Safetex)	Y	Y	Y	N	2.05	7.2	0.069	Transparent
Sheik Elite Non-Lubricated Mint Scented (Schmid)	Y	N	N	N	2.05	7.5	0.07	Neutral
Sheik Elite Ribbed (Schmid)	Y	Y	Y	N	2.05	7.5	0.07	Transparent
Sheik Elite Sensi-Creme (Schmid)	Y	Y	N	N	2.05	7.5	0.07	Transparent
Sheik Elite Spermicidal (Schmid)	Y	Y	Y	N	2.05	7.5	0.07	Neutral
Sheik Super Thin Lubricated (Schmid)	Y	Y	N	N	2.05	7.5	0.04	Neutral
Sheik Super Thin Spermicidal (Schmid)	Y	Y	Y	N	2.05	7.5	0.04	Neutral
Touch From Protex Lubricated (Schmid)	Y	Y	N	N	2.05	7.5	0.07	Transparent

(continued)

Table 7-1 A consumer's guide to condoms *(cont.)*

Brand (Manufacturer)	Reservoir End	Lubri- cated	Sperm- icide	Pre- Shaped	Width (in.)	Length (in.)	Thickness (mm)	Color
Latex Condoms (Continued)								
Touch From Protex Ribbed (Schmid)	Y	Y	N	N	2.05	7.5	0.07	Transparent
Touch From Protex Sunrise Colors (Schmid)	Y	Y	N	N	2.05	7.5	0.07	Assorted
Touch From Protex Thins (Schmid)	Y	Y	N	N	2.05	7.5	0.04	Neutral
Touch From Protex Non-Lubricated (Schmid)	Y	N	N	N	2.05	7.5	0.07	Transparent
Touch From Protex Spermicidal (Schmid)	Y	Y	Y	N	2.05	7.5	0.07	Neutral
Trojan Assortment (Carter-Wallace)	Y	Y	N	Y	2.0	7.0	NA	Gold
Trojan Assortment With Spermicidal Lubricant (Carter-Wallace)	Y	Y	Y	Y	2.0	7.0	NA	Neutral
Trojan-Enz (Carter-Wallace)	Y	N	N	N	2.0	7.0	0.06	Neutral
Trojan-Enz Lube (Carter-Wallace)	Y	Y	N	N	2.0	7.0	0.06	Neutral
Trojan-Enz With Spermicidal Lubricant (Carter-Wallace)	Y	Y	Y	N	2.0	7.0	0.06	Neutral
Trojan-Enz Large Lubricated (Carter-Wallace)	Y	Y	Y	N	2.3	7.5	0.06	Neutral
Trojan-Enz Large Spermicidal Lubricant (Carter-Wallace)	Y	Y	Y	N	2.3	7.5	0.06	Neutral
Trojan Extra Strength Lubricated (Carter-Wallace)	Y	Y	N	N	2.0	7.0	0.06	Gold
Trojan Extra Strength With Spermicidal Lubricant (Carter-Wallace)	Y	Y	Y	N	2.0	7.0	0.06	Gold
Trojan Naturalube (Carter-Wallace)	Y	Y	N	N	2.0	7.0	0.06	Neutral
Trojan Plus (Carter-Wallace)	Y	Y	N	Y	2.0	7.0	0.06	Gold
Trojan Plus2 (Carter-Wallace)	Y	Y	Y	Y	2.0	7.0	0.06	Gold

(continued)

Table 7-1 A consumer's guide to condoms *(cont.)*

Brand (Manufacturer)	Reservoir End	Lubri-cated	Sperm-icide	Pre-Shaped	Width (in.)	Length (in.)	Thickness (mm)	Color
Latex Condoms (Continued)								
Trojan Regulars (Carter-Wallace)	N	N	N	N	2.0	7.0	0.06	Neutral
Trojan Ribbed (Carter-Wallace)	Y	Y	N	N	2.0	7.0	0.06	Gold
Trojan Ribbed With Spermicidal Lubricant (Carter-Wallace)	Y	Y	Y	N	2.0	7.0	0.06	Gold
Trojan Very Sensitive Lubricated (Carter-Wallace)	Y	Y	N	Y	2.5	7.9	0.08	Transparent
Trojan Very Sensitive With Spermicidal Lubricant (Carter-Wallace)	Y	Y	Y	Y	2.5	7.9	0.08	Transparent
Trojan Very Thin Lubricated (Carter-Wallace)	Y	Y	N	N	2.0	7.0	0.05	NA
Trojan Very Thin Spermicidal (Carter-Wallace)	Y	Y	Y	N	2.0	7.0	0.05	NA
Yellow Circle Coin (Safetex)	Y	N	N	Y	2.05	7.0	0.069	Yellow
Natural Membrane Condoms								
Fourex (Schmid)	N	Y	N	N	2.05	7.0	0.07	Neutral
Fourex Spermicidal (Schmid)	N	Y	Y	N	2.05	7.0	0.07	Neutral
Naturalamb (Carter-Wallace)	Y	Y	N	N	2.0	7.0	0.08	Neutral
Naturalamb With Spermicidal Lubricant (Carter-Wallace)	N	Y	Y	N	2.0	7.0	0.08	Neutral

Source: U.S. condom manufacturers.

Note: The lengths of Ansell and Carter-Wallace condoms do not include the 0.5-in. reservoir end.

or absence of reservoir-tip or nipple-ends. Condoms can be straight-sided or tapered toward the closed end, textured (*e.g.*, ribbed) or smooth, colored or nearly translucent, and odorless or scented. Lubricated condoms are coated on both the inner and outer surfaces with silicone, wet jellies, or spermicides. Unlubricated (*i.e.*, dry) or scented condoms present a good option for oral intercourse. Most condoms are about 170 mm

(7 in.) long, 50 mm (2 in.) wide, and 0.03 mm–0.10 mm (0.001 in. -0.004 in.) thick.

As the public's awareness of AIDS and other STDs has grown, condom manufacturers have continued to improve the condom to make it more appealing and more effective. Several innovations in condoms are currently being researched. The development of the female condom (intravaginal pouch) represents the most dramatic change in condom design. As implied by its name, the female condom is worn by the woman during intercourse. Three types of female condoms undergoing clinical testing for FDA approval[19,49] are further discussed in Chapter 9.

Enhancement of Acceptability

Other changes in condom design have been implemented to increase acceptability. For example, a special applicator "hood" and inner ring of adhesive are featured in the Mentor condom (Carter-Wallace) to reduce the incidence of slippage and breakage, although the condom is considerably more expensive than most.[8] The Pleasure Plus condom (Reddy Health Care) has a bulbous pouch near the condom's tip that provides a looser fit on the distal shaft and glans of the penis.[43] Both of these condoms are currently available on the U.S. market. The Spiral Scientific condom (Thornton International) contains a series of curved helix ribs to increase sensitivity and may be available later this year.[40]

Latex-Sensitivity

Two other condoms undergoing extensive testing will provide an alternative for persons allergic to latex products and for whom latex condoms are contraindicated.[31] (See section on latex allergy under Disadvantages and Cautions.) Given that natural membrane condoms have been found to permit viral passage, no viable option exists for STD or HIV prevention among latex-sensitive persons until other non-latex condoms are FDA-approved.

The first non-latex condom, the Tactylon condom (Tactyl Technologies), is a latex-free (NRL) natural rubber, non-allergenic product. Tactylon material is a synthetic thermoplastic elastomer that is manufactured from the same material used in the company's FDA-approved non-allergenic examination gloves.[32] A comparative clinical study of U.S. couples found no overall differences in the breakage rates and levels of user preference between the Tactylon condom and a leading condom on the market.[42] The Tactylon condom is expected to be available in the United States within the next year.[16] The second latex-free condom is the polyurethane condom (Family Health International), made of a thin, flexible transparent plastic. This condom is anticipated to be available within the next few years.[50] Both non-latex condoms will offer latex-sensitive users protection from pregnancy and sexually transmitted infections, including HIV.

EFFECTIVENESS

Condoms can be very effective at preventing unintended pregnancy when used consistently *and* correctly. Method failure of the condom is relatively uncommon. The estimate of the failure rate for the first year of use among perfect users of condoms (*i.e.*, those who use condoms consistently and correctly) is about 3% (see Table 7-2). The proper interpretation of the condom's failure rate is key to one's decision to use condoms as a method of birth control. The 3% perfect user failure rate does *not* indicate that three of every 100 condoms used will lead to unintended pregnancy. The rate is based on computations using couples, rather than condoms, as the measured denominator. Thus, the 3% failure rate means that of 100 couples who use condoms perfectly for 1 year, only three couples will experience an accidental pregnancy. If each of the 100 couples had intercourse an average of twice per week, then the 100 couples would have had sexual intercourse 10,400 times over the course of a year. Three pregnancies resulting from 10,400 acts of condom use during sexual intercourse is a remarkably low pregnancy rate (0.03%) *when calculated on a per-condom basis.* A summary of individual studies of condom failure rates is presented in Table 27-9 on page 671.

Table 7-2 First-year failure rates* for couples using condoms, withdrawal, diaphragm, and pill

Method (1)	% of Women Experiencing an Accidental Pregnancy Within the First Year of Use		% of Women Continuing Use at One Year (4)
	Typical Use (2)	Perfect Use (3)	
Withdrawal	19	4	
Diaphragm Without Spermicide	18	6	58
Condom			
Male	12	3	63
Female (Reality)	21	5	56
Pill	3		72
Progestin Only		0.5	
Combined		0.1	

* See Table 5-2 for first-year failure rates of all methods.

Emergency Contraceptive Pills: Treatment initiated within 72 hours after unprotected intercourse reduces the risk of pregnancy by at least 75%.

Unlike male and female sterilization, Norplant, and Depo-Provera, condoms and other barrier methods tend to be used inconsistently and incorrectly. The first-year failure rate among typical users of condoms averages about 12% and includes pregnancies resulting from errors in condom use. This is lower than the rates for typical users of other barrier methods (range: 18%-36%) but higher than the typical user failure rates associated with sterilization and hormonal methods (range: 0.09%-3.0%). Thus, the condom provides only moderately effective protection against accidental pregnancy for the *typical user*. The difference in condom failure rates between typical and perfect users results from misuse and nonuse, although nonuse probably accounts for the majority of this variation.

CONCOMITANT USE WITH A SECOND METHOD

When used consistently and correctly, condoms alone offer excellent protection from pregnancy and infection. When condoms are used concurrently with another contraceptive method (and both methods are used consistently and correctly), the couple is provided additional protection against pregnancy and possible increased protection against infection, depending on the other method used. Many couples can be encouraged to use condoms in addition to another method of birth control. The 1991 Ortho Survey of 7,805 women aged 15-50 found that condoms were used as a concomitant method of birth control by 54% of women using foam, 52% of women using the sponge, 42% of women using the diaphragm, 21% of women using oral contraceptives, 6% of women using spermicidal vaginal suppositories, 5% of couples with male or female sterilization, and 9% of women using other methods.[34]

The concomitant use of condoms and spermicides enhances effectiveness. A recent mathematical modeling of the effectiveness of simultaneous use of condoms and separately applied vaginal spermicides concluded that the annual probability of contraceptive failure for couples during perfect use of both condom and intravaginally applied spermicide was 0.1% (see Chapter 5), the same as that associated with perfect use of the combined pill.[24]

If spermicide use is desired as a backup method to the condom for pregnancy prevention, use of an intravaginally applied spermicide is recommended,[7] not spermicide applied to the surface of the condom or use of a commercially sold spermicidal condom. Unlike spermicidal condoms, use of *intravaginally applied spermicide* guarantees its presence in the vaginal region in the unlikely case of condom breakage or leakage. Although laboratory studies have shown sperm to become quickly inactivated when injected into spermicidally lubricated condoms,[9] the dose of active ingredient delivered by a spermicidally lubricated condom is much less than that provided by a separate vaginal spermicide (*e.g.*, vaginal cream, foam, or suppository). Despite their increased cost, spermicidally lubricated condoms are unlikely to be more effective than regular condoms in the prevention of STDs or pregnancy. One study found the concentration of active ingredient in spermicidal condoms insufficient to minimize the risk of HIV transmission. In that study, nearly 50% of the concentration of the spermicide in the lubricant leached into the condom.[41]

CONDOM BREAKAGE

In addition to condom failure rates, rates of condom breakage and condom slippage deserve attention. Two studies evaluating the frequency of condom breakage and slippage demonstrated the effectiveness of the condom to remain intact throughout intercourse. Most condoms (94%-98%) were found neither to break nor to fall completely off the penis during intercourse.[27,42]

Vaginal Intercourse

Not every condom break leads to pregnancy or infection. One U.S. survey of family planning patients, reproductive health employees, and university students found only 1 pregnancy reported for every 23 condom breaks.[18] Table 7-3 presents results of prospective studies of condom breakage for vaginal intercourse in developed countries. Most studies indicate rates of breakage of less than 1 or 2 condoms per 100 condoms used, some of which can be attributed to condom misuse. Some users have tested condoms for holes by filling them with air or water.[12,43] Other men have been found to unroll the condom before use and then slide it on like a sock.[12] All of these events can increase the probability of breakage.

Perhaps the most common user error is the use of oil-based lubricants (*e.g.*, mineral oil) with condoms, which, unlike water-based lubricants, have been shown to reduce condom integrity[48] and may increase the likelihood of breakage. The confusion with proper lubricant use lies in the definitions of "oil-based" and "water-based." Oil-based products such as Vaseline petroleum jelly, Johnson's Baby Oil, and Vaseline Intensive Care and Nivea hand lotions have been viewed in some studies as acceptable lubricants for use because they readily wash off with water.[43,46] Many products that wash off with water actually contain oil as a major ingredient. Table 7-4 lists lubricants that are safe and unsafe to use with condoms. When prescribing any product as a condom lubricant, particularly vaginal medications, abstinence or the use of another contraceptive in addition to a condom should be recommended.

Not all condom breaks pose equal risks. Both the timing and the location of the break are important in the estimation of actual risk. Breakage occurring during removal of the condom from the package or during placement on the penis is much less likely to result in pregnancy than breakage occurring during intercourse or withdrawal. In two U.S. studies, 0.7% and 2.4% of condoms, respectively, were reported to have broken before the initiation of intercourse, which presumably would not increase the risk of pregnancy.[42,43]

Table 7-3 Prospective studies of condom breakage during vaginal intercourse – developed countries: a review of the literature

Reference*	Description	Total Subjects	Total Condoms Used	% Users Reporting Break	% Condoms Broken
Free et al., 1980	Planned Parenthood, U.S.	6	36	0	0.0
Leeper & Conrardy, 1989	4-month study of female prostitutes in brothel, Sydney	4	605		0.5
Richters et al., 1988	Clinical research testing laboratory, U.S.	49	147		0.7
Trussell et al., 1992(a)	21-day study of self-selected women recruited to family planning clinic	49	241	10	1.2 (Tactylon)
	10 unlubricated reservoir-tipped condoms each (5 per brand), U.S.		237		1.3 (Trojan-Enz)
Trussell et al., 1992(b)	16-day study of self-selected women recruited to family planning clinic	68	203	10	1.5 (Pleasure Plus)
	6 lubricated reservoir-tipped condoms each (3 per brand), U.S.		202		2.0 (Trojan-Enz)
Gotzsche & Harding, 1988	Female prostitutes and hospital staff of both sexes, 10 condoms per participant randomized to one of two brands, Denmark	40	385	18	5.0
Russell-Brown et al., 1992	Six-week study of locally recruited men, 8 silicone-lubricated reservoir-tipped condoms each, U.S.	45	358	36	6.7
Totals		**261**	**2,414**	**0%–36%**	**0.0%–6.7%**

Source: Family Health International (1992).

*Full reference listed in original article by FHI.

Table 7-4 Lubricants and products that are safe or unsafe to use with condoms

Safe	Unsafe
Aloe-9	Baby Oils
Aqua-Lube	Burn Ointments
Aqua-Lube Plus (Spermicidal)	Coconut Oil/Butter
Astroglide	Edible Oils
Carbowax	(e.g., Olive, Peanut, Corn, Sunflower)
Condom-Mate	Fish Oils
Contraceptive Foams	Hemorrhoidal Ointments
(e.g., Emko, Delfen, Koromex)	Insect Repellants
Contraceptive Creams and Gels	Margarine/Dairy Butter
(e.g., Prepair, Conceptrol, Ramses)	Mineral Oil
Duragel	Palm Oil
Egg White	Petroleum Jelly
ForPlay Lubricant	(e.g., Vaseline)
Glycerin U.S.P.	Rubbing Alcohol
H-R Lubricating Jelly	Suntan Oil
Intercept	Vaginal Creams/Spermicides
Koromex Gel	(e.g., Monistat, Estrace, Femstat, Vagisil,
Lubafax	Premarin, Rendell's Cone, Pharmatex Ovule,
Lubrin Insert	Vagisil)
Norform Insert	Some Sexual Lubricants
Ortho-Gynol	(e.g., Elbow Grease, Hot Elbow Grease,
Personal Lubricant	and Shaft)
PrePair Lubricant	
Probe	
Saliva	
Semicid	
Silicones DC 360	
Transi-Lube	
Water	

Adapted from Waldron (1989).

Restricting the definition of breakage to that occurring during vaginal intercourse or in the process of withdrawal (during which exposure to risks of pregnancy and infection are most likely to occur), these studies also reported low rates of rupture, ranging from 1.2% to 2.0%. Further, a study of female prostitutes in Australia reported only three breaks in 605 acts of vaginal intercourse (0.5%), all of which were discovered before ejaculation.[36]

The location of rupture on the condom's surface may also affect the likelihood of pregnancy or infection. Tears occurring at the rim or along the sides of the condom may not release much semen. There has been some evidence that a substantial proportion of condom breakage may occur in these less risky areas. A prospective study of men in North Carolina found that only one-third of condom breaks occurred at the tip of the condom.[29]

Anal Intercourse

Only limited research exists on breakage rates during anal intercourse, but available data suggest that these rates may not be higher than the breakage rates reported for vaginal intercourse. One prospective study of breakage during anal intercourse followed 30 Australian male prostitutes[52] and reported a breakage rate of 0.5% (3 of 664 condoms), which was comparable to the 0.5% (3 of 605) breakage rate associated with vaginal intercourse in that study.[36] A similarly low 1% breakage rate during anal intercourse (1 in 105) was calculated from a survey of heterosexual and homosexual readers by *Consumer Reports*,[8] although both of these rates are lower than those reported in other retrospective studies.[5] Condom breakage may be more likely to occur during intercourse because of the possibility of increased friction. Additional research is needed on rates of breakage during anal intercourse before more definite conclusions can be made.

CONDOM SLIPPAGE

Condom slippage has also been mentioned as a potential problem for condom users.[26,27,42,43] Studies indicate that condoms rarely slip completely off during intercourse; however, they may slip down the shaft of the penis without falling off. One study distinguishing condoms that slipped off from condoms that merely slipped down reported only 0.6% (3 of 478) condoms fell off during intercourse or withdrawal.[42] However, 1 in 10 condoms slipped down during intercourse and 1 in 6 condoms slipped down during withdrawal, the latter presumably because men did not hold the condom against the base of the penis while withdrawing. In contrast, a study of 49 U.S. women found that only 2.0% of condoms slipped down without completely falling off.[27] Given these findings, research is needed to determine whether slippage places the woman at greater risk of pregnancy (due to possible semen leakage from the open end of the condom) or either partner at greater risk of acquiring a sexually transmitted infection (either due to semen leakage or due to contact of the penile shaft and the female genitalia). Slippage during withdrawal, classified as user error, may be minimized if the rim of the condom is held against the base of the penis during withdrawal, soon after ejaculation.

CONDOM TESTING

In the United States, manufacturers follow the voluntary performance standards for condoms established by the American Society for Testing and

Materials (ASTM) and recommended by the U.S. Food and Drug Administration (FDA). Before commercial distribution in the United States, each condom is tested electronically for holes and weak points.[29]

Samples of condoms from each batch passing electronic testing undergo a series of laboratory tests. In the tensile and elongation test, a segment of a condom is stretched to its breaking point and measured for breaking force. The water leakage test is conducted on condoms sampled from randomly selected batches manufactured domestically and imported for sale in the United States.[2] In this test, each condom is filled with 300 ml of water and evaluated for holes. Any moisture detected on the outside of the condom is considered a failed test. Batches with more than 4 failed tests per 1,000 condoms are not permitted for sale in the United States. The air burst test, a third laboratory test used extensively in other countries, has recently been proposed for adoption in the United States.[29] Although the validity of these tests to accurately predict breakage during intercourse has been questioned,[47] Table 7-3 indicates low rates of condom breakage in most U.S. studies.

COST

The condom is among the most inexpensive of contraceptives. In the late 1980s, U.S. consumers paid an average price of 50 cents per condom.[29] Based on the average coital frequency per U.S. couple of twice per week, the cost to a couple using condoms with every act of intercourse amounts to $52 annually.

U.S. condom manufacturers often make condoms available in bulk to nonprofit family planning facilities at a reduced cost (often as low as 5–10 cents per condom) so that they may be distributed to patients. Chapter 28 lists names and telephone numbers of condom manufacturers in the United States.

ADVANTAGES AND INDICATIONS

Perhaps condoms would be a great deal more popular if some of the noncontraceptive benefits and other advantages of condoms received greater emphasis, thereby offsetting the stigma often associated with condom use (*e.g.*, promiscuity, prostitution).

1. **Accessible.** Usage does not require examination, prescription, or fitting. Further, condoms can be obtained by men or women from drug stores, family planning clinics, barber shops, vending machines, gas stations, restaurants, bars, mail order services, or other sources.
2. **Inexpensive.** Not only is the retail cost low, but condoms may also be purchased in large numbers by public family planning programs at very low cost and may even be obtained for free.

3. **Male participation.** Men actively participate in contraception and protection from infection.

4. **Erection enhancement.** Condoms can help users maintain an erection longer and prevent premature ejaculation. The prolonged plateau phase may be desirable both for the man wearing the condom and for his partner.[8] In addition, some men may find the rim of the condom to have a slight tourniquet effect, helping to maintain erection.[13]

5. **Hygienic.** Messy postcoital discharge of semen from the vagina, a very annoying aftermath for some women, is avoided by using condoms.

6. **Prevention of sperm allergy.** Women have very occasionally been allergic to the sperm or semen of their partner; urticarial and even anaphylactic reactions have occurred. Condom use would obviously prevent these allergies. In some infertile couples where the woman's body produces antibodies to her partner's sperm, condom use for 3–6 months can prevent the release of sperm antigens into the vagina (the length of time depends on the level of antibody titer and how long it remains elevated).

7. **Proof of protection.** Condoms furnish immediate, visible proof of effectiveness as ejaculate is contained within the condom.

8. **Personal concerns.** Some women and men do not wish to have the penis in direct contact with the vagina. If this concern exists, the condom is an effective barrier that may make intercourse more pleasurable.

9. **Portable.** Condoms can be easily and discretely carried by men or women.

PREVENTION OF STDS AND HIV

Condoms, used as a single method, can effectively prevent transmission of HIV infection. However, no studies have demonstrated a protective effect for spermicides when used without condoms in the prevention of HIV.[39] A potential risk of any spermicide use is the possible causal association between vaginal irritation and an increased likelihood of HIV infection after viral exposure.[5,39] These findings should be considered preliminary until more studies are conducted. Further, the simultaneous use of a condom and spermicide is estimated to be 99.9% effective in reducing the risk of STD transmission per act of intercourse.[24]

Condoms have been shown in laboratory studies to be effective barriers against herpes simplex virus, *Chlamydia trachomatis*, cytomegalovirus, *N. gonorrhoeae*, HBV, and HIV.[5] In actual use during intercourse, condoms have been shown to protect against gonorrhea, ureaplasma infection, herpes simplex virus, and HIV infection (summarized in Tables 7-5 and 7-6). Condoms may also diminish the likelihood of infertility or cervical intraepithelial neoplasia in some women by diminishing the risk of sexually transmitted infections.[13]

A collaborative cohort study of HIV transmission among serodiscordant couples found that individuals who consistently used condoms were significantly less likely to seroconvert than those who did not. Among 24 couples who consistently used condoms for HIV prevention, none of the partners of HIV-positive persons was infected. Conversely, among the 44 couples reporting inconsistent condom use, six female partners were found to be HIV-positive.[11] Consistent use of the condom is obviously key to its effectiveness.

Protection Against HIV, STDs During Oral and Anal Intercourse

Use of condoms or other barriers can also be encouraged for orogenital and anogenital intercourse. Very few cases of HIV transmission have been reported in which the only known form of intimate contact between two persons was oral sex.[22,28,37,38] However, mouth-to-penis contact (fellatio) can transmit gonorrhea, syphilis, hepatitis B virus, oral or genital herpes simplex virus, and chlamydia; mouth-to-vulva contact (cunnilingus) can transmit herpes and syphilis.

For protection from infection during mouth-to-penis contact, non-lubricated (dry) latex condoms are an excellent barrier and generally preferred to lubricated condoms. A spermicidal condom is not recommended for use during oral sex because it is unlikely to provide better protection than a non-spermicidal condom and its taste is unpleasant. The condom can be put on before mouth-to-penis contact occurs and is not recommended for more than a single use.

For protection during mouth-to-vulva contact, household plastic wrap can be used, although it has neither been manufactured, tested, nor approved for medical applications.[2] Dental dams and condoms cut to form a barrier sheet have been proposed; however, their limited size may allow potentially infectious fluids to roll off onto adjacent tissues.

For protection during anal intercourse, latex or other synthetic condoms are recommended, although studies of their effectiveness are limited. For couples having anal intercourse (or rigorous vaginal intercourse), the use of two condoms at once, use of a thicker condom, or use of a water-based lubricant (*e.g.*, K-Y jelly) may help to minimize the increased potential for breakage.

Table 7-5 Studies investigating the efficacy of condoms in preventing STDs

Reference*	Description	Outcome Measure	Relative Risk (95% C.I.)
Men			
Cross-Sectional			
Pemberton et al., 1972	STD clinic clients, Belfast	Urethral gonorrhea	0.51 (0.33-0.80)
McCormack et al., 1973	College volunteers, U.S.	Urethral Ureaplasma urealyticum	0.33 (0.16–0.68)
Barlow, 1959	STD clinic clients, London	Urethral gonorrhea	0.25 (0.11–0.59)
Cohort			
Hart, 1974	Australian soldiers, Vietnam	Self-reported STDs	0.00
Hooper et al., 1978	Naval crewmen, Phillipines	Urethral gonorrhea	0.00
Darrow, 1989	STD clinic clients, U.S.	Urethral gonorrhea	0.34 (0.10–1.13)

(continued)

Table 7-5 Studies investigating the efficacy of condoms in preventing STDs *(cont.)*

Reference*	Description	Outcome Measure	Relative Risk (95% C.I.)
Women			
Cross-Sectional			
Oberle et al., 1989	Controls from case-control study of cervical cancer, Costa Rica	Herpes 2 seropositivity	0.60 (0.40–0.80)
Case–Control			
Austin et al., 1984	STD clinic clients, U.S.	Cervical gonorrhea	0.87 (0.64–1.19)
Syrjanen et al., 1984	Ob/Gyn clinic clients, Finland	Cervical human papillomavirus	1.35 (0.72–2.78)
Rosenberg et al., 1992	STD clinic clients, U.S.	Cervical gonorrhea	0.66 (0.52–0.84)
		Vaginal trichomoniasis	0.70 (0.55–0.89)
		Cervical chlamydia	0.97 (0.60–1.57)
		Bacterial vaginosis	1.11 (0.86–1.45)
Kelaghan et al., 1982	Hospital patients, U.S.	Pelvic inflammatory disease	0.60 (0.40–0.90)
Cramer et al., 1987	Women seeking infertility services, U.S.	Tubal infertility	0.70 (0.50–1.10)
Cohort			
Cameron et al., 1991	Commercial sex workers, STD clinic clients, Kenya	Genital ulcers (Adjusted for HIV infection)	0.18 (0.10–0.88)

Source: Cates (1992).

*Full reference listed in original article by Cates.

Table 7-6 Studies investigating the efficacy of condom use in preventing HIV infection in heterosexuals

Reference*	Description	Measure of Use	Outcome Measure	Measure of Effect
Cross Sectional				
Mann et al., 1987	Commercial sex workers, Zaire	> = 50% vs. <50% > 50% vs. none	Seropositivity	0.0 (p = 0.046) 0.0 (p = 0.09)
Padian, 1987	Partners of HIV+ men, U.S.	?	Seropositivity	0.6 (0.30–1.30)
Quinn et al., 1988	STD clinic clients, U.S.	Always vs. never	Seropositivity	0.6 (0.00–4.10)
Smiley et al., 1988	Partners of hemophiliacs, U.S.	Routine vs. none	Seroconversion	0.5 (p = 0.5)
Roumelioutou-Karayannis et al., 1988	Partners of HIV+ men, Greece	Regular vs. none	Seropositivity	0.0 (p< 0.0)
Musicco et al., 1991	Partners of HIV+ men, Italy	Always vs. other	Seropositivity	0.2 (0.00–0.70)
Guimaraes et al., 1991	Partners of HIV+ men, Brazil	Use vs. non-use	Seropositivity	0.3 (0.10–0.90)

(continued)

Table 7-6 Studies investigating the efficacy of condom use in preventing HIV infection in heterosexuals *(cont.)*

Reference*	Description	Measure of Use	Outcome Measure	Measure of Effect
Cohort				
Fischl et al., 1987	Partners of AIDS patients, U.S.	Regular use	Seroconversion	0.1 (0.00–0.40)
Ngugi et al., 1988	Commercial sex workers, Kenya	Any vs. none	Seroconversion	0.3 (0.13–0.92)
Laurian et al., 1989	Partners of hemophiliacs, France	Always vs. other	Seroconversion	0.0 (p = 0.015)
Kamenga et al., 1991	Partners of HIV+ men, Zaire	Sporadic	Seroconversion	HIV incidence = 1.9 per women-year
Allen et al., 1991	Women attending pediatric/prenatal clinic, Rwanda	Sporadic	Seroconversion	Decreased from 4.6% per year to 3.4% per year after increase in condom use
Musicco et al., 1991	Partners of HIV+ men, Italy	Always vs. other	Seroconversion	0.3 (0.10–1.50)
DeVincenzi et al., 1991	Serodiscordant couples, Europe	Systematic	Seroconversion	0.0 (p = 0.0009)
Moss et al., 1991	Serodiscordant couples, Kenya	?	Seroconversion	"Not Associated" HIV incidence = 18% per year

Source: Cates and Stone (1992).

*Full reference listed in original article by Cates.

Table 7-7 Condoms for women's health

Four key points are essential for understanding the importance of condoms for STD prevention:

1. Bacterial and viral sexually transmitted diseases (STDs) such as gonorrhea and chlamydia are biologically sexist illnesses that are typically more damaging to the reproductive tract of the woman than to the man.

2. Infected men transmit bacterial lower genital tract infections (e.g., gonorrhea) to two out of three female sex partners. Infected women transmit these STDs to one out of three male sex partners.

3. Condoms help protect women from unplanned pregnancy, ectopic pregnancy, vaginitis (lower tract infection), pelvic inflammatory disease (upper tract infection), infections that can harm a fetus during pregnancy or delivery, tubal infertility, genital cancer, and HIV infection.

4. It is a woman's right to insist on condom use. It is a woman's right to say no to intercourse if her partner says no to condoms.

DISADVANTAGES AND CAUTIONS

Condom use has few disadvantages:

1. **Reduced sensitivity.** Men often comment that the condom reduces glans sensitivity, although no objective data prove whether this is true. In order to provide a perception of increased sensitivity, the man may wish to use a textured, ultra-thin, or transparent condom.

2. **Interference with erection.** Occasionally a man cannot maintain an erection when the condom is used. If this occurs repeatedly, condom use becomes impossible. Integrating the placement of the condom on the penis as a routine part of foreplay may help overcome this obstacle.

3. **Interruption.** Often couples object to the interruption of foreplay to put on the condom. In this instance, the woman can be encouraged to put the condom on the man as part of foreplay. Women with long fingernails or sharp rings should be careful.

4. **Decreased pleasure.** In some instances, a woman enjoys intercourse less when the man's penis is covered.

5. **Allergy.** In rare cases, a man or a woman may be allergic or sensitive to latex condoms. While skin condoms may be used for pregnancy prevention, their use is probably contraindicated for prevention of sexually transmitted infection. Several non-latex condoms impervious to small viruses are currently being researched. The

non-latex Tactylon condom (Tactyl Technologies; Phoenix, AZ), is anticipated to become available in the United States soon. (The prevalence of latex sensitivity is increasing, particularly among workers with repeated exposure to latex medical devices and latex consumer products,[45] including condoms. An estimated 1%-3% of the general U.S. population is latex-sensitive. Among surgical workers, who have more frequent exposure to latex, 6%-7% experience reactions from repeated latex contact.)

6. **Male involvement.** In some instances a man will not accept the responsibility for birth control or infection prevention, thus making condom use impossible.

7. **Embarrassment.** Some men and women are extremely embarrassed to suggest or initiate condom use with their partner. Some people also find it embarrassing to purchase condoms or to go to a clinic to obtain them.

8. **Breakage.** Condoms can break (see section on Effectiveness). However, estimates of the probability of HIV infection resulting from a single exposure (*e.g.*, post-ejaculatory condom break) range from one in 10 to less than one in 1,000, depending on type of transmission (male-male, male-female, and female-male) and the presence of genital ulcers.[29]

PROVIDING CONDOMS
Innovative Programs

Innovative programs have been shown to dramatically increase the use of condoms. One important feature of successful distribution programs is the provision of large numbers (50-100) of condoms to each client. Providing 3-6 condoms is a very short-term solution for clients who find the health care system to be inaccessible or who find it embarrassing to return repeatedly for condoms. Some creative marketing/public awareness efforts are as follows:

- The Beyond condom package, created by Okamoto, contains six condoms in a stylish royal blue container that intentionally resembles a make-up compact. This product appeals to the woman who is afraid to carry easily noticed, exposed condoms.

- In Britain and Italy, condoms are packaged in cigarette-shaped boxes and sold in vending machines.[29]

- In Cambridge, MA, the city government requires all businesses (including theaters, bars, restaurants, motels and hotels) to put condom machines on the premises.[29]

- In Portland, OR, Project Action—an HIV/AIDS prevention program for young adults—has developed a social marketing program to encourage condom use through strategic placement of condom vending machines and a television campaign.[1]

Schools

Among the existing policy issues are questions as to where condoms should be made readily available for the prevention of infection to young men and women, who may be too embarrassed to purchase or otherwise obtain condoms. A survey of college and university health services found that condoms were dispensed by 23 of 24 contacted schools and are also available at other sites on campus.[17]

In contrast, there is a lack of availability of condoms in high schools and a virtual absence of condoms in middle schools where many youth are sexually active. A recent national survey of risk behaviors for HIV infection among high school students found:

- The median age of first intercourse to be 16.1 years for males and 16.9 years for females.
- Nearly 1 in 5 students reported more than four lifetime sexual partners.
- Only 45% of sexually active students reported using a condom at last intercourse.[6]

Some public high schools have adopted programs to make condoms more obtainable for students. In New York City, as part of an expanded HIV prevention program, condoms were made available to 120 public high schools through school-based clinics and trained teachers, staff, and counselors.[23] There also appears to be considerable community support for condom distribution in schools. A nationally representative U.S. survey found that 64% of adults favored availability in high schools while 47% favored availability in middle schools.[25]

Useful print materials have been prepared for teenage and college-age students. See Chapter 28 for a description of *Sexual Etiquette 101* and other resources.

COUNSELING ISSUES

Many family planning providers have had the experience of offering condoms to a woman only to hear the reply, "You might as well not give me any of those. I know he won't use them!" It seems to be the view of this woman that if she votes "yes" on condoms and he votes "no," then "no" wins. In those cases it becomes critical for family planning providers to help her believe in the authority and the carrying power of her "yes" vote, and to teach her skills for using condoms to take care of her health and fertility.

Find out what the patient thinks her partner will say when he objects to condoms, and help her practice her reply so that she can insist on condom use in a firm, clear manner that doesn't cause her partner to feel attacked (see Table 7-8).

When counseling patients on the use of condoms, discuss with the patient the many advantages and few disadvantages condoms offer. Instructions are available in print and on audiotape ("Listen Carefully"); see Chapter 28 for a description of these resources. Try to obtain a history of patients who do not use condoms and determine whether they are unable or unwilling to use them and why. Note the specific problems or obstacles they are experiencing. Encourage patients to share their fears and problems associated with condom use. Provide enough condoms so that the patient will not have to visit the clinic frequently to get more condoms. Convey that the condom must be used correctly with every act of intercourse. Do not assume that the patient knows how to correctly use a condom, regardless of the patient's past condom experience—the patient may be using them incorrectly each time. In one study, men who acquired gonorrhea despite condom use put the condoms on after starting intercourse instead of at the time of initial genital contact.[10] The counseling session presents the ideal opportunity for recognizing and correcting potential misuse. You may wish to ask questions about the patient's experience with condom breakage, condom slippage, and use of lubricants. Are the condoms too big? Too small? Too dry? Is the patient using petroleum jelly as a lubricant? Finally, offer to demonstrate proper application of a condom on a model of a penis (or other similarly shaped object) and encourage the patient to try this as well.

Table 7-8 Anticipatory guidance for getting partners to agree to use condoms[15]

He:	"I won't feel as much if I have a condom on."
She:	"You won't feel anything if you don't have a condom on."
He:	"I don't have any condoms and we don't want to go out and get some."
She:	"Well, I just happen to have some condoms with me. What color do you like best?"
He:	"I know I'm clean (disease-free); I haven't had sex with anyone in a number of months."
She:	"Thanks for telling me. As far as I know, I'm disease-free too. But I'd still like to use a condom since either of us could have an infection and not know it."
He:	"It will interrupt sex."
She:	"Let me put it on for you. You'll love it."
He:	"Condoms are unnatural, fake, a total turn-off."
She:	"There's nothing great about genital infections either. Please let's try to work this out; either give the condom a try or let's look for alternatives."

Be cautious when strongly urging the simultaneous use of two methods of birth control to patients. Concomitant use may be overly complicated and counterproductive for some couples; thus, the use of a condom plus another contraceptive method should be advised with a degree of caution. Requiring compliance with multiple methods may lead the couple to opt for use of no method of birth control as the easier alternative.

INSTRUCTIONS FOR USING CONDOMS

The condom provides a barrier between the penis and the vagina and represents the most effective contraceptive at reducing the risk of sexually transmitted infection. Couples using the most effective approaches to contraception such as Norplant, pills, IUDs, or sterilization may also choose to use condoms consistently to gain protection versus infection. For extra contraceptive protection with use of the condom, use a back-up method of birth control such as a diaphragm; vaginally applied spermicide, contraceptive foam, gel, or suppositories; the spong;, or the pill.

Practice makes perfect, especially if you have never tried the condom before. First practice unrolling a dry condom onto a banana. Notice the importance of placing the condom on the right way. Try with your eyes open, and then again in the dark. Men can also practice on themselves alone. Condoms may be used by a man having intercourse with another man and may be used at the time of oral-genital sex or anal-genital sex.

WHO CAN USE CONDOMS?

Because condoms rarely cause side effects, they can be used by nearly any sexually active couple to provide protection from pregnancy and infection. A woman at high risk for sexually transmitted infections may wish to use condoms consistently during pregnancy to protect the fetus, her partners, and herself. Each postpartum woman may also wish to use a condom for STD protection for 3 months after delivery because this is when she is at greatest risk for puerperal infection (postpartum endometritis).[33]

WHY SHOULD YOU USE CONDOMS?

1. To enjoy sexual intercourse more by helping some men to last longer (which is fun!) and by helping some women to achieve orgasm.
2. To prevent an unwanted pregnancy.
3. To protect yourself and your partner against sexually transmitted infections including AIDS (synthetic condoms only).

4. To protect the woman against infertility and cervical cancer.
5. To protect the woman and her fetus during pregnancy against AIDS, gonorrhea, herpes, chlamydia, trichomonas, and genital warts (synthetic condoms only).
6. To protect the postpartum woman from infection during the first 3 months after delivery, the time in her life when she is most likely to develop a pelvic infection.

WHEN SHOULD YOU USE CONDOMS?

EVERY time you have intercourse, even during pregnancy, when sexually transmissible infection is a concern for any reason.

1. Use the condom *every* time, with *every* act of intercourse.
2. Before penetration, carefully unroll the condom onto the erect penis, all the way to the base of the penis.
3. During withdrawal of the penis after ejaculation (while the penis is still erect), hold the rim of the condom against the base of the penis.

HOW DO YOU USE CONDOMS?

1. Put the condom on the erect penis (either partner can do this) *before* the penis comes in contact with the woman's genitals.
2. Condoms can tear before use when being removed from the package and placed on the penis. Since it is possible to tear a hole in a condom with your fingernail, be careful. Do not try to fill your condom with liquid or air as a test for holes; every condom is pretested before distribution.
3. Unroll the condom a short distance over a finger before placing it onto the penis to ensure the condom is being properly unrolled. The rolled rim should always remain on the outside of the condom. Again, be careful with long fingernails.
4. Unroll the condom down to the base of the erect penis. If the condom has been unrolled incorrectly (backwards), it is recommended that you remove the condom from the penis and throw it away, starting over with a new condom. (If unrolled incorrectly, the condom's outer surface may come in direct contact with pre-ejaculatory fluid or infectious organisms on the penis. If the same condom is then unrolled correctly on the penis, your partner may be unintentionally exposed.

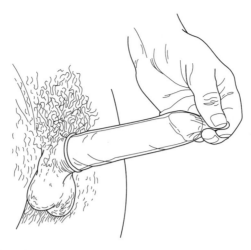

Figure 7-1 Condom, leave 1/2-in. empty space at tip

Although the risk of pregnancy from pre-ejaculate is unlikely, recent studies have suggested the presence of HIV in the pre-ejaculatory fluid of HIV-infected men.[21,35] Whether exposure to this amount of HIV is sufficient to cause infection has not been established.)

5. It is often recommended to leave 1/2-in. of empty space at the tip of the condom. This step may or may not be necessary to prevent breakage. To do this, pinch the tip of the condom as you unroll it down the penis.

6. Ensure adequate lubrication (natural or artificial) before penetration. A condom may be more likely to tear if the vagina or anus is dry.

7. For extra lubrication, use products such as water, K-Y jelly, or spermicidal creams, jellies, foam, or suppositories. Do NOT use oil-based products such as cold cream, mineral oil, cooking oil, petroleum jelly, shortening, lotions, massage oil or baby oil, which can degrade the quality of the condom. See Table 7-4 for a listing of recommended and non-recommended lubricants.

8. If at any time during intercourse you or your partner believe the condom may have torn or slipped off, stop and check the condom. If the condom is damaged or has slipped off, replace with a new condom before continuing intercourse.

9. During withdrawal of the penis *soon* after ejaculation and while the penis is still erect, hold the rim of the condom against the base of the penis. This technique should help to prevent condom slippage and the spillage of semen.

10. When your penis is clearly away from your partner's genitals (after withdrawal), slowly slide the condom off the penis without spilling semen.

11. Check the condom for visible damage (*e.g.,* holes), then wrap it in tissue and throw it away. It is strongly recommended that condoms not be used more than once for oral, vaginal, or anal intercourse. You may wish to keep at least two condoms with you in case the first condom is damaged or torn.

12. If the condom has torn (or slipped off):
    • Immediately insert spermicidal foam or gel into the vagina (if available and you have not yet done so). If no spermicidal product is available, immediately wash both penis and vagina with soap and water to minimize any risk of conception or infection.
    • Postcoital contraception may be used to reduce the risk of pregnancy. The simplest and best studied regimen is to take two combined estrogen and progestin birth control pills orally (Ovral) as soon as possible following, but within 72 hours of unprotected intercourse, and then take two more Ovral tablets 12 hours later (see Chapter 16). Consult your health care worker as soon as possible.

13. Store condoms in a cool, dry, and dark place away from sunlight. Heat may cause the rubber to weaken, so condoms should not be stored in a place that becomes very hot. Although placing condoms in wallets has been discouraged in the past because of the presumed increase risk of breakage due to mechanical stress and excessive heat, recent studies suggest it is safe to use a condom that has been carried in a wallet for up to 1 month.[14]

14. Each condom packet contains either a manufacture date or an expiration date. If the date is an expiration date, it should be marked as such.[3] Otherwise, the date should be considered to be the manufacture date. Condoms that are kept dry, sealed, and away from heat, sunlight, humidity, and fluorescent light can probably be used up to 5 years past the indicated manufacture date.

REFERENCES

1. Anonymous. Population Services International (PSI). Personal communication to David Lee Warner. May 1993.
2. Arrowsmith-Lowe T. Personal communication to David Lee Warner. January 1993.
3. ASTM (American Society for Testing and Materials). Annual book of ASTM standards: section 9, rubber. Volume 09.02 Rubber Products, Industrial Specifications and Related Test Methods; Gaskets; Tires. Philadelphia PA: American Society for Testing and Materials, 1989.

4. Casanova J. Memoires de Jacques Casanova de Seingalt. Brussells: J. Rosez, 1872.
5. Cates W, Stone KM. Family planning, sexually transmitted diseases and contraceptive choice: a literature update – Part I. Fam Plann Perspect 1992;24(2): 75-84.
6. Centers for Disease Control and Prevention. Selected behaviors that increase risk for HIV infection among high school students—United States, 1990. MMWR 1992;41(14):231,237-240.
7. Centers for Disease Control and Prevention. 1993 STD treatment guidelines. MMWR 1993;42(RR-14):1-73.
8. Consumers Union. Can you rely on condoms? Consum Rep 1989;March: 135-142.
9. Dale E. A laboratory investigation of the anti-spermatozoal action of condoms treated with a spermicidal preparation. Schmid Products Company, 1982.
10. Darrow W. Condom use and use-effectiveness in high-risk populations. Sex Transm Dis 1989;16(3):157-160.
11. European Study Group. Comparison of female to male and male to female transmission of HIV in 563 stable couples. BMJ 1992;304(6830):809-813.
12. Family Health International. How human use affects condom breakage. Network 1991;12(3):10-14.
13. Free MJ. Condoms: the rubber remedy. In: Corson SC, Derman RJ, Tyrer LB (eds). Fertility control. Boston MA: Little, Brown & Co., 1985.
14. Glasser G, Hatcher RA. The effect on condom integrity of carrying a condom in a wallet for three months [abstract]. American College of Obstetricians and Gynecologists District IV Conference, November, 1992, San Juan, P.R.
15. Grieco A. Cutting the risks for STDs. Med Aspects Hum Sex 1987;21(3):70-84.
16. Hamann C. Personal communication to David Lee Warner. May 1993.
17. Hatcher RA, Atkinson A, Cates D, Glasser L, Legins K. Sexual etiquette 101. Atlanta GA:Bridging the Gap Communications, Inc., 1992.
18. Hatcher RA, Hughes MS. The truth about condoms. SIECUS Report 1988;17(2): 1-9.
19. Hatcher RA, Warner DL. New condoms for men and women, diaphragms, cervical caps, and spermicides: overcoming barriers to barriers and spermicides. Curr Opin Obstet Gynecol 1992;4(4);513-521.
20. Himes NE. Medical history of contraception. New York NY: Gamut Press, 1963.
21. Ilaria G, Jacobs JL, Polsky B, Koll B, Baron P, Maclow C, Armstrong D. Detection of HIV-1 DNA sequences in pre-ejaculatory fluid. Lancet 1992;340(8833):1469.
22. Keet IPM, Van Lent NA, Sandfort TGM, Coutinho RA, Van Griensven GJP. Orogenital sex and the transmission of HIV among homosexual men. AIDS 1992;6(2):223-226.
23. Kerr DL. Condom availability in New York City schools. Sch Health 1991;61(6):279-280.
24. Kestelman P, Trussell J. Efficacy of the simultaneous use of condoms and spermicides. Fam Plann Perspect 1991;23(5):226-7,232.
25. Kirby D. School-based programs to reduce sexual risk-taking behaviors. J Sch Health 1992;62(7):280-286.
26. Kirkman RJE, Morris J, Webb AMC. User experience: Mates v. Nuforms. Br J Fam Plann 1990;15:107-111.
27. Leeper MA, Conrardy M. Preliminary evaluation of REALITY, a condom for women to wear. Adv Contracept 1989;5(4):229-235.

28. Lifson AR, O'Malley PM, Hessol NA, Buchbinder SP, Cannon L, Rutherford GW. HIV seroconversion in two homosexual men after receptive oral intercourse with ejaculation: implications for counseling concerning safe sexual practices. Am J Publ Health 1990;80(12):1509-1511.
29. Liskin L, Wharton C, Blackburn R, Kestelman P. Condoms: now more than ever. Popul Rep 1990;8:Series H.
30. London KA, Mosher WD. What is current use of a contraceptive? Hyattsville MD: National Center for Health Statistics,1990.
31. Mason V (ed). Latex allergies create two-pronged problem for clinics. Contraceptive Technology Update 1992;13(7):109-111.
32. Mason V (ed). New contraceptive methods: the good, the bad, & the ugly. Contraceptive Technology Update 1992;13(7):101-105.
33. National Family Planning and Reproductive Health Association. Policy statement on condoms and pregnant women, 1988.
34. Ortho Pharmaceutical Corporation. Report on the 1991 Ortho Annual Birth Control Study. Raritan NJ: Ortho Pharmaceutical Corporation, 1991.
35. Pudney J, Oneta M, Mayer K, Searge G (III), Anderson D. Pre-ejaculatory fluid as potential vector for sexual transmission of HIV-1. Lancet 1992;340(8833):1470.
36. Richters J, Donovan B, Gerofi J, Watson L. Low condom breakage rate in commercial sex [letter]. Lancet 1988;2(8626/8627):1487-1488. Correction by John Gerofi in personal communication to Philip Kestelman, July 1989.
37. Rozenbaum W, Gharakhanian S, Cardon B, Duval E, Coulaud JP. HIV transmission by oral sex. Lancet 1988;1ii(8599):1395.
38. Spitzer PG, Weiner NJ. Transmission of HIV infection from a woman to a man by oral sex. N Engl J Med 1989;320(4):251.
39. Stone KM, Peterson HB. Spermicides, HIV, and the vaginal sponge. JAMA 1992;268(4):522-523.
40. Thornton T. Personal communication to David Lee Warner. March 1993.
41. Trap R, Trap B, Petersen CS. Evaluation of the amount of nonoxynol available in condoms for the inhibition of HIV using a method based on HPLC. Int J STD AIDS 1990;1(6):449.
42. Trussell J, Warner DL, Hatcher RA. Condom performance during vaginal intercourse: comparison of Trojan-Enz and Tactylon condoms. Contraception 1992;45(1):11-19.
43. Trussell J, Warner DL, Hatcher RA. Condom slippage and breakage rates. Fam Plann Perspect 1992;24(1):20-23.
44. Turjanmaa K, Reunala T. Condoms as a source of latex allergen and cause of contact urticaria. Contact Dermatitis 1989;20(5):360-364.
45. U.S. Food and Drug Administration. Allergic reactions to latex-containing medical devices. March 29, 1991; Publication #MDA91-1.
46. Voeller B. Persistent condom breakage. Topanga CA, Mariposa Educational Foundation, 1989. (Mariposa Occasional Paper No. 12), 9 pp.
47. Voeller B. Relevance of condom testing. In Alexander NJ, Gabelnick HL, Spieler J (eds). The heterosexual transmission of AIDS. CONRAD 2nd International Workshop. New York NY: Alan R. Liss Publishing Company, 1990.
48. Voeller B, Coulson A, Bernstein GS, Nakamura R. Mineral oil lubricants cause rapid deterioration of latex condoms. Contraception 1989;39(1):95-101.
49. Waldron T. Female condoms scheduled to reach U.S. market this year. Contraceptive Technology Update 1991(a);12(8):117-127.

50. Waldron T. Newer, innovative condoms may help increase compliance. Contraceptive Technology Update 1991(b);12(11):171.

51. Waldron T. Tests show commonly used substances harm latex condoms. Contraceptive Technology Update 1989;10(2):20-21.

52. Richters J, Watsun L, Gerofi J, Donovan B. In search of the perfect condom. Healthright 1989;9(1):16-19.

Vaginal Spermicides

- Spermicides are simple, free of systemic side effects, available without prescription, and can be used intermittently, with little advance planning required.
- Spermicides are an integral component of vaginal barrier methods (diaphragm, sponge, and cap; see Chapter 9).
- Using spermicide reduces transmission of important STDs including gonorrhea and chlamydia infection. The effect of spermicide on HIV risk, however, is uncertain.

Spermicide products can be purchased without prescription in pharmacies and supermarkets. They can be used alone, with a vaginal barrier method, or as an adjunct to any of the other contraceptive methods for added protection from both pregnancy and some sexually transmitted infections.

MECHANISM OF ACTION

Spermicidal preparations consist of two components:

- Base or carrier (foam, cream, jelly, film, suppository, or tablet)
- Spermicidal chemical that kills the sperm

For some products, the carrier also helps assure dispersion and, in the case of foam, may provide an additional barrier effect. Nonoxynol-9 is the active agent in most spermicide products available in the United States (see Table 8-1); both

Table 8-1 Spermicides

Representative Products (Brand Names)	Spermicidal Agent	Comments
Film	Contraceptive protection begins 15 minutes after insertion; remains effective no more than 1 hour.	
VCF (Vaginal Contraceptive Film)	Nonoxynol-9	Small, thin sheets
Foam	Contraceptive protection is immediate; remains effective for at least 1 hour.	
Delfen, Emko, Koromex	Nonoxynol-9	Aerosol container
Emko Because, Emko Prefil	Nonoxynol-9	Small container
Jellies and Creams	Contraceptive protection is immediate. When used alone remains effective at least 1 hour; used with diaphragm or cap remains effective at least 6–8 hours.	
Conceptrol, Delfen, Koromex Jel, Ortho Gynol II, Ramses	Nonoxynol-9	Reuseable applicator
Koromex Cream, Ortho Gynol	Octoxynol	Reuseable applicator
Conceptrol Jel, Milex Shur Seal Jel	Nonoxynol-9	Single-use packets
Suppositories and Tablets	Contraceptive protection begins 10–15 minutes after insertion; remains effective no more than 1 hour.	
Encare, Intercept, Koromex Inserts, Prevent, Semicid	Nonoxynol-9	

nonoxynol-9 and octoxynol, the only two options in the United States, are surfactants that destroy the sperm cell membrane. Other surfactant products, including menfegol and benzalkonium chloride, are widely used in other parts of the world.

Foam. Foam is marketed for use alone, but can be used satisfactorily with a diaphragm or with a condom.

Creams and gels. Creams and gels are commonly marketed for use with a diaphragm, but also can be used alone. One application of foam, cream, or gel provides 80mg–150 mg of spermicide, depending on the product; spermicide concentration is 12.5% in foam and ranges from 1% to 5% in gels and creams.

Suppositories. Spermicide suppositories are intended for use alone or with a condom. Suppositories contain 2.3%–8.3% spermicide, and provide 100–150 mg of spermicide. Adequate time between insertion and intercourse (10–15 minutes depending on the product) is essential to allow the spermicide to disperse. Incomplete dissolution of the suppository may reduce contraceptive efficacy and may cause an uncomfortable gritty sensation or friction for the woman or the man.

Film. Vaginal contraceptive film (VCF) can be used alone or with a diaphragm or condom. Each 2″ × 2″ paper-thin sheet of film is 28% spermicide, and contains 72 mg of nonoxynol-9. The sheet must be inserted on or near the cervix (or inside the diaphragm) at least 5 minutes before intercourse to allow time for the sheet to melt and spermicide to disperse. Placing film on the tip of the penis for insertion is not recommended because the film will not have adequate time to dissolve and because the film may not end up covering the cervical os.

Spermicidal condoms. Latex condoms with nonoxynol-9 already covering the surface, have been available in the United States since 1983. (More detail on spermicidal condoms is presented in Chapter 7.)

EFFECTIVENESS

Failure rates reported in studies of spermicide efficacy range from 0% to more than 50% for typical users. Unfortunately, clinical trials of spermicide used alone do not meet modern standards for study design and analysis. Therefore, meaningful comparisons between spermicide efficacy and the efficacy of other methods, or between one spermicide preparation and another, are impossible to make. Analysis and estimates used for Table 8-2 are described in Chapter 27. *Consistent use is the most important factor in minimizing failure with spermicides.*

Table 8-2 First-year failure rates* for women using spermicides and barriers

Method (1)	% of Women Experiencing an Accidental Pregnancy Within the First Year of Use		% of Women Continuing Use at One Year (4)
	Typical Use (2)	Perfect Use (3)	
Spermicides	21	6	43
Sponge			
Parous Women	36	20	45
Nulliparous Women	18	9	58
Diaphragm	18	6	58
Condom			
Male	12	3	63
Female (Reality)	21	5	56

* See Table 5-2 for first-year failure rates of all methods.

Emergency Contraceptive Pills: Treatment initiated within 72 hours after unprotected intercourse reduces the risk of pregnancy by at least 75%.

Table 8-3 Perfect, simultaneous use of spermicide and condoms

	Contraceptive Failure within One Year (%)
Condoms used alone	3
Spermicide used alone	6
Spermicide and condom used together	0.01

Source: Kestelman and Trussell (1991).

Greater contraceptive efficacy can be achieved by the use of latex or synthetic condoms along with spermicide either all the time or for 1 week each month, beginning 5 days before ovulation is expected. When condoms and spermicide are used together, consistently and correctly with every act of intercourse, a couple can expect extremely efficacious contraceptive protection[17] (see Table 8-3). See also Chapter 5 for a discussion of protection provided by the concomitant use of two methods.

Correct placement of spermicide and correct timing of insertion are important for success. The spermicide applicator, tablet, suppository, or film need to reach the cervix, which for most women is deep in the vagina. Suppositories, foaming tablets, and films require adequate time for dissolution and dispersion. Slightly differing method characteristics (timing, degree of lubricating effect, delay for suppository melting) also may be important. A couple is most likely to succeed with a method that meets their non-contraceptive needs.

Douching is not a reliable contraceptive, even when a spermicide is used in the douching solution, because sperm enter the cervical canal too quickly—as soon as 15 seconds after ejaculation. Cola beverages, commonly believed to be spermicidal, are not effective,[11] and douching is statistically associated with increased risk for pelvic infection and for ectopic pregnancy (see Chapters 4 and 20). A woman who has used a vaginal spermicide for contraception, and chooses to douche following sexual intercourse, should wait at least 6-8 hours after intercourse to avoid washing away the spermicide prematurely.

C OST

The overall cost of this method depends on intercourse frequency. Retail prices for supplies range from less than $0.35 (for discount suppositories or gel) to $1.30 (for single-use gel packets). Users must make a small initial investment, however, to purchase a full container of foam ($12.00), a package of film ($9.25 for 12 sheets), a package of suppositories ($4.00 for 12 suppositories), or a full tube of gel or cream ($12.00).

ADVANTAGES AND INDICATIONS

Spermicides are an important contraceptive option in many temporary situations and may be a reasonable long-term choice for couples who use them consistently.

1. For women who are not at risk for STD, spermicide use, backed up by abortion in case of failure, is comparable in medical safety to consistent use of vaginal barrier methods or condoms.

2. Spermicides can be purchased over-the-counter without any encounter with the medical system.

3. Spermicide can be used by the woman without the necessity for partner involvement in the decision or in the implementation.

4. Spermicide can be kept available for immediate protection whenever it is needed, no matter how long the interval between uses.

5. Spermicides are a simple back-up option for a woman who is waiting to start oral contraceptives or have an IUD inserted, for a woman who forgets two or more pills or runs out of pills, or for an IUD user who suspects her IUD has been expelled.

6. Spermicides can be used consistently or at midcycle to augment the effectiveness of condoms, an IUD, or fertility awareness methods.

7. Spermicides can be used as an emergency measure if a condom breaks. An application of spermicide should be quickly inserted in this instance.

8. Spermicides can be used to provide lubrication during intercourse and can appropriately be used for lubrication with a condom.

PROTECTION AGAINST STDS AND HIV

In the laboratory, nonoxynol-9 is lethal to organisms that cause gonorrhea, genital herpes, trichomonas, syphilis and AIDS.[1,3,7,9,16,21,32,34] *In vitro* microbicide activity, however, does not mean that spermicides can provide reliable protection against STD transmission. Especially for intracellular organisms such as HIV, the organism's location inside an infected cell may shield it from exposure to spermicide.[20] Also, transmission from one partner to another may be influenced by other factors such as access of an infected cell to the intracervical or endometrial environment, or to open lesions denuded of protective epithelium, where macrophages are present to ingest the infected intruder cell and its contents. Similarly, alterations in vaginal flora or pH, or the presence of inflammation caused by spermicide, could alter HIV infectivity.[35]

Protection against sexually transmitted disease is potentially the most important noncontraceptive benefit of spermicide use. Unfortunately, uncertainty about spermicide impact on HIV risk clouds this issue. On one hand, reducing risks for gonorrhea and chlamydia infection may in turn reduce HIV susceptibility,[36] and spermicide products are lethal to HIV virus in laboratory tests.[1,7,9,34] On the other hand, spermicide chemicals are toxic to normal epithelial cells and can cause vaginal irritation. Damage to the vaginal epithelium could increase HIV susceptibility.[19]

Until the relationship between spermicide use and HIV risk is better understood, we hesitate to recommend spermicide use, especially frequent or prolonged use, when HIV exposure is a concern. In this situation, the safest choice is to avoid intercourse altogether. Prevention messages should stress the importance of thoughtful decisions in choosing a sexual partner, and the behavioral characteristics associated with high risk for HIV such as use of illegal, injection drugs and previous male homosexual relationships. Sexually active people also need to know that reduced HIV risk has been well documented with correct, consistent use of latex, male condoms.

Vaginal damage has been documented for women exposed to frequent use of spermicides,[24,26] and one study found increased HIV seroconversion among commercial sex workers who used spermicide-containing sponges.[19] Using nonoxynol-9 spermicide suppositories, however, reduced the risk for HIV seroconversion in two other studies.[10,37] Researchers have postulated that the lower dose of spermicide (100 mg in the suppositories as compared with 1,000 mg in sponges), and the shorter duration of exposure (sponges in the sex worker study were worn for many hours daily) might have minimized the undesirable, toxic effects found in the sponge study.

Unlike HIV, the beneficial impact of spermicide use on more common STDs is clear-cut. Clinical studies have shown that women who use nonoxynol-9 products derive significant protection against gonorrhea and against chlamydia. Some evidence suggests that risks for cervical cancer and for sexual transmission of hepatitis B virus also may be reduced.[4,25,27,28] The relative risk for gonorrhea in one study of nonoxynol-9 gel was 0.75;[15] similar reductions in both gonorrhea and chlamydia infection were found in another study of nonoxynol-9 spermicide used alone.[22] Using nonoxynol-9 reduced gonorrhea and chlamydia risk, although not as effectively as condom use, in another study.[24] In studies of PID and of tubal infertility, risk reduction was greatest when both a mechanical barrier and a spermicide were used together.[5]

The importance of actual use on STD protection deserves emphasis. Latex male condoms provide excellent protection when used consistently, but their use is low among women at highest risk for STD. Some evidence suggest that methods women can use autonomously may, in net, result in equal or better protection because of better compliance.[27,28] Yet the science on this topic is still unclear. If male condoms are not being used, and female condoms are not feasible, then use of spermicide or a vaginal barrier method with spermicide is reasonable notwithstanding the current uncertainty about HIV risk impact. This is especially true for women who do not have very frequent intercourse that would involve repeated or prolonged spermicide exposure.

D ISADVANTAGES AND CAUTIONS

Spermicide is not a reasonable choice in the following circumstances:

- Allergy or sensitivity to the spermicidal agent or to ingredients in the base
- Inability to learn correct insertion technique
- Abnormal vaginal anatomy (such as vaginal septum, prolapse, double cervix) that interferes with appropriate placement or retention of spermicide

Irritation and common dislikes. Temporary skin irritation involving the vulva or penis caused by sensitivity or allergy is the most common problem associated with spermicide use. Vaginal irritation can also occur, especially with frequent or prolonged exposure. When allergy or sensitivity is suspected, changing to another product may be an alternative. Some couples find the taste of spermicide unpleasant with oral-genital sex; some women find that the effervescence of foaming vaginal suppositories is unpleasant or that vaginal suppository products do not melt or disperse as intended.

Yeast vaginitis. Women who use sponges have an increased incidence of symptomatic candidiasis.[19,29] Increased vaginal colonization with *Candida* species has been documented after use of a diaphragm with spermicide.[12] *Candida* is much more resistant to the microbicidal effects of nonoxynol-9 than are other normal, desirable, vaginal organisms such as *Lactobacillus*,[18] and nonoxynol-9 exposure increases adherence of some *Candida* strains to vaginal epithelial cells.[23] Spermicide use, therefore, can encourage selective colonization of the vagina with uropathogens relatively resistant to nonoxynol-9.[12] A similar mechanism may also explain the increased incidence of urinary tract infection reported among diaphragm users; wearing this device entails prolonged spermicide exposure for some women.

Systemic effects. Serious adverse reactions have not been reported for the spermicide products now marketed in the United States. In 1980, an FDA panel reviewed published information and information from manufacturers and approved them as safe and effective. However, toxicology studies to determine the degree of vaginal absorption and to detect possible systemic effects are limited. In animal studies, intravaginal exposure to large doses of nonoxynol-9 have been associated with abnormalities such as liver toxicity and embryotoxic effects.[2]

Spermicide use and pregnancy. One study reported a statistical association between medical record evidence of spermicide purchase during the 2 years before pregnancy and the occurrence of a diverse range of fetal abnormalities.[14] Two other studies, published in 1982, also reported possible adverse associations between spermicide exposure and birth defects.[13,30] Serious methodologic problems have been identified in these studies. Subsequent researchers have failed to confirm adverse fetal effects in several large, carefully designed studies,[6,8,31,33] Thus, experts believe that no true association exists between spermicide use and fetal defects.[6,8,31]

PROVIDING SPERMICIDES

When providing spermicides in a clinical setting, reinforce instructions for proper use and remind users about common errors that can lead to unintended pregnancy (see Instructions for Using Spermicides). Warn women who have abnormalities of vaginal anatomy such as a septate vagina or severe prolapse, which may interfere with proper spermicide placement, that spermicide use may not be effective for them.

MANAGING PROBLEMS AND FOLLOW-UP

Spermicide use does not require any special follow-up surveillance. Women who experience irritation may seek care. If symptoms persist more than a day or two after discontinuing spermicide exposure, evaluate the underlying factors. An exam is essential if STD exposure is possible, and may be needed to identify yeast vaginitis. If irritation occurs immediately after insertion of spermicide, sensitivity rather than true allergy is the likely diagnosis. Changing to an alternative product, with different carrier constituents, or changing to a less concentrated product, may help. Some women who are sensitive to nonoxynol-9 are able to use octoxynol products (see Table 8-1).

Women who have initiated sponge use on their own may not be aware of the substantial failure rate for parous, as opposed to nulliparous, users of this method. Review with them other similar contraceptive options such as the diaphragm.

INSTRUCTIONS FOR USING SPERMICIDES

1. **Use spermicide every time you have intercourse.** Be sure that spermicide is in place before your partner's penis penetrates your vagina.

2. **If you have problems** with vaginal or penile irritation and may be at risk for a sexually transmitted infection, see your clinician promptly. Otherwise, you may want to try a different spermicide product. You could switch to condoms or see your clinician for another method of birth control.

3. **You can use condoms** along with spermicide if you wish. By using this combination, birth control protection is more effective and your risk of sexually transmitted infection is greatly reduced.

COMMON ERRORS IN SPERMICIDE USE

Common errors can lead to unintended pregnancy:

- Failing to use spermicide or an alternative method such as condoms each and every time intercourse occurs, even when menstrual bleeding is present.
- Failing to wait long enough after insertion for suppositories or film to dissolve and disperse.
- Failing to use another application of spermicide if more than 1 hour has elapsed between insertion and intercourse.
- Using too little spermicide or foam, or failing to shake the foam can vigorously enough.
- Failing to use another applicator with every repeated act of intercourse.
- Failing to recognize that the foam bottle or spermicide tube is empty.
- Failing to have spermicide available.

BEFORE INTERCOURSE

1. **Check to be sure you have all the supplies you need**—enough to last until you can obtain more. If you are using foam, cream, or jelly, you also need a plastic applicator. If you use foam, keep an extra full container on hand. You may not be able to tell when your current container is running low.

2. **Read the package instructions** to be sure you understand the time rules for your product.

3. **Plan ahead about when to insert your method.** Try to find a routine that is comfortable for you. Foam is effective immediately. If you are using suppositories, cream, jelly or film, a waiting period between insertion and intercourse is essential to allow the product to melt and spread inside your vagina. The package instructions explain the exact time required. One dose of spermicide remains effective for 1 hour. If a longer time has passed, or if you have intercourse again, you must use a new dose of spermicide.

For Insertion

1. Wash your hands carefully with soap and water.

2. **Foam.** Shake the foam container vigorously at least 20 times then use the nozzle to fill the plastic applicator.
   Jelly or cream. Fill the applicator by squeezing the spermicide tube. Next insert the applicator into your vagina as far as it will comfortably go; then, holding the applicator still, push the plunger to release the foam, cream, or jelly. The spermicide should be deep in your vagina, close to your cervix.
   Suppository. Remove the wrapping and slide the suppository into your vagina. Push it along the back wall of your vagina as far as you can so that it rests on or near your cervix.
   Film. Be sure your fingers are completely dry. Place one sheet of film on your finger tip and slide it along the back wall of your vagina as far as you can so the film rests on or near your cervix.

3. **Repeated intercourse.** Apply a new application of spermicide each time you have intercourse. Alternatively, you can switch to condoms for repeated intercourse if you wish.

4. **After intercourse.** Leave spermicide in place for at least 6–8 hours after intercourse; do not douche or rinse your vagina. Douching later is not recommended, but if you choose to douche you must wait at least 6–8 hours.

Caring for Spermicide Supplies

1. Store your spermicide in a convenient location that is clean, cool, and dark.

2. Wash your spermicide inserter after each use with plain soap and warm water. Do not use talcum powder on your inserter.

REFERENCES

1. Alexander NJ. In: Alexander NJ, Gabelnick HL, Spieler JM. Heterosexual Transmission of AIDS. New York, NY:Wiley-Liss Publishers, 1990.

2. Anonymous. Vaginal spermicides. Med Let Drugs Ther 1986;5:13-16

3. Benes S, McCormack WM. Inhibition of growth of *Chlamydia trachomatis* by nonoxynol-9 in vitro. Antimicrob Agents Chemother 1985;27:724-726.

4. Celentano DD, Klassen AC, Weisman CS, Rosenshein NB. The role of contraceptive use in cervical cancer: the Maryland Cervical Cancer Case-Control Study. Am J Epidemiol 1987;126(4):592-604.

5. Cramer DW, Goldman MB, Schiff I, Belisk S, Albrecht B, Stadel B, Gibson M, Wilson E, Stillman R, Thompson I. The relationship of tubal infertility to barrier method and oral contraceptive use. JAMA 1987;257(18):2446-2450.

6. Einarson TR, Koren G, Mattice D, Schechter-Tsafriri O. Maternal spermicide use and adverse reproductive outcome: a meta-analysis. Am J Obstet Gynecol 1990;162(3):655-660.

7. Elias CJ, Heise L. The development of microbicides: a new method of HIV prevention for women. The Population Council, Working Papers, No.6, 1993. The Population Council, One Dag Hammarskjold Plaza, New York, NY 10017.

8. FDA. Data do not support association between spermicides, birth defects. FDA Drug Bulletin 1986;11:21.

9. Feldblum PJ, Fortney JA. Condoms, spermicides, and the transmission of human immunodeficiency virus: a review of the literature. Am J Publ Health 1988;78(1):52-54.

10. Feldblum P. Efficacy of spermicide use and condom use by HIV-discordant couples in Zambia. (Abstract No. WeC 1085). VIII International Conference on AIDS. Amsterdam, The Netherlands, 1992.

11. Hong CY, Shieh CC, Wu P, Chiang BN. The spermicidal potency of Coca-Cola and Pepsi-Cola. Hum Toxicol 1987;6(5):395-396.

12. Hooton TM, Fennell CL, Clark AM, Stamm WE. Nonoxynol-9: differential antibacterial activity and enhancement of bacterial adherence to vaginal epithelial cells. J Infect Dis 1991;164:1216-1219.

13. Huggins G, Vessey M, Flavel R, Yeates D, PcPherson K. Vaginal spermicides and outcome of pregnancy: findings in a large cohort study. Contraception 1982;25(3):219-230.

14. Jick H, Walker AM, Rothman KJ, Hunter J, Holmes LB, Watkins RN, Dewart DC, Danford A, Madsen S. Vaginal spermicides and congenital disorders. JAMA 1981;245(13):1329-1332.

15. Jick H, Hannan MT, Stergachis A, Heidrich F, Perera DR, Rothman KJ. Vaginal spermicides and gonorrhea. JAMA 1982;248(13):1619-1621.

16. Kelly JP, Reynolds RB, Stagno S, Louv WC, Alexander WJ. In vitro activity of the spermicide nonoxynol-9 against *Chlamydia trachomatis*. Antimicrob Agents Chemother 1985;27(5):760-762.

17. Kestelman P, Trussell J. Efficacy of the simultaneous use of condoms and spermicides. Fam Plann Perspect 1991;23(5):226-227,232.

18. Klebanoff SJ. Effects of the spermicidal agent nonoxynol-9 on vaginal microbial flora. J Infect Dis 1992;165(1):19-25.

19. Kreiss J, Ngugi E, Holmes K, Ndinya-Achola J, Waiyaki P, Roberts PL, Ruminjo I, Sajabi R, Kimata J, Fleming TR, Anzala A, Holton D, Plummer F. Efficacy of nonoxynol-9 contraceptive sponge use in preventing heterosexual acquisition of HIV in Nairobi prostitutes. JAMA 1992;268(4):477-482.
20. Levy JA. The transmission of AIDS: the case of the infected cell. JAMA 1988;259(20):3037-3038.
21. Liskin L, Blackburn R, Maier JH. AIDS—a public health crisis. Popul Rep 1986;Series L(6).
22. Louv WC, Austin H, Alexander WJ, Stagno S, Cheeks J. A clinical trial of nonoxynol-9 for preventing gonococcal and chlamydial infections. J Inf Dis 1988;158(3):518-523.
23. McGroarty JA, Soboh F, Bruce AW, Reid G. The spermicidal compound nonoxynol-9 increases adhesion of *Candida* species to human epithelial cells in vitro. Infect Immun 1990;58(6):2005-2007.
24. Niruthisard S, Roddy RE, Chutivongse S. The effects of frequent nonoxynol-9 use on the vaginal and cervical mucosa. Sex Transm Dis 1991;18(3):176-179.
25. Peters RK, Thomas D, Hagan DG, Mack TM, Henderson BE. Risk factors for invasive cervical cancer among Latinas and non-Latinas in Los Angeles County. JNCI 1986;77(5):1063-1077.
26. Rekart M. The toxicity and local effects of the spermicide nonoxynol-9. J Acq Immuno Def Syn 1992;5(4):425-426.
27. Rosenberg MJ, Davidson AJ, Chen JH, Judson FN, Douglas JM. Barrier contraceptives and sexually transmitted diseases in women: a comparison of female-dependent methods and condoms. Am J Publ Health 1992;82(5):669-674.
28. Rosenberg MJ, Gollub EL. Commentary: methods women can use that may prevent sexually transmitted disease, including HIV. Am J Public Health. 1992;82(11):1473-1478.
29. Rosenberg MJ, Rojanapithayakorn W, Feldblum PJ, Higgins JE. Effect of the contraceptive sponge on chlamydial infection, gonorrhea, and candidiasis: a comparative clinical trial. JAMA 1987;257(17):2308-2312.
30. Rothman M. Spermicide use and Down's syndrome. Am J Publ Health 1982;72(4):399-401.
31. Simpson JL, Phillips OP. Spermicides, hormonal contraception and congenital malformations. Adv Contracept 1990;6(3):141-167.
32. Stone KM, Grimes DA, Magder LS. Personal protection against sexually transmitted diseases. Am J Obstet Gynecol 1986;155(1):180-188.
33. Strobino B, Kline J, Warburton D. Spermicide use and pregnancy outcome. AJPH 1988;78(3):260-263.
34. Voeller B. Spermicides for controlling the spread of HIV. AIDS 1992;6(3):341-342.
35. Voeller B, Anderson DJ. pH and related factors in the urogenital tract and rectum that affect HIV-1 transmission. Mariposa Occasional Paper #16. Topanga CA: The Mariposa Education and Research Foundation, 1992.
36. Wasserheit JN. Epidemiological synergy: interrelationships between human immunodeficiency virus infection and other sexually transmitted diseases. Sex Transm Dis 1992;19(2)61-77.
37. Zenkeng L. HIV infection and barrier contraceptive use among high risk women in Cameroon. Paper presented at the International Society for Sexually Transmitted Disease Research: Banff, Canada. October, 1991.

9

The Diaphragm, Contraceptive Sponge, Cervical Cap, & Female Condom

- Vaginal barriers are simple to use and non-invasive.
- Women who use a diaphragm, sponges, spermicides, or male condoms have reduced risks for gonorrhea and chlamydia, and for serious sequelae including pelvic inflammatory disease and ectopic pregnancy. For diaphragm users and for spermicide users, a reduced risk for cervical neoplasia also is documented. It is likely that female condoms also provide protection against infection.

- The impact of vaginal barriers on HIV risk is not known. When HIV risk is a consideration, abstinence is the safest choice, and using latex male condoms can reduce risk.
- Unlike male condoms or spermicide, a woman can use a vaginal barrier without the direct cooperation of her partner, and correct use does not require an interruption in lovemaking.
- Consistent and correct use is essential for success with vaginal barrier methods; most failures occur because the method is not used.

Vaginal contraceptives have been used since antiquity, with natural sea sponges probably among the most ancient. In 1983, the FDA approved the vaginal contraceptive sponge for use in the United States.

When Margaret Sanger and Emma Goldman visited Europe in the early 1900s, they found a wide variety of cap and diaphragm models. The diaphragm soon became "the" modern contraceptive method in the United States In 1925, Sanger's husband established Holland Rantos, the first U.S. diaphragm manufacturer.[8] Except for improvements in spermicides used with it, diaphragm technology changed little during its first 60 years in the

United States. The most recent development was the 1983 introduction of a new model, the wide-seal style. This product features a soft latex flange attached to the inner side of the rim, intended to create a better seal with the vaginal wall.

Compared with the diaphragm, the cap has been less widely known in the United States. Caps used earlier in this century were made of silver, copper, or more recently, of impermeable plastic. Inserted and removed by the woman's physician, they were left in place for as long as 3–4 weeks. These have been replaced by latex caps now manufactured in England. In 1977, after the Food and Drug Administration (FDA) gained jurisdiction over medical devices, cap importation from England was temporarily restricted to centers participating in FDA-approved research. A study comparing the experience of 581 cap users with 572 diaphragm users, concluded that both methods provide equivalent contraceptive protection.[3] Based on the results of this research, the Prentif cavity-rim cervical cap was approved by the FDA in 1988 for general use in the United States.

The first female condom, called Reality, was approved by the FDA in 1993 for over-the-counter sale in the United States. Its approval, after more than 5 years of review and negotiation with the FDA, was based on results of a multi-center study designed to evaluate contraceptive efficacy. For ethical reasons, women at risk for STD were not included in the trial, so study results provide only indirect evidence of its likely efficacy in reducing STD risk. Its design and physical properties, however, are appropriate to the task. The same device, manufactured in England, has been approved and marketed in Switzerland, Austria, The Netherlands, and the United Kingdom, as Femidom, and also has been approved for sale in Canada.

MECHANISM OF ACTION

The female condom provides a physical barrier that lines the vagina entirely and partially shields the perineum. The other vaginal barriers combine two contraceptive mechanisms: a physical barrier to shield the cervix and a chemical to kill sperm. The presence of the device also may help to hold spermicide in place against the cervix, and in the case of the sponge, absorb and trap sperm.

VAGINAL BARRIER OPTIONS

Female condom. The Reality Female Condom is a thin (0.05 mm) polyurethane sheath, 7.8 cm in diameter and 17 cm long. The soft, loose-fitting sheath contains two flexible polyurethane rings. One ring lies inside, at the closed end of the sheath, and serves as an insertion mechanism and internal anchor. The other ring forms the external, open edge of the device and remains outside the vagina after insertion (see Figure 9-1). The external

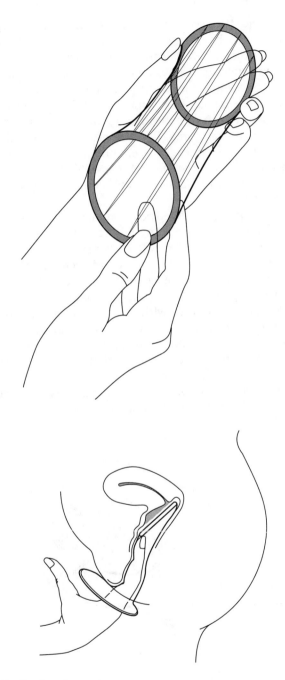

Figure 9-1 Reality female condom

Mechanism of Action   **193**

portion of the device thus covers part of the perineum and provides protection to the labia and the base of the penis during intercourse. The sheath is pre-lubricated on the inside with a silicone-based lubricant. Additional lubricant is provided with the device. Reality, approved for over-the-counter sale without prescription, is intended for one-time use. It does not contain spermicide and should not be used in conjunction with use of a latex male condom.

The polyurethane used in the sheath is a soft, impermeable material with good heat-transfer characteristics. It is stronger than latex and less likely to tear or break. It is not susceptible to deterioration with exposure to oil-based products and is less susceptible than latex to deterioration during storage.

Product labeling specifies that the female condom can be inserted up to 8 hours before intercourse.

Contraceptive sponge. The Today vaginal contraceptive sponge is a small, pillow-shaped polyurethane sponge that contains 1 gram of nonoxynol-9 spermicide. The Today Sponge has a concave dimple on one side that is intended to fit over the cervix and decrease the chance of dislodgement during intercourse (see Figure 9-2). The other side of the sponge incorporates a woven polyester loop to facilitate removal. The sponge is available in one size, over-the-counter, without prescription. It is moistened with tap water prior to use and inserted deep into the vagina.

The sponge provides continuous protection for up to 24 hours, no matter how many times intercourse occurs. After intercourse, the sponge must be left in place for at least 6 hours before it is removed and discarded. Wearing the sponge for longer than 24–30 hours is not recommended because of the possible risk of toxic shock syndrome.

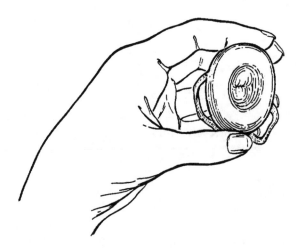

Figure 9-2 Contraceptive sponge

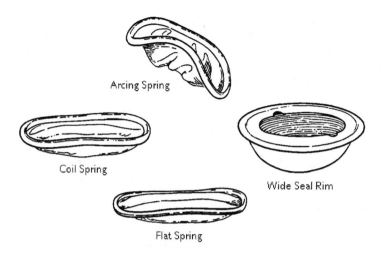

Arcing Spring

Coil Spring

Wide Seal Rim

Flat Spring

Figure 9-3 Types of diaphragms

Diaphragm. This dome-shaped rubber cup has a flexible rim; it is inserted into the vagina before intercourse so that the posterior rim rests in the posterior fornix and the anterior rim fits snugly behind the pubic bone. The dome of the diaphragm covers the cervix; spermicidal cream or jelly applied to the dome before insertion is held in place near the surface of the cervix. Diaphragm purchase requires a prescription.

Once in position, the diaphragm provides effective contraceptive protection for 6 hours. If a longer interval has elapsed, insertion of additional, fresh spermicide with an applicator (without removing the diaphragm) is recommended. Labeling for contraceptive jelly and cream also recommends an additional applicator-full of spermicide whenever intercourse is repeated. After intercourse, the diaphragm must be left in place for at least 6 hours. Wearing it for longer than 24 hours is not recommended because of the possible risk of toxic shock syndrome.

Diaphragms are available in sizes ranging from 50 to 95 (diameter in mm) and in several styles (see Figure 9-3). Styles differ in the inner construction of the circular rim, and in the case of the wide-seal style, the presence of a flexible flange attached to the inner edge of the rim. The thin, flat spring rim has a gentle spring strength that is comfortable for women with very firm vaginal muscle tone. The sturdy coil spring rim has a firm spring strength suitable for a woman with average muscle tone and an average pubic arch depth. A plastic diaphragm introducer can be used with coil or flat spring styles. The very sturdy and firm arcing spring folds into an arc shape that facilitates correct insertion; it can maintain correct position despite lax muscle. Wide-seal diaphragms are available with either an arcing spring rim or a coil spring rim.

Cervical Cap. The Prentif Cavity Rim Cervical Cap is a deep, soft rubber cup with a firm round rim (see Figure 9-4). A groove along the inner circumference of the rim improves the seal between the inner rim of the cap and the surface of the cervix. The Prentif cap fits with its rim snugly around the base of the cervix, close to the junction between the cervix and the vaginal fornices. Spermicide, used to fill the dome 1/3 full prior to insertion of the cap, is held in place against the cervix until the cap is removed.

The Prentif cap provides continuous protection for 48 hours, no matter how many times intercourse occurs. Additional spermicide is not necessary for repeated intercourse. Because of the possible risk of toxic shock syndrome, also wearing it for longer than 48 hours is not recommended. Some women experience odor problems with prolonged use.

Future barrier devices. Several new vaginal barrier devices are on the horizon. Disposable, single-use diaphragms, packaged with spermicide, could offer helpful convenience with little additional development or research required. A hat-shaped silicone rubber cap called FemCap, and an oval silicone rubber device called Lea's shield, have shown initial success in contraceptive efficacy testing. Other cap devices made of polymers that release spermicide are also being developed, as are modifications of the contraceptive sponge. A sponge with a spermicide other than nonoxynol-9, or a combination of spermicide and germicide, could have significant advantages, especially as STD protection becomes increasingly important.

BARRIER METHOD DIFFERENCES

Vaginal barriers differ somewhat in efficacy (see following section) and also differ in rules for their use. These differences may make one option or another easier or more appealing for a specific woman. Since consistent use is so important for success with vaginal barriers, a comfortable match between the method and the woman's personal needs and sexual patterns may improve efficacy. For example, a woman whose life involves sexual intimacy only on weekends may find the diaphragm method cumbersome because of the need for extra spermicide with repeated intercourse and the 24-hour recommended time

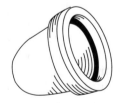

Prentif Cavity Rim Cervical Cap

Figure 9-4 Cervical cap

limit. For her, a cap or a sponge that can be left in place with no additional spermicide required may be easier to use correctly. Similarly, the necessity to wash and store a diaphragm or cap and to have a tube of spermicide available may be cumbersome for a women who is not at her own home.

A woman who finds spermicide irritating or does not like the messiness of other vaginal barriers may prefer the female condom. Also, unlike other vaginal barrier methods, the female condom prevents contact between semen and the vagina. Its use does not require the precise timing in relation to erection and intercourse that is necessary with male condoms, so some couples may find the female condom easier to use or that it involves less interruption in lovemaking.

Origins of barrier use rules. Rules for use of vaginal barrier methods (Table 9-1) are based on decisions by FDA and device manufacturers. They have attempted to balance concerns about possible toxic shock syndrome (TSS) risk, the need to assure good inherent spermicide efficacy, and the need to make the method convenient for users. The research basis for these rules is woefully inadequate. For example, how duration of wear may influence TSS risk is not known. No data exist for specifying a safe duration, or for prohibiting an unsafe duration of wear. Similarly, optimal spermicide dose and concentration, as well as duration of spermicide efficacy, are unknown. Whether an extra application of spermicide for repeated intercourse improves efficacy for diaphragm users is not known.

The official rules also do not necessarily replicate the protocol rules used in efficacy studies that were the basis for the FDA approval process. In the cap/diaphragm study, for example, use instructions allowed cap wear for as long as 3 days (72 hours).[3] Most women in the study, however, reported actual wear of less than 40 hours, so the reviewers decided that cap efficacy with longer wear had not been documented, and a 48-hour maximum was chosen for the labeling.

STD risk. Methods that are managed by women may be more effective than condoms in relation to STD prevention when use efficacy is considered.[37] Some studies that have compared STD risks for women who rely on condom use with the risks for vaginal barrier users have found lower risk among barrier users.[37] Presumably, the greater theoretical protection against STDs afforded by condom use was more than balanced in these studies by better use-effectiveness of vaginal barriers in actual practice. The fact that these methods can be entirely managed by the woman no doubt makes them more efficacious than condoms in some circumstances. Carefully consider how to make these methods as easy and as pleasant as possible to use so use is optimal. Because of the possibility that spermicide irritation may adversely affect susceptibility to HIV transmission, providing adequate, but not excessive, spermicide is prudent (see Disadvantages and Cautions section later in this chapter).

Table 9-1 Vaginal barrier methods–rules for use

	Diaphragm	Cap	Sponge	Female Condom
Pelvic Exam Required for Fitting	Yes	Yes	No	No
Spermicide Needed	Yes	Yes	Yes	No
Spermicide Supplies Needed with Insertion	Yes	Yes	No	No
Additional Spermicide Needed for Repeated Intercourse	Yes	No	No	No
Supplies Needed to Add Spermicide After Initial Insertion	Yes	No	No	No
Equipment Needed for Storage After Use	Yes	Yes	No	No
Can Be Used During Menses	Yes	No	No	Yes
Duration of Protection After Insertion	6 hours	48 hours	24 hours	8 hours
Longest Wear Recommended	24 hours	48 hours	30 hours	8 hours

E FFECTIVENESS

For nulliparous women, the female condom, diaphragm, cervical cap, and sponge all provide similar contraceptive efficacy during typical use; with perfect use, the female condom and diaphragm are somewhat more effective than the cap or sponge. For parous women, the sponge and the cap are substantially less effective than the diaphragm or female condom (see Table 9-2).[48]

Efficacy and diligence. Reanalysis of data from two, randomized studies[3,11] has provided new information on failure rates during perfect use (*i.e.,* both consistent and correct) for the sponge, diaphragm, and cap.[47] This information is especially helpful for a woman who is deciding among contraceptive options. To make an informed choice, she needs to understand what correct use of the method requires, and what success she can expect if she is able to use it consistently and correctly.

In most studies of vaginal barrier efficacy, approximately half of the women who conceived reported that their pregnancy occurred in a context of misuse. *The other half experienced method failure despite correct use.* From 5%–9% of nulliparous users and from 5%–26% of parous users of these methods will become pregnant during the first year of perfect use. So it is misleading to teach patients that all conscientious barrier users can achieve excellent success. The difference between low failure rates reported in some studies and high rates reported in others is not accounted for entirely by patient diligence. The wide range reflects the profound effect of differences

Table 9-2 First-year failure rates* for women using vaginal barrier methods

Method (1)	% of Women Experiencing an Accidental Pregnancy Within the First Year of Use		% of Women Continuing Use at One Year (4)
	Typical Use (2)	Perfect Use (3)	
Cap			
Parous Women	36	26	45
Nulliparous Women	18	9	58
Sponge			
Parous Women	36	20	45
Nulliparous Women	18	9	58
Female Condom	21	5	56
Diaphragm	18	6	58

*See Table 5.2 for first-year failure rates of all methods.

Emergency Contraceptive Pills: Treatment initiated within 72 hours after unprotected intercourse reduces the risk of pregnancy by at least 75%.

between study populations in fertility characteristics as well as in patient compliance. Differences in study design and analysis methods also are important factors.

Efficacy and fertility characteristics. A woman who uses a diaphragm with typical diligence but has characteristics associated with high fertility, such as age less than 25 years and frequent intercourse (three times weekly or more), is more likely to experience contraceptive failure than is the average woman. In effect, the failure rate for her is greater than the 18% overall "typical-user" rate for the diaphragm. On the other hand, citing an 18% failure rate significantly overestimates the pregnancy risk for a 30-year-old diaphragm user who has intercourse less often. Available research data are limited, but they do show that the effect of such factors is substantial. For example, in the diaphragm/cap comparison study, women who used the diaphragm consistently, and had intercourse three times weekly or more, were almost three times as likely to experience failure compared to women who had intercourse less than three times weekly (see Table 9-3).

Efficacy and research design. Because it is so often cited as evidence that conscientious diaphragm users can achieve highly effective contraceptive protection, the 1976 study by Lane et al., deserves special comment.[26] Lane reported an overall failure rate of 2.1% for 2,168 women using the diaphragm for 1 year. At the time this rate was calculated, however, the accepted procedures for data analysis were somewhat different than those used

Table 9-3 Intercourse frequency and diaphragm failure

	Contraceptive Failure Within One Year (%)
Consistent diaphragm user Intercourse less than 3 times weekly	3.4
Consistent diaphragm user Intercourse 3 times weekly or more	9.7

Source: Trussell et al., (1993).

in more recent studies. Subjects who were no more than 2 months late for a follow-up visit were assumed to be continuing, successful users. Consequently, up to 14 months of successful diaphragm use were counted for women who had been enrolled in the study and were no more than 2 months late for their follow-up visit (a 1-year visit) when the study ended. Data analysis procedures used in more recent studies would have credited months of successful use only for patients who actually did return for follow-up. Using current analysis methods, Lane would have reported a substantially higher failure rate.

THE CLINICIAN'S ROLE IN BARRIER EFFICACY

The clinician can play an important role in helping women to decide wisely about vaginal barrier methods and use them successfully:

1. Help the woman assess her own risk of failure. If her risk is low, do not discourage her confidence in vaginal barriers. If her risk is high, however, a vaginal barrier may not be a wise solo method choice. Characteristics that may be associated with higher than average risk of failure include:
   - Frequent intercourse (three times or more weekly)
   - Age less than 30 years
   - Personal style or sexual patterns that make consistent use difficult
   - Previous contraceptive failure (any method)
   - Ambivalent feelings (patient or partner) about the current desirability of pregnancy
   - Intention to delay (rather than prevent) next pregnancy[40]
2. Help the woman assess her risk of STD exposure. If the risk is high, she needs to know that abstinence is the safest option. Encourage her to use condoms along with her diaphragm, sponge, or cap if possible. (Female condoms should not be used simultaneously with male condoms because the two condoms may stick together.)
3. If unintended pregnancy would be personally devastating for the woman, or if she is at high risk for vaginal barrier failure, encourage

her to consider using a combination of methods such as a diaphragm, sponge, or cap plus male condoms or oral contraceptives along with any of the vaginal barriers.

4. Be sure that every vaginal barrier user has an accurate understanding of ovulation timing and knows that high-risk days for conception begin approximately 4 days before ovulation.

5. Be sure that every vaginal barrier user is aware of emergency, post-coital treatment and knows how to obtain it if a contraceptive emergency arises. If possible, provide her with a kit, containing an instruction sheet and a supply of oral contraceptive pills sufficient for one or more emergency treatment regimens (see Chapter 16).

6. If a user becomes pregnant, help her determine whether incorrect use or method failure was the culprit. In many cases women assume that incorrect use was responsible when in fact it was not (*i.e.,* estimated pregnancy duration does not match the date of unprotected intercourse). A woman who has one method failure (any method) is probably at high risk for a method failure in the future and would be wise to consider using two methods simultaneously.

COST

The cost for obtaining a diaphragm or cap ranges from $50 to $150, depending on the fee for the necessary medical visit and device fitting. Purchase of a cap or diaphragm alone is approximately $22; replacement is recommended every 3 years. The only ongoing cost for these methods is for spermicide, which depends on intercourse frequency. Cream or jel cost is minimal, approximately $0.25 per application. Sponges cost $1.25 to $1.50 each. Reality female condoms cost $2.50 each.

ADVANTAGES AND INDICATIONS

Vaginal barrier methods have many advantages that make them reasonable both for temporary and for long-term contraception. Apart from STD risk, the overall medical safety of these methods, backed up by abortion in case of failure, is comparable to consistent use of condoms. They do not cause systemic side effects and do not alter a woman's hormone patterns. For many women, relying on a partner to use condoms is not a realistic option, so the fact that vaginal barrier methods do not require partner involvement in the decision to use them or in their implementation may be particularly important. For women who need contraception only intermittently, these methods are also attractive. A vaginal barrier can be available for immediate protection whenever needed, no matter how long the interval between uses. No doubt many pregnancies have been prevented because a woman had available a diaphragm, cap, or sponge obtained long before.

Potentially, the most important noncontraceptive benefit of vaginal barrier use is protection against spread of sexually transmitted diseases (STDs). Unfortunately, uncertainty about the affect of spermicide on HIV risk clouds this issue (see Chapter 8). Use of vaginal barrier methods with spermicide does

Table 9-4 STD protection with use of vaginal barrier methods

Reference[a]	STD Studied	Relative Risk (95% Confidence Interval)	
Rosenberg (1992)	Gonorrhea	0.35	(0.16–0.75)
Colorado STD Clinic*	Trichomoniasis	0.29	(0.15–0.58)
Diaphragm	Chlamydia	0.28	(0.05–1.54)
	Bacterial Vaginosis	0.99	(0.63–1.55)
Kjaer (1990)	Cervical HPV	1.00	(0.70–1.40)
Greenland and Denmark**	Herpes 2 Seropositivity	0.90	(0.60–1.30)
Condom or Diaphragm			
Magder (1988)	Gonorrhea	Protective (p < 0.001)	
Colorado STD Clinic	Chlamydia	0.00	(0.00–0.20)
Diaphragm**			
Cramer (1987)	Tubal Infertility	0.50	(0.30–0.70)
US Infertility Centers*			
Diaphragm			
Rosenberg (1987)	Gonorrhea	0.67	(0.42–1.07)
Thailand Prostitutes***	Chlamydia	0.31	(0.16–0.60)
Sponge			
Quinn (1985)	Gonorrhea	0.11	(0.08–0.17)
Tennessee STD Clinic***			
Diaphragm or Condom			
Austin (1984)	Gonorrhea	0.45	(0.12–1.67)
Alabama STD Clinic*			
Diaphragm			
Kelaghan (1982)	Pelvic Inflammatory	0.40	(0.20–0.70)
U.S. Hospitals*	Disease		
Diaphragm			
Berger (1975)	Gonorrhea	0.53	(0.18–1.59)
Louisiana Family			
Planning Clinic**			
Diaphragm or			
Condom, with Foam			

Source: Cates et al. (1992b).

* Case-control study; **Cross-sectional study, ***Randomized study

[a] Full reference listed in original article by Cates.

reduce risks for important STDs including gonorrhea and chlamydia infection, and also cervical neoplasia risk related to HPV infection (see Table 9-4). Studies of HIV risk, however, are contradictory. Some studies suggest a protective effect while others suggest that HIV risk could be increased for spermicide users (see Disadvantages and Cautions section). Women at risk for any STD are also at increased risk for HIV. So until the HIV risk issue is clarified, caution will be needed in making recommendations about vaginal barrier use when STD risk is a concern.

SEXUALLY TRANSMITTED DISEASE PROTECTION

The female condom lines the vagina completely, preventing contact between the penis and vagina. Semen is trapped within the condom and then discarded. Polyurethane is a well-known, widely used material. Medical examination gloves made of polyurethane, for example, have been used for many years. Polyurethane is strong and impermeable to organisms as small as the HIV virus.[10] In a study of postcoital leakage designed to detect pinholes and tears after actual condom use, 3.5% of male latex condoms showed leakage when tested after use compared with 0.6% of Reality condoms.[27] Unless the condom slips out of place or is torn, it should provide protection against STD exposure that is as least as good as that provided by latex male condoms. Research documentation, however, is not yet available to demonstrate STD protection for this new device.

With the exception of the female condom, available vaginal barrier methods all involve use of spermicide. Laboratory research shows that nonoxynol-9 is lethal to the organisms that cause gonorrhea, genital herpes, trichomoniasis, syphilis, and AIDS (see Chapter 8). Unfortunately nonoxynol-9's lethal effect on free organisms does not mean that infection risk is eliminated for couples who choose spermicide or vaginal barrier methods. The importance of consistent use is self-evident. Even if the products are used correctly, however, it is possible that they could fail to protect. Factors such as even dispersion of spermicide in the vagina, or thorough mixing of semen and vaginal fluids with the spermicide, may influence infection protection. Also, some organisms may be more difficult than others to eliminate. It is possible that intracellular organisms such as human immunodeficiency virus (HIV) may not be as susceptible to spermicide effects.[29] Spermicide use also may alter vaginal flora or acidity, which could affect HIV infectivity. Some researchers are concerned that vaginal irritation caused by nonoxynol-9 could increase HIV susceptibility (see Disadvantages and Cautions section).

Gonorrhea, chlamydia, trichomoniasis, and sequelae. For gonorrhea, chlamydia, and trichomoniasis, the degree of risk reduction with use of vaginal barrier methods differs in different studies. Some have found very effective protection, with infection risk for users reduced to only 10% of that faced by couples not using the method. In most studies, however, the reduction is less dramatic—overall perhaps a 50% reduction in risk.[37] Protection against STD consequences such as pelvic inflammatory disease (PID) and tubal infertility has also been documented for diaphragm users.[9,23] The magnitude of protection against PID is substantial; diaphragm users have about half the risk noncontraceptors face. In both the PID study and in the tubal infertility study, risk reduction was greatest when spermicide was used along with a mechanical barrier. Neither condoms used alone nor spermicide used alone provided protection comparable to the barrier/spermicide combination.[6]

Cervical neoplasia risk. Diaphragm use confers protection against cervical neoplasia. A lower risk of cervical dysplasia and/or cancer has been reported for women using the diaphragm as well as for condom users and spermicide users in several studies (see Table 9-5). Because cervical infection with certain strains of human papillomavirus has been implicated as an important factor in cervical neoplasia, the role of diaphragm use here may be similar to its protective effect against other STDs.

D ISADVANTAGES AND CAUTIONS

Few serious medical problems are associated with use of vaginal barriers, and most women are medically appropriate candidates for their use. Toxic shock syndrome and pregnancy complications in the aftermath of method failure are potentially life-threatening, but very rare. Increased susceptibility to acquiring HIV infection also would be a serious disadvantage, if this proves to be a consequence of spermicide-induced irritation.[24] Using vaginal barrier methods also increases the risk for urinary tract infection, bacterial vaginosis, and vaginal candidiasis. Concerns about Pap smear abnormalities, systemic effects, and exposure during pregnancy are discussed at the end of this section.

The following conditions may preclude satisfactory use or make vaginal barrier methods inadvisable:

1. Allergy to spermicide, rubber, latex, or polyurethane
2. Abnormalities in vaginal anatomy that interfere with satisfactory fit or stable placement of a sponge, diaphragm, or cap
3. Inability to learn correct insertion technique
4. History of toxic shock syndrome
5. (For the diaphragm) Repeated urinary tract infections that persist despite efforts to refit the diaphragm

Table 9-5 Contraceptive method and cervical neoplasia risk

Study and Method	Risk Estimate
	Relative Risk (RR) / Use of Barrier Method
Parazzini (1989)	(Condom or Diaphragm)
Never Used Barrier	1.0
Used Less Than 2 Years	0.86
Used 2 Years or More	0.57
Celentano (1987)	Odds Ratio / Ever Used Method
Oral Contraceptives	0.48
Diaphragm	0.29
Vaginal Spermicides	0.28
	Matched Risk / Duration of Use
Peters (1986)	(Use Less Than 2 Years = RR 1.0)
Oral Contraceptives, 2-9 Years	1.0
Oral Contraceptives, 10 Years or More	1.1
Diaphragm, 2-9 Years	0.7
Diaphragm, 10 Years or More	0.3
Spermicide Alone, 2-9 Alone	0.7
Spermicide Alone, 10 Years or More	0.2
Condoms, 2-9 Years	0.5
Condoms, 10 Years or More	0.4
Vessey (1978)	Neoplasia Incidence / 1,000 Woman-Years
All Women	0.73
Oral Contraceptives	0.95
IUD Users	0.87
Diaphragm Users	0.17

Sources: Celentano et al. (1987).
Parazzini et al. (1989).
Peters et al. (1986).
Vessey (1978).

6. (For the diaphragm and cap) Lack of trained personnel to fit the device and/or lack of clinical time to provide instruction in use

7. (For the cap and sponges) Full-term delivery within the past 6 weeks, recent spontaneous or induced abortion, or vaginal bleeding from any cause, including menstrual flow

8. (For the cap) Known or suspected cervical or uterine malignancy, an abnormal Pap smear result, or vaginal or cervical infection.

Common minor problems. Problems are not common with use of the female condom. Among 360 women in the efficacy study, one discontinued using the method because of vaginal discomfort and one because her partner experienced penile irritation.

The most common problem associated with the use of vaginal barriers that involve the concomitant use of spermicide is local skin irritation. Some patients are allergic or sensitive to nonoxynol-9, in which case changing to a spermicide product that contains octoxynol may be helpful. Some women have cramps, bladder pain, or rectal pain when wearing a diaphragm or cap, and partners occasionally report penile pain during intercourse. For diaphragm users, refitting with an alternative size or rim type resolves the problem in some cases.

Problems with sponge removal are fairly common. Some women have difficulty with vaginal dryness when they use a sponge. Foul odor and vaginal discharge are likely to occur if a diaphragm, cap, or sponge is inadvertently left in the vagina for more than a few days. Symptoms abate promptly when the device is removed. Rare cases of vaginal trauma, including abrasion and laceration, have been reported with use of the Prentif cap and the diaphragm.[3]

Spermicide irritation and HIV risk. Nonoxynol-9, a detergent, can cause local irritation on the surface of exposed vaginal and cervical tissue.[30,35] Irritation could adversely affect transmission risk, and results of some studies are worrisome. The rate of HIV seroconversion in a group of Nairobi prostitutes who used nonoxynol-9 sponges was higher than the rate for a comparison group using placebo suppositories.[24] Genital ulcers were also more common among the nonoxynol-9 users in the Nairobi study. In another study, vaginal irritation was observed among prostitutes in Vancouver who used nonoxynol-9 lubricated condoms.[35] Subjects in both of these studies had unusually high exposure to spermicide and to the trauma of intercourse. In other studies, however, results suggest a protective effect for nonoxynol-9 suppositories. Some evidence suggests that the occurrence of vaginal irritation may depend on the dose and/or frequency of exposure to spermicide.[13,16,51] So it is possible that nonoxynol-9 might be helpful rather than harmful in regard to HIV susceptibility when used under noncommercial, less extreme circumstances.[44] Nevertheless, further research is needed before it will be possible to determine how spermicide use, and therefore also vaginal barrier method use, affect HIV risk.[45]

Vaginal and urinary tract infections. Sexual intercourse is followed by increased vaginal colonization with *Escherichia coli*. The shift in vaginal flora is prolonged among women who use spermicide alone or in combination with condoms, and even more prolonged among diaphragm users, when compared with women using oral contraceptives.[20,38] This finding is of concern because bacterial vaginosis may be associated with increased risk for upper genital tract infection,[5] and because it may account for the increased risk of urinary tract infection (UTI) observed among diaphragm users.[17,18,50] The pressure a diaphragm rim places on the urethra also may contribute to the risk of developing UTI for some women.

Toxic shock syndrome. Toxic shock syndrome (TSS) is a rare but serious disorder caused by toxin(s) released by some strains of *Staphylococcus aureus* bacteria (see Chapter 20). Most TSS occurs in association with tampon use during menses; nonmenstrual TSS risk is increased for women who use vaginal barrier methods.[41] The overall health risks attributable to TSS, however, are very low. Two or three cases of TSS per year can be expected for every 100,000 women using vaginal barrier methods.[41] These cases would result in 0.18 death annually for every 100,000 vaginal barrier users, while complications of pregnancy that occur as a result of method failure would cause almost 10 times this many deaths (1.2 deaths per 100,000 users).

Nevertheless, patients using vaginal barriers need to be aware of the TSS danger signs, and instructions for using the method should be consistent with recommended TSS precautions.

Pap smear abnormalities. Pap smear abnormalities were an issue of special concern in the FDA's review of data for the Prentif cap. The cap/diaphragm comparison study, which was the basis for FDA approval of the device, found an unusually high incidence of abnormal Pap smears among both cap and diaphragm users.[3] Four percent of cap users and 2% of diaphragm users had Class I Pap results at the enrollment visit and Class III results at the 3-month follow-up visit. This difference was not statistically significant, but was of sufficient concern that the FDA mandated special Pap screening and surveillance for cap users. Cap product labeling requires normal Pap results before providing a cap, to exclude patients who may have evidence of HPV infection. A repeat Pap smear after 3 months of cap use is also recommended. If the 3-month Pap smear result is abnormal, cap use must be discontinued. If the Pap smear result is normal, annual testing thereafter is sufficient.[34]

A subsequent reanalysis of the cap/diaphragm study data found no statistically significant differences in Pap smear result distributions between the cap group and the diaphragm group either at 3 months or throughout the first year of use.[19] And other cap researchers have not found Pap smear problems. In the largest cap study, a much lower abnormal Pap rate was reported.[36] Among 1,835 cap users who had Pap smears repeated during the first 6 months of use, only 0.2% developed Class III abnormalities.

Protection against cervical neoplasia is an important benefit for diaphragm users (see earlier discussion).

Systemic effects and pregnancy exposure. No serious systemic side effects have been reported in association with human use of nonoxynol-9, although systemic effects following large doses have been reported in animal studies.[2] Safety concerns have centered on the issue of spermicide use during early pregnancy. Although studies in 1981 and 1982 suggested a possible link between spermicides and birth defects,[21,22,39] subsequent studies have not confirmed this finding. Experts in the field have concluded that no true association exists between spermicide use and fetal defects.[12,15,43,46]

PROVIDING VAGINAL BARRIER METHODS

Help the woman choose which of the available barrier options is most likely to meet her needs. For parous women, the diaphragm and female condom provide more effective contraceptive protection than the sponge or cap. For nulliparous women, the difference in efficacy is less striking. Female condoms or sponges do not require a fitting, or even a pelvic exam. If possible, however, the new user may benefit from an opportunity to insert her device and have its position verified by the clinician. Make sure that the woman does not have an unusual anatomic anomaly such as septate vagina or duplicate cervices that might make sponge use inadvisable. For a woman who wishes to use a diaphragm or cervical cap, select a device that fits well, or determine that a satisfactory fit is not possible so that the patient can choose another contraceptive method. Additional clinical tasks in providing a vaginal barrier method include:

1. Ensure that the patient is able to insert and remove her device correctly. Check placement and reaffirm the correct size after the patient herself has inserted her device.

2. Reinforce instructions for proper use, especially:
   - The importance of consistent, correct use
   - Rules for use of spermicide with the barrier chosen
   - The important of removing the female condom promptly and carefully after intercourse, or for women using a diaphragm, sponge, or cap, the importance of waiting at least 6 hours after intercourse before removing the device or douching.

3. Remind each user to watch for toxic shock syndrome danger signs (see Instructions for Patients section).

4. Discuss the possibility of using two methods such as condoms plus a sponge.

5. Teach each user to identify ovulation timing and her cycle days of maximal fertility: the midcycle week beginning four postcoital days before ovulation.

6. Confirm that the user is aware of emergency postcoital hormone treatment and knows how to obtain it. If possible, provide the barrier user with an instruction sheet and a supply of oral contraceptive pills sufficient for one or more emergency regimens. (See Chapter 16.)

Be sure that each patient has an opportunity to practice inserting and removing her device. Check the fit and placement after the patient has inserted it to verify that its position is correct and that the fit is good. Most patients find that inserting a cap is somewhat more difficult than inserting a diaphragm, and removal can be tricky. New cap users should try the cap initially while still using another method of birth control, such as condoms or oral contraceptives, to be sure that the cap remains in position after intercourse.

PRACTICAL CAUTION: AVOID OIL-BASED LUBRICANTS AND MEDICATIONS

Lubricants such as mineral oil, baby oil, suntan oil, vegetable oil, and butter; and vaginal medications such as Femstat cream, Monistat cream, estrogen cream, and Vagisil have a rapid, deleterious effect on latex.[1] Significant damage has been demonstrated for latex condoms exposed to such oil-based products. Their effects on diaphragm or cap integrity has not been studied, but it is reasonable to warn vaginal barrier users to avoid oil products. If additional lubrication is needed, a vaginal spermicide or a product intended for use with latex condoms would be reasonable options.

FITTING A DIAPHRAGM

Choosing a style to try. The first step in fitting a diaphragm is to select an initial diaphragm style (rim type) to try. Most women find that the arcing rim style is easier than the other rim styles to insert correctly; it is quite difficult to insert an arcing style incorrectly. The gentle spring strength of the coil and flat spring types, however, is often more comfortable, and these styles can be inserted with a diaphragm introducer (see Figure 9-5).

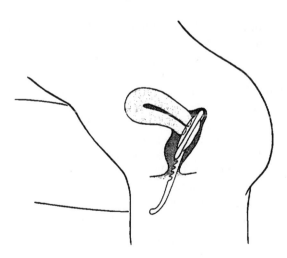

Figure 9-5 Some women prefer to use a plastic introducer for diaphragm insertion

Diaphragm manufacturers produce sets of fitting rings that are sample diaphragm rims with no dome. Whole diaphragms are preferable for fitting so that the patient can practice insertion and removal with the sample diaphragm. Fitting rings are not adequate for patient practice. Different products differ somewhat in rim spring strength, so prescribe precisely the same brand and rim type as was used in fitting. Coil and arcing diaphragms are widely available. Flat spring diaphragms may not be stocked in all drugstores, however, and wide-seal diaphragms are distributed directly to physicians and clinics. Products available are:

Flat Spring Rim: This diaphragm has a thin, delicate rim with gentle spring strength and is intended for a woman with a very firm vaginal muscle tone (nulliparous) or a shallow notch behind the pubic bone. The flat spring folds flat for insertion. Products available: Ortho-White Diaphragm, sizes 55-95, latex.

Coil Spring Rim: The coil spring has a sturdy rim with a firm spring strength intended for women with average vaginal muscle tone and average pubic arch notch. It folds flat for insertion. Products available: Koromex Diaphragm, sizes 50-95, latex; Ortho Diaphragm (coil spring), sizes 50-95, latex; and Ramses Flexible Cushioned Diaphragm (coil spring), sizes 50-95, gum rubber.

Arcing Spring Rim: This diaphragm has a very sturdy rim with firm spring strength. Most women are able to use the arcing rim comfortably. It can often be used despite a rectocele and/or a cystocele or lax vaginal muscle tone. Products available: Koroflex Diaphragm, sizes 60-95, latex; Allflex Diaphragm (Ortho), sizes 55-95, latex; and Ramses Bendex Diaphragm, sizes 65-95, gum rubber.

The Allflex (Ortho) arcing diaphragm folds at any point along its rim and is slightly less rigid than the Koroflex (Holland Rantos) or the Ramses Bendex (Schmid) products. The Koroflex and Bendex fold at two points only (a hinge or bow-bend construction). Many women find that the bow-bend rim is easier to insert because the fold compresses to a narrow leading edge and the two stiff halves of the arc can be held in the folded position close to either end of the arc, whereas the Allflex must be held in the middle.

Wide-seal Rim: The wide-seal rim has a flexible flange approximately 1.5 cm wide attached to the inner edge of the rim of this diaphragm. The flange is intended to hold spermicide in place inside the diaphragm and to create a better seal between the diaphragm and the vaginal wall. Wide-seal diaphragms are available in two different rim styles, arcing and coil spring. The arcing model folds at two points (bow-bend) but is similar in rigidity to the lighter Allflex arcing spring. The coil spring model folds at any point on the rim, but because of the inner flange, assumes a slight arc shape unlike other coil spring diaphragms that are flat when folded. Products available: Milex Wide-seal arcing diaphragm, sizes 60-95, latex; and Milex Wide-seal Omniflex coil spring diaphragm, sizes 60-95, latex.

Choosing a diaphragm size. To estimate the diaphragm size that will be needed:

1. Insert your index and middle fingers into the vagina until your middle finger reaches the posterior wall of the vagina.
2. Use the tip of your thumb to mark the point at which your index finger touches the pubic bone.
3. Extract your fingers.
4. Place the diaphragm rim on the tip of your middle finger. The opposite rim should lie just in front of your thumb.

Insert a sample diaphragm of the size you have selected into correct position in the patient's vagina. The device should rest snugly in the vagina, its rim in contact with the lateral walls and posterior fornix, but without tension against the vaginal walls. There should be just enough space to insert one finger tip comfortably between the inside of the pubic arch and the anterior edge of the diaphragm rim.

Choose the largest rim size that is comfortable for the patient. Try more than one rim size or type before making a final selection. Do not choose a size that is too small, because vaginal depth increases during sexual arousal (3-5 cm in nulliparous women), and a too-small diaphragm may fail to maintain its position covering the cervix. A diaphragm that is too large, however, may cause vaginal pressure, abdominal pain or cramping, or vaginal ulceration, and may be a factor in recurrent urinary tract infection.

FITTING A CERVICAL CAP

Prentif Cavity-Rim cervical caps are available in sizes 22 mm, 25 mm, 28 mm, and 31 mm (internal rim diameter). They are manufactured by Lamberts (Dalston) Ltd. in Luton, England, and can be purchased from the U.S. distributor: Cervical Cap Ltd., P.O. Box 38003-292, Los Gatos, California 95031.

Because of variations in normal anatomy and the limited number of cap sizes available, it will not be possible to fit every patient properly. Factors such as average parity in each patient population affect the frequency of fitting problems; 6%–10% of subjects could not be fitted in the large U.S. cap studies.[3,36]

When a Prentif cap is fitted correctly, the inner diameter of the cap rim must be almost identical to, or just a few millimeters larger than, the diameter of the base of the cervix. The rim forms a seal with the cervical surface that helps maintain the cap's position. The rim should rest at the base of the cervix so that the vaginal walls surround the outer side of the rim. The cervix should be completely covered. The dome of the cap should be deep enough so that it does not rest on the cervical os.

A Prentif cap that is too tight can cause cervical trauma, and one that is too loose or fails to make a secure seal over the entire circumference of the cervix, will be more likely to dislodge. Dislodgement during intercourse is also more likely if, during thrusting, the penis bumps the cap's side or rim rather than the dome. For this reason, a woman whose uterus is acutely ante-flexed, so that her cervical portio faces downward toward the back of her vagina, may find that her cap dislodges.

Estimating cap size. Perform a bimanual exam to determine the position and size of the uterus and cervix. Next, inspect the woman's cervix to estimate the proper cap size. The cervix must be fairly symmetrical, without extensive laceration or scarring that could interfere with uniform contact between the cap rim and cervix around its full diameter. The cervix must also be long enough to accommodate the height of the cap. A cervix that is flush or partially flush with the vaginal vault cannot be fit with the Prentif cap. Try two or more cap sizes to determine the fit.

Inserting, checking, and removing a cap. To insert the cap, fold the rim and compress the cap dome so that when it is released in place over the cervix, the unfolding dome can create suction between the rim of the cap and the cervix. After inserting the cap, check it with one finger around its entire circumference to be sure that no gaps occur between the cap rim and the cervix. Next the check stability by noting its resistance to dislodgement when the cap and cervix are probed with a finger tip.

Check for evidence of suction after the cap has been in place for a minute or two. Pinch the cap dome and tug gently. The dome should remain collapsed, and the cap should resist the tug and not slide off easily. Finally, try to rotate the cap in place on the cervix. If it does not rotate at all, it is too tight; if it rotates too easily or comes off the cervix, it is too large. To be considered a good fit, the cap must cover the cervix completely, with no gaps between the rim and the cervix. It must have good suction and not dislodge easily when the dome is probed with a finger tip.[8]

To remove the cap, probe the rim with the end of your index finger; tip the cap rim to break the seal, then gently pull the cap down and out.

DISINFECTING DIAPHRAGM AND CAP FITTING SAMPLES

Scrupulously attend to hygiene when fitting sample diaphragms and caps, as well as when cleaning and disinfecting them after each patient use. Wash devices used for fitting with soap and water and then immerse them in an alcohol solution (70% isopropanol or 80% ethanol) for at least 20 minutes after each use.[28] Alcohol reliably kills bacterial pathogens as well as some viruses, including those responsible for hepatitis and AIDS. Chlorine bleach solution (1 part bleach to 3 parts water), another effective antibacterial and antiviral agent, is recommended for disinfection of caps.[34]

M ANAGING PROBLEMS AND FOLLOW-UP

FDA-approved patient labeling recommends a follow-up Pap smear after the first 3 months of cap use. Otherwise, women using vaginal barriers need no special follow-up. Labeling for the diaphragm recommends refitting at each annual exam, after weight gain or loss of 10 pounds or more, after abortion, and after full-term pregnancy.[31] Weight change does not commonly require a new diaphragm size, nor does abortion.[25] Women using vaginal barriers should be reminded to avoid wearing them for the last 2 or 3 days before routine exams, if possible, to provide optimal conditions for Pap screening.

When a barrier user returns for a routine exam, ask an open-ended question about how the method is working out. If the woman is finding it inconvenient or uncomfortable, offer her an opportunity to consider an alternative method. Refitting with a different size or rim style may also be helpful.

Problems caused by these methods may require clinical intervention. Recurrent vaginal or introital irritation, with no evidence of vaginal infection, may indicate allergy or sensitivity to spermicide or to latex. Recurrent urinary tract infection (UTI) may be associated with diaphragm use, and recurrent yeast infection or bacterial vaginosis with use of contraceptive sponges or a diaphragm.

If a diaphragm user experiences recurring UTIs, consider refitting with a smaller diaphragm size, alternative rim style, or with a cervical cap. If UTI problems persist despite these measures, changing to an alternative method of birth control may be advisable.

A vaginal barrier user who develops toxic shock syndrome (TSS) signs or symptoms requires urgent and intensive evaluation and treatment. Vaginal culture can confirm the presence of *Staphylococcus aureus*. Treat the patient with antibiotics, and follow her carefully. If her symptoms are severe, she may need hospitalization for surveillance. Since TSS risk is increased for a woman who has had TSS in the past, the woman should avoid use of vaginal barrier methods in the future.

I NSTRUCTIONS FOR BARRIER USERS

1. **Use your method every time you have intercourse.** Be sure that your sponge, or your diaphragm or cap with spermicidal cream or jelly, is in place before your partner's penis enters your vagina.

2. **If you are using a sponge, diaphragm, or cap, learn the danger signs for toxic shock syndrome** and watch for them. If you have a high fever and one or more of the danger signs, you may have early toxic shock syndrome. Remove the sponge, diaphragm, or cap and contact your clinician.

Toxic Shock Syndrome Danger Signs

Caution

- ■ Sudden high fever
- ■ Vomiting, diarrhea
- ■ Dizziness, faintness, weakness
- ■ Sore throat, aching muscles and joints
- ■ Rash (like a sunburn)

3. Wash your hands carefully with soap and water before inserting, checking, or removing your female condom, sponge, cap, or diaphragm. This precaution may reduce your risk for toxic shock syndrome and for other infections as well.

4. If you are having problems with vaginal or penile irritation, try a different spermicide product. If you have problems with recurring bladder infections or vaginal yeast infections, discuss these with your clinician.

5. If you feel unsure about the proper fit or placement of your diaphragm, cap, or sponge use male condoms until you see your clinician to be sure that your insertion technique is correct.

6. **Douching after intercourse is not recommended.** If you are using a diaphragm, sponge, or cap and choose to use a douche, wait at least 6 hours after intercourse to avoid washing away essential spermicide.

7. **You can use male condoms** along with your diaphragm, sponge, or cap if you wish. Using this combination, you will have extremely effective protection against pregnancy and sexually transmitted infection.

No conclusive studies show just how long spermicide is fully active or exactly how long the diaphragm, cap, or sponge must be left in place after intercourse. The most important thing is having your device in place, protecting your cervix—not in your drawer. So, if you need to vary the length of time you leave the device in place, do that rather than "take a chance" just once.

Before Intercourse

1. Check that you have all the supplies you need.
   - **Female condoms.** You need enough new, unopened condoms to last until you can obtain more.
   - **Sponges.** You need clean water and enough fresh, unopened sponges to last until you can obtain more. You may also need a supply of condoms to use instead of sponges if you have intercourse while you are having a menstrual period.

- **Diaphragm.** You need fresh spermicidal cream or jelly, a plastic applicator for inserting additional spermicide, and a diaphragm. Check your diaphragm to be sure it has no holes, cracks, or tears.
- **Cap.** You need fresh spermicidal cream or jelly and a cap. Check your cap to be sure it has no holes, cracks, or tears. You may also need a supply of condoms to use instead of your cap while you are having a menstrual period.

2. Plan ahead about when to insert your method. Try to find a routine that is comfortable for you.
   - **Female condoms.** You can insert the female condom for immediate protection just before intercourse or as long as 8 hours ahead of time if you prefer. It provides effective birth control protection for just one act of intercourse.
   - **Sponges.** You can insert the sponge for immediate protection just before intercourse, or ahead of time. It provides effective birth control protection for 24 hours, no matter how many times you have intercourse.
   - **Diaphragm.** The diaphragm may be inserted just before intercourse, or up to 6 hours beforehand.
   - **Cap.** The cap can be inserted just before intercourse, or ahead of time if you wish. Some cap experts recommend that you allow 30 minutes between insertion and intercourse, if possible, so that a good suction develops. The cap provides effective birth control protection for 48 hours, no matter how many times you have intercourse.

INSERTION

1. **Wash your hands carefully with soap and water.**
2. Insert your method carefully; it must be in the proper location in your vagina to be maximally effective.
   - **Female condom.** Remove the Reality condom from its package and check to be sure the inner ring is at the bottom, closed end of the pouch. Follow the directions for insertion in the package; the illustrations can help you. Hold the pouch with the open end hanging down. Use the thumb and middle finger of one hand to squeeze the inner ring into a narrow oval for insertion; place your index finger between your thumb and middle finger to guide the Reality during insertion. With your other hand, spread the lips of your vagina. Insert the inner ring and the pouch of Reality into the vaginal opening and with your index finger, push the inner ring with the pouch the rest of the way up into the vagina. The outside ring lies against the outer lips when Reality is in place; about 1 inch

of the open end will stay outside your body. Once the penis enters, the vagina will expand and the slack will decrease.

- **Sponges.** Remove the sponge from its package, moisten it with about 2 tablespoons of clean water, and squeeze it once. Then insert the sponge into the vagina and slide it along the back wall of the vagina until it rests against your cervix. The dimple side should face your cervix, with the loop away from your cervix. Check with your finger to be sure you can feel your cervix covered by the sponge.

- **Diaphragm.** First apply spermicidal jelly or cream. Hold the diaphragm with the dome down (like a cup). Squeeze the jelly or cream from the tube into the dome (use about 1 teaspoon); spread a little bit around the rim of the diaphragm with your finger. To insert the diaphragm hold it with the dome down (spermicide in the dome) and squeeze opposite sides of the rim together so that the diaphragm folds. Hold it folded in one hand between your thumb and fingers. Spread the opening of your vagina with your other hand, and insert the folded diaphragm into your vaginal canal. This can be done standing with one foot propped up (on the edge of a chair, a bathtub, or a toilet), squatting, or lying on your back.

Push the diaphragm downward and along the back wall of your vagina as far as it will go. Then tuck the front rim up along the roof of your vagina behind your pubic bone. Once it is in place properly, you should not be able to feel the diaphragm except, of course, with your fingers. If it is uncomfortable, then most likely it is not in the correct position; take it out and reinsert it.

After insertion, check placement. When correctly placed, the back rim of the diaphragm is below and behind the cervix, and the front edge of the rim is tucked up behind the pubic bone. Often you may not be able to feel the back rim. You should check to be sure that you can feel that your cervix is covered by the soft rubber dome of the diaphragm and that the front rim is snugly in place behind your pubic bone. The spermicidal cream (inside the dome of the diaphragm) should be next to your cervix.

- **Cap.** Before insertion, fill the dome of the cap 1/3 full with spermicidal cream or jelly. Next, find your cervix with your finger. It feels like a short, firm nose projecting into the vagina. This can be done standing, with one foot propped up (on the edge of a chair, a bathtub, or a toilet), squatting, or lying on your back. Separate the lips of your vagina with one hand. With the other hand, squeeze (fold) the rim of the cap between your thumb and index finger. Slide the cap into your vagina, and push it along the rear wall of the vagina as far as it will go. Using your finger to locate your cervix, press the rim of the cap around the cervix until it is completely covered. Finally, check the cap position by pressing the dome of the cap to make sure your cervix is covered. Sweep your finger around the cap rim. The cervix should not be felt outside the cap.

REPEATED INTERCOURSE

- **Female condoms.** Use a new Reality condom for each act of intercourse.
- **Sponges.** The sponge provides continuous protection for up to 24 hours, no matter how many times you have intercourse.
- **Diaphragm.** If you have intercourse more than once within the 6 hour time that your diaphragm must remain in place, an additional dose of spermicidal cream or jelly is recommended. **Do not remove your diaphragm**; use the plastic applicator to insert fresh jelly or cream in front of the diaphragm.
- **Cap.** Use of additional spermicide for repeated intercourse with the cap is optional. **Do not remove your cap**. If you wish to add spermicide, use the plastic introducer to insert fresh cream or jelly in front of the cap.

AFTER INTERCOURSE

1. **Remove your female condom immediately after intercourse,** before you stand up. Squeeze and twist the outer ring to keep semen inside the pouch. Pull Reality out gently and discard it in a trash can. Do not try to flush a used Reality down the toilet. Do not try to reuse the Reality condom.

2. **Leave the cap, diaphragm, or sponge in place for at least 6 hours after intercourse.** Douching is not recommended, but if you choose to douche, wait at least 6 hours.

3. Your sponge, diaphragm, or cap should not interfere with normal activities. Urination or a bowel movement should not affect its position, but you can check its placement afterward if you wish. It is fine to shower or bathe with a sponge, diaphragm, or cap in place.

4. Before removing a cap, diaphragm, or sponge, wash your hands carefully with soap and water.

5. Check the position of the device. If it is dislodged, or seems not to be in correct position, you may want to contact your clinician about emergency postcoital contraception.

    - **Sponges.** Grasp the loop on the sponge with one finger and pull it gently to remove the sponge. Check to be sure the sponge is intact, then throw it away. If it is torn, remove all the pieces from the vagina.

- **Diaphragm.** Locate the front rim of the diaphragm with your finger. Hook your finger over the rim or behind it, then pull the diaphragm down and out. Wash the diaphragm with plain soap and water, and dry it. Hold it up to the light to check for holes, tears, or cracks.

- **Cap.** Locate the cap rim on your cervix. Press on the cap rim until the seal against your cervix is broken, then tilt the cap off the cervix. Hook your finger around the rim and pull it sideways out of the vagina. Wash the cap with plain soap and water, and dry it. Check the cap for holes, tears or cracks.

TAKING CARE OF YOUR SPERMICIDE SUPPLIES, SPONGES, DIAPHRAGM, OR CAP

1. Store your supplies in a convenient location that is clean, cool, and dark.

2. Wash your spermicide inserter, diaphragm, or cap after each use. Plain soap is best; avoid deodorant soap or perfumed soap. Do not use talcum powder on your diaphragm or cap, or in the case.

3. **Contact with oil-based products can deteriorate a diaphragm or cap.** Do not use oil-based vaginal medications or lubricants when you are using a diaphragm or cap. Some examples include petroleum jelly (Vaseline), mineral oil, hand lotion, vegetable oil, cold cream, and cocoa butter as well as common vaginal yeast creams and vaginal hormone creams. If you need extra lubrication for intercourse, contraceptive jelly is a good choice, or you can try a water soluble lubricant specifically intended for use with condoms.

REFERENCES

1. Anonymous. Tests show commonly used substances harm latex condoms. Contraceptive Technology Update 1980;10:20-21.
2. Anonymous. Vaginal spermicides. The Medical Letter 1986;5:13-16.
3. Bernstein GS, Clark V, Coulson AH, Frezieres RG, Kilzer L, Moyer D, Nakamura RM, Walsh T. Use effectiveness of cervical caps. Final report. Washington DC: National Institute of Child Health and Human Develpment, Contract No. 1-HD-1-2804, July, 1986.
4. Cates W Jr, Stewart FH, Trussell J. Commentary: the quest for women's prophylactic methods—hopes vs. science. Am J Public Health 1992;82(11): 1479-1482.
5. Cates W Jr, Stone KM. Family planning, sexually transmitted diseases and contraceptive choice: a literature update—Part I. Fam Plann Persp 1992;24(2): 75-84.

6. Cates W Jr. Tubal infertility: an ounce of (more specific) prevention. JAMA 1987;257(18):2480.

7. Celentano DD, Klassen AC, Weisman CS, Rosenshein NB. The role of contraceptive use in cervical cancer: the Maryland cervical cancer case-control study. Am J Epidemiology 1987;126(4):592-604.

8. Chalker R. The complete cervical cap guide. New York: Harper & Row Publishers, 1987.

9. Cramer DW, Goldman MB, Schiff I, Belisle S, Albrecht B, Stadel B, Gibson M, Wilson E, Stillman R, Thompson I. The relationship of tubal infertility to barrier method and oral contraceptive use. JAMA 1987;257(18):2446-2450.

10. Drew WL, Blair M, Miner RC, Conant M. Evaluation of the virus permeability of a new condom for women. Sex Transm Dis 1990;17(2):110-112.

11. Edelman DA, McIntyre SL, Harper J. A comparative trial of the Today contraceptive sponge and diaphragm. Am J Obstet Gynecol 1984;150(7): 869-876.

12. Einarson TR, Koren G, Mattice D, Schechter-Tsafriri O. Maternal spermicide use and adverse reproductive outcome: a meta-analysis. Am J Obstet Gynecol 1990;162(3):655-60.

13. Elias CJ, Heise L. The development of microbicides: a new method of HIV prevention for women. The Population Council, Working Papers, No.6, 1993. The Population Council, One Dag Hammarskjold Plaza, New York, NY 10017.

14. Farr G, Gabelnick H, Sturgen K. The Reality ® female condom: efficacy and clinical acceptability of a new barrier contraceptive. Durham NC: Family Health International, 1993.

15. Food and Drug Administration. Data do not support association between spermicides, birth defects. FDA Drug Bulletin 1986;11:21.

16. Feldblum PJ, Fortney JA. Condoms, spermicides, and the transmission of human immunodeficiency virus: a review of the literature. Am J Public Health 1988;78(1):52-54.

17. Fihn SD, Latham RH, Roberts P, Running K, Stamm WE. Association between diaphragm use and urinary tract infection. JAMA 1985;254(2):240-245.

18. Foxman B. Recurring urinary tract infection: incidence and risk factors. Am J Pub Health 1990;80(3):331-33.

19. Gollub EL, Sivin I. The Prentif cervical cap and Pap smear results: a critical appraisal. Contraception 1989;40(3):343-349.

20. Hooten TM, Hillier S, Johnson C, Roberts PL, Stamm WE. Escherichia coli bacteriuria and contraceptive method. JAMA 1991;265(1):64-69.

21. Huggins G, Vessey M, Flavel R, Yeates D, McPherson K. Vaginal spermicides and outcome of pregnancy: findings in a large cohort study. Contraception 1982;25(3):219-230.

22. Jick H, Walker AM, Rothman KJ, Hunter JK, Holmes LB, Watkins RN, D'Ewart DC, Danford A, Madsen S. Vaginal spermicides and congenital disorders. JAMA 1981;245(13):1329-1332.

23. Kelaghan J, Rubin GL, Ory HW, Layde PM. Barrier-method contraceptives and pelvic inflammatory disease. JAMA 1982;248(2):185.

24. Kreiss J, Ngugi E, Holmes K, Ndinya-Achola J, Waiyaki P, Roberts PL, Ruminjo I, Sajabi R, Kimata J, Fleming TR, Anzala A, Holton D, Plummer F. Efficacy of nonoxynol-9 contraceptive sponge use in preventing heterosexual acquisition of HIV in Nairobi prostitutes. JAMA 1992;268(4):477-482.

25. Kugel C, Verson H. Relationship between weight change and diaphragm size change. J Ob Gyn Nursing 1986;15(2):123-129.
26. Lane M, Arceo R, Sobrero AJ. Successful use of the diaphragm and jelly by a young population: report of a clinical study. Fam Plann Perspect 1976;8(2):81-86.
27. Leeper MA, Conrardy M. Preliminary evaluation of Reality, a condom for women to wear. Adv Contracept 1989;5(4):229-235.
28. Lettau LA, Bond WW, McDougal JS. Hepatitis and diaphragm fitting [letter to editor]. JAMA 1985;254(6):752.
29. Levy JA. The transmission of AIDS: the case of the infected cell. JAMA 1988;259(20):3037-3038.
30. Niruthisard S, Roddy RE, and Chutivongse S. The effects of frequent nonoxynol-9 use on the vaginal and cervical mucosa. Sex Transm Dis 1991;18(8):176-179.
31. Ortho Diaphragm. FDA-approved product literature, 1993.
32. Parazzini F, Negri E, LaVecchia C, Fedele L. Barrier methods of contraception and the risk of cervical neoplasia. Contraception 1989;40(5):519-530.
33. Peters RK, Thomas D, Hagan DG, Mack TM, Henderson BE. Risk factors for invasive cervical cancer among Latinas and non-Latinas in Los Angeles County. JNCI 1986;77(5):1063-1077.
34. Prentif cavity-rim cervical cap. FDA-approved product literature, 1988.
35. Rekart ML. The toxicity and local effects of the spermicide nonoxynol-9. J Acq Imm Def Syndromes 1992;5(4):425-526.
36. Richwald GA, Greenland S, Gerber MM, Potik R, Kersey L, Comas MA. Effectiveness of the cavity-rim cervical cap: results of a large clinical study. Obstet Gynecol 1989;74(2):143-148.
37. Rosenberg MJ, Gollub EL. Commentary: methods women can use that may prevent sexually transmitted disease, including HIV. Am J Public Health 1992;82(11):1473-1478.
38. Rosenberg MJ, Rojanapithayakorn W, Feldblum PJ, Higgins JE. Effect of contraceptive sponge on chlamydial infection, gonorrhea, and candidiasis. JAMA 1987;257(17):2308-2312.
39. Rothman M. Spermicide use and Down's syndrome. Am J Public Health 1982;72(4):329-401.
40. Schirm AL, Trussell J, Menken J, et al. Contraceptive failure in the United States: the impact of social, economic and demographic factors. Fam Plann Perspect 1982;14(2):68-75.
41. Schwartz B, Gaventa S, Broome CV, Reingold AL, Hightower AW, Perlman JA, Wolf PH. Nonmenstrual toxic shock syndrome associated with barrier contraceptives: report of a case-control study. Reviews of Infections Diseases 1989;2(1):S43-S49.
42. Shiata AA, Trussell J. New female intravaginal barrier contraceptive device: preliminary clinical trial. Contraception 1991; 44(1):11-19.
43. Simpson JL, Phillips OP. Spermicides, hormonal contraception and congenital malformations. Adv Contracept 1990;6(3):141-167.
44. Stein Z. Editorial: the double bind in science policy and the protection of women from HIV infection. Am J Publ Health 1992;82(11):1471-1472.
45. Stone KM, Peterson HB. Spermicides, HIV, and the vaginal sponge [editorial]. JAMA 1992;268(4):521-523.
46. Strobino B, Kline J, Warburton D. Spermicide use and pregnancy outcome. Am J Public Health 1988;78(3):260-263.

47. Trussell J, Strickler J, Vaughan B. Contraceptive efficacy of the diaphragm, sponge and cervical cap. Fam Plann Persp 1993;25(3):101-105,135.

48. Trussell J, Sturgen K, Strickler J, Dominik R. Contraceptive efficacy of the Reality female condom: comparison wtih other barrier methods. Fam Plann Perspect 1994;26(2).

49. Vessey MP. Contraceptive methods: risks and benefits. Brit Med J 1978; 2(6139):721-722.

50. Vessey MP, Metcalfe MA, McPherson K, Yeates D. Urinary tract infection in relation to diaphragm use and obesity. Intl. J. Epidem 1987;16(3):441-444.

51. Zenkeng L. Barrier contraceptive use and HIV infection among high risk women in Cameroon. JAIDS 1993. In press

The Pill: Combined Oral Contraceptives

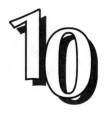

- Pills may be used throughout the reproductive years by most women.
- Pills provide no protection against sexually transmitted infections including HIV infection.

- Women at any risk of becoming infected with HIV (or of infecting a man with HIV) should use condoms consistently and correctly.

The combined oral contraceptive (OC) pill is a safe and effective method of birth control. It is one of the most extensively studied medications ever prescribed. Since its approval by the FDA in 1960, the pill has played an important role in contraception. In many countries, pills are now available without a prescription. The overall risks and benefits of pills suggest that it would be appropriate for combined oral contraceptives to be available to women in the United States without a prescription.

In this text, we use the terms birth control pills, combined oral contraceptives, oral contraceptives, and OCs when referring to pills containing both an estrogen and a progestin. These terms do not refer to progestin-only pills which may also be called minipills; progestin-only contraceptives are discussed in Chapter 11.

MECHANISM OF ACTION

Combined OCs prevent pregnancy primarily by suppressing ovulation through the combined actions of estrogen and progestin. Estrogens and progestins affect many different organ systems and produce a broad range of symptoms.

Estrogenic effects

In some women, less suppression of endogenous estrogen production may occur, particularly as the dosage of exogenous estrogen is lowered. Therefore, in each woman taking OCs, the total estrogenic effect will be the result of estrogen from an oral contraceptive and endogenous estrogen from the ovaries and adipose tissue.

- Ovulation is inhibited in part by the suppression of FSH and LH. In a sense, the pituitary gland is fooled into thinking a woman is already pregnant and therefore does not release hormones to stimulate the ovary.[31]
- Secretions within the uterus are altered as is the cellular structure of the endometrium leading to the production of areas of edema alternating with areas of dense cellularity.
- Ovum transport is accelerated.
- Luteolysis, the degeneration of the corpus luteum, may occur as high levels of estrogen alter local prostaglandins.[73]

Progestational effects

Progestins vary in both their inherent estrogenicity and their anti-estrogenic properties. Progestins vary in their androgenic effects.

- Ovulation is inhibited in part by suppression of luteinizing hormone (LH).
- A thick cervical mucus is created, hampering the transport of sperm.
- Capacitation, the activation of enzymes that permit the sperm to penetrate the ovum, may be inhibited.
- Ovum transport may be slowed, or fallopian tube secretions altered.
- Implantation is hampered by production of a decidualized endometrial bed with exhausted and atrophied glands.[72]

COMBINED PILL OPTIONS

Estrogens.   Only two estrogenic compounds are used in current U.S. oral contraceptives: ethynyl estradiol (EE) and mestranol. Ethinyl estradiol is pharmacologically active, whereas mestranol must be converted into ethinyl estradiol by the liver before it is pharmacologically active.

Ethinyl estradiol has been marketed in oral contraceptives in dosages ranging from 100 mcg (Oracon, a sequential pill) down to 20 mcg (Loestrin 1/20). The most recent year in which a mestranol-containing OC was introduced to the market was 1968 when both Ortho-Novum 1/50 and Norinyl 1+50 were first marketed. No oral contraceptive containing less than 50 mcg of mestranol has ever been marketed in the United States.

Progestins. Several progestogenic compounds are available in pills: norethindrone, norethindrone acetate, ethynodiol diacetate, norgestrel, levonorgestrel, and norethynodrel. The new progestins include desogestrel and norgestimate. Gestodene is marketed in Europe.

POTENCY

Figure 10-1 depicts estimates of the hormonal potency in many of the pills currently on the U.S. market. Pills containing the new progestins are not included. Statements about relative potency of an estrogen or a progestin tend to be based on hormonal effects on one or two organ systems or biochemical changes, not on all the functions influenced by the hormone. Therefore, statements about the overall potencies of an estrogen or progestin tend to be oversimplifications. For example, Dorflinger's summary (column 3 of Figure 10-1) of the relative potency of progestins in OCs suggests that norethindrone, norethindrone acetate, and ethynodiol diacetate are approximately equipotent, whereas norgestrel is about five times and levonorgestrel 10 times more potent in terms of altering high density lipoprotein (HDL) cholesterol in the presence of an equal amount of estrogen.[20] When determined by the delay of menses in normal women, levonorgestrel ranges from being two to 60 times more potent than norethindrone.

Figure 10-1 depicts ethinyl estradiol to be 1.2–1.4 times stronger than mestranol on a microgram-to-microgram basis, although the actual conversion factor is not known.[38] In mouse uterus assays and the rat vaginal cell assays, mestranol had 67% of the potency of ethinyl estradiol.[19] When 100 mcg of mestranol is combined with 2.5 mg of norethynodrel, as in the oral contraceptive called Enovid-E, the effectiveness is very close to 100%; however, when the amount of mestranol is lowered to 36 mcg while leaving the norethynodrel dose at 2.5 mg, the efficacy of this combination as a contraceptive drops from 100% to 71%.[22,51] It has not been possible to lower the mestranol dosage to 50 mcg while maintaining an efficacy of over 99%.

Even more vague is the relative potency of the progestins. Progestational potency shown in Figure 10-1 is based on delay of menses assay. (New progestins are not included in this figure.) Potency differs when other tests for progestational potency are employed. Therefore, the clinical significance of various relative potency rankings is uncertain. Levonorgestrel and dextronorgestrel are the two isomers of norgestrel. Levonorgestrel is the active component. Lo/Ovral contains 0.3 mg of norgestrel, of which only 0.15 mg is said to be in the active state. Nordette contains 0.15 mg of levonorgestrel, all of which is in the active state. Leaving out the inactive isomer should have little, if any, clinical effect. However, the spotting patterns described later in the chapter seem to indicate a difference in the pharmacologic effects of the progestin in these two pills.

Progestin (mg)					Estrogen (mcg)	
Greenblatt (1967) Relative Potency	Swyer (1982) Relative Potency	Dorflinger (1985) Relative Potency	Dose of Progestin (mg)	Name(s) of Pills	Dose of Estrogen (mcg)	Relative Potency
0.35	0.35	0.35	Norethindrone 0.35	Micronor / Nor-QD		1
2.2	0.15–0.22	0.375–0.75	Norgestrel 0.075	Ovrette		2
2.0	0.5	1.0	Norethindrone Acetate 1.0	Loestrin 1/20	Ethinyl Estradiol 20	0.7–0.8 — 3
1.0	1.0	1.0	Norethindrone 1.0	Norinyl 1/50 / Ortho 1/50 / Genora 1/50	Mestranol 50	1.0 — 4
3.0–7.5	0.10–0.375	0.5–2.5	L-Norgestrel 0.05/0.075/0.125	Triphasil / Tri-Levien	Ethinyl Estradiol 30/40	1.0–1.2 — 5
9.0	0.3–0.45	1.5–3.0	L-Norgestrel 0.15	Nordette / Levien	Ethinyl Estradiol 30	1.0–1.2 — 6
9.0	0.6–0.9	1.5–3.0	Norgestrel 0.3	Lo/Ovral	Ethinyl Estradiol 30	1.0–1.2 — 7
3.0	0.75	1.5	Norethindrone Acetate 1.5	Loestrin 1.5/30	Ethinyl Estradiol 30	1.0–1.2 — 8
0.4	0.4	0.4	Norethindrone 0.4	Ovcon 35	Ethinyl Estradiol 35	1.2–1.4 — 9
0.5	0.5	0.5	Norethindrone 0.5	Brevicon / Modicon	Ethinyl Estradiol 35	1.2–1.4 — 10
0.5–1.0	0.5–1.0	0.5–1.0	Norethindrone 0.5/1.0/0.5	Ortho 10/11	Ethinyl Estradiol 35	1.2–1.4 — 11
0.5–1.0	0.5–1.0	0.5–1.0	Norethindrone 0.5/1.0/0.5	Tri-Norinyl	Ethinyl Estradiol 35	1.2–1.4 — 12
0.5–1.0	0.5–1.0	0.5–1.0	Norethindrone 0.5/0.75/1.0	Ortho 7/7/7	Ethinyl Estradiol 35	1.2–1.4 — 13
1.0	1.0	1.0	Norethindrone 1.0	Norinyl 1/35 / Ortho 1/35 / Genora 1/35 / N.E.E. 1/35	Ethinyl Estradiol 35	1.2–1.4 — 14
15	0.5	1.0	Ethynodiol Diacetate 1.0	Demulen 1/35	Ethinyl Estradiol 35	1.2–1.4 — 15
1.0	1.0	1.0	Norethindrone 1.0	Norinyl 1/80 / Ortho 1/80	Mestranol 80	1.6 — 16
1.0	1.0	1.0	Norethindrone 1.0	Ovcon 50	Ethinyl Estradiol 50	1.7–2.0 — 17
2.0	0.5	1.0	Norethindrone Acetate 1.0	Norlestrin 1/50	Ethinyl Estradiol 50	1.7–2.0 — 18
2.0	2.0	2.0	Norethindrone 2.0	Norinyl 2 / Ortho 2	Mestranol 100	2.0 — 19
2.7	2.5		Norethindrone 2.5	Enovid-E	Mestranol 100	2.0 — 20
5.0	1.25	2.5	Norethindrone Acetate 2.5	Norlestrin 2.5/50	Ethinyl Estradiol 50	1.7–2.0 — 21
15	1.5	2.5 / -5	Norgestrel 0.5	Ovral	Ethinyl Estradiol 50	1.7–2.0 — 22
15	0.5	1.0	Ethyndiol Diacetate 1.0	Demulen 1/50	Ethinyl Estradiol 50	1.7–2.0 — 23
15	0.5	1.0	Ethynodiol Diacetate 1.0	Ovulen	Mestranol 100	2.0 — 24

15 10 5   0 2.0 1.5 1.0 0.5 0 5 4 3 2 1
Potency Units

0   1.0   2.0
Potency Units

Sources: Dorflinger (1985).
Greenblatt (1967).
Swyer (1982).
Heinen (1971).

Figure 10-1 Relative potency of estrogens and progestins in currently available oral contraceptives reflecting the debate about the strength of the progestins

E FFECTIVENESS

If combined estrogen-progestin pills are used perfectly (when pills are taken at the same time every day as directed and other instructions regarding concomitant drug use or diarrhea or vomiting are followed), only about 1 in 1,000 women is expected to become pregnant within the first year (see Tables 10-1 and 27-11). Failure rates during typical use is determined by the extent and type of imperfect use. Among OC users in the United States, about 3% become pregnant during the first year of typical use.[78] (See also Chapter 27.)

An important factor decreasing the use-effectiveness failure rate of the pill is the high rate of discontinuation among OC users. Many pregnancies occur when women discontinue pills, fail to begin another method of contraception, and have unprotected intercourse. Usually no more than 50%–75% of women who start pills are still using them after 1 year. Most women who discontinue pills do so for nonmedical reasons. That is, they have not developed a complication or major side effect. Because of these high discontinuation rates, we recommend that every woman receiving the pill be provided with a second method of birth control. She should be instructed how to use the back-up method and encouraged to practice using it. She should know of the availability of emergency hormonal contraception (postcoital pills) should she have unprotected intercourse.

Table 10-1 First-year failure rate* of combined pills compared to other hormonal contraceptives

Method (1)	% of Women Experiencing an Accidental Pregnancy Within the First Year of Use		% of Women Continuing Use at One Year
	Typical Use (2)	Perfect Use (3)	(4)
Pill	3		72
Progestin Only		0.5	
Combined		0.1	
IUD			
Progesterone T	2.0	1.5	81
Copper T 380A	0.8	0.6	78
LNg 20	0.1	0.1	81
Depo-Provera	0.3	0.3	70
Norplant (6 Capsules)	0.09	0.09	85

* See Table 5-2 for first-year failure rates of all methods.

COST

As of 1992, pills cost the pharmacist from $5.95–$34.35 per cycle. Women pay that cost plus whatever markup is charged by the pharmacist.[4] In the autumn of 1989, the price paid for one cycle of OCs in five Atlanta pharmacies ranged from $12.89–$16.89 for Ortho 7/7/7 (the pill most commonly prescribed for new patients at this time). For Ovral, one of the most expensive pills and the only pill commonly prescribed as a postcoital pill, the price of one package ranged from $14.25–$22.55. In subsidized clinics, pills are sold to women for $1.00–$11.00 per cycle. Generic pills cost women approximately half as much as nongeneric pills when bought from a drugstore. On an annual basis, generic pills cost a woman $100–$130; nongeneric pills cost $200–$300 per year. Public clinics may pay as little as 30 cents to $1 per cycle of pills and pass these low prices to clients.

A survey of 24 college and university health services in the summer of 1992 found a wide range in the price charged women per cycle of OCs. In eight health services, the cost was $5 or less per cycle; in three it was $10 or more per cycle. Some colleges do not dispense pills, and the prescriptions they write will cost women an average of $18–$20 per cycle of pills. Depending on the college a woman attends, she could pay from $14.73–$260 per year for birth control pills.[35]

ADVANTAGES AND INDICATIONS

1. **Effectiveness.** When taken consistently and correctly, pills are a very effective contraceptive which give women control over their own fertility. Some women find it fairly easy to remember to take pills on schedule for long periods of time.

2. **Safety.** Pills are very safe for most women. In the United States, it is safer to use pills than to deliver a baby, unless a woman is over 35 years of age and smokes more than 35 cigarettes a day. Consider the following illustration of pill safety: If you were to draw a line 215 meters high (the height of a 70-story building) to represent 100,000 young nonsmoking pill users, and then were to draw a line beside it to represent the number of pill users in the United States who die each year from complications related to higher-dose pills, that second line would be about 0.5 centimeters high. In comparison, the line representing the number of U.S. women who would die of pregnancy-related problems would be just under 2.5 centimeters high. A line representing maternal mortality in developing countries would be 25 centimeters to 1.5 meters tall.[74] The risk of death from birth control

pills is very low, and would be even lower if heavy smokers over 35 years of age did not take pills.[34] It is reassuring for women to learn that although there are still some unanswered questions about oral contraceptives, pills are one of the best-studied medications ever prescribed.

3. **Option throughout reproductive years.** Most women can safely use pills throughout their reproductive years as long as they do not have specific reasons to avoid use of pills. Age is not a reason to avoid pills in very young women or in women toward the end of the reproductive life span. Furthermore, pills may be used for a number of years cumulatively or consecutively without increasing a woman's risk for complications. *A rest period every few years is definitely not recommended for women wishing to continue using pills.*

4. **Reversibility.** A pill user will not experience loss of fertility caused by oral contraceptives, although she may take longer to become pregnant after taking pills than after using other contraceptives. Advice for women seeking to become pregnant after taking birth control pills[36] is summarized in Table 10-2.

5. **Beneficial menstrual cycle effects.**
   - Pills tend to decrease menstrual cramps and pain. Some women consider this to be the most desirable effect of pills. Indeed, many women use OCs exclusively for their beneficial effects on menstrual pain. Pills may relieve menstrual cramps or pain that has been resistant to therapy with prostaglandin inhibitors.
   - Pills prevent ovulation in most women and thus eliminate the midcycle pain some women experience at the time of ovulation (mittelschmerz).
   - Pills suppress the androgens produced by the ovaries of many hirsute women and are a standard part of the management of hirsutism.[73]
   - Pills decrease the number of days of bleeding and the amount of blood loss, thereby decreasing a woman's likelihood of developing iron deficiency anemia. Pills decrease menstrual flow by 60% or more in normal uteri.[73]
   - Women can avoid menstrual periods on weekends or vacations by taking extra pills from a separate package.
   - For retarded women with severe hygienic problems, pills may be used to decrease menstrual bleeding to one period every 90 days. This change may be accomplished by having the woman take four consecutive packages of 21 pills. After 84 consecutive days of taking a pill, the woman does not take a pill for 6 days
   - Because OCs suppress stimulation of the ovaries by FSH and LH, the incidence of functional ovarian cysts among women using

Table 10-2 Pregnancy after birth control pills

Advice for the woman who knows that she will want to become pregnant after using pills:

1. Pills are a good option for women who want to become pregnant in the future.

2. By preventing causes of infertility such as pelvic infections, uterine fibroids, ectopic pregnancies, ovarian cysts, endometrial cancer and possibly endometriosis, OCs may improve a woman's future ability to become pregnant.

3. If your periods are irregular prior to taking pills, they may again become irregular after you stop taking pills.

4. Return of fertility is *not* improved by periodically taking a break from pills.

5. *You may experience some delay (an average of 2–3 months) in becoming pregnant* compared to the amount of time it would have taken if you had not taken the pills.

6. Between 1% and 2% of women will not menstruate for 6 months or more after taking pills. However, it is not certain that this lack of menses is caused by birth control pills.

7. Because most women conceive soon after stopping pills, you should use another method of contraception right away if you don't want to become pregnant.

pills is reduced by 80%-90%.[31,57] Triphasic and other very low-dose pills provide less protection against functional ovarian cysts than do earlier, higher potency pills.[31]

- Some women note a reduction in premenstrual symptoms such as anxiety, depression, headaches, and fluid retention.[31] For other women, these symptoms definitely become worse. However, premenstrual symptomatology most often improves among women using the current low-dose pills. Monophasic pills may be better than triphasic pills in managing PMS.

6. **PID protection.** The pill has a protective effect against pelvic inflammatory disease (PID), a major cause of female infertility.[34,66] Pill users are less likely to develop more severe forms of PID than are users of other contraceptives. The mechanisms that have been postulated include the following:

- Pills decrease the average amount of menstrual blood a woman loses each month. Menstrual blood may act as culture medium, facilitating the development of PID in some women.

- Pills cause a woman's cervical mucus to become scanty, thick, and difficult to penetrate, thereby discouraging the ascent of sperm from the vagina into the uterine cavity and the fallopian tubes. It has been shown that bacteria attached to the surface of sperm gain entry to the upper genital track through the ascent of sperm.

- Pills cause the cervical canal to be less dilated, principally because the volume of cervical secretions and menstrual blood diminishes.
- Pills decrease the strength of uterine contractions throughout the cycle, thereby decreasing the likelihood of spreading an infection from the uterine cavity into the fallopian tubes.

Although numerous articles have noted a decreased risk of severe PID for women using oral contraceptives, current information does not permit the generalization that oral contraceptives protect against all forms of PID, especially the more chronic, subclinical type caused by *Chlamydia trachomatis*. Epidemiologic and biologic evidence indicates that cervical infections with *C. trachomatis* are enhanced by oral contraceptives, possibly offsetting the protective effects of OCs against PID.[81]

7. **Prevention of ovarian and endometrial cancer.**[9,10,11,30,34] When compared with never-users, women who have used combined oral contraceptives for 4 years or less are 30% less likely to develop ovarian cancer; for 5-11 years, 60% less likely; and for 12 or more years, 80% less likely to develop ovarian cancer. Women who start using OCs at an early age and continue for a long time may be more strongly protected than women starting pills at an older age.[34]

   The risk of endometrial cancer among women who have used OCs for at least 2 years is about 40% less than among women who have never used pills. This protective effect increases to 60% in women who have used pills for 4 or more years.[34]

   The protective effect of oral contraceptives against ovarian and endometrial cancer is even greater in nulliparous women. The protective effect of using pills appears to persist long after pills are discontinued.

8. **Decreased risk for benign breast disease.** Long-range studies have repeatedly documented that pill users are less likely to develop benign breast tumors than are women who are not using the pill.[57] Unfortunately, pills do not appear to have a protective effect against benign breast lesions caused by ductal atypia, which is thought to be premalignant.

9. **Ectopic pregnancy prevention.** By stopping ovulation, pills prevent almost all conceptions, including those that implant outside the uterus, thus preventing ectopic pregnancies, an important cause of maternal mortality throughout the world.

10. **Acne improvement.**[31,72] Combined OCs lower serum testosterone levels through a number of mechanisms.

11. **Enhanced sexual enjoyment.** Probably because the fear of pregnancy is diminished, many couples enjoy sexual intimacy more. In some women the effect is the opposite.

12. **Improvement of other medical conditions.**
    - Symptoms of estrogen deficiency may be improved. Pills have been shown to have similar beneficial effects in preventing osteoporosis as other forms of estrogen replacement therapy.
    - Pills have been used in the prevention and treatment of endometriosis.[31,72,73]
    - The use of combined oral contraceptives prevents more hospitalizations than it causes, as shown in Figure 10-2. An estimated 1,614 per 100,000 current pill users avoid being hospitalized each year due to the protective effects of pills. This may be compared with an estimated 133 per 100,000 women who require hospitalization as a result of a condition that occurs more commonly in pill users than in other women at risk for an unintended pregnancy.[34] Pills also prevent a number of less-serious conditions that do not usually lead to hospitalization, including menstrual pain, anemia, fibroid tumors, and benign breast masses.

13. **Emergency hormonal contraception.** Combined oral contraceptives may be used as postcoital contraceptives. Widespread availability of this postcoital therapy could prevent as many as 2.3 million unintended pregnancies and 1.0 million induced abortions annually in the United States.[79] (See Chapter 16.)

INDICATIONS

Certain situations make pills an extremely attractive contraceptive option for women:

- Sexually active young women and adolescents
- Nulliparous women
- Couples using birth control for spacing
- Nonlactating postpartum women
- Need for short- or long-term reversible birth control
- Women with endometriosis who are not ready to get pregnant
- Need for postcoital birth control
- Immediate postabortion period
- Acne
- Heavy, painful, or irregular menstrual periods
- Recurrent ovarian cysts
- Family history of ovarian cancer
- Past experience using pills correctly
- Women experiencing anxiety due to irregular periods

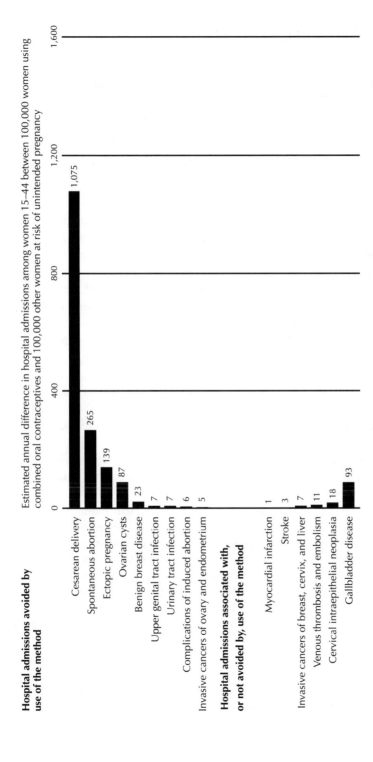

Hospital admissions avoided by use of the method

Estimated annual difference in hospital admissions among women 15–44 between 100,000 women using combined oral contraceptives and 100,000 other women at risk of unintended pregnancy

Cesarean delivery — 1,075
Spontaneous abortion — 265
Ectopic pregnancy — 139
Ovarian cysts — 87
Benign breast disease — 23
Upper genital tract infection — 7
Urinary tract infection — 7
Complications of induced abortion — 6
Invasive cancers of ovary and endometrium — 5

Hospital admissions associated with, or not avoided by, use of the method

Myocardial infarction — 1
Stroke — 3
Invasive cancers of breast, cervix, and liver — 7
Venous thrombosis and embolism — 11
Cervical intraepithelial neoplasia — 18
Gallbladder disease — 93

Source: Harlap et al. (1991) with permission of the Alan Guttmacher Institute.

Figure 10-2 Use of combined oral contraceptives prevents many more hospital admissions than it adds.

Advantages and Indications **233**

DISADVANTAGES AND CAUTIONS

Infection with the HIV virus is a greater threat to the health of many sexually active individuals than is an unplanned pregnancy. Pills provide no known protection against HIV infection. Condoms should be used instead of or in addition to pills if protection against HIV is desired in an intimate sexual relationship. Abstinence and a long-term mutually faithful relationship are the safest approaches to avoiding HIV infections transmitted by intercourse.

1. **Pills must be taken daily.** Taking pills is complicated, and compliance is poor for many individuals. Pills must be taken every day. When pill use is inconsistent or incorrect, failure rates rise to high levels.

2. **Expense.** The high cost of pills in many pharmacies may prompt some women to discontinue pills.

3. **Unwanted menstrual cycle changes.** Pills may be associated with menstrual changes including missed periods, very scanty bleeding, spotting, or breakthrough bleeding.

4. **Nausea or vomiting.** Nausea may occur in the first cycle or so of pill use or, less commonly, in subsequent cycles.

5. **Headaches.** Headaches may start in a woman who has not previously had headaches or may become worse than they were before starting pills. Rarely, changes in vision accompany these headaches.

6. **Depression.** Depression (sometimes severe) and other mood changes may occur in women on pills.

7. **Decreased libido.** Some women experience a decreased interest in sex or a decreased ability to have orgasms. Decreased libido may be due to decreased levels of free testosterone caused by oral contraceptives.

8. **Cervical ectopia and *Chlamydia* infection.** Chlamydial cervicitis is more common in women on pills.[72,81] Pills can cause cervical ectopia, a condition in which part of the cervical surface near the opening of the canal becomes covered by the delicate mucus-secreting columnar cells that normally line the cervical canal. With an ectropion, the cervix of the pill user is more vulnerable to *Chlamydia trachomatis* infection, although no evidence exists that this increased risk places women using OCs at greater risk for pelvic inflammatory disease (salpingitis).

9. **Other infections...possibly.** Although urinary track infections occurred at an increased rate in women using pills in the Royal College of General Practitioners Study, this link was not found in the Oxford/FPA Study.[64,72] Women using pills tend to have intercourse

more frequently and it is difficult to know if infections are due to intercourse-induced cystitis or to effects of pills.[31] Other early studies found that women using pills appeared to have a slightly higher incidence of bronchitis, viral illness such as chickenpox, cervical ectropion, or vaginal discharges.

10. **Thrombophlebitis, pulmonary emboli, and other cardiovascular disease**. The most serious complications attributable to oral contraceptive use have been circulatory system diseases.[31,34,72,74,82] Cardiovascular disease (CVD) is most likely to occur in women who are:

Smokers

Sedentary

Overweight

Over 50 years of age

Hypertensive, diabetic, or have a history of heart or vascular disease

Diabetic or have a family history of diabetes or heart attack in a person under the age of 50 years (particularly heart attack in a female relative)

Have an elevated cholesterol level or a high LDL/HDL cholesterol ratio

These characteristics, which are totally unrelated to the use of oral contraceptives, are far more important in determining a woman's risk for cardiovascular disease than are the possible effects of low-dose combined oral contraceptives on blood pressure, lipids, or coagulation. Because current low-dose pills have minimal effect on blood pressure, carbohydrate metabolism, and atherogenesis and less effect on blood clotting than earlier pills, serious cardiovascular system disease attributable to pills is rare in women placed on low-dose pills.

Hospitalizations associated with, or not avoided by, use of combined pills occur with approximately the frequency shown in Table 10-3.[34] The possibly increased risks for cardiovascular system diseases are placed into context with other hospitalizations attributable to and

Table 10-3 Hospitalizations for cardiovascular conditions

Condition	Incidence per 100,000 Women on Pills
Myocardial infarction:	1
Stroke:	3
Venous thrombosis/embolism:	11

Source: Harlap et al. (1991).

Table 10-4 Circulatory diseases attributable to pills

Diagnosis	Location of Pathology	Symptoms
Thrombophlebitis	Lower leg	Calf pains, swelling, heat or tenderness
Thrombophlebitis	Thigh	Pain, heat, or redness
Pulmonary embolism	Lung	Cough, including coughing up blood, chest pains; shortness of breath
Myocardial infarction (Heart attack)	Heart	Chest pains, left arm and shoulder pain, shortness of breath, weakness
Thrombotic stroke	Brain	Headache, weakness or numbness, visual problem, sudden intellectual impairment
Hemorrhagic stroke, including subarachnoid hemorrhage	Brain	Headache, weakness or numbness, visual problem, sudden intellectual impairment
Retinal vein thrombosis	Eye	Headache, complete or partial loss of vision
Mesenteric vein thrombosis	Intestines	Abdominal pain, vomiting, weakness
Pelvic vein thrombosis	Pelvis	Lower abdominal pain, cramps

Source: Stewart et al. (1987).

prevented by pills in Figure 10-2.[34] The location and symptoms of the major circulatory disorders possibly associated with OCs are summarized in Table 10-4.

Clinically significant hypertension has been associated with both the estrogen and the progestin in pills but is rare in women using low-dose pills. One large study of over 25,000 African-American women in the southeastern United States did not find blood pressure changes in pill users that differed significantly from changes in nonusers.[8] When blood pressure elevations do occur, they are usually mild, not life-threatening, and usually vanish within a few weeks after pills are discontinued. Rarely, an individual has an idiosyncratic reaction to the hormones in OCs and becomes hypertensive. This emphasizes the importance of periodic blood pressures in women even if on low-dose pills.[31,72] Both estrogens and progestins may affect blood pressure.[82] If a woman's blood pressure rises to over 90 mm Hg on several visits, her pills should be discontinued or changed to a lower dose.

It may be appropriate to switch to a progestin-only pill, because the dosage of the progestin in progestin-only pills is less than in combined OCs.

Hypercoagulability is associated with exogenous estrogens. The estrogen component of pills appears to be the component of combined OCs capable of activating blood clotting mechanisms. Low-dose pills appear to have fewer deleterious effects on blood clotting than did earlier higher dose pills. Heavy smoking is clearly a risk factor for thrombosis in OC users. Other individuals at greater risk for blood clots include: women with high or abnormal blood lipids; women with severe diabetes who already have signs of damage to arteries, kidneys, or ophthalmologic complications; women with consistently elevated blood pressure; and women weighing more than 50% above ideal body weight.[31] Although tests can help a clinician to predict who will not clot, no tests predict who will clot abnormally while taking pills. Traditionally, it has been recommended that women should discontinue OCs for 1 month prior to surgery. The more major the surgery, the more strongly this recommendation has been made. Some clinicians do not discontinue pills for the month prior to small surgical procedures such as tubal sterilization, in part because of the concern that pregnancy is a greater potential risk. Another alternative prior to surgery is a progestin-only contraceptive such as progestin-only pills or Depo-Provera. Because of their greater tendency to develop deep vein thrombosis, women with polycythemia vera should not be provided combined OCs. Should a woman develop a deep vein thrombosis while using OCs, carefully evaluate clotting factors. Women who are anticoagulated and women who bleed heavily because of a bleeding disorder are generally considered to be excellent candidates for pill use; indeed, some clinicians consider these to be *indications for the use of pills.*

Atherogenesis is prevented by estrogens and may be encouraged by some progestins. Estrogens tend to have desirable effects on lipids: increasing high-density lipoproteins (HDLs) and decreasing low-density lipoproteins (LDLs). Androgens and some progestins have just the opposite effect on HDLs and LDLs. Recent changes in OC formulations have therefore involved efforts to lower the progestins in OCs and to find new formulations capable of producing a more favorable lipoprotein pattern than a woman had before initiating use of pills. Of the pills available for the past decade, Ovcon-35, Modicon, and Brevicon produce the best pattern of HDL and LDL cholesterol.[26,44,45] These pills have now been joined by the "new progestin" pills that also lead to a positive lipid pattern. (The exact role of triglycerides as an independent predictor of coronary heart disease [CHD] is uncertain; it appears that elevated triglycerides are not associated with an increased risk for CHD so long as HDL levels are also high.[27])

11. **Glucose intolerance.** Carbohydrate metabolism is not affected to an important degree in most women using most of our current low-dose pills. Studies of OCs providing higher doses than are now generally used demonstrate increased glucose levels, increased plasma insulin levels, and a slightly decreased glucose tolerance. However, the early literature of OCs and carbohydrate metabolism demonstrated that following discontinuation of OCs, normal glucose tolerance rapidly returns to normal. Impairment of glucose tolerance with accompanying changes in insulin tolerance are significantly affected by both the estrogen and the progestin in a combined OC.[87] Some evidence suggests that progestins and progesterone itself produce an increase in tissue resistance to insulin by decreasing the number of insulin receptors.[87]

Of the progestins, norgestrel appears to have the greatest insulin-antagonizing activity.[71,85] A long-term study of women taking an OC containing 30 mcg of ethinyl estradiol and 150 mcg of levonorgestrel (marketed as Nordette in the United States) demonstrated a significant and progressive deterioration of glucose tolerance, concluding that this preparation is too strongly progestogenic for continuous use in a combined pill.[88] A 1986 study found significantly less effect on carbohydrate metabolism in women on an OC with 20 mcg of ethinyl estradiol and 1 mg of norethindrone acetate (Loestrin 1/20).[87] A 1988 study found no impairment in carbohydrate metabolism in women on 0.4 mg of norethindrone and 35 mcg of ethinyl estradiol (Ovcon-35) in postpartum gestational diabetics; in this study, women on Triphasil had significantly elevated insulin levels at 3 and 6 months.[67]

Other studies of a number of low-dose combined OCs have shown minimal or no change in glucose tolerance, plasma insulin, or insulin binding to erythrocytes and monocytes in low-dose combined OCs.[68,71,87] One major study found less effect on the carbohydrate metabolism of women on low-dose norethindrone than on low-dose levonorgestrel.

Low-dose combined pills (including the new progestin pills), both triphasics and monophasics, may be provided to some gestational diabetics, to some women with a family history of diabetes, and in some instances, to women with insulin-dependent diabetes. The use of OCs by gestational diabetics, diabetics being controlled by diet alone, and insulin-dependent diabetics would depend upon the alternative contraceptives available to a woman. Such women should be followed closely. Some clinicians maintain that any increase in the amount of insulin a diabetic might require as a result of using an OC is far outweighed by the potential adverse effects of a pregnancy.

12. **Gallbladder disease.** Gallbladder disease was positively associated with pill use in some early studies. Recent studies conclude that OCs are not an important risk factor for the development of gallstones or gallbladder cancer. While pills do not cause gallstones, it is now thought that OCs may accelerate the development of gallbladder disease for women who are already susceptible so that problems become evident earlier.[32,72,82]

13. **Hepatocellular adenomas.** Benign liver tumors have been associated with use of combined OCs. Although histologically benign, these tumors may lead to rupture of the capsule of the liver, extensive bleeding, and death. Abdominal pain often continues for months before this rare tumor is diagnosed. Long-term users of OCs have an estimated annual incidence of hepatocellular adenomas (HCA) of 3–4 per 100,000. Women on over age 30 using higher potency pills may have an increased risk. In women aged 16-30 years who have used OCs for 24 months or less, HCA develops at an annual rate of about 1.0 per million compared with 1.3 per million for women 31-44 years of age. In 1977, about 320 hepatocellular adenomas were diagnosed each year in the United States, of which 282 (88%) were attributable to OC use. A small group of women may be genetically predisposed to developing HCA after long-term OC use.[63] With the current low-dose pills, the risk for liver tumors is either nonexistent or very much lower than with higher-dose pills.

14. **Cancer**. The most controversial question surrounding pill use since their arrival on the contraceptive scene in 1960 has been "Do oral contraceptives cause cancer?" A 1985 Gallup Poll commissioned by the American College of Obstetricians and Gynecologists (ACOG) found that both men and women regard cancer as the most significant OC risk.[25] Because of the long latency period between exposure to a carcinogen and clinical manifestations of cancer, the final word is still not in on pills and cancer. A recent model estimated that every 100,000 pill users would experience 44 *fewer* lifetime reproductive cancers than would women who did not use pill. This model assumed that 5 years or more of pill use was associated with a 20% increase in breast cancer diagnosed before age 50, 20% increase in cervical cancer, and 50% decrease in ovarian and endometrial cancer.[14]

Breast cancer. Numerous epidemiologic studies have been performed on the risk of breast cancer in pill users.[12,13,14,34,60,84] It remains to be seen whether an increased risk can be repeatedly shown for any specific subgroup of women. It is also possible that OCs may have a breast cancer promoting effect on a specific subgroup of women that would lead to an earlier diagnosis of cancer which would have otherwise become clinically apparent at an older age. In view of the statistical power of the large studies showing no overall increased risk for breast cancer in women using OCs, it is highly likely that if a subgroup of women—for example young, nulliparous women using pills for a number of years—is found to be at *increased* risk for breast cancer because of OCs, then another group of women—for example, women above age 50 who used pills for a number of years—will be found to be at *decreased* risk for breast cancer.

Ovarian and endometrial cancer. At least nine epidemiologic studies have demonstrated a decreased relative risk of ovarian cancer in pill users (approximately 0.5 risk).[11,30,34] Pills protect women from endometrial cancer (approximately 0.5 risk).[10,30,34] The decreased risk of both endometrial and ovarian cancer in women who have used OCs persists for at least 10 years after pills have been discontinued. Since ovarian epithelial cancer is more likely to occur in some families,[49] a strong family history for this type of ovarian cancer might be considered an indication for using OCs.

Cervical cancer. Although a causal relationship between oral contraceptive and cervical cancer has not been established, five of 13 epidemiologic studies have found a significantly increased risk of cervical neoplasia in oral contraceptive users, whereas seven found no statistically increased risk.[65] In a large British study, invasive cervical cancer, carcinoma-in-situ, and dysplasia occurred more frequently in parous women using OCs than in parous women using an IUD. The risk of cervical neoplasia increased with longer OC use. All 13 cases of invasive cancer occurred in women using OCs; nine of those women had used OCs for more than 6 years.[80] It may be that the regular Pap smears taken from women who use OCs is one reason why the epidemiologic picture regarding cervical cancer and pills is not in sharper focus; early dysplasia is more likely to be recognized and treated in women using OCs. Another confounding variable is that pill users tend to have more sexual partners.

Melanoma. In contrast to earlier findings, the largest case-control study indicates no increased incidence of melanoma in OC users.[39]

Hepatocellular carcinoma. Although a link between OCs and benign hepatocellular adenomas has been established for several years,[63] an association between OCs and hepatocellular carcinoma (HCC) is less certain. Trends in mortality due to HCC in the United States and Australia and two recent reviews cast considerable doubt on a positive association between OC use and HCC.[28,75] However, two large tumor registries in Los Angeles[40] and in Great Britain[23] suggest an association. In a series of 1,300 controls and 26 women who developed

HCC in noncirrhotic livers, women who had used OCs for a median of 8 years had an increased relative risk of developing HCC.[55] Their most common symptom was upper abdominal pain or right-side chest pain. In only three of 18 OC users who developed HCC were the tumors resectable. In a 1986 case-control study of OC use among women who died from liver cancer, use of OCs for 8 or more years was associated with a 20-fold increased risk of dying from HCC. This study concluded that liver cancer in young women is still exceptionally rare in Britain, but that a substantial proportion of the few cases that do occur in noncirrhotic livers are attributable to OC use.[24] Because liver cancer is extremely rare in developed countries, the absolute number of cases of liver cancer caused by pills would be small if there is any increased attributable risk caused by pills.

15. **Other side effects.** The estrogenic, progestational, and androgenic effects of OCs affect a number of organs and tissues throughout the body (skin, uterus, ovaries, brain, breasts, arteries, veins, etc.). A birth control pill may stimulate a given end-organ in a given woman quite differently than do the endogenous hormones that the woman produced before using oral contraceptives. A specific birth control pill may affect two different women quite differently.

Estrogenic effects. Most of the women using pills with less than 50 mcg of ethinyl estradiol do not experience one of the estrogen-mediated side effects. However, if one's therapeutic goal is to minimize the risk of a specific side effect that is usually related to the estrogenic component of pills, such as nausea or breast tenderness, the clinician may again choose the pill with lowest amount of ethinyl estradiol. Side effects which may be caused by the estrogen in pills are listed below:[19,32]

- Nausea
- Increased breast size (ductal and fatty tissue)
- Stimulation of breast neoplasia
- Fluid retention
- Cyclic weight gain due to fluid retention
- Leukorrhea
- Cervical erosion or ectopia
- Thromboembolic complications
- Pulmonary emboli
- Cerebrovascular accidents
- Hepatocellular adenomas
- Hepatocellular cancer

- Rise in cholesterol concentration in gallbladder bile
- Growth of leiomyomata
- Telangiectasia

Progestogenic effects. Both the estrogenic and the progestational components of oral contraceptives may contribute to the development of the following adverse effects:

- Breast tenderness
- Headaches
- Hypertension
- Myocardial infarction

Androgenic effects. All low-dose combined pills tend to have a beneficial effect on acne and oily skin because they all suppress a woman's production of testosterone. The progestin component of OCs, which in some instances has androgenic as well as progestational effects, may be associated with the following adverse effects:[19]

- Increased appetite and weight gain
- Depression, fatigue, tiredness
- Decreased libido and enjoyment of intercourse
- Acne, oily skin
- Increased breast size (alveolar tissue)
- Increased LDL cholesterol levels
- Decreased HDL cholesterol levels
- Diabetogenic effect
- Pruritus
- Decreased carbohydrate tolerance

The new progestins appear to be suitable options to minimize androgenic effects such as hirsutism, oily skin, sebaceous cysts, pilonidal cysts, or weight gain. (See following discussion on New Progestins.)

CAUTIONS

Certain words trigger such vivid images that they virtually block out all rational communication about anything else. To a certain extent, *contraindication* is such a trigger word. Health educators, journalists, clinicians, and clients need only hear the word contraindication and all attempts to qualify the degree of contraindication are virtually futile. Hence, in this and the following chapters, *precautions* replaces contraindications to various methods. Table 10-5 describes the precautions in the provision of combined oral contraceptives.

Table 10-5 Precautions in the provision of combined oral contraceptives (OCs)

Refrain from providing combined oral contraceptives for women with the following diagnoses:

Precautions	Rationale/Discussion
Thrombophlebitis or thromboembolic disorder or a history thereof	Estrogens promote blood clotting, therefore, women with other risk factors for excess blood clotting are at risk for future blood clotting problems with OCs. However, thromboembolic events related to known trauma or an intravenous needle are not necessarily a reason to avoid use of pills.
Cerebrovascular accident or a history thereof	Estrogens promote blood clotting. Women with other risk factors for excess blood clotting are at risk for future blood clotting problems with OCs.
Coronary artery or ischemic heart disease or a history thereof	Women with angina, heart attacks, or congestive heart failure may have valvular heart disease, coronary artery disease, kidney failure, or other serious disease. These women are at high risk for fatal complications during pregnancy and should strongly consider voluntary surgical contraception, or a reliable progestin-only method like Norplant or injectables. If these are not acceptable, the risks associated with low-dose OCs are almost certainly lower than the risks associated with pregnancy.
Known or strongly suspected breast cancer or a history of breast cancer	In theory, the hormones in OCs might cause some lumps to grow. Some clinicians and some clinical protocols suggest that women found to have a breast mass should not be provided combined OCs until cancer of the breast has been ruled out. Other clinicians are comfortable prescribing pills while the cause of the breast mass is being evaluated. Lumps which are suspicious should be evaluated.
Known or strongly suspected estrogen-dependant neoplasia or a history thereof	It is generally accepted that exogenous estrogens should not be provided to women with cancer of the reproductive organs. Estrogens may stimulate the growth of some cancers of the reproductive organs.

(continued)

Table 10-5 Precautions in the provision of combined oral contraceptives (OCs) *(cont.)*

Refrain from providing combined oral contraceptives for women with the following diagnoses:

Precautions	Rationale/Discussion
Pregnancy or pregnancy quite strongly suspected	Pregnancy would not be strongly suspected in a woman who had taken her last cycle of pills on schedule and has gone through 21 active pills and her 7 placebo pills without bleeding. In this instance the next package of pills should be started on schedule.
	Current data do NOT show that hormonal contraceptives taken during pregnancy cause any significant risk of birth defects because the doses are so low. However, since exposing the fetus to any medication could in theory cause birth defects, hormonal contraceptives should not be given to pregnant women. Ideally, women who have missed pills should be tested for pregnancy before continuing their cycles.
Benign hepatic adenoma or liver cancer or a history thereof	Progestins and estrogens affect the general functioning of the liver and should not be used during acute hepatitis. Use of OCs is associated with a higher risk of a rare benign liver tumor (hepatocellular adenoma). However, recent studies in the developing world by WHO found no evidence that combined OC use causes liver cancer.
Markedly impaired liver function at present time	Progestins and estrogens affect the general functioning of the liver and should not be used during acute hepatitis. Some clinicians suggest that combined pills should not be used in patients with hepatitis until liver function tests have returned to normal.

(continued)

Table 10-5 Precautions in the provision of combined oral contraceptives (OCs) *(cont.)*

Exercise caution *if combined oral contraceptives are used or considered in the following situations and carefully monitor for adverse effects:*

Precautions	Rationale/Discussion
Over 35 years old and currently a heavy smoker (15 or more cigarettes a day)	Cigarette smoking is the most important risk factor for vascular disease in women. Women over age 35 who smoke are at increased risk of heart attack, stroke, and other blood clotting problems. The mechanisms of this increased risk are not proven, but both estrogen and smoking increase the body's tendency to form blood clots. All smokers should be warned of this risk and all women should be advised to stop smoking.
Migraine headaches that start after initiation of oral contraceptives	Migraine headaches have been associated with an increased risk of stroke; however, some women report an improvement in their headaches with OCs.
Hypertension with resting diastolic blood pressure of 90 or greater or a resting systolic blood pressure of 140 or greater on three separate visits, or an accurate diastolic measurement of 110 or more on a single visit	A woman under 35 who is otherwise healthy and whose blood pressure is controlled by medication can elect to use oral contraception. For women who are over 35, the progestins and estrogens in combined oral contraceptives can slightly increase blood pressure. Women who have high blood pressure are already at increased risk for heart problems; using OCs can increase this risk.
Diabetes mellitus	Women with diabetes are at increased risk of heart disease and stoke, particularly if the woman smokes. Estrogens and progestins may slightly decrease glucose tolerance but this is unlikely to happen with low-dose OCs. Women with uncontrolled diabetes are also at high risk for poor pregnancy outcome, and need a very reliable contraceptive.
Elective major surgery or major surgery requiring immobilization planned in next 4 weeks	With the current low-dose pills, the problems associated with pill use and elective surgery have decreased.

(continued)

Table 10-5 Precautions in the provision of combined oral contraceptives (OCs) *(cont.)*

Exercise caution *if combined oral contraceptives are used or considered in the following situations and carefully monitor for adverse effects:*

Precautions	Rationale/Discussion
Undiagnosed abnormal vaginal/uterine bleeding	Although oral contraceptives are often used to manage heavy bleeding, clinicians should be sure that the cause of the bleeding is known before prescribing oral contraceptives. The causes of irregular bleeding include: intrauterine and ectopic pregnancy, breast feeding, pelvic inflammatory disease, cancer of the reproductive tract, early or premenopause, hypo- or hyperthyrodism, and other gynecological problems.
Sickle cell disease or sickle C disease	Patients with sickle cell trait can use oral contraception. Progestins stabilize the red blood cell membrane. The risk of thrombosis in women with sickle cell disease or sickle C diseases is theoretical (and medical-legal).
Lactation	Estrogen very slightly decreases the quality and the quantity of breast milk, while progestins are galactogens, promoting breast milk production. Breast feeding alone is an adequate contraceptive when the mother is still amenorrehic and not substituting other foods or liquids for breast feeding meals. Thus OC use is only indicated when breast feeding is no longer adequate, and when other methods are unacceptable. Some experts advise against combined pills entirely when other alternatives such as the mini-pill are available.[32] If estrogen-containing contraceptives are the only available option, breast feeding should be well established (at least 6 weeks' postpartum) before low-dose estrogen-containing pills are introduced.

(continued)

Exercise caution *if combined oral contraceptives are used or considered in the following situations and carefully monitor for adverse effects:*

Precautions	Rationale/Discussion
Gestational diabetes	Low-dose formulations do not produce a diabetic glucose tolerance response in women with previous gestational diabetes, and there is no evidence that oral contraception increases the incidence of overt diabetes mellitus. It is believed that women with previous gestational diabetes can use oral contraception with annual assessment of the fasting glucose level.[72]
Active gallbladder disease	OCs may accelerate the development of gallbladder disease in woman already susceptible to it. The mechanism is unclear, but it probably relates to effects of the pill on cholesterol metabolism.
Congenital hyperbilirubinemia (Gilbert's disease)	Women with this condition can be started on OCs but monitored carefully for jaundice hyperbilirubinema.
Over 50 years of age	Women over 50 are at increased risk for heart and cerebrovascular disease. Estrogens promote blood clotting. Women with other risk factors for blood clotting, particularly women age 35 or older, are at risk for future blood clotting problems with OCs. Women over 50 should consider using lower-dose estrogen replacement therapy.
Completion of term pregnancy within the past 10–14 days	When a woman starts OCs during the third postpartum week, she safely avoids the hypercoaguable state that occurs immediately after delivery (10–14 days).
Cardiac or renal disease or history thereof	These women are at high risk for fatal complications during pregnancy and should strongly consider voluntary surgical contraception, or a reliable progestin-only method like Norplant or injectables. If these are not acceptable, the risks associated with low-dose OCs are almost certainly lower than the risks associated with pregnancy.
Conditions likely to make it very difficult for a woman to take OCs consistently and correctly	Mental retardation, major psychiatric illness, alcoholism, or other chemical abuse, and/or a history of repeatedly taking oral contraception or other medications incorrectly, make compliance with taking OCs difficult.

(continued)

Table 10-5 Precautions in the provision of combined oral contraceptives (OCs) *(cont.)*

Exercise caution if combined oral contraceptives are used or considered in the following situations and carefully monitor for adverse effects:

Precautions	Rationale/Discussion
Family history of hyperlipidemia	Hyperlipidemia increases a woman's risk for atherosclerotic heart disease.
Family history of death of a parent or sibling due to myocardial infarction before age 50	Myocardial infarction in a mother or sister is especially significant and indicates a need for lipid evaluation.

Source: Angle (1992).

PROVIDING COMBINED PILLS

Although for most women the advantages of birth control pills outweigh the risks and disadvantages, negative misinformation about oral contraceptive pills is rampant. No contraceptive option is without disadvantages. It is important for clinicians balance the risks and benefits of pill use for each individual:

- Teach women the pill warning signals at each visit.
- Avoid pills for women who have important reasons to avoid pill use.
- Encourage women at risk for HIV infection to consider using condoms instead of or in addition to pills. Approximately 21% of pill users do concomitantly use condoms.[56]
- Encourage women to inform any clinician they see for a medical or psychological problem that they are on birth control pills.
- Measure blood pressure and use a checklist to evaluate clients on an annual basis.
- Avoid using pills with more than 35 mcg of estrogen.
- Prescribe pills with low dosages of progestin.
- Encourage all smokers to stop smoking.
- Provide women with clear instructions on how to use pills, what side effects to expect, and what to do if problems with the pill should occur. Included in the instructions she takes home might be a well-balanced answer to the most commonly asked question about pills: "Do the pills cause cancer?" See pill instructions on page 276.
- Inform women about the noncontraceptive benefits they may experience from pill use.

Initial Visit

Weight, blood pressure, Pap smear, and pelvic examination should be done at the time of the initial examination and at each annual exam. In women at high risk for cardiovascular disease, perform a lipid profile and a fasting blood sugar when pills are started and annually thereafter. Baseline mammography is recommended for women once between the ages of 35 and 40 and every other year from ages 40–50. Contact the American Cancer Society regarding frequency of mammography procedures. Pill instructions are available on audiotape. See "Listen Carefully," Chapter 28.

Women over 35 years of age.   Experts in the field of family planning and reproductive health now recommend that healthy women who are non-smokers and have no cardiovascular disease may continue use of oral contraceptives well into their 40s.[32,54,72] This trend is the consequence of a reanalysis of data from earlier studies, the availability and use of lower-dose pills, and recognition that it is primarily smoking and not pills which increases the risk of older women for cardiovascular complications. In prescribing OCs to women over 35, the following steps may be helpful at the time pills are initiated:

- Check for reasons to refrain from using pills (see Table 10-5).
- Ask about the client's history of diabetes or hypertension.
- Ask about a family history of premature cardiovascular disease and diabetes.
- Measure blood pressure.
- Perform breast exam and order mammography.
- Obtain total cholesterol and triglyceride level and fasting blood sugar tests.

The frequency of these procedures has been debated; some clinicians suggest annually. The pill prescribed should contain 35 mcg estrogen or less.

Women over 35 are often eager to discontinue taking daily OCs and also to stop using barrier contraceptives. Tubal sterilization and vasectomy are the contraceptives most often chosen in this age group. If a woman wants to use pills until she is 50, has no risk factors other than age for the use of combined oral contraceptives, is not a smoker, and experiences no side effects from pills, OCs may be an appropriate option for her. The non-contraceptive benefits of OCs in mature women (prevention of ovarian cancer and endometrial cancer; prevention of osteoporosis; and prevention of menopausal symptoms of women aged 35-50 years) must be evaluated more extensively in future research projects.

Smokers.   All women should be discouraged from smoking. However, it is not rational to withhold pills from all young women who are heavy smokers but have no other contraindications to pill use. If OCs are prescribed to a woman who is a smoker, explain to her that cigarette smoking has been recognized to have a synergistic effect with OC use to increase a woman's risk of myocardial infarction, stroke, and thromboembolic injury. *During each visit, teach her the pill warning signals and ask if she has developed any of these symptoms.* Encourage her to stop smoking.

Teenagers and college students. When can a young teenager start taking birth control pills? Ideally, she would have had from 6–12 regular periods before starting pills. However, if a young teenager is already sexually active, the medical and social risks of pregnancy exceed the risks of taking OCs, even if she has not started having menstrual periods.

A teenager who has had very irregular periods or very late onset of menses will have more regular menses, but when she stops her OCs in the future to become pregnant, her periods may become irregular again. Even though very little, if any, permanent loss of fertility follows use of OCs, an earlier pill study demonstrated that about 25% of pill patients (teenagers and adults, patients with regular as well as irregular menses) require at least 12 months, and 10% of pill patients need at least 24 months, to conceive.[46] Some clinicians tell a woman with a history of irregular periods to discontinue pills and use an alternative contraceptive for 6–12 or even 18 months before she would like to conceive.

We have no evidence that the estrogen in our current low-dose OCs can limit height due to premature closure of the epiphyses, even in premenarchal teens. In menstruating teens, epiphyseal closure is well under way.

Teen pill users may be more likely to abandon pills because of minor side effects such as nausea or spotting, so take all minor side effects in teenagers seriously. If acne is a particular concern use of one of the new progestin pills may be indicated. New progestin pills raise the level of sex hormone binding globulin (SHBG) and lower the level of free testosterone. Other pills to consider for the woman with acne are Ovcon-35, Brevicon, Modicon, and Demulen-35. If nausea is a problem, prescribe the 20 mcg pill, Loestrin 1/20, or a progestin-only-pill.

Teens can read about the pill and other contraceptive options in two small books written especially for them called *Sexual Etiquette 101* and *The Quest for Excellence.* (See Chapter 28.)

Postpartum/lactating women. Pills may cause a decrease in the amount of milk a breastfeeding woman produces. The FDA-approved pill labeling recommends that pill use begin only after the baby has been weaned. A better choice than a combined pill is probably a progestin-only pill. Contraceptive choice for the breastfeeding women is discussed extensively in Chapter 17 on Postpartum Contraception and Lactation and in Chapter 11 on Norplant, Depo-Provera, and Progestin-Only Pills.

STDs. Oral contraceptives provide no protection against STDs, including HIV infection. Clinicians should seriously raise the question of concomitant use of condoms on a regular basis until a woman becomes committed to a long-term, mutually faithful relationship. Consider writing a prescription for both an oral contraceptive and a specific condom.

Choosing a Combined OC: Which Pill to Prescribe

Too many pill options exist in the United States. Figure 10-3 is designed to assist clinicians in deciding which pill to prescribe for a woman requesting birth control pills. The following selection considerations are keyed to this figure.

Price (Step 3).   It is appropriate for price to enter the picture in choosing a pill. In many public family planning settings, decisions about which pill to provide are influenced by the cost of pills to that program. Local and national bids for OCs determine which pills are available for the clinician to prescribe in a given setting. In a very similar vein, the clinician in private practice often decides which low-dose combined OC to prescribe to a new pill patient on the basis of the availability of free samples to give to his or her patient.

If data clearly indicated greater safety, effectiveness, or patient acceptability of one low-dose OC over all the rest, then it would be important that this pill be chosen by both the public and the private sectors to the exclusion of other OCs even if it were not the least expensive. The data, however, do not support the conclusion that a single OC is clearly better than all the rest.

Lowest dose (Step 3).   Any of the sub-50 microgram (mcg) pills may be used by most women. If all the present brands of OCs were to be available to a clinician and to his or her patients at the same cost, how might the clinician determine which sub-50 mcg pill is best? *One approach is to prescribe the very lowest dose OC first:*

- Loestrin 1/20 with 33.3% less ethinyl estradiol than a woman receives in a 30 mcg OC and 43% less ethinyl estradiol than a woman receives in all the 35 mcg OCs.
- Ovcon-35 with a total of 8.4 mg of norethindrone or Modicon or Brevicon with a cycle total of 10.5 mg of norethindrone as compared with Ortho-Novum 7/7/7 with 15.75 mg of norethindrone or Tri-Norinyl with 15 mg of norethindrone or the even higher-dose OCs, such as Norinyl 1+35 or Ortho-Novum 1+35 with 21 mg of norethindrone per cycle.
- Triphasil or Tri-Levlen with a total of 1.925 mg of levonorgestrel per cycle, 39% less than the amount of levonorgestrel in Nordette (Levlen).
- All the new progestin pills contain low doses of progestin. The two new progestin pills with desogestrel (Desogen and Ortho-Cept) are also low estrogen, containing but 30 mcg of ethinyl estradiol.

The lowest-dose pills will probably offer the same noncontraceptive benefits. Documentation of most of the noncontraceptive benefits of pills has been primarily in women using higher-dose pills. Pills dramatically decrease dysmenorrhea. Pills decrease menstrual irregularities. Pills have been used

Figure 10-3 Choosing a combined oral contraceptive

Start by determining if the woman can safely use estrogen

Step 1	Step 2

Can this individual be ⟶ prescribed a pill with estrogen?

YES, she can use ⟶ an estrogen.

Definitely refrain from ⟶ prescribing a pill with estrogen to women with a history of a cerebro-vascular accident; ischemic heart disease; uncontrolled hypertension; insulin dependent diabetes with vascular disease; classic migraine with neurologic impairment which has increased with estrogen; breast cancer; estrogen dependent neo-plasia; active hepatic disease with impaired liver function at the present time; benign or malignant liver tumor; or deep vein thrombosis. Some clinicians would make an exception and provide combined OCs to women following postpar-tum pelvic vein thrombosis or women whose thrombophlebitis was due to trauma or IV. Also, in most instances refrain from provid-ing combined pills to women over 35 who smoke. Breast feeding women, in general, should avoid estrogen.

NO, it would be best if she did not use an estrogen. Therefore, you can consider:

- Progestin-only pills, such as:
  - Micronor (0.35 mg norethindrone daily)
  - NOR QD (0.35 mg nonrethindrone daily)
  - Ovrette (0.075 mg nogestrel daily)
  - Norplant (5-year levonorgestrel implants)
  - Depo-Provera (150 mg medroxyprogestrone acetate injection every 3 months)

- Intrauterine device
  - Copper T 380-A
  - Progestasert System

- Condoms (male or female)
- Diaphragm, Cervical Cap
- Foam, VCF Film, Suppository
- Sponge

© Robert A. Hatcher, MD, MPH
April 1993

The following individuals assisted in the develpment of this flow chart:
Marcia Angle, MD, MPH, Program for International Training and Health (INTRAH)
James Bellinger, PAC, Emory University School of Medicine
Robert A. Hatcher, MD, MPH, Emory University School of Medicine
Michael Policar, MD, MPH, Planned Parenthood Federation of America
Sharon Schnare, CNM, MSN, FNP, Harbor-UCLA Women's Health Care
Gary S. Stewart, MD, MPH, Planned Parenthood of Sacramento Valley
Susan Wysocki, RNC, BSN, NP, National Association of Nurse Practitioners in Reproductive Health
Graphic Design: Anne Atkinson and Beth Coffey

Most women who can safely use estrogen may use any of the sub-50 microgram pills

Step 3

Therefore, you may choose between any of the following OCs based on:

- Number of micrograms of ethinyl estradiol
- Availability of pill
- Ease of remaining on schedule because of pills
- Price of pills to clinic
- Price of pills to client
- Prior experience of this individual woman or the clinician caring for this woman with a special pill

Pills are listed from the lowest to the highest number of micrograms of ethinyl estradiol:

Combined Pill	Estrogen (mcg)	Availability/Cost In Your Clinic	Company
Loestrin 1/20	20	_____	Parke-Davis
Loestrin 1.5/30	30	_____	Parke-Davis
Desogen	30	_____	Organon
Lo-Ovral	30	_____	Wyeth
Nordette	30	_____	Wyeth
Levlen	30	_____	Berlex
Ortho-Cept	30	_____	Ortho
Tri-Levlen	30/40/30	_____	Berlex
Triphasil	30/40/30	_____	Wyeth
Ovcon 35	35	_____	Mead Johnson
Demulen 1/35	35	_____	Searle
Ortho-Cyclen	35	_____	Ortho
Ortho Tri-Cyclen	35	_____	Ortho
Ortho Novum 777	35	_____	Ortho
Ortho-Novum 1/35	35	_____	Ortho
Modicon	35	_____	Ortho
Brevicon	35	_____	Syntex
Norinyl 1/35	35	_____	Syntex
Tri-Norinyl	35	_____	Syntex
Norcept-E 1/35**	35	_____	Syntex
Nelova 0.5/35**	35	_____	GynoPharma
Nelova 1/35**	35	_____	Warner-Chilcott
NEE 0.5/35	35	_____	Lexis
NEE 1/35	35	_____	Lexis
Genora 0.5/35**	35	_____	Rugby
Genora 1/35	35	_____	Rugby
Jenest	35	_____	Organon
NEE 10/11	35	_____	Lexis
Norethin 1/35E	35	_____	Schiaparelli-Searle

On December 11, 1992, **The Medical Letter** published the cost to pharmacists for a one-month cycle of OCs based on "Average Wholesale Price Listing in Drug Topics Red Book 1992" and its November Update. The four pills costing pharmacists less than $10.00 per cycle were Norcept E ($5.72); Nelova 0.5/35; Nelova 1/35 ($6.25); and Genora 0.5/35 ($8.23). The cost of most pills to pharmacists was $17.00 to $22.33 per cycle. In some clinics, pills may be purchased at prices as low as $0.50 to $1.00 per cycle. These low prices are usually reflected in the prices clinics charge women.

Step 4

Other clinical considerations that might help in OC choice:

A. To minimize the risk potential for *thrombosis* due to estrogen in a woman 40–50 years of age or a woman at increased risk for thrombosis due to another cause (e.g., diabetic or heavy smoker), prescribe:
- Loestrin 1/20

B. To minimize *nausea, breast tenderness, vascular headaches*, and estrogen-mediated side effects, prescribe:
- Loestrin 1/20
Or a 30 mcg pill, such as:
- Desogen
- Levlen
- Loestrin 1.5–30
- Lo-Ovral
- Nordette
- Ortho-Cept

C. To minimize *spotting and/or breakthrough bleeding*, prescribe:
- Lo-Ovral, Nordette, or Levlen
- A new progestin pill: Desogen, Ortho-Cept, Ortho-Cyclen, or Ortho Tri-Cyclen

D. To minimize androgen effects such as *acne, hirsutism, oily skin, sebaceous cysts, pilonidal cysts, or weight gain*, prescribe:
- Desogen, Ortho-Cept
- Ortho Tri-Cyclen
- Ortho Cyclen
- Ovcon-35, Brevicon, or Modicon (of norethindrone pills)
- Demulen-35 (of ethnodiol diacetate pills)

E. To produce the most *favorable lipid profile*, prescribe:
- Ortho Cyclen or Ortho Tri-Cyclen
- Desogen or Ortho-Cept
- Ovcon-35, Brevicon, or Modicon (of norethindrone pills)

Contraceptive Technology 1994–1996

as replacement therapy for women whose ovaries have been removed or whose ovaries are not functioning. And pills are used to treat dysfunctional uterine bleeding, endometriosis, acne, hirsutism, benign breast disease, and functional ovarian cysts. Pills have also been shown to prevent anemia, ovarian and endometrial cancer, uterine fibromyomata, and pelvic inflammatory disease. Most of the noncontraceptive benefits of combined OCs appear to occur in women using low-dose pills.

Most of the oral contraceptives currently prescribed to new patients contain either 30 or 35 mcg of ethinyl estradiol. If a clinician were to limit his or her use of oral contraceptives to ethinyl estradiol-containing pills, some of the confusion could be eliminated as to the relative potency of ethinyl estradiol and mestranol. If a clinician uses both ethinyl estradiol and mestranol preparations, pill potency cannot be compared on a milligram-for-milligram basis.

Thrombosis (Step 4.A.).   The most serious of the complications to avoid is thrombophlebitis. The clinician faced with a client already at an increased risk for thrombophlebitis may want to use the 20 microgram pill.

Estrogenic side effects (Step 4.B.)   Provision of a low-estrogen pill may minimize the likelihood of any of the side effects or complications positively associated solely with the estrogen in pills or positively associated with either the estrogen or the progestin in a birth control pill.

Spotting (Step 4.C.).   To minimize spotting and/or breakthrough bleeding (BTB), several specific pills are suggested in Figure 10-3. However, this subject is very complex because definitions of spotting and BTB vary from study to study.

- Spotting has increased with all the lower-dose pills in comparison with the higher dose pills of 30 years ago. Spotting and BTB are two of the trade-offs for safer pills.

- Pill discontinuation due to spotting may be minimized by thoughtful counseling.

- Spotting and BTB tend to diminish dramatically over the first few months of pill use with all the combined pills.

- If one pill does not lead to an acceptable pattern of bleeding, another pill may.

Androgenic effects (Step 4.D.).   There have been studies of the benefits of new progestin pills in treating hirsutism, chronic anovulation with the syndrome of polycystic ovarian disease, and acne.[17,62] In one study, acne improved in women on a desogestrel pill and in women on a levonorgestrel pill, but was greater in women on the desogestrel pill; in this study, the rise in sex hormone binding globulin (SHBG) was greater and the fall in free testosterone was greater in women on the desogestrel pill than the women on a levonorgestrel pill.[58] Long before the entry of the new progestins, it was known that the lowest norethindrone combined pill (Ovcon 35) was associated with a 270% increase in SHBG and a decrease in free testosterone levels. Clinical evidence from several trials also confirms that SHBG levels increase and plasma androgen levels decrease in women taking levonorgestrel pills.[48,89] Some women may find it undesirable to have lower free testosterone levels, although this has not been reported. Consider the extensive use of androgens by postmenopausal women in response to a decrease in interest in sex due to lowered testosterone levels. New progestin pills also appear to have as good or better patterns of weight gain as other low-dose pills.

Lipids (Step 4.E.).   To produce the most positive lipid profile, prescribe one of the new progestin pills, which will tend to increase HDL cholesterol and decrease LDL cholesterol. Of the norethindrone pills, prescribe the pill with 0.4 mg of norethindrone, Ovcon-35, or one of the 0.5mg norethindrone pills. The clinical revelance of the lipid profile produced by the new progestin pills is not known at this time.

Other Considerations in Pill Choice

Higher dose estrogens.   Even if a woman is a satisfied user of an 80mcg or 100 mcg pill, she should be switched to a lower-dose pill. There are, however, several clinical situations when a 50 mcg pill may be helpful:

- Occasionally spotting or the absence of withdrawal bleeding cannot be managed on a lower dose pill and the woman must switch to a 50 mcg pill.
- Acne, dysfunctional uterine bleeding, ovarian cysts, and endometriosis have all been treated occasionally with OCs containing 50 mcg of estrogen. Dysfunctional bleeding has been treated by prescribing a variety of OCs in the following regimen: one tablet four times a day for 5-7 days. Ovarian cysts less than 6 cm in diameter in the childbearing-aged woman have been treated with combined monophasic pills.
- Low-estrogen symptoms of menopause may rarely occur in a woman taking a 20, 30, or 35 mcg pill. These symptoms may be eliminated by a 50 mcg pill.
- Contraceptive method failure despite perfect use of a 30-35 mcg pill perfectly may signal that the user is a candidate for a 50 mcg pill such as Ovcon-50, the only 50 mcg (ethinyl estradiol) pill with norethindrone. A second approach, which may be preferable, is to decrease the number of pill-free days from 7 to 4 or 5 (21 active pills followed by only 4, 5, or 6 days of no oral contraceptives before beginning a new package of pills).
- Rifampin and Dilantin (phenytoin) both accelerate the breakdown of estrogens in OCs, and women on these medications should probably be started on a 50 mcg pill.[5]

New progestins. For many new contraceptors, the new progestin pills may be the pills to start. The new progestins have several potential advantages over pills previously available:

- Higher HDL cholesterol and lower LDL cholesterol levels. While it might be expected that this biochemical profile would be beneficial to women over time, no clinical studies to date demonstrate clinical advantages. In one study of a desogestrel pill, the specific subfraction of HDL-2 fell, which has a beneficial effect in terms of cardiovascular disease; it has been suggested that a rise in HDL-3 is not associated with any cardiovascular benefits.[26]

- Lower free testosterone levels, higher sex hormone binding globulin (SHBG) levels, and greater affinity to progesterone binding sites (rather than to androgen binding sites). Sex hormone binding globulin (SHBG) is increased more by desogestrel (DSG) pills than by levonorgestrel (LNG) pills.[7,16,33,42,43,47,58,69] In two studies, free testosterone levels fell more in women on DSG pills than in women on LNG formulations.[7,58] In one study SHBG was increased more by the DSG pill than by the LNG pill, but the fall in free testosterone was identical in women using the two progestins.[41] In another study, SHBG rose more in women on the DSG pill than the LNG pill but there was an insignificant difference in the fall in total testosterone with the slightly greater fall in women on the LNG pill.[69]

- Reduced amenorrhea. There appear to be no women who go 2 months without a withdrawal bleed. This may be an important advantage for women who repeatedly miss several cycles on other low-dose OCs and feel uncertain or uncomfortable about this degree of menstrual irregularity.

In terms of beneficial effects on androgenic symptoms and beneficial effects on HDL cholesterol, the new progestin pills do not appear to have major advantages over Ovcon-35, Modicon, or Brevicon. The new progestins are an evolution, not a revolution. Satisfied users of previously available pills may best be left on those pills. For some women, a pill with just 20 micrograms of ethinyl estradiol may be preferable to any of the new progestin pills (see Figure 10-3). The disadvantages of the new progestin pills are that they may increase the confusion over the many pill options; the lowering of free testosterone may have negative effects on women although preliminary evidence has not demonstrated this effect; and the price of some of the new progestins may be higher than the price of other pills.

Norgestimate (Ortho-Cyclen, Ortho Tri-Cyclen) has less androgenic effect than previously available progestins.[59] With ethinyl estradiol, norgestimate raises SHBG, reduces free testosterone, and elevates HDL cholesterol. It produces a more favorable LDL-to-HDL ratio over a 2-year period than do levonorgestrel and norethindrone and does not adversely affect clinical coagulation profiles.

Desogestrel (Desogen, Orhto-Cept) has metabolic effects similar to norgestimate.

Gestodene (Minulet, Tri Minulet) has many of the advantages of norgestimate and desogestrel. It had not been approved for use in the United States when this edition went to press.

MANAGING PROBLEMS AND FOLLOW-UP

Clear and concise self-administered questions can protect the pill user from continuing to use pills when she has developed medical problems or is experiencing one of the pill warning signals. It has generally been recommended that women initiating OC use should be reevaluated during the first 3–6 months. After a woman has used the pill for 3–6 months, is having no problems, and wants to continue the pill, seven packets (a 6-month supply) may be provided. After a woman has used pills for 1 year (cumulative year of pill use), a full year's supply of pills may be provided in an effort to decrease pill discontinuation rates.

(The following problems are listed in alphabetical order.)

ACNE OR OILY SKIN

History should include questions about family history, age of onset, duration and progression of symptoms, and relationship to taking pills. Ask about cyclicity of flare-ups before pill use and while using pills. Oligomenorrhea and acne before pill use, hirsutism, and inability to become pregnant may suggest chronic anovulation associated with polycystic ovarian disease. Determine whether stressful situations, dietary patterns, or medications (including different oral contraceptive formulations) have made acne worse or better.

Look for location, size, number, and color of lesions. Observe amount, thickness, and distribution of hair. Look for ovarian enlargement or cysts. Consider ordering serum testosterone/DHAS levels.

The differential diagnosis of acne or oily skin while using pills may include:

- Use of an oral contraceptive with high androgenic potency.
- High endogenous ovarian or adrenal androgenic production.
- Dietary, allergic, hygienic, familial, or other factors.
- An androgen-producing ovarian or adrenal tumor.

The plan for the management of acne if a woman is on combined pills may include the following:

- Provide a low-androgen pill that may suppress ovarian androgenic production while providing the least exogenous androgen. As noted in Step 4, section D on Figure 10.3, the pills you may want to consider include the new progestin pills, Ovcon-35, Brevicon, Modicon or Demulen-35.

- Increase the amount of estrogen in the oral contraceptive to increase the sex hormone binding globulin (SHBG), thus decreasing free serum testosterone levels and improving acne.

- Consider alternative approaches to treatment of acne including use of a broad spectrum antibiotic such as tetracycline, dietary changes, good hygiene, use of special soaps or skin cleansers, or use of the vitamin A analogue, Accutane.

- Women taking Accutane must use a reliable contraceptive. A high percentage of infants born to mothers taking Accutane in early pregnancy have severe neurological defects. Contraception should continue for at least 30 days after Accutane is discontinued.

- Discontinue the pill (remember that pills are more likely to improve acne than to make it worse).

- Refer the patient to a dermatologist or endocrinologist for further assessment.

AMENORRHEA (MISSED PERIODS)

As strength of pills has fallen over the years, missed periods have become more common. The cyclic build up of the uterine lining is almost always less in women using pills than in women experiencing natural cycles. The amount of vaginal bleeding in the 7 pill-free days may be minimal, or no bleeding at all may occur. Women should be told in advance to anticipate a decrease in bleeding.

Determine if the patient has had any bleeding or spotting (while taking pills) or a total absence of bleeding. Ask about staining of underwear. History should include questions about missing pills, patterns of sexual intercourse, date of last sexual intercourse, the symptoms of pregnancy (including enlarging breasts, breast tenderness, and nausea), breast discharge, vigorous exercise, increased stress, weight changes, major life changes, recreational drug use, periods prior to taking oral contraceptives, and use of drugs causing rapid clearance of estrogens from the blood stream, such as rifampin or phenobarbital. Ask the patient what she would do were she to become pregnant while using oral contraceptives (*e.g.*, carry the pregnancy to term or seek an abortion). Ask if the patient has performed a home pregnancy test.

Determine whether the patient is pregnant. When doing physical assessment, look for uterine enlargement, softening of the cervix, and other signs of pregnancy. If the basal temperature is elevated, it would indicate the possibility of pregnancy. Further tests include serum or sensitive urine pregnancy tests.

The most important differential diagnosis of missed periods or prolonged amenorrhea while using pills is usually between: pregnancy (intrauterine or ectopic) and inadequate buildup of endometrium due to use of a low-dose oral contraceptive.

Missed menses or prolonged amenorrhea in a woman on combined pills may be managed by using one or more of the following approaches:

- Most important of all, *warn low-dose pill users in advance of the possibility of very scanty bleeding or no bleeding at all.* This side effect is a result of lowering the potency of oral contraceptives to attain a desirable effect: greater safety.
- Consider having the client check her basal body temperature on three consecutive "off day" mornings. A temperature below 98° F on three consecutive mornings during "off days" suggests that ovulation and pregnancy have not occurred.
- Rule out the possibility of pregnancy with a sensitive beta-HCG test if the patient has two or more missed periods. Rule out the possibility of pregnancy if the patient has a single missed period, the patient has missed taking pills, and abortion would not be the patient's choice if she were pregnant.
- Provide a pill with higher progestin potency to produce greater endometrial buildup. Because women using the new progestin pills virtually never miss two consecutive menstrual periods, it may now be possible to manage amenorrhea in women on other pills by switching them to one of the new progestin preparations.

BREAKTHROUGH BLEEDING AND SPOTTING BETWEEN PERIODS

Although spotting and breakthrough bleeding are less likely to occur among women taking low-dose pills than among women who are not taking pills, both spotting and breakthrough bleeding are more common among users of low-dose OCs than among users of high-dose pills. Although breakthrough bleeding is not harmful, it can be annoying and is a frequent reason for women discontinuing the pill. Patients must be informed of this possible side effect and reassured of its benign nature.

History should include questions about duration of pill use, dosage, regularity of taking pills, duration and amount of spotting, most recent period, symptoms of pregnancy, past history of gynecologic problems, pelvic pain, chills, fever, malaise, pain during intercourse, recent new sexual partners, vaginal discharge, use of other drugs that may interact with oral contraceptives (such as rifampin, phenytoin, phenobarbital, carbamazepine, ampicillin, or tetracycline), history of nausea and vomiting, diarrhea, or other intestinal or liver problems.

Look for signs of pregnancy (intrauterine or ectopic), pelvic infection (consider obtaining cultures for chlamydia and gonorrhea), myomata, cervical inflammation or polyp, or endometriosis. Obtain a hematocrit.

The differential diagnosis of breakthrough bleeding or spotting while using pills may include inadequate estrogenic stimulation of endometrial activity; inadequate progestin effect on endometrium; missing pill(s) or altering the time of taking birth control pills; threatened abortion; spontaneous abortion; ectopic pregnancy; pelvic inflammatory disease; endometriosis; leiomyomata, particularly submucous myoma; endometrial cancer; cervical inflammation, condylomata, or cancer; and a cervical or endometrial polyp. *In young women, it is always important to remember the possibility of chlamydia as the cause of spotting or breakthrough bleeding, particularly if she has had a recent change in sexual partners.*

After the possibility of pregnancy, pelvic inflammatory disease, and other gynecologic causes of bleeding (other than pills) have been eliminated, plans that may be appropriate include informing the patient initiating pills that breakthrough bleeding decreases dramatically over the first 4 months of pill use; reassuring and encouraging her when breakthrough bleeding occurs; informing her that lowering the potency of OCs has increased their safety but has also increased the breakthrough bleeding associated with their use.

Most clinicians now increase the progestin potency of the pill if they make a switch in pills as a response to BTB or spotting. Lo/Ovral may be more powerful than Nordette and less likely to result in spotting. However, rates of spotting and breakthrough bleeding come from different studies, conducted by different investigators at different times and in different patient populations.

A second type of switch in pill potency is to increase the estrogenic potency of the pill while leaving the progestin unchanged. This is most easily accomplished by supplementing the estrogen in OCs for one to three cycles with exogenous estrogen in the form of 17-beta estradiol (*e.g.,* Estrace 1 mg or 2 mg daily taken 12 hours after OC is taken, ethinyl estradiol (20 mcg per day), or conjugated estrogen (Premarin 0.625 mg daily).

Another intervention that may benefit a woman is to have her try a prostaglandin inhibitor. Prostaglandin inhibitors decrease both menstrual bleeding and menstrual cramps and pain.

BREASTFEEDING PROBLEMS

Pills appear to diminish both the volume and protein content of breast milk in some lactating women. In addition, small amounts of the hormones in birth control pills are present in the breast milk. Although some studies have shown normal weight gain in infants whose mothers were using OCs while nursing, many experts who have reviewed this subject suggest that women use an alternative to combined oral contraceptives during lactation.[32,72,82] If combined OCs are initiated postpartum, they should not be used until after a woman has established a good flow of breast milk. Progestin-only OCs and other progestin-only contraceptives are a better choice than combined OCs for lactating women. See Chapter 17 on Postpartum Contraception and Lactation.

BREAST FULLNESS OR TENDERNESS (MASTALGIA)

Lowering the amount of estrogen provided in each pill tends to reduce breast tenderness. Pregnancy, benign breast masses, and breast cancer also cause breast tenderness. History should include questions about duration and severity, when during the cycle discomfort occurs, severity prior to use of pills, symptoms of pregnancy, progression of symptoms, cyclic changes in weight, change in bra size, breast discharge, past history of benign breast disease, biopsies or mammography, and family history of breast cancer.

Look for local or generalized tenderness, difference in fullness, nodularity or masses, and nipple fluid. Note comparative size of the two breasts. Look for signs of early pregnancy. Further tests may include mammography, microscopic or cytologic evaluation of breast discharge, fine-needle aspiration of masses for cytologic study, biopsy, urine or serum pregnancy tests, or prolactin level. *Draw blood to obtain a prolactin level before examining the breast because breast stimulation immediately raises the serum prolactin level.*

The differential diagnosis of breast fullness or tenderness includes actual growth of breast tissue; cyclic edema due to either the estrogen or the progestin; early pregnancy; masses or tenderness due to benign breast disease, fibroadenomata, or breast cancer; or an elevated prolactin level.

After ruling out the possibility of pregnancy and breast cancer, recommend that the client change to a pill with less estrogen or less progestin. Switch to the 20 mcg pill, or to a progestin-only pill. Inform her that her symptoms may improve if she avoids vigorous exercise (which shakes breast tissue) during times of most discomfort. Some women have benefitted from decreasing intake of methylxanthines found in coffee, tea, chocolate, and soft drinks.

Some women have also benefitted from vitamin E, 400 IU two times a day, to relieve the symptoms of fibrocystic breast tenderness. Recommend good bra support for symptomatic relief. Bromocriptine or Danocrine may be of benefit to some women who have severe tenderness. Bromocriptine should not be used with diuretics or hypotensive drugs. Even if a breast mass is not palpable, order baseline mammography if the woman is 35-40 years of age or older, has family history of breast cancer, or simply expresses a desire to have a mammogram.

CHLOASMA OR THE MASK OF PREGNANCY

Darkening of skin pigment usually occurs on the upper lip, under the eyes, and on the forehead. Although not dangerous, chloasma may cause a woman a great deal of concern because the increased pigmentation may be slow to fade when pills are discontinued. Increased pigmentation may even be permanent.

Other skin conditions that may occur in pill users include telangiectasia, neurodermatitis, erythema multiforme, erythema nodosum, eczema, photosensitivity, and loss of hair. Occasionally, women note increased hair growth or the appearance of darker hair on the body and face. However, usually hirsutism, acne, and oily skin improve when a woman is on pills.

DEPRESSION AND OTHER MOOD CHANGES

In some instances, pills produce a deficiency of pyridoxine (vitamin B_6). While premenstrual irritability and depression are more likely to decrease in women taking low-dose pills, some women experience more severe premenstrual symptoms.

The history should include questions about onset of depression relative to initiating the current pill, depression while using other pills, depression prior to pill use, severity of depression, past history of suicide attempts, thoughts of suicide, changes in appetite, weight change, ability to sleep, changes in life situation, fear of AIDS and other sexually transmitted diseases, relationship with partner(s), physical abuse, job satisfaction, and illnesses. Ask about changes in the frequency of intercourse, libido, the ability to have orgasm, and use of diazepam and other mood-altering drugs that may interact with pills.

Look for signs of depression including lethargy, depressed mood, and expressions of inability to cope. Severe depression may need to be evaluated by a mental health professional.

Accurately diagnosing the cause of depression in a pill user may be extremely difficult. The onset of depression may be quite insidious. It may be diagnosed by a person's acquaintances before it is recognized by the patient herself. Determine the severity of depression and if the depression began or became worse after starting pills. Possible mechanisms of pill-induced depression including the following:

- Depression, lethargy, and tiredness related to progestin in the pill
- Depression caused by a pill-induced decrease in pyridoxine (B_6) levels

- Depression associated with cyclic fluid retention caused by the estrogen or the progestin in an oral contraceptive
- Interaction with diazepam. The half-life of diazepam (Valium) is increased from 47 to 60 hours by oral contraceptives and the dosage of diazepam may need to be lowered for the woman on pills.[1]

If the depression is severe, discuss with the patient immediate sources of psychiatric help. Take severe depression seriously, regardless of its etiology. If the depression is clearly temporally related to pill use and bothersome to the patient, the easiest approach is to provide an alternative method and discontinue pills completely for three to six cycles and see what happens.

Lowering the estrogen or the progestin (or both) may benefit all types of pill-induced depression except for depression actually due to the low estrogen in a woman's pill (and this is very rare). Depression is more likely to be due to progestin excess.

Consider providing the patient with 20 mg of vitamin B_6 daily. If the patient discontinues pills, be sure that she is counseled to use a different method acceptable to her and her partner. If depression is related, in part to fear of becoming infected with HIV, encourage condom use or clarification of the source of her anxiety.

EYE PROBLEMS (BLURRED OR LOSS OF VISION)

Eye problems may accompany headaches and transient ischemia. On rare occasions, pills may cause inflammation of the optic nerve with loss of vision, double vision, or swelling or pain in one or both eyes. Women using OCs are at an increased risk for retinal artery and retinal vein thrombosis. Pill-related fluid retention may cause corneal edema, leading to an increased likelihood of discomfort or even corneal damage among contact lens users, although modern soft contact lenses and low-dose OCs have diminished this problem. Loss of vision may also indicate the need for glasses. There is no evidence that pills cause or aggravate glaucoma. If a patient has experienced transient, total, or partial loss of vision, discontinue pills immediately and refer her to a neurologist. If visual symptoms accompany migraine headaches which have become worse, discontinue pills immediately.

GALACTORRHEA

History should include questions about stimulation of breast by suckling, duration and amount of discharge, and past history of galactorrhea. Ask about symptoms of pregnancy such as nausea, breast fullness or tenderness, change in appetite, missed menses, weight gain. Ask when last sexual intercourse occurred. Ask if the patient has experienced headaches or changes in vision. Galactorrhea associated with excessive estrogen in birth control pills is most noticeable in the pill-free week.[72]

Determine if secretions can be expressed from breasts. Describe the quantity and quality of any discharge. Look at the discharge under a microscope (fat globules, white blood cells, etc.)

The differential diagnosis of galactorrhea in a woman using pills may include suppression of PIF (prolactin inhibiting factor) by OCs, galactorrhea secondary to breast suckling, or prolactin secreting tumor.

The plan for a woman experiencing galactorrhea may include the following:

- If discharge can be expressed from breast, send it to cytology after fixing as you would fix Pap smear of cervix (unless galactorrhea is felt to be due to breast suckling).

- Draw blood for serum prolactin level. Breasts cannot have been examined before blood is drawn because this immediately raises serum prolactin levels; wait until the next day if breast examination has already been performed. If an elevated level is found, consider whether a breast examination occurred immediately prior to obtaining blood or whether breasts were stimulated the previous night.

- Perform a sensitive pregnancy test if pregnancy is a possibility.

- Consider discontinuing pills if galactorrhea is of concern to the woman. Initiate alternative contraceptive if she is sexually active. Galactorrhea caused by excessive estrogen is less common now with lower dose pills. However, if galactorrhea is due to pills, it will disappear within 3-6 months after discontinuing pills.[72]

If galactorrhea is felt to be due to breast suckling during lovemaking, discuss how much galactorrhea is bothering the patient; consider recommending less intense breast stimulation.

HEADACHES

Headaches may be mild, severe, recurrent, or persistent. Women may note an increase (or a decrease) in the severity of migraine headaches. Pill-induced headaches are sometimes associated with blurred vision, loss of vision, nausea, vomiting, or weakness in an extremity. Because severe headaches may be an early warning of a stroke, they need to be evaluated carefully.

History should include questions about age at onset of headaches, severity, duration, stress, location of pain, cyclicity, jaw pain, and the relationship of headaches to taking pills. Ask if the headaches are unilateral, throbbing, or associated with nausea, vomiting, dizziness, scotomata or blurred vision, watering of the eyes, or loss of vision. Ask about history of sinusitis or postnasal drip. Find out what medications have made the headaches better or worse. Ask about alcohol use, caffeine intake, and take a drug history. Ask if headaches have ever been diagnosed as migraine and if a family history of migraine headaches exists. Determine if the patient is able to function during the time when headaches are most severe. Ask if she has ever had loss of speech, weakness, numbness, or tingling associated with a headache.

Check the patient's blood pressure and perform a funduscopic exam. Look for localized tenderness at sites on the face, head, and neck. A complete neurological exam may be indicated. If the patient's headaches are severe or accompanied by neurological symptoms, get a CAT scan.

After taking a good history and the above physical exam, the differential diagnosis of headaches in a patient using pills may include the following:

- Transient ischemic attacks, migraine headaches, vascular headaches associated with oral contraceptive use, or cerebrovascular accident
- Hypertension
- Headache associated with cyclic fluid retention that may be induced by the estrogen or progestin components of an oral contraceptive
- Tension or stress-induced headaches
- Headaches following use of alcohol, caffeine withdrawal, or other drugs
- Sinusitis, viremia, sepsis, or headaches associated with a dental problem, or with seasonal allergies
- Temporomandibular joint (TMJ) disorder
- Central nervous system tumor

Take headaches in a pill user seriously, because they are the major warning signal that precedes cerebrovascular accidents. Pay particular attention if symptoms are increasing. Definitely consider discontinuing pills if headaches are becoming worse.

If the headache is clearly temporally related to initiation of oral contraceptive use, discontinue or change to a preparation with lower estrogenic or lower progestational activity. Reevaluate after a cycle or two.

DECREASED LIBIDO OR SEX DRIVE

Perhaps due to decreased androgen production by the ovary, some women experience a decreased libido. Some women also experience decreased vaginal lubrication, making sexual intercourse less comfortable (and occasionally painful); this is possibly an estrogen deficiency effect. Other pill users enjoy sex more because the fear of pregnancy is removed by pills. It has been demonstrated that free testosterone levels fall dramatically in women on the new progestin OCs. Whether this is associated with significant problems in terms of decreased libido remains to be seen.

Nausea

Nausea most often occurs during the first cycle of birth control pills or during the first few pills of each new package. Nausea is less of a problem in lower dose pills. Vomiting is rare. Many women can control nausea by taking their pills after eating a meal or snack or at bedtime. When nausea occurs for the first time after months or years of taking pills, look for signs of early pregnancy. Nausea may also be caused by flu or another acute infection. Further tests in the evaluation of nausea may include sensitive urine or serum pregnancy tests and diagnostic tests for HIV, hepatitis, mononucleosis, or gallbladder disease.

Consider changing to a combined pill with less estrogen or to a progestin-only pill containing no estrogen. A 20 mcg pill dramatically decreases nausea for many women although it may also lead to more spotting and breakthrough bleeding. Inform the client that nausea often decreases after the first few cycles or becomes limited to the first day or so of each cycle. Recommend that the patient consistently take the pill at the time of the evening meal. Taking the pill at bedtime has proven helpful for some women. Inform the patient that should she vomit within 1 hour of taking a pill, she should take an extra pill from a separate pack to replace the pill she took just prior to vomiting. Counsel the patient to "catch up" by taking pills at 12-hour intervals rather than two at a time. Very disturbing nausea or vomiting may occur when a woman doubles up after missing two or three pills.

Pregnancy

Although uncommon, pregnancy may occur even if pills have been taken perfectly. History should include questions about duration of pill use; menstrual periods in past while taking OCs, including missed periods; history of missing oral contraceptives from the past two packages of pills; date(s) of the patient's last sexual intercourse, to attempt to identify the time of fertilization; history of nausea, vomiting, breast tenderness, enlarging breasts; history of all medications and drugs, including alcohol taken during the time of the pregnancy; history of abnormalities in previous pregnancies, miscarriages, and abortions; date of most recent HIV test and result. Determine HIV risk.

Determine whether or not the patient is pregnant. Ask the patient what she would want to do if she were to become pregnant while using OCs (carry pregnancy to term or seek an abortion). Ask the patient if she has performed a home pregnancy test. Look for signs of pregnancy on physical exam. Perform sensitive pregnancy test.

The plan for a woman who may possibly be pregnant while using OCs may include the following:

- Inform the patient that little if any increased risk of birth defects exists as a result of pill use during pregnancy.
- Discontinue pills if a diagnosis of pregnancy is made.
- Discontinue pills if the patient would not want an abortion and an early gestation cannot be ruled out. If OCs are discontinued, be sure to offer alternative contraception, such as condoms, sponge, foam, or diaphragm.
- Refer the patient for an abortion if she does not wish to be pregnant and wants to have pregnancy termination procedure.
- Refer the patient for prenatal care if she wishes to continue pregnancy. Have her immediately begin prenatal vitamins and stress the importance of care during pregnancy.

WEIGHT CHANGE

In most instances, weight change is minimal and is unrelated to pill use. History should include questions about the relationship of weight gain to the initiation of current oral contraceptives, weight change on any other birth control pills, change in appetite, cyclicity of weight gain, symptoms of early pregnancy, and patient recall of previous weights. Current work, sleep, and exercise habits, signs of depression, and any changes in lifestyle may be significant factors in weight gain.

Look for edema, the amount and distribution of fat, uterine enlargement, and signs of pregnancy. Further tests may include sensitive urine or serum pregnancy tests, or 2-hour postprandial glucose. Record weight and note previous weights in chart.

Approximately as many women lose weight as gain weight while taking OCs. In some women, however, weight gain is definitely caused by oral contraceptives. Rarely, pills can cause a gain of 10–20 pounds or more.

The differential diagnosis of weight gain in a woman using oral contraceptives may include the following:

- Fluid retention due to either the progestin or the estrogen in an oral contraceptive. This pattern of weight gain occurs in the month or so after initiating pills.
- Estrogen-induced weight gain due to increased subcutaneous fat, particularly in the hips, thighs, and breasts. This type of weight gain is noted after several months on pills.
- Increased appetite and increased intake of food (anabolic effect) occurs over several years.
- Depression may be accompanied by concomitant increase in caloric intake.

- Increased availability of high-caloric foods and a change in pattern of eating, or decreased exercise.

Weight gain usually responds to decreasing caloric intake and increasing exercise. Inform the patient who has experienced weight gain that using pills is a possible cause. Therapy for weight gain may include one of the following interventions:

- Switch to a pill with decreased androgenic potency if the patient has experienced an anabolic effect and persistent weight increase over time. It may be necessary to discontinue pills.
- Decrease the estrogen, progestin, or both, or discontinue the pills if the patient has clearly been experiencing cyclic weight change.
- Switch to a pill with decreased estrogenic potency if the patient has had weight gain due to increased breast tissue and subcutaneous fat, particularly in the thighs or hips.

Obese women can be started on low-dose combined OCs just as one would prescribe them for women of normal weight. The protective effect of combined OCs against endometrial cancer may be particularly desirable in overweight women whose risk of endometrial cancer is increased. OCs may be prescribed for women who are obese. There is no evidence that overweight women need to be prescribed a higher-dose pill for oral contraceptives to be effective. Strongly consider performing a lipid profile and 2-hour postprandial glucose test, particularly if the patient has a family history of diabetes or of heart disease at a young age. Carefully teach an obese woman the pill warning signals. *Use of one of the new progestin OCs, Ovcon-35, Modicon, or Brevicon may improve the lipid profile of a young obese women who will be on OCs for a number of years.*

PILL INTERACTIONS

Hormonal contraceptives affect many organ systems, and the metabolism of OCs is altered by a number of drugs a woman may be taking. The trend toward lower dosages of hormones in OCs has been dramatic. The lower the dose of the estrogen or the progestin provided to a woman as a contraceptive, the greater must be one's concern with regard to several factors that may decrease the effectiveness of a contraceptive pill, injection, implant, or vaginal ring. Table 10-6 summarizes the effects of taking oral contraceptives in combination with a number of drugs and the metabolic effects felt to cause these adverse effects. A woman placed on a medication that may decrease the effectiveness of her OCs should be informed of this possible effect and offered the option of using a back-up contraceptive, such as condoms.

Effectiveness of a very low-dose hormonal contraceptive may be lowered through the following mechanisms:

- A second medication may induce liver enzymes that cause breakdown of an estrogen or progestin (microsomal liver enzyme induction). The anticonvulsants most likely to have this effect are phenobarbital, phenytoin, carbamazepine, primidone, and ethosuximide (the anticonvulsant sodium valproate does not have this effect).[5] Several investigators have suggested that pregnancy may occur more often in low-dose OC users on anticonvulsants.[5,18] The contraceptive efficacy of OCs can be restored by using higher dosage OCs.[18] Women receiving long-term phenobarbital therapy may initially be placed on an OC containing 50 mcg of ethinyl estradiol, and the dose increased should breakthrough bleeding occur. Rifampin also has potent enzyme-inducing effects and the antifungal drug griseofulvin may have similar but less powerful enzyme-inducing properties.

- A second medication may increase plasma sex hormone binding globulin (SHBG) levels, thereby decreasing the amount of biologically active free steroid.

- A second medication may decrease the amount of hormone absorbed initially or reabsorbed following passage through the liver. It has been suggested that antibiotics could decrease OC effectiveness by decreasing enterohepatic recirculation, increasing fecal or urinary excretion of steroids, or increasing liver degradation. In spite of anecdotal case reports of contraceptive failure in OC users on antibiotics, no firm pharmacokinetic evidence exists linking antibiotic use to altered steroid blood levels.[6]

- Side effects of medication may cause nausea, diarrhea, or drowsiness or may cause a woman to fail to take OCs. Women on low-dose hormonal contraceptives who miss a pill may compromise contraceptive protection more than women on higher dosages.

- Spotting or breakthrough bleeding may lead to patient concern and either several missed pills or discontinuation of the method, both of which could lead to unplanned pregnancy.

While each of the above changes may decrease pill effectiveness, one intervention may increase the amount of ethinyl estradiol absorbed in the digestive system. It is quite common for people to take high doses of vitamin C each day to prevent colds, in the (unproven) belief that this practice will prevent or treat the common cold. *Taking 1 gram of vitamin C daily to prevent or treat colds is not recommended for women on pills.*[31] High-dose vitamin C (ascorbic acid) has been shown to increase the serum concentration of steroids by inhibiting the liver enzymes that conjugate ethinyl estradiol and by increasing the amount of ethinyl estradiol absorbed.[6,31] One gram of vitamin C increases the serum ethinyl estradiol level by 50% in OC users.[6] This in effect changes a low-dose pill into a high-dose pill. Intermittent use

Table 10-6 Pill interactions with other drugs

Interacting Drugs	Adverse Effects (Probable Mechanism)	Comments and Recommendations
Acetaminophen (Tylenol and others)	Possible decreased pain-relieving effect (increased metabolism)	Monitor pain-relieving response
Alcohol	Possible increased effect of alcohol	Use with caution
Anticoagulants (oral)	Decreased anticoagulant effect	Use alternative contraceptive
Antidepressants (Elavil, Norpramin, Tofranil, and others)	Possible increased antidepressant effect	Monitor antidepressant concentration
Barbiturates (phenobarbital and others)	Decreased contraceptive effect	Avoid simultaneous use; use alternative contraceptive for epileptics
Benzodiazepine Tranquilizers (Ativan, Librium, Serax, Tranxene, Valium, Xanax, and others)	Possible increased or decreased tranquilizer effects including psycho-motor impairment	Use with caution. Greatest impairment during menstrual pause in oral contraceptive dosage
Beta-blockers (Corgard, Inderal, Lopressor, Tenormin)	Possible increased blocker effect	Monitor cardiovascular status
Carbamazepine (Tegretol)	Possible decreased contraceptive effect	Use alternative contraceptive
Corticosteroids (cortisone)	Possible increased corticosteroid toxicity	Clinical significance not established
Griseofulvin (Fulvicin, Grifulvin V, and others)	Decreased contraceptive effect	Use alternative contraceptive
Guanethidine (Esimil, Ismelin)	Decreased guanethidine effect (mechanism not established)	Avoid simultaneous use
Hypoglycemics (Tolbutamide, Diabinese, Orinase, Tolinase)	Possible decreased hypoglycemic effect	Monitor blood glucose
Methyldopa (Aldoclor, Aldomet, and others)	Decreased antihypertensive effect	Avoid simultaneous use

(continued)

Table 10-6 Pill interactions with other drugs *(cont.)*

Interacting Drugs	Adverse Effects (Probable Mechanism)	Comments and Recommendations
Penicillin	Decreased contraceptive effect with ampicillin	Low but unpredictable incidence; use alternative contraceptive
Phenytoin (Dilantin)	Decreased contraceptive effect	Use alternative contraceptive
	Possible increased phenytoin effect	Monitor phenytoin concentration
Primidone (Mysoline)	Decreased contraceptive effect	Use alternative contraceptive
Rifampin	Decreased contraceptive effect	Use alternative contraceptive
Tetracycline	Decreased contraceptive effect	Use alternative contraceptive
Theophylline (Bronkotabs, Marax, Primatene, Quibron Tedral, Theor-Dur, and others)	Increased theophylline effect	Monitor theophylline concentration
Troleandomycin (TAO)	Jaundice (additive)	Avoid simultaneous use
Vitamin C	Increased serum concentration and possible increased adverse effects of estrogens with 1 g or more per day of vitamin C	Decrease vitamin C to 100 mg per day

Source: Rizack (1985).

of a 1-gram dose of vitamin C has been found to cause spotting when the vitamin is discontinued. Discontinuing the vitamin is like switching from a high- to a low-dose pill, which is often accompanied by spotting.[31] It has been suggested that if a woman is a strong believer in the use of vitamin C and insists on taking it, that she take it at a different time than her birth control pills—at least 4 hours apart. If no vitamin C is taken in the hours before or after taking birth control pills, then the amount of ethinyl estradiol absorbed will not be increased by the vitamins.

Use of OCs may also affect the pharmacokinetics of other drugs a woman is taking. Studies have suggested that OCs decrease clearance of benzodiazepines such as diazepine, nitrazepine, chlordiazepoxide, and alprazolam, and that lower doses of these medications may be indicated for women on pills.[1,6] Use of OCs and anti-inflammatory corticosteroids may increase the effects of the latter by decreasing their clearance and increasing their half-life. Lower doses of steroids may be indicated in OC users.[6] Clearance of bronchodilating drugs such as theophylline and amino-phylline, as well as the closely related drug, caffeine, may be reduced by 30% to 40% in pill users.[6] Questions remain as to the effects of OCs on analgesics, antihypertensive agents, and cyclosporin.[6]

Oral contraceptives can alter the results of several laboratory tests. Notify the laboratory if requesting results on an OC user. Table 10-7 lists many of the laboratory tests that may have increased or decreased values as a result of the influence of oral contraceptives.

INSTRUCTIONS FOR USING COMBINED PILLS

Birth control pills do not protect you from AIDS or other sexually transmitted infections. Consider all the approaches you have heard to preventing HIV infection. If you decide to have intercourse, use a male or a female condom every time that sexual intercourse may expose you or your partner to infection.

1. The pill works primarily by stopping ovulation (release of an egg). Pills are very effective if swallowed at the same time every day and if other instructions regarding concurrent drug use or use during episodes of diarrhea or vomiting are followed. In addition to preventing pregnancy, pills decrease your risk for ovarian cancer, cancer of the lining of the uterus, benign breast masses, and ovarian cysts. Pills decrease menstrual blood loss and menstrual cramps. Pills also decrease your chance of having an ectopic pregnancy—a pregnancy outside of the uterus.

2. **Choose a back-up method of birth control** (such as condoms or foam) to use with your first pack of pills because the pills may not fully protect you from pregnancy during this first cycle. A back-up method is probably not necessary if you start taking pills on the first day of bleeding (see instruction #3 below). Keep this back-up method handy all the time and learn to use it correctly in case you:

   • Run out of pills

   • Forget to swallow your pills

   • Experience a serious pill warning signal and discontinue pill use

   • Want protection from sexually transmitted infections, most notably the virus that causes AIDS (condoms provide the best protection.)

   • Have repeated episodes of breakthrough bleeding

3. You may start taking your pills according to one of several different schedules. The possible schedules are:
   - Starting on the first day of menstrual bleeding
   - Starting on the first Sunday after your period begins
   - Starting today if you are certain that you are not pregnant

   Check with your clinician to see how long you should use a back-up method.

4. Take one pill a day until you finish the pack. Then:
   - If you are using a 28-day pack, begin a new pack immediately. Skip no days between packages.
   - If you are using a 21-day pack, stop taking pills for 1 week and then start your new pack.

5. **Try to associate taking your pill with something else that you do at about the same time every day,** like going to bed, eating a meal, or brushing your teeth. A regular routine may make it easier to remember your pills. Pills work best if you take one about the same time every day in order to keep a steady level of hormones in your system.

6. **Check your pack of birth control pills each morning** to make sure you took your pill the day before.

7. If you have bleeding between periods, try to take your pills at the same time every day. If you have spotting (light bleeding between periods) for several cycles, you may want to call your clinician to see whether you need a different pill. Spotting is more likely to occur with the current low-dose birth control pills. Because spotting is generally not a sign of any serious problem in young women, your clinician may take a "watch-and-wait" approach if you are not concerned or inconvenienced. If you suddenly begin to have bleeding between periods, and have not previously had this problem, or have not missed pills or taken pills late, consider having your doctor check you for an infection. Spotting between periods may also signal decreased pill effectiveness. Some clinicians recommend a back-up contraceptive for women experiencing spotting on pills, especially if the woman is taking a medication that may lower pill effectiveness.

8. The effectiveness of birth control pills may be slightly decreased by a number of drugs that change liver function or decrease the ability of the body to absorb the hormones in birth control pills. Be sure to tell your clinician if you are using rifampin, Dilantin (phenytoin) or carbamazepine, or ampicillin or tetracycline. Use a back-up contraceptive. Taking vitamin C may actually increase the level of estrogen in your blood and may lead to increased spotting.[31]

9. **If you forget to take your birth control pill or you start your pack late,** follow the instructions below:

   • **If you miss one pill,** take that tablet as soon as you remember it. Take your next tablet at the regular time. You probably will not get pregnant but just to be sure, you may want to use a back-up method for 7 days after the missed pill.

   • **If you miss two pills in a row,** then take two tablets as soon as you remember and take two tablets the next day. Then return to your regular schedule but use a back-up method of birth control for 7 days after two missed tablets.

   • **If you miss three pills in a row** you will probably begin your period. Whether or not you are menstruating throw away the rest of your pack and begin your next pack as you did when you first started the method. For example, if you are a "Sunday starter" begin your next pack on Sunday. If you started on any other day, you may simply start your next pack immediately.
     Use a back-up method of birth control until you have been back on pills for 7 days.

   • **If the only pills you miss are from the *fourth* *week*** of a 28-day pill pack, simply throw away the missed pills. Then continue taking pills from your current package of pills on schedule. The pills in this fourth week do not contain hormones. So missing these pills does not increase your risk for pregnancy at all.

10. **If you have diarrhea or vomiting,** use your back-up method of birth control until your next period. Start using a back-up method on your first day of diarrhea or vomiting. Many women experience nausea the first month they take pills. This tends to go away in the next cycle or so. If nausea continues, switching to the lowest estrogen pill may be very helpful. See your clinician, your doctor, nurse or physician assistant.

11. Women taking pills note that periods tend to be short and scanty, and you may see no fresh blood at all. **A drop of blood, or a brown smudge on your tampon or on your underwear, is considered a period when you are on the pill.**

12. **If you do not have your menstrual period** when expected while taking birth control pills, you may want to consult your clinician.

    • **If you have not missed any pills and you miss one period** without any other signs of pregnancy, pregnancy is very unlikely. Many women taking birth control pills occasionally miss one period. Call the clinic if you are worried. You are fairly safe and can start a new package of pills at the regularly scheduled time. There is a simple way to help confirm that you are not pregnant: If your period does not appear during the last few days on pills or during the first 3 days of the pill-free interval, take your basal body temperature (BBT); if BBT is below 98° F for 3 days in a row, you are probably not pregnant.

- **If you forget one or more pills and miss a period**, you should stop taking pills and use another method of birth control. Contact your clinic for a pelvic examination or a sensitive pregnancy test. Ordinary 2-minute urine tests available in drug stores will not be positive this early in a possible pregnancy.

- **If you miss two periods in a row**, come to the clinic for a pregnancy test immediately, even if you took your pills every day. Bring a sample of your first-morning urine in a clean container.

13. **If you do become pregnant** while taking birth control pills, you must decide whether you want to have a child at this time or, alternatively, whether abortion is an option for you. The risk of having a baby with birth defects does not seem to be increased in pill users who become pregnant. The American College of Obstetricians and Gynecologists recently concluded that pills do not increase the risk for birth defects: "There is no evidence that there is an increased risk of fetal anomalies for previous pill users, from inadvertent exposure early in pregnancy, or in pregnancies occurring immediately after discontinuation of oral contraceptives."[2]

14. **If you decide you want to become pregnant**, stop taking pills. You may wish to use another reliable method of birth control until you have two or three normal menstrual periods off the pill so that when you become pregnant, your date of delivery might be accurately calculated. The American College of Obstetricians and Gynecologists recently concluded that "There is no evidence that oral contraceptive use decreases subsequent fertility. After oral contraceptive use is stopped, there may be a short delay of 1-2 months in the reestablishment of menses and ovulation."[2]

15. If you see a clinician for any reason or are hospitalized, be sure to mention that you are taking birth control pills.

16. **If you notice any pronounced mood changes**—depression, irritability, change in sex drive—see your clinician. Switching pill brands may help if your mood changes are pill-related. Your clinician can help in assessing what to do to help you.

17. Read the new pill package insert for women on pills. We know that it is very complicated and technical. But it contains much information that may help you. It provides a balanced picture of the risks and benefits of pills.

18. Learn the pill warning signals. Any one of these symptoms may mean that you are in serious trouble. Note that the first letter of each symptom spells out the word "ACHES."

Early Pill Warning Signs

Caution

A ■ Abdominal pain (severe)
C ■ Chest pain (severe), cough, shortness of breath
H ■ Headache (severe), dizziness, weakness, or numbness
E ■ Eye problems (vision loss or blurring), speech problems
S ■ Severe leg pain (calf or thigh)

See your clinician if you have any of these problems, or if you develop depression, yellow jaundice, or a breast lump.

See your clinician if you have any of these problems or if you develop depression, yellow jaundice, a breast lump, a bad fainting attack or collapse, a seizure (epilepsy), difficulty speaking, a blood pressure above 160/95, a severe allergic skin rash, or if you are immobilized after an accident or major surgery. Most of these warning signs usually have an explanation other than pills, but you should be checked out to be sure.

If you smoke, stop smoking. If you can't, it is all the more important that you watch for the pill warning signals. If you smoke you should probably STOP taking pills at age 35, and definitely by age 40.

Do not ignore these problems or wait to see if they disappear. Contact your nurse practitioner or doctor immediately to tell them about your problem. Birth control pills are safer when you get help as soon as problems arise.

THE MOST COMMONLY ASKED QUESTION ABOUT PILLS

Do Birth Control Pills Cause Cancer?

Although the final word is still not in, we have learned more and more as we have gained experience with pills:

Good News:

Pills make women less likely to develop three types of cancer:

- Ovarian cancer
- Endometrial cancer
- Choriocarcinoma, also called trophoblastic disease or molar pregnancies

Pills also make women less likely to develop several benign tumors or masses:

- Benign breast masses (fibroadenomas and cysts)
- Fibroids (leiomyomata)
- Ovarian cysts

Bad News:

There is no type of *cancer* definitely known to be more common in pill users. However, one benign tumor of the liver called a hepatic adenoma is more likely to develop in women using pills. The increased risk for this tumor is one of the reasons why women using pills are encouraged to contact their clinicians if they develop upper abdominal pain. Fortunately, benign liver tumors are very rare and combined pills are probably not associated with an increased risk for liver cancer.[83]

Neither Harmful Nor Beneficial Effect:

Pills probably have no effect on a woman's likelihood of developing a malignant melanoma; kidney, colon, or gall bladder cancer; or pituitary tumors.[34,53]

Still Not Sure—The Jury Is Still Out:

- **Breast cancer.** By age 55, women who have used pills are just as likely to be diagnosed with breast cancer as women who have not used pills.[34,84] It appears that there is a group of young women who have used pills and who are at increased risk for having breast cancer diagnosed before the age of 35.[34,84]
- **Cervical cancer.** It is known that barrier contraceptives and spermicides protect women against cervical cancer. Pills do not have this protective effect. Some studies have shown an increased risk for cervical cancer among pill users; others have not. Women taking pills should have a Pap smear once a year.
- **Cancer of the liver.** Some studies have shown an increased risk for hepatocellular cancer.[23,40,55] Others, including a large WHO study, have not.[28,75,83]

If we add up all the good news, the bad news, and the uncertain news, we can say in balance that by age 55, a woman is less likely to be diagnosed with cancer if she has used pills than if she used no method.[34] Women using barrier or spermicidal contraceptives are also less likely to develop cancer by age 55, but the protective effect is less than in women using pills.[34] In general, a number of factors have conspired to make reproductive cancers many times more common among modern-day women than among women living thousands of years ago.[21]

Table 10-7 Potential effects of oral contraceptives on the results of a selected group of laboratory tests

	Specific Tests and Potential Alteration of Lab Value	
Group	**Increased**	**Decreased**
Carbohydrate Metabolism	FBS and 2 hr. pp Insulin level	Glucose Tolerance
Hematologic/Coagulation	Coagulation factor II, VII, XIII, IX, X, XII Erythrocyte sedimentation rate Euglobulin lysis Fibrinogen Leukocyte count Partial thromboplastin time Plasma volume, plasmin, and plasminogen Platelet count, platelet aggregation, and platelet adhesiveness Prothrombin time	Antithrombin III Erythrocyte count (total) Hematocrit Prothrombin time
Lipid Metabolism*	Cholesterol Lipoproteins (prebeta, beta, and alpha) Phospholipids, total Total lipids Triglycerides	
Liver Function/GI Tests	Alkaline phosphatase Bilirubin, SGOT, SGPT Cephalin flocculation Formiminoglutamic acid excretion after histidine (urine) Gamma-Glutamyl trans-peptidase Leucine aminopeptidase Protoporphyrin, coproporphyrin excretion (urine), uroporphyrin excretion (urine) Sulfobromophthalein retention	Alkaline phosphatase Etiocholanolone excretion (urine) Haptoglobin (serum) Urobilinogen excretion (urine)

(continued)

Table 10-7 Potential effects of oral contraceptives on the results of a selected group of laboratory tests *(cont.)*

Specific Tests and Potential Alteration of Lab Value		
Group	**Increased**	**Decreased**
Metals	Copper and ceruloplasmin Iron, iron binding capacity and transferrin	Magnesium Zinc
Thyroid Function	Butanole extractable iodine Protein bound iodine Thyroid-binding globulin Triiodothyronine (serum)	Triiodothyronine resin (serum) Free thyroxin
Vitamins	Vitamin A (blood and plasma)	Folate (serum) Vitamin B_2 (RBC and urine excretion) Vitamin B_6 Vitamin B_{12} Vitamin C
Other Hormones/Enzyme Measurements	Aldosterone (blood and urine) Angiotensinogen Angiotensin I and II Cortisol (blood and urine) Growth hormone Prolactin Testosterone (serum) Total estrogens	Estradiol and Estriol FSH (urine), LH (blood and urine) Gonadotropin excretion (urine) 17-Hydroxycorticosteroid excretion (urine) 17 Ketosteroid excretion (urine) Pregnanediol excretion (urine) Renin (serum) Tetrahydrocortisone
Miscellaneous Laboratory	Alpha-1 antitrypsin Antinuclear antibody Bilirubin Complement-reactive protein Globulins a-1, a-2 Lactate Lupus erythematosus cell preparation Pyruvate Sodium	Albumin Alpha amino nitrogen Calcium (serum) and calcium excretion (urine) Complement-reactive protein Immunoglobulin A, G, and M

Sources: Maile (1974).
The Medical Letter (1979).

*HDL Cholesterol is increased with estrogens and decreased with progestins.

REFERENCES

1. Abernethy DR, Greenblatt DJ, Divoll M, Arendt R, Ochs HR, Shader RI. Impairment of diazepam metabolism by low-dose estrogen-containing oral contraceptive steroids. N Engl J Med 1982;306(13):791-792.
2. American College of Obstetricians and Gynecologists. Oral contraceptives. ACOG Bulletin No. 106; July, 1987.
3. Angle M, Murphy C. Guidelines for clinical procedures in family planning. A reference for trainers. Program for International Training in Health. Chapel Hill NC; 1992.
4. Anonymous. Choice of contraceptives. Med Lett Drugs Ther 1992;34(885):111-114.
5. Back DJ, Bates M, Bowden A, Breckenridge AM, Hall MJ Jones H, MacIver M, Orme-M, Perucca E, Richens A, Rowe PH, Smith E. The interaction of phenobarbital and other anticonvulsants with oral contraceptive steroid therapy. Contraception 1980;22(5):495-503.
6. Back DJ, Orme ML'E. Pharmacokinetic drug interactions with oral contraceptives. Clin Pharmacokinet 1990;18(6):472-484.
7. Bergink W, Bos ES, Kloosterboer HJ, Lund L, Nummi S, Van Der Vies J. Comparison of the metabolic effects of desogestrel and levonorgestrel in low-dose oestrogen oral contraceptives. In: Van Keep PA, Kopera H (eds). Oral contraceptives and lipoproteins. Geneva: Int Health Foundation 1983:52-63.
8. Blumenstein BA, Douglas MB, Hall WD. Blood pressure changes and oral contraceptive use: a study of 2,676 black women in the southeastern United States. Am J Epidemiol 1980;112(4):539-552.
9. Casagrande JT, RK, Louie EW, Roy S, Ross RK, Henderson BE. Incessant ovulation and ovarian cancer. Lancet 1979;2(8135):170-173.
10. Centers for Disease Control and Prevention. Oral contraceptive use and the risk of endometrial cancer. The Centers for Disease Control Cancer and Steroid Hormone (CASH) study. JAMA 1983;249(12):1600-1604.
11. Centers for Disease Control and Prevention. Oral contraceptive use and the risk of ovarian cancer. The Centers for Disease Control Cancer and Steroid Hormone (CASH) study. JAMA 1983;249(12):1596-1599.
12. Centers for Disease Control and Prevention. The cancer and steroid hormone (CASH) study of the Centers for the Disease Control and the National Institute of Child Health and Human Development: oral contraceptive use and the risk of breast cancer. N Eng J Med 1986;315(7):405-411.
13. Chilvers C, McPherson K, Peto J, Pike MC, Vessey MP. Oral contraceptive use and breast cancer risk in young women. Lancet 1989;1(8645):973-982.
14. Coker AL, Harlap S, Fortney JA. Oral contraceptives and reproductive cancers: weighing the risks and benefits. Fam Plann Perspect 1993;25(1):17-22,36.
15. Conney AH. Pharmacological implications of microsomal enzyme induction. Pharmacol Rev 1967;19(3):317-366.
16. Crona N, Silverstolpe G, Samsioe G. Changes in serum apo-lipoprotein AI and sex-hormone-binding globulin levels after treatment with two different progestins administered alone and in combination with ethinyl estradiol. Contraception 1984;29(3):261-270.
17. Dewis P, Petsos M, Anderson DC. The treatment of hirsutism with a combination of desogestrel and ethinyl oestradiol. Clin Endocrin 1985;22(1):29-36.

18. Diamond MP, Greene JW, Thompson JM, Van Hooydonk JE, Wentz AC. Interaction of anticonvulsants and oral contraceptives in epileptic adolescents. Contraception 1985;31(6):623-632.
19. Dickey RP. Managing contraceptive pill patients. 4th ed. Durant OK: Creative Infomatics, Inc., 1985.
20. Dorflinger LJ. Relative potency of progestins used in oral contraceptives. Contraception 1985;31(6):557-570.
21. Eaton SB, Pike MC, Short RV, Lee NC, Trussell J, Hatcher RA, Wood JW, Worthman CM, Jones NB, Konner MJ, Hill K, Bailey R. Women's reproductive cancers in evolutionary context. Atlanta GA: Department of Radiology, West Paces Ferry Hospital, 1993.
22. Eckstein P, Waterhouse JAH, Bond GM, Mills WG, Sandilands DM, Shotton DM. The Birmingham oral contraceptive trial. Br Med J 1961;2(5261);1172-1178.
23. Forman D, Doll R, Peto R. Trends in mortality from carcinoma of the liver and use of oral contraceptives. Br J Cancer 1983;48(3):349-354.
24. Forman D, Vincent TJ, Doll R. Cancer of the liver and the use of oral contraceptives. Br Med J 1986;292(6532):1357-1361.
25. Gallup Organization, Inc. Attitudes toward contraception. Princeton NJ; March 1, 1985:4.
26. Godsland IF, Wynn V. Does the new progestagen desogestrel have metabolic advantages? Lancet 1984;2(8398):359-360.
27. Godsland IF, Crook D, Simpson R, Proudler T, Felton C, Lees B, Anyaoku V, Devenport M, Wynn V. The effects of different formulations of oral contraceptive agents on lipid and carbohydrate metabolism. N Engl J Med 1990;323(20):1375-81.
28. Goodman ZD, Ishak KG. Hepatocellular carcinoma in women probable lack of etiologic association with oral contraceptive steroids. Hepatology 1982;2(4):440-444.
29. Greenblatt RB. Progestational agents in clinical practice. Med Science 1967;18(5):37-49.
30. Grimes DA. The safety of oral contraceptives: epidemiologic insights from the first 30 years. Am J Obstet Gynecol 1992:166(6-2):1950-1954.
31. Guillebaud J. The pill and other hormones for contraception, f4th ed. Oxford: Oxford University Press, 1991.
32. Guillebaud J. Contraception: your questions answered. New York NY: Pitman, 1985.
33. Hammond GL, Langley MS, Robinson PA, Nummi S, Lund L. Serum steroid binding protein concentrations, distribution of progestogens, and bioavailability of testosterone during treatment with contraceptives containing desogestrel or levonorgestrel. Fertil Steril 1984;42(1):44-51.
34. Harlap S, Kost K, Forrest JD. Preventing pregnancy, protecting health: a new look at birth control choices in the United States. New York and Washington DC; The Alan Guttmacher Institute;1991.
35. Hatcher RA, Atkinson A, Cates D, Glasser L, Legins K. Sexual etiquette 101. Atlanta GA: Bridging the Gap Communications, 1992.
36. Hatcher RA, Kowal D, Guest F, Trussell J, Stewart F, Stewart G, Bowen S, Cates W. Contraceptive technology: international edition. Atlanta: GA Printed Matter, Inc., 1989.
37. Hatcher RA. Choosing a combined oral contraceptive with less than 50 mcg of estrogen (in press).

38. Heinen G. The discriminating use of combination and sequential preparations in hormonal inhibition of ovulation. Contraception 1971;4(6):393-400.
39. Helmrich SP, Rosenberg L, Kaufman DW, Miller DR, Schottenfeld MD, Stolley PD, Shapiro S. Lack of an elevated risk of malignant melanoma in relation to oral contraceptive use. J Natl Cancer Inst 1984;72(3):617-620.
40. Henderson BE, Preston-Martin S, Edmondson HA, Peters RL, Pike MC. Hepatocellular carcinoma and oral contraceptives. Br J Cancer 1983;48(3): 437-440.
41. Jung-Hoffman C, Kuhl H. Divergent effects of two low-dose oral contraceptives on sex hormone-binding globulin and free testosterone. Am J Obstet Gynecol 1987;156(1):199-203.
42. Kauppinen-Makelin R, Kuusi T, Ylikorkala O, Tikkanen MJ. Contraceptives containing desogestrel or levonorgestrel have different effects on serum lipoproteins and post-heparin plasma lipase activities. Clin Endocrinol 1992;36(2): 203-209.
43. Kloosterboer HJ, Van Wayjen RGA, Van Den Ende A. Effects of three low-dose oral contraceptive combinations on sex hormone binding globulin, corticosteroid binding globulin and antithrombin III activity in healthy women. Acta Obstet Gynecol Scand Suppl 1987;144:41-44.
44. Krauss RM, The effects of oral contraceptives on plasma lipids and lipoproteins. Int J Fertil 1988;33 (Suppl 2):35-42.
45. Krauss RM, Drauss RM, Roy S, Mishell DR, Casagrande J, Pike MC. Effects of two low-dose oral contraceptives on serum lipids and lipoproteins: differential changes in high-density lipoprotein subclasses. Am J Obstet Gynecol 1983;145(4):446-452.
46. Linn S, Schoenbaum SC, Monson RR, Rosner B, Ryan KJ. Delay in conception for former "pill" users. JAMA 1982;247(5):629-632.
47. Liukko P, Erkkola R, Bergink EW. Progestagen-dependent effect on some plasma proteins during oral contraception. Gynecol Obstet Invest 1988;25(2):118-122.
48. Lobo RA. The androgenicity of progestational agents. Int J Fertil 1988;33 (Suppl 2):6-12.
49. Lynch HT, Albano WA, Lynch JF, Lynch PM, Campbell A. Surveillance and management of patients at high genetic risk for ovarian carcinoma. Obstet Gynecol 1982;59(5):589-596.
50. Miale JB, Kent JW. The effects of oral contraceptives on the results of laboratory tests. Am J Obstet Gynecol 1974 120(2):264-272.
51. Mears E. Clinical trials of oral contraceptives. Br Med J 1961;5261(2): 1179-1183.
52. The Medical Letter. Effects of oral contraceptives on laboratory test results. Med Lett Drugs Ther 1979;21(13):54-56.
53. Milne R, Vessey M. The association of oral contraception with kidney cancer, colon cancer, gallbladder cancer (including extrahepatic bile duct cancer) and pituitary tumours. Contraception 1991;43(6):667-693.
54. Mishell DR. Use of oral contraceptives in women of older reproductive age. Am J Obstet Gynecol 1988;158(6-2):1652-1657.
55. Neuberger J, Forman D, Doll R, Williams R. Oral contraceptives and hepatocellular carcinoma. Br Med J 1986;292(6532):1355-1357.
56. Ortho Pharmaceutical Laboratories. 1991 Ortho annual birth control study. Raritan NJ.

57. Ory HW, Forrest JD, Lincoln R. Making choices: evaluating the health risks and benefits of birth control methods. New York NY: The Alan Guttmacher Institute, 1983.
58. Palatsi R, Hirvensalo E, Liukko P, Malmiharju T, Mattila L, Riihiluoma P, Ylostalo P. Serum total and unbound testosterone and sex hormone binding globulin (SHBG) in female acne patients treated with two different oral contraceptives. Acta Derm Venereol 1984;64(6):517-523.
59. Phillips A. The selectivity of a new progestin. Acta Obstet Gynecol Scand Suppl 1990; 152:21-24.
60. Pike MC, Henderson BE, Krailow MD, Duke A, Roy S. Breast cancer in young women and use of oral contraceptives: possible modifying effect of formulation and age of use. Lancet 1983;2(8356):926-930.
61. Rizack MA, Hillman CDM. The Medical letter handbook of adverse drug interactions. New Rochell NY: The Medical Letter, 1985.
62. Rojanasakul A, Chailurkit L, Sirimongkolkasem R, Chaturachinda K. Effects of combined desogestrel-ethinylestradiol treatment on lipid profiles in women with polycystic ovarian disease. Fertil Steril 1987;48(4):581-585.
63. Rooks JB, Ory HW, Ishak KG, Strauss LT, Greenspan JR, Hill AP, Tyler CW. Epidemiology of hepatocellular adenoma. The rule of oral contraceptive use. JAMA 1979;242(7):644-648.
64. Royal College of General Practitioners. Oral contraceptives and health: report of Royal College of General Practitioners. New York NY: Pitman Publishing Corporation, 1974.
65. Rubin GL, Peterson HB. Oral contraceptive use and cancer. Contraceptive Technol Update 1985;6(1):1-24.
66. Senanayake PL, Kramer DG. Contraception and the etiology of pelvic inflammatory disease: new perspectives. Am J Obstet Gynecol 1980;138(7-2): 852-860.
67. Shoupe D, Bopp B. Contraceptive options for the gestational diabetic woman. Int J Fertil 1991;(Suppl 2):80-86.
68. Skouby SO, Anderson O, Kuhl C. Oral contraceptives and insulin receptor binding in normal women and those with previous gestational diabetes. Am J Obstet Gynecol 1986,155(4):802-807.
69. Song S, Chen JK, Yang PJ, He ML, Li LM, Fan BC Rekers H, Fotherby K. A crossover study of three oral contraceptives containing ethinyloestradiol and either desogestrel or levonorgestrel. Contraception 1992;45(6):523-532
70. Reference removed.
71. Spellacy WN, Buhi WC, Birk SA. Prospective studies of carbohydrate metabolism in "normal" women using norgestrel for 18 months. Fertil Steril 1981;35(2):167-171.
72. Speroff L, Darney P. A clinical guide for contraception. Baltimore MD: Williams & Wilkins, 1992.
73. Speroff L, Glass RH, Kase NG. Clinical gynecologic endocrinology and infertility. 4th ed. Baltimore MD: Williams & Wilkins, 1989.
74. Stewart FH, Guest F, Stewart G, Hatcher RA. Understanding your body. New York NY: Bantam, 1987.
75. Stricker BH, Spoelestra P. Drug induced hepatic injury. In: Dukes MNG (ed.) Drug induced disorders. Volume I. Amsterdam: Elseveir, 1985:237-241.
76. Reference removed.
77. Swyer GI. Potency of progestogens in oral contraceptives—further delay of menses data. Contraception 1982;26(1):23-27.

78. Trussell J, Hatcher RA, Cates W, Stewart FH, Kost K. Contraceptive failure in the United States: an update. Stud Fam Plan 1990;21(1):51-54.
79. Trussell J, Stewart F, Guest F, Hatcher RA. Emergency contraceptive pills (ECPs): a simple proposal to reduce unintended pregnancies. Fam Plann Perspect 1992;24(6):269-273.
80. Vessey MP, Lawless M, McPherson K, Yeates D. Neoplasia of the cervix uteri and contraception: a possible adverse effect of the pill. Lancet 1983;2(8356):930-934.
81. Washington AE, Gove S, Schachter J, Sweet RL. Oral contraceptives, *Chlamydia trachomatis* infection, and pelvic inflammatory disease. A word of caution about protection. JAMA 1985;253(15):2246-2250.
82. Wharton C, Blackburn R. Lower-dose pills. Popul Rep 1989;Series A(7):1-31.
83. World Health Organization Collaborative Study of Neoplasia and Steroid Contraceptives, Combined Oral Contraceptives and Liver Cancer. Int J Cancer. 1989;43(2):254-259.
84. Wingo PA, Lee NC, Ory HW, Beral V, Peterson HB, Rhodes P. Age-specific differences in the relationship between oral contraceptive use and breast cancer. Obstet Gynecol 1991;78(2):161-170.
85. Wynn V. Effect of progesterone and progestins on carbohydrate metabolism. In: Bardin CW, Milgrom E, Mauvais-Jarvis P (eds). Progesterone and progestins. New York NY: Raven Press, 1983:395-410.
86. Wynn V, Niththyananthan R. The effect of progestins in combined oral contraceptives on serum lipids with special reference to high-density lipoproteins. Am J Obstet Gynecol 1982;142(6-2):766-771.
87. Wynn V, Godsland I. Effects of oral contraceptives on carbohydrate metabolism. J Repro Med 1986;31(Suppl 9):892-897.
88. Wynn V, Niththyananthan R. The effect of progestogens in combined oral contraceptives on serum lipids with special reference to high-density lipoproteins. Am J Obstet Gynecol 1982;142(6-2):766-772.
89. Upton GV, Corbin A. The relevance of the pharmacologic properties of a progestational agent to its clinical effects as a combination oral contraceptive. Yale J Biol Med 1989;62:445-457.

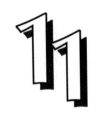

Norplant, Depo-Provera, and Progestin-Only Pills (Minipills)

- Progestin-only contraceptives tend to cause menstrual irregularities.
- The success of a program offering Norplant, Depo-Provera, progestin-only pills, or a progestin-elaborating intrauterine device hinges on counseling women in advance about possible menstrual changes.
- Contraceptive efficacy of Norplant and Depo-Provera is very high.
- Lactating women may use progestin-only contraceptives.
- Progestin-only methods provide no protection against sexually transmitted infections, including HIV.

Norplant.   When a woman decides to have Norplant implants inserted, a single decision may provide her with 5 years of effective birth control. At the time of insertion, assure the client that she can have the method reversed at any time, by having the capsules removed. As of the end 1992, Norplant had been approved for use in 27 countries. Formal approval in the United States occurred on December 10, 1990. It is estimated by the Population Council that approximately 1.8 million women worldwide will have had Norplant implants inserted as of the end of 1992.[29]

Depo-Provera (DMPA).   Depo-Provera is the most commonly employed injectable progestin. DMPA is extremely effective in part because it is forgiving should a woman return several days to 2 weeks late for an injection. DMPA has been used by more than 15 million women worldwide. Depo-medroxyprogesterone acetate, or DMPA, is approved for use in more than 90 countries including the United States where it was finally approved in late 1992. Approval was delayed in the United States because of its effect on dogs (see section on "Providing Depo-Provera" for more discussion). Its approval in the United States will facilitate distribution worldwide through the U.S. Agency for International Development (USAID).

Minipills. The marketing of progestin-only pills (POPs, sometimes referred to as minipills) began about 10 years after combined OCs were introduced. A number of preparations are currently available using a variety of progestins. Progestin-only pills are taken every day with no pill-free interval. Progestin-only pills account for no more than 8% of the oral contraceptive market in the United Kingdom.[15] They account for an even lower percentage in most other countries.

MECHANISM OF ACTION

Progestin-only contraceptives may be administered via different routes: by mouth, injection, and implants, as well as by intrauterine devices and vaginal rings. The effects of these delivery systems are summarized in Table 11-1.[15] Progestin-only contraceptives may prevent pregnancy via several mechanisms:

- Inhibition of ovulation
- Thickening and decreasing the amount of cervical mucus (making it more difficult for sperm to penetrate)
- Creation of a thin, atrophic endometrium
- Premature luteolysis

Norplant. This long-acting contraceptive takes advantage of the tissue compatibility of the nonbiodegradable silicone rubber capsules. The contraceptive steroid levonorgestrel slowly diffuses through six slender, flexible capsules. (See Figure 11-1.) When the capsules are removed, the contraceptive effect wears off quickly. Each of six match-sized capsules is 34 mm long, with a diameter of 2.4 mm. Each set of Norplant capsules contains 35 mg of levonorgestrel, which is released at a low, steady rate of 85 mcg daily initially decreasing to 50 mcg at 9 months and 35 mcg at 18 months, with a further decline thereafter to 30 mcg per day.

Depo-Provera. A deep intramuscular injection of 150 mg of DMPA is given every 3 months. DMPA injections inhibit ovulation by suppressing FSH and LH levels and eliminating the LH surge. The pituitary gland remains responsive to GNRH, suggesting that the site of action of DMPA is the hypothalamus.[30] Other contraceptive actions include the development of a shallow and atrophic endometrium and the development of a thick cervical mucus that decreases sperm penetration. One of the reasons the failure rate is so low is that each 150 mg injection actually provides more than 3 months of protection.[52] A long-term user of DMPA has a 2-week "grace period" (longer in many instances) during which she can be late for her next shot but still not be at much risk of becoming pregnant.

Table 11-1 Delivery systems for progestin-only contraceptives and combined pills

	Injectable	Implant	Oral	
	Depo-Provera	**Norplant**	**Progestin-only Pill**	**Combined OC**
Administration				
Frequency	Every 3 months	5 years	Daily	Daily
Progestin dose	High	Ultra-Low	Ultra-Low	Low
Blood levels	Initial peak then decline	Constant	Rapidly Fluctuating	
1st pass through liver	No	No	Yes	Yes
Major Mechanisms of Action				
Ovary: ↓ovulation	+++	++	+	+++
Cervical mucus: ↓sperm penetrability	Yes	Yes	Yes	Yes
Endometrium: ↓receptivity to blastocyst	Yes	Yes	Yes	Yes
First-year failure rate (perfect use)	0.3	0.09	0.5	0.1
Menstrual pattern	Very irregular	Very irregular	Often irregular	Regular
Amenorrhea during use	Very common	Common	Occasional	Rare
Reversibility				
Immediate termination possible	No	Yes	Yes	Yes
By woman herself at any time	No	No	Yes	Yes
Median time to conception from first omitted dose, removal	6 months	c.1 month	<3 months	3 months

Adapted from Guillebrand (1985), and Table 5-2.

* By several mechanisms – LH and FSH surges suppressed; preovulatory follicles suppressed

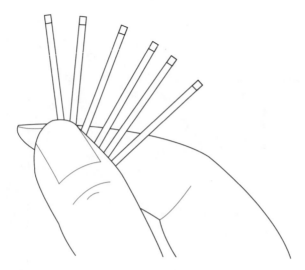

Figure 11-1 The 6-capsule Norplant system

Minipills. The effectiveness of progestin-only pills is highest if ovulation is consistently inhibited. When this happens, a woman tends to be amenorrheic or to have prolonged periods of time between menstrual bleeding episodes. *In other words, effectiveness is greatest when the "normal" bleeding pattern is most disturbed.* If ovulation is not suppressed, the progestin-only pills have no effect on the cyclicity of bleeding, and menstrual bleeding occurs as it had before the woman started progestin-only pills.

EFFECTIVENESS
NORPLANT

Norplant failures are rare. (See Tables 11-2 and 27-14.) Population Council data based on 2,470 women in a multicountry trial indicate that the proportion experiencing an accidental pregnancy in the first year of use is 0.2%.[46,47] If the women who were already pregnant when the device was implanted are removed from this calculation, the proportion failing falls to 0.09%. The Population Council further reported failure rates of 0.5%, 1.2%, 1.6%, and 0.4% in the second, third, fourth, and fifth years of use respectively.[56] The cumulative probability of failing at the end of 5 years of use is therefore only 3.7%.

In three of the five pregnancies in the first year, conception preceded implantation of the device. To avoid Norplant insertion in women who are already pregnant, insert Norplant implants within 7 days of onset of menstruation or immediately postpartum or within 3 weeks after a delivery. A negative sensitive pregnancy test will also help to minimize the number of insertions in women who are already pregnant.

Table 11-2 First-year failure rates* for women using progestin–containing contraceptives

Method (1)	% of Women Experiencing an Accidental Pregnancy Within the First Year of Use		% of Women Continuing Use at One Year (4)
	Typical Use (2)	Perfect Use (3)	
Pill	3		72
Progestin Only		0.5	
Combined		0.1	
IUD			
Progesterone T	2.0	1.5	81
Copper T 380A	0.8	0.6	78
LNg 20	0.1	0.1	81
Depo-Provera	0.3	0.3	70
Norplant (6 Capsules)	0.09	0.09	85

* See Table 5-2 for first-year failure rates of all methods.

The failure rates in the previous paragraph were based on clinical trials that contained two different types of Norplant capsules: the original hard capsules and newer soft capsules. Cumulative failure rates through the end of 5 years were three times higher among women with the hard capsules (4.9%) than among women with soft ones (1.6%).[47] The Finnish company that produces all the Norplant implants used throughout the world, Leiras Oy, now produces implants only with the new soft tubing.[29]

In those Population Council studies that led to FDA approval of Norplant, a higher failure rate was noted in women who weighed more than 154 lbs. The 1990 Wyeth package insert states that the cumulative pregnancy rate after 5 years for women weighing 154 lbs or more is 8.5%, falling to 5.0% for women weighing 131-153 lbs, to 3.4% for women weighing 110–130 lbs, and to 0.2% for women under 110 lbs. However, women in those studies used both soft and hard Norplant capsules. Failures in heavier women using soft Norplant capsules are far lower than in those using hard capsules. The cumulative failure rate through the end of 5 years among those women weighing more than 154 lbs is 9.3% for hard capsules but only 2.4% for soft capsules; among those weighing 131-153 lbs, the corresponding rates are 4.5% for hard capsules but only 1.5% for soft.[47]

Because failures increase in the sixth year, Norplant capsules should be removed at the end of the fifth year. In a study in Chile, 19 pregnancies were observed during 18,530 woman-months of use; however, 11 of the 19 pregnancies occurred during years 6 through 8 of treatment. The failure rate during years 6 through 8 was six times that during the first 5 years.[10] An

Indonesian study found a net cumulative pregnancy rate at 5 years of 1.8%. However, six of the eight pregnancies occurred in the last month of the fifth year.[2] It is important to remember that Norplant is approved as a 5-year method. The tendency for failure rate to increase undoubtedly reflects gradually diminishing release rates of levonorgestrel. If a woman wishes to continue using Norplant, another set of implants can be inserted at the visit when the first set is removed.

Norplant continuation. Continuation rates for Norplant users reported by the Population Council for Norplant are high: Approximately 85% continued after 1 year.[46] About half of the women continued Norplant use for 3 years.[24] Other studies have reported higher first-year continuation rates ranging from 87% to 95%.[24] In five studies around the world, 76%–90% of users completed 1 year of use, and 33%–78% completed 5 years.[29] Proportions continuing use of Norplant at the end of 1 year were taken from the results of the Norplant (6-capsule) trial shown in Table 27-14.[46]

DEPO-PROVERA

Depo-Provera is an extremely effective contraceptive option (see Table 11-2). The first-year probability of failure is only 0.3% (see Tables 5-2 and 27-13). These failure rates apply to injections providing 150 mg of DMPA per 1 cc.

Questions have been raised as to the effectiveness of injections of 150 mg of DMPA each 3 months when DMPA is constituted in much less expensive solutions providing 400 mg of DMPA per 1 cc of this medication. It is very difficult to provide exactly the correct volume of DMPA in solution (0.37 cc), and the injection and absorption of DMPA from this very concentrated solution is not approved as a contraceptive. An unpublished Upjohn-sponsored trial of 400 mg/ml (administered as 1 ml of the 400 mg/ml formulation) every 6 months did not demonstrate suitable contraceptive efficacy; failures occurred throughout the 6-month treatment period, not just at the end.[4] The concentrated form of DMPA is also more painful. Pain has been overcome by diluting the very concentrated form of DMPA with an equal volume of 1% xylocaine.

In the largest U.S. study, continuation rates for women on DMPA were 59.4% at 1 year, 41.5% at 2 years, 30.2% at 3 years, and 24.1% at 4 years.[40] Proportions continuing use of Depo-Provera at the end of 1 year were calculated from the results of the two WHO trials of the 150 mg dose injected every 90 days shown in Table 27-13.

MINIPILL

Progestin-only pills are generally less effective than combined OCs. The proportion of women becoming pregnant in the first year of typical use ranges from 1.1% to 13.2% (see Tables 11-2 and 27-10). If minipills are used correctly and consistently, only 5 in 1,000 women would become pregnant in the first year (see Table 5-2). A multicenter, double-blind study compared progestin-only oral contraceptives containing levonorgestrel (0.03 mg) and norethindrone (0.35 mg) with two combined OCs containing mestranol (50 mcg) and norethindrone (1 mg) or ethinyl estradiol (30 mcg) and levonorgestrel (0.15 mg). The pregnancy rates for the progestin-only pills were only slightly higher than the rates for the combined pills, and at 670 days the pregnancy rate for progestin-only pills containing levonorgestrel was actually lower than the rate for the mestranol/norethindrone combined pill (9.5% vs. 12.9%).[41]

In lactating women, the progestin-only pill is nearly 100% effective.[15] Moreover, progestin-only pills do not alter the quantity of milk, so they represent an effective form of contraception for the lactating woman.[4,15,44] Combined pills, in contrast, may have an adverse effect upon the quantity of milk produced and the duration of lactation. It is particularly important that progestin-only pills not be taken even a few hours late, because of the loss of effectiveness. Figure 11-2 illustrates how the sperm penetration of cervical mucus increases if the time interval between progestin-only pills is more than 24 hours.

COST

Norplant. In the United States, each set of Norplant implants costs the health care provider from $365–$375. (Programs in developing countries pay US $23 per set of six implants.)[29] The cost to the client for insertion (which may include a physical exam and some laboratory tests such as a sensitive pregnancy test) ranges from $500–$700. Implants may be paid for by Medicaid, which covers the cost of insertion and removal in all 50 states; by the Norplant Foundation; or by a client's health plan. As of August 1992, 46 of the 58 major health maintenance programs in the United States had decided to pay part or all of the cost of Norplant insertion and private insurance programs will also cover the cost of Norplant insertion and removal in some instances.[29] The Norplant Foundation, (703) 706-5933, provides free Norplants to women who do not qualify for Medicaid but who cannot afford the cost of Norplant insertion. Removal takes more time and the charge is usually greater than that charged for insertion. *If a woman wants her implants removed, this must be done regardless of her ability to pay.*

Depo-Provera. Each vial containing 150 mg of DMPA in a 1 cc injection will cost the provider $29. If the client is charged $35 per injection then the annual cost will be $140, plus the cost of her annual examination, routine laboratory tests, transportation, and the loss of work necessitated by repeat visits. No laboratory tests are specifically indicated unless a woman is more than 2 weeks late for her shot and may therefore need a pregnancy test.

Minipills. Minipills cost women between $100 and $300 per year, depending on whether they are generic or brand name. Public clinics and college health services often pass lower prices on to their clients.

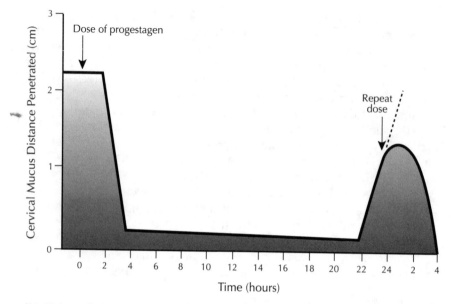

Note: Minimum reduction in sperm penetration between 4 hours and 22 hours after a single dose of megestrol acetate (0.5 mg). Unlike the rest of the figure, the effect of a repeat dose is presumed, not experimental.

Source: Guillebaud (1985).

Figure 11-2 Sperm penetration test following progestin-only pill

ADVANTAGES AND INDICATIONS

The following advantages hold for all progestin-only contraceptives.

1. **No estrogen.** Because progestin-only contraceptives contain no estrogen, they do not cause the serious complications attributable to estrogenic agents (including thrombophlebitis and pulmonary embolism). Studies thus far have not shown any serious short- or long-term effects of DMPA.[13,14,31,36,52]

2. **Noncontraceptive benefits.** Norplant, Depo-Provera, and progestin-only pills offer several noncontraceptive benefits, including the following:

   • Scanty menses or no menses
   • Decreased anemia
   • Decreased menstrual cramps and pain
   • Suppression of pain associated with ovulation (mittelschmerz)
   • Decreased risk of developing endometrial cancer, ovarian cancer, and pelvic inflammatory disease

- Management of pain associated with endometriosis

The magnitude of these noncontraceptive benefits needs careful evaluation.

3. **Reversibility.** Norplant and minipills are immediately reversible. Contraception must be initiated the same day as Norplant implants are removed or minipills are stopped. Depo-Provera is reversible but return of fertility is not as rapid as with Norplant or progestin-only-pills.[34] No surgical procedure is necessary to stop using Depo-Provera or progestin-only pills and from this viewpoint it is easier to discontinue these methods than it is to discontinue Norplant. However, once injected DMPA cannot be discontinued immediately.

4. **Long-term effective contraception.** Norplant implants and long-acting injections are extremely effective long-term contraceptives. In the case of Norplant (and the Levonorgestrel IUD, see Chapter 14), a single decision leads to long-term contraception. The efficacy of implants and injections is not dependent on any day-to-day responsibility. DMPA provides excellent short-term contraception for women who require maximum protection following rubella immunization, are awaiting sterilization, or are partners of men undergoing vasectomy. Women appearing late for their injection of DMPA have a period of grace during which they will not become pregnant. The package insert defines this period as 2 weeks; others suggest that the grace period is 4 weeks.

5. **Low risk of ectopic pregnancy.** Norplant and DMPA reduce a woman's risk for having an ectopic pregnancy compared with women using no contraceptive at all. Ectopic pregnancy is less likely to occur among women using Norplant (1.3 per 1,000 woman years) than among women who use no contraceptive (6.5 per 1,000 woman-years). Ectopic pregnancy may be more common in heavier women or may increase with longer use of Norplant (which reinforces the importance of removal after 5 years of use).[29] Ectopic pregnancy is also very unlikely to occur in women receiving DMPA injections. Progestin-only pills are less protective against ectopic pregnancies than are combined pills, Norplant, or DMPA.

6. **Amenorrhea.** Progestin-only contraceptives cause amenorrhea in some women. The absence of bleeding may be considered an advantage by some users. During the first year of DMPA use, for example, 30%-50% of women are amenorrheic; by the end of the second year, 70% are amenorrheic; and by the end of the fifth year, 80%.[31] Most women consider amenorrhea an advantage. Over time, amenorrhea occurs less frequently in women using Norplant.

Norplant

7. **Continuation rates.** Norplant has higher continuation rates than do other hormonal contraceptives. The percentage of women continuing to use Norplant at 1 year is 85%. The continuation rate is about 15% less for women using pills and Depo-Provera (see Table 5-2).

8. **Not coitus dependent.** Norplant (and to a lesser extent, long-acting injections) is an excellent contraceptive option for women who have difficulty remembering to take pills or use coitus-dependent methods. For example, Norplant may be a particularly attractive option for a women who abuses drugs and will have difficulty taking pills but definitely wants to avoid pregnancy.

Depo-Provera

9. **Culturally acceptable.** In some cultures, receiving medications by injection is considered desirable. In some cultures, a woman may wish to use a contraceptive without the knowledge of her partner, husband, or family.

10. **No drug interaction.** Thus far there has been no demonstrated interaction between Depo-Provera and antibiotics or enzyme-inducing drugs.[52] The only drug that decreases the effectiveness of DMPA is aminoglutethimide (Cytadren,) which is usually used to suppress adrenal function in selected cases of Cushings syndrome. DMPA is given parenterally; therefore, effectiveness is not dependent on normal GI function.

11. **Fewer seizures.** DMPA has been found to decrease the frequency of seizures.[25,26,55,56] Improvement in seizure control is probably due to the sedative properties of progestins.

Minipills

12. Because they take the same type of pill every single day (same color and hormone content), some women may find it easier to remember minipills.

INDICATIONS

Breastfeeding women.   Norplant, Depo-Provera, and minipills do not have adverse effects on lactation. Some studies suggest that milk volume may increase.[21,28] Although progestins can be transferred through breast milk, the dose consumed by the infant is small. No data and no biologic reasoning support the concern about a deleterious effect on child growth and development.[1,9,19,21,23,28,32,35] (See Chapter 17.) Opinions vary about whether Norplant and Depo-Provera should be provided immediately postpartum. A prudent approach would be to wait until breastfeeding has been well established.

Norplant. If a breastfeeding woman is unlikely to return for a postpartum visit and requests Norplant before leaving the hospital after delivery, the real long-term contraceptive benefit of using this method seems likely to exceed the theoretical risks, especially if she plans to supplement the infant's diet relatively soon after birth. In studies of Norplant, however, the method has not been started until at least 30 days postpartum. In one Egyptian study, Norplant was inserted between 30 and 42 days postpartum in 50 lactating women. There was no difference in lactational performance between the Norplant group and two control groups. In all three groups, infant growth was above average for Egyptian infants. Among exclusively breastfed infants, weight gains in the early postpartum months were slightly but statistically significantly lower in the Norplant group.[43] In a second Egyptian study, Norplant was inserted between 30 and 49 days postpartum in 120 lactating women. There was no difference in breast-feeding performance between the women using Norplant and women in the control group. Moreover, there was no difference in growth or in mental development between infants of the Norplant users and infants of the women in the control group.[42] In a Chilean study, Norplant was inserted between 52 and 58 days postpartum in 100 lactating women. There were no important differences in lactational performance between Norplant users and women in the control group. Among exclusively breastfed infants during the first year postpartum, average weights were slightly lower in the Norplant group than in the control group, but the difference was statistically significant only for the fourth through the sixth month. Average monthly weight gains did not significantly differ between the two groups in the first 6 months postpartum among exclusively breastfed infants.[9] In an Indonesian study, Norplant was inserted 4–6 weeks after delivery in 60 lactating women. The weight and height growth curves were very similar among infants in the control and Norplant groups through the first 6 months postpartum.[1]

Depo-Provera. Studies of Depo-Provera started 1-4 days postpartum or at 7 days postpartum[27] or within 6 weeks postpartum[22] have found no adverse effects. Because the contraceptive benefit to the lactating woman in obtaining Depo-Provera immediately postpartum is smaller and the theoretical risks might be higher (hormonal levels are relatively high in the immediate post-injection days) than for Norplant, a case would be less compelling for injecting Depo-Provera before breastfeeding is well established.

Minipills. Studies of minipills have demonstrated no adverse effects on lactation or infant growth even when started in the first week postpartum.[28,32]

Older women. For older women, Norplant, Depo-Provera (and other long-acting injections) and progestin-only pills are desirable because of their safety and low failure rates. A woman may have Norplant inserted when she is fairly certain she wants no more children. Then, after 3-4 years when she is absolutely certain she wants no more children, she may have a tubal ligation (or her partner/husband may have a vasectomy) followed by Norplant removal. For a woman who will be deciding about sterilization in the next 3-12 months, DMPA may be a better option than Norplant. Progestin-only pills are also an excellent option for women who are late in their reproductive years; they are more effective for older women.[5] The absence of thrombotic complications makes Depo-Provera, Norplant, and progestin-only pills advantageous for older women and for women who are going to having an operative procedure done that might increase her risk for thrombophlebitis.

Young women. For younger women, Norplant is desirable because of its extremely low failure rate and its ready reversibility. The production of a thick cervical mucus throughout the time implants are in place also causes them to have a protective effect against pelvic inflammatory disease. Depo-Provera is less readily reversible but has a very low failure rate and probably has a protective effect against PID.

Women who cannot take estrogen. Progestin-only pills, as well as the other progestin-only methods, are particularly desirable for women who want to use an oral contraceptive but have contraindications to combined pills. Women who have developed severe headaches or hypertension while taking combined OCs or prior to initiating use of hormonal contraceptives may be candidates for progestin-only pills. Lactating women who desire a hormonal contraceptive should be advised that minipills are an excellent option.

D ISADVANTAGES

The progestin-only methods have few serious disadvantages. Listed below are those disadvantages that apply to implants, injections, and minipills. The precautions for prescribing are listed under the following sections on how to provide each of the methods (see Tables 11-4, 11-6, and 11-9).

1. **Menstrual cycle disturbance.** Progestin-only contraceptives change women's menstrual cycles and this is one of the most frequent reasons for discontinuation of each of these methods. Many women experience an increased number of days of light bleeding. Some women experience amenorrhea, which is most likely to occur in the first year of Norplant use. (See Table 11-3.) It is during the first year of Norplant use when anovulation is most likely to occur. *While missed menstrual periods become less common over time among women using Norplant, amenorrhea becomes more common over time in Depo-Provera users.* On the other hand, some women using Norplant or DMPA experience an increased number of days of heavy bleeding. Bleeding changes are usually *not* asso-

ciated with increased blood loss in users of progestin-only contraceptives. Women using any of the progestin-only methods should be counseled to expect changes in their cycles. If these changes are bothersome, administration of oral contraceptives, oral estrogens, prostaglandin inhibitors, or a combination of these therapeutic approaches can improve bleeding patterns. Counseling is the key to minimizing discontinuation of progestin-only methods due to bleeding irregularities.

Table 11-3 Bleeding patterns over 5-year period among women using Depo-Provera injections and Norplant implants

	DMPA Injections		Norplant Implants	
	1 Yr.	5 Yr.	1 Yr.	5 Yr.
Regular cycles*	30	17	27	67
Amenorrhea	25	80	5	9

Sources: Shoup et al., (1991).
Depo-Provera NDA 20-246

* Regular cycle – Norplant: 21–35 days
  Regular cycle – DMPA: 25–34 days

During the first year of use, Depo-Provera often increases the number of days the user has very light spotting or breakthrough bleeding. The longer a woman is on Depo-Provera, the greater the likelihood of amenorrhea. Amenorrhea may be viewed very positively by women if it is explained well and if women are prepared for this change in advance. Heavy bleeding is uncommon. Bleeding disturbances are the most common reason for discontinuation of DMPA.

2. **Weight gain.** Some women using progestin-only methods gain weight or complain of feeling bloated. Others experience breast tenderness. The weight gain is probably due to increased appetite rather than fluid retention.[52] The World Health Organization monograph on injectable contraceptives notes that a weight gain of 1 kg (2.2 pounds) annually "is reported in nearly all women using injectable contraceptives."[52]

Over 5 years of use, weight gain in Norplant users averages just under 5 pounds, which is very close to the average weight gain for women in their early to mid-reproductive years. Weight gain is less of a problem in women on progestin-only pills than in women on combined OCs.

Disadvantages **297**

3. **Breast tenderness.** Breast tenderness has been noted in some women using Norplant and Depo-Provera. Occasionally breast tenderness is very painful. Always rule out pregnancy as the cause.

4. **Interaction with anticonvulsants.** Anticonvulsants (all except valproic acid) make Norplant failure rates rise to unacceptable levels; this would probably be true for progestin-only pills.

5. **Bone density decrease.** Decreased bone density has been reported in a retrospective study of 30 women using Depo-Provera for long periods of time.[7] Decreased bone density was as likely to be found in thin as in heavier women and was reversible when DMPA was stopped. Women were matched for age and body mass, but not for parity or history of smoking. There were more smokers among the DMPA users (40%) than among the premenopausal control women (10%). Another criticism of this study is that the bone density of DMPA users and control women was not determined prior to initiation of DMPA injections. Although this one study does not mean that women should be counseled to avoid long-term use of DMPA, the results sound a cautionary note suggesting that osteoporosis and other effects of low estrogen need to be carefully analyzed in women using DMPA, Norplant, and progestin-only pills. *Very low serum estradiol levels below 20 picograms/ml have occurred in some DMPA users. Avoid falsely reassuring women about the possible long-term effects of amenorrhea in association with very low serum estradiol levels.*

Norplant

6. **Difficult removal.** Both insertion and removal require a minor surgical procedure. Removal is particularly likely to be difficult if insertion of an implant is too deep. Discontinuation of Norplant requires a clinic visit, and occasionally, removal requires more than one visit.

7. **Higher initial cost.** The initial cost of Norplant is high in the United States, and if the implants are removed soon after insertion, then this method is extremely expensive per month of contraception provided. Recently, Wyeth Laboratories made the decision to replace Norplant implants or refund the amount paid if a woman's implants were removed in less than 180 days. Removals can be minimized by explaining in advance the menstrual cycle changes that are likely to occur, by avoiding Norplant insertion for the woman who may change her mind quickly and want to become pregnant in the near future, and by avoiding insertions for women who are already pregnant. The cost of Norplant over a 5-year period compares favorably with the cost of most other hormonal contraceptives.

8. **Extremely low-dose contraceptive.** Because its low dose, Norplant's effectiveness is more significantly lowered by antiseizure medicines (except for valproic acid) and by rifampin than are other hormonal contraceptives. Norplant failure rates increase to unacceptable levels if a woman is on certain drugs including:[16,33]

carbamazepine	primidone
phenytoin (Dilantin)	phenylbutazone
phenobarbital	rifampin

All antiseizure medications are strong inducers of the hepatic enzymes that break down of levonorgestrel. If a Norplant user begins one of these medications, she should use a back-up contraceptive.

9. **Local inflammation or infection at site of implants.** A pooled analysis of 2,674 first-year users in seven countries found that 0.8% experienced infection, 0.4% experienced expulsion of a capsule, and 4.7% had skin irritation at the insertion site. Complications did not always occur immediately after insertion. Some 35% of infections and 64% of expulsions occurred after the first 2 months of use.[20] Norplant implants are slightly visible under the skin of some women. Slightly increased pigmentation of the skin occasionally appears over the site of the implants.

10. **Ovarian cysts.** Norplant suppresses the hypothalamic pituitary axis, particularity FSH, less than combined OCs do. Most ovarian cysts regress spontaneously. Cysts do not need to be evaluated sonographically or laparoscopically unless they become large and painful or fail to regress.[48]

Depo-Provera

11. **No immediate discontinuation.** Weight gain, depression, breast tenderness, and menstrual irregularities may continue until the DMPA is cleared from a woman's body about 6-8 months after her last injection. Fortunately, anaphylactic reactions to DMPA and allergic reactions of any kind are rare. There is a delay in return of fertility of an average of 6 months to 1 year after ceasing to use Depo-Provera.[52]

12. **Return visits every 3 months.** Some individuals find the requirement of repeated injections unacceptable. Approximately 70% of women continue to use DMPA at 1 year (see Table 5-2).

13. **Lipid changes.** High density lipoprotein cholesterol levels fall significantly in women using DMPA.[31] Adverse changes in lipids do not occur in women using Norplant.

Minipills

14. **Vulnerable efficacy.** The disadvantages of progestin-only pills may include the need for obsessive regularity in pill-taking and attention to timing. Moreover, there is a greater risk of pregnancy in women whose menstrual cycles are ovulatory and whose cycles are least disturbed.[15]

15. **Less available.** Minipills are less likely to be stocked by pharmacies, family planning clinics, and hospital formularies.

16. **Less experience.** Clinicians are less likely to have had experience prescribing progestin-only pills, and may be less comfortable in counseling patients.

17. **Ovarian cysts.** Users experience an increased risk of functional ovarian cysts.

18. **Ectopic pregnancy.** Ectopic pregnancy is more likely among minipill failures.

N ORPLANT IMPLANTS

PROVIDING NORPLANT

Norplant implants produce few side effects or complications. Nonetheless, some women are not ideal candidates. Table 11-4 describes the precautions in the provision of Norplant implants. These precautions replace the outmoded concept of contraindications.

Although hormonal methods are not considered the method of first choice for women who are breastfeeding, Norplant implants may be inserted for breastfeeding women. See the section on Indications in this chapter and the discussion in Chapter 17 on Postpartum Contraception and Lactation.

NORPLANT INSERTION: 20 HELPFUL HINTS

Norplant insertion is a minor surgical procedure done under local anesthesia. Using a trocar, the clinician places Norplant implants under the skin on the inside of a woman's upper arm in a fan-shaped configuration (see Figure 11-1). It is recommended that Norplant implants be replaced after 5 years.

Each Norplant kit distributed in the United States comes with detailed step-by-step instructions and diagrams. Wyeth Laboratories also makes available at no cost two excellent videos—one for clinicians and one for clients. A two-capsule Norplant system is being developed. This system will simplify both insertion and removal.

Table 11-4 Precautions in the provision of Norplant implants

Refrain from providing Norplant for women with the following diagnoses:

Precautions	Rationale/Discussion
Known or suspected pregnancy	Although current data do not show any increased risk for birth defects caused by taking hormones during pregnancy, it is best to avoid any exposure of the fetus to hormones. It is recommended that Norplant implants be removed if a pregnant woman wishes to continue her pregnancy to term.[37]
Unexplained abnormal vaginal bleeding	Use of Norplant usually leads to irregular menses, increased days of light bleeding or spotting, heavy bleeding, or amenorrhea. These Norplant-induced changes in menses may mask an underlying problem such as pelvic inflammatory disease, cancer of the reproductive tract, or pregnancy. Therefore until a diagnosis of the cause of unexplained vaginal bleeding is reached by the clinician, Norplant implants should not be inserted.[37]
Contraindicated drugs	
Antiseizure medications: phenytoin (Dilantin) phenobarbital carbamazepine primidone phenylbutazone Antibiotic: rifampin/rifampicine	Medications for epilepsy (except valproic acid) cause the liver to metabolize progestins more rapidly, decreasing already low blood levels of levonorgestrel. This increases a woman's risk for pregnancy. If Norplant implants are inserted for a woman already on one of these drugs, she must be told to use a back-up contraceptive, such as condoms, consistently.
Active thrombophlebitis or pulmonary emboli	Although progestins are not known to increase a woman's risk for thrombophlebitis, Norplant insertion should be avoided if a woman has active thrombophlebitis. If thrombophlebitis develops after implants have been in place, it is probably advisable to inform a woman that progestins are not known to have any specific effect on the course of thrombophlebitis but that her implants will be removed immediately she wishes. Women with a past history of thromboembolic or cardiovascular disease can probably use low-dose progestin-only methods such as Norplant safely.

(continued)

Table 11-4 Precautions in the provision of Norplant implants (cont.)

Precautions	Rationale/Discussion
Known or strongly suspected breast cancer or a history of breast cancer. (Evidence is insufficient to include known or strongly suspected cervical or endometrial cancer as a reason not to use Norplant).	Norplant does NOT cause breast cancer. However, some breast cancers are sensitive to progestins and estrogens. Hormones should be avoided in women with breast cancer. Suspicious masses should be evaluated.

Exercise caution if Norplant implants are used or considered in the following situations and carefully monitor for adverse effects:

Precautions	Rationale/Discussion
Intolerance of irregular bleeding due to cultural or personal reasons	The pattern of menstrual bleeding does change for women using Norplant. This side effect must be discussed particularly well with women for whom irregular bleeding may be bothersome and with all teenagers considering Norplant.
Migraine or other headaches	Headaches may become more or less severe following Norplant insertion. Patients with a history of headaches should be forewarned of this potential side effect in order to monitor any change in their headaches.
Heart lesions that predispose to sub-acute bacterial endocarditis	Bacteria may be introduced into the blood stream at the time of insertion. Strongly consider use of prophylactic antibiotics at the time of insertion or removal of implants. Careful attention to sterile technique is important for all insertions and removals.
History of heart attack; chest pain due to diagnosed heart disease; stroke; thrombo-phlebitis; pulmonary embolism or blood clots in the eye; women with diabetes, which predisposes to cardiovascular disease	Warnings related to cardiovascular complications (in the Wyeth package inserts for patients and for physicians, December, 1990) are based on past experience with higher-dose combi-nation (progestin plus estrogen) oral contraceptives, not on data suggesting that Norplant users are at increased risk for the diseases or diabetes. Women with active or past history of cardiovascular disease and women with diabetes have a greatly increased risk of complications during pregnancy and may want to consider voluntary surgical contraception. If sterilization is not acceptable, Norplant should be considered because of its low failure rate.

(continued)

Table 11-4 Precautions in the provision of Norplant implants (cont.)

Precautions	Rationale/Discussion
History of allergic reaction such as erythema nodosum, angioneurotic edema, or generalized pruritus while using pills, if levonorgestrel was a component of the pill used when the allergic reaction developed	Allergic reactions to hormones are rare. If it is possible that a woman is allergic to levonorgestrel, provide her levonorgestrel in the progestin-only pill Ovrette for a cycle or so prior to Norplant insertion.
History of acne becoming worse while using combined pills; concern that current acne will become worse while using Norplant	Acne is the most common skin complaint in Norplant users. Levonorgestrel may have some androgenic effects and it may also decrease sex hormone binding globulin (SHBG) leading to increased circulating levels of free levonorgestrel and testosterone. If a woman is extremely concerned about acne, provide her with several cycles of oral levonorgestrel in the progestin-only pill Ovrette to evaluate her response to this hormone. When acne does develop in Norplant users it can usually be managed using topical treatments (Retin-A cream, gel, or liquid), antibiotics (1% clindamycin solution, or gel, or topical erythromycin), good skin hygiene with soap or cleansers, dietary change, or exogenous estrogens (Premarin or Estrace).[48]

Source: Angle and Murphy (1992).

NORPLANT INSERTION, CONTINUED

1. Use the arm model to practice insertion. If this is the first, second, or third time you have inserted Norplant implants, take 3-5 minutes to insert a set of implants into an arm model.

2. Fear of pain at the time of insertion is the number one concern of women considering Norplant. Therefore, it is very helpful to have someone who has already had Norplant implants inserted reassure your new client that insertion is not painful.

3. Raise the head of the exam table. Your patient will be more comfortable.

4. Use the width of four fingers if you are a man, or five fingers if you are a woman, to measure up from the crease of the elbow to decide where to place your incision. Mark this site.

5. Use a template and a pen every time you insert a set of Norplant implants. Make no exceptions. These marks will help you to put your

local anesthetic at the precise site your trocar will be placed. They will also make removals easier as you will know more accurately where to look for implants.

6. Add sodium bicarbonate to the local anesthetic to decrease stinging as the local anesthetic is injected into the insertion sites. Use 0.5 cc of NaHCO$_3$ for every 5 cc of 1% xylocaine (a 1:10 ratio). Xylocaine comes in a 30 cc bottle. By adding 3 cc of NaHCO$_3$, you will have enough local anesthetic for a number of Norplant insertions in a single session. Throw away any remaining anesthetic at the end of each insertion session, because the NaHCO$_3$ destabilizes the xylocaine over time. Mix up only as much of the 1:10 solution as you will need in a day.

7. Inject the local anesthetic slowly. The patient will feel less discomfort. A slow injection is particularly helpful if you are injecting xylocaine with no sodium bicarbonate. By the time the injection has been made for the sixth implant, the local anesthesia will be almost ready for the incision to be made.

8. Save 1 cc of local anesthetic for the sixth implant insertion site. If the anesthetic runs out, the client may experience significant pain during insertion of the last implant.

9. The incision can be very small—about 2-3 mm. With a small insertion, the scar will be smaller. It is possible to make the incision with the trocar itself, with no increased risk for pain, tenderness, edema, ecchymosis, or extensive scarring.[11] Making a small incision with a scalpel eases introduction of the trocar.

10. Proper subdermal insertion of implants is the most important goal of the entire insertion process. Implants inserted deeper in the tissue layers cause more difficulty upon removal. However, insertions should not be too superficial. Some Norplant insertions have actually been too superficial (intradermal) and have been associated with increased visibility of implants and some transient discomfort.

11. Do not move the inner plunger as you withdraw the outer part of the trocar. Do not push on the inner plunger with your thumb or retract the inner plunger. The plunger should remain fixed.

12. The trocar should remain inside of the incision (under the skin) between insertion of each individual implant.

13. Once you have inserted an implant, hold it in place while you advance the trocar to insert the next implant. By holding the implant in place, you will prevent the trocar from catching and misplacing an already inserted implant.

14. Locate the distal tips of all six implants following insertion. If an implant is 5 mm to 1 cm further from the incision than the others,

it is often possible to push the implant with your fingernail toward the incision before wrapping the arm. This will simplify removal.

15. Gently clean the area with an alcohol swab prior to bandaging your client's arm.

16. Show the client the incision site before you put on the butterfly bandage or gauze. She will be reassured seeing the very small incision.

17. Roll the gauze/bandage over 4" × 4" folded pad. Do not wrap it too tightly. Suggest that your client leave the gauze wrapping on her arm for 3-5 days to avoid having people touch the area while it is still tender.

18. Warn your client that she may have a large bruise when her bandage is removed. Tell her that the bruise will change colors before going away completely.

19. After insertion, inform the client if any implant has been inserted too deeply, too far, or if the proximal end of one implant was pulled distally.

20. After insertion, provide your phone number to your client and encourage her to call if she has questions or problems. Remind her that Norplant will cause a change in her menstrual cycle and that she should call if her new pattern of bleeding is bothersome. Remind her that medications can improve patterns of bleeding.

Norplant Removal: 20 Helpful Hints

Wyeth Laboratories provides clinicians with written materials, a brief video, and an arm model to practice removal.

1. Use the arm model to practice removal. Wyeth Laboratories provides a plastic sheathing into which the implants are placed. The clinician may practice cutting the plastic sheath to remove implants.

2. If possible, perform your first Norplant removal with someone at your side who has experience removing Norplant implants. Schedule adequate time. Your first few removals may take 45-60 minutes. As you gain experience, the time of removal decreases to 20-30 minutes.

3. The Emory method of Norplant removal can ease the procedure. Some clinicians are able to average less than 15 minutes per removal by using the following three techniques:[39]

   • Use 6-8 cc of local anesthesia rather than 3 cc

   • Make a 8 mm to 1 cm incision rather than a 4 mm incision

   • Vigorously disrupt adhesions for 30 seconds by repeatedly opening a small curved hemostat in the tissue near the end of the implants prior to attempting removal of implants.[39]

4. Remind the client that removal may be more difficult than insertion. Inform her that removal may take 30 or more minutes and could require a second visit.

5. Raise the head of the examining table. The patient will be more comfortable.

6. Be sure you are comfortable as you begin the removal. You may be more at ease sitting rather than standing and leaning over her arm.

7. Identify both the proximal and distal end of each of the six implants. Mark the ends with a pen.

8. Add sodium bicarbonate to the local anesthetic to decrease stinging. This procedure is described in suggestion #6 in the section on Norplant insertion.

9. Inject the local anesthetic slowly under the proximal 1/3 of the implants. Wyeth instructions recommend that you initially inject approximately 3 cc of 1% xylocaine. Have an additional 3-5 cc of xylocaine available to provide additional anesthesia in case you need it later. An alternative approach is to inject 8-10 cc of local anesthesia to permit a longer incision (1 cm) and more vigorous breaking up of adhesions with a small curved hemostat.[39]

10. Rather than making your incision at exactly the same site as the location of the incision used to insert implants, make the incision 3-5 mm up the arm from the original incision site. This procedure makes the removal incision closer to the proximal tips of the six implants.

11. The incision for removal may need to be a bit longer (8 mm to 1 cm) than the incision used for insertion.

12. Make a second incision if one implant is far from the other implants.

13. Throughout the procedure, ask the client if she feels any pain. Provide additional local anesthetic if needed.

14. An assistant may be helpful during the removal procedure, although removal may be accomplished by one person.

15. With your finger, apply pressure to the distal end of each implant as you remove it. Push the implant toward the incision.

16. With a sharp blade or a gauze pad, remove the scar tissue covering the implants.

17. Do not pull an implant too hard. It may break.

18. Warn your client that she may develop a bruise after removal, but that it will go away completely.

19. Advise your client that a prostaglandin inhibitor may be helpful if she has pain in her arm following removal.

20. Remind your client that she may become pregnant immediately following Norplant removal. If she does not want to become pregnant, discuss contraception.

MANAGING NORPLANT PROBLEMS AND FOLLOW-UP

A number of side effects may occur in women using Norplant implants. During the first year of Norplant use, certain side effects have been noted:[29]

Table 11-5 Norplant side effects during first year of use

Side Effect	Norplant Users	
	Study 1	Study 2
Headaches	16.7	18.5
Ovarian enlargement	3.1	11.6
Dizziness	5.6	8.1
Breast tenderness	6.2	6.8
Nervousness	6.2	6.8
Nausea	5.1	7.7
Acne	4.5	7.2
Dermatitis	3.8	8.2
Breast discharge	3.5	5.1
Change in appetite	3.5	6.2
Weight gain	3.3	6.2
Hair growth or loss	1.8	2.6

Source: McCauley (1992).

A variety of treatments have been used to improve these symptoms. Occasionally, Norplant implants must be removed to eliminate these complications. The physiological basis of many Norplant side effects needs clarification and is an important research priority.

Menstrual disturbances, such as changes in pattern of menstrual bleeding, are the most common reason for removal of Norplant implants during years 1 and 2. Counseling can minimize removals for this side effect. Inform women in advance to expect a change in the pattern of bleeding. Over 80% of women will note a change.[7] The three most common patterns are an increased number of days of amenorrhea, very light bleeding, or heavy bleeding. Fortunately, the third pattern is not common. Inform women that several medications can improve bleeding patterns associated with Norplant implants. It is very reassuring for women to know in advance or at the first sign of a bleeding problem, and that something can be done to help them. Clinicians may find several therapeutic approaches helpful:

- Several cycles of a low-dose combined OC
- Prostaglandin inhibitors
- Exogenous estrogens such as oral 17-beta estradiol, (Estrace), ethinyl estradiol (Estinyl), or conjugated estrogens (Premarin)

Be sure to inform women that the irregular pattern of bleeding may return when treatment is stopped.

Headaches may be associated with pregnancy and use of oral contraceptives and Norplant implants. If severe headaches associated with blurred vision and papilledema develop as a new symptom following Norplant insertion, removal of Norplant implants may need to be done quickly. In December of 1992, Wyeth Laboratories sent a letter to physicians describing severe headaches, papilledema, and a pseudotumor cerebri-like syndrome in 14 women using Norplant implants. Whether or not Norplant is causally related to the development of these symptoms is not yet clear. If a client's headaches can be explained by causes other than Norplant and if headache symptoms are not severe, it may not be necessary to perform a fundoscopic exam.

Breast tenderness may occur in some women. Recommended treatments have included Vitamin E (600 units/day), bromocriptine (2.5 mg/day), tamoxifen (20 mg/day), or danazol (200 mg/day).[48]

Weight gain may accompany Norplant use, although weight gain is usually due to other causes. Occasionally it has been necessary to discontinue this method because of client complaints of weight gain.

Hair loss has been noted in a small number of women, occasionally requiring Norplant removal.

Acne has been a problem for some women on Norplant. Usually it is possible to manage acne without removing Norplant.

Suitability Test

"Should I prescribe a minipill containing levonorgestrel to a woman for several months to see if she is going to tolerate Norplant?" This question is asked repeatedly at Norplant training sessions. Several side effects that could potentially lead to Norplant removal might be anticipated if a woman used a levonorgestrel progestin-only pill (Ovrette, in the United States) for a month or two prior to Norplant insertion.

Possible indications for the use of Ovrette as a test of suitability for Norplant are a past history on pills of – or extreme patient concern about –

- Acne
- Weight gain
- Severe headaches
- Depression
- Allergy to levonorgestrel

In contrast, changes in the menstrual cycle a Norplant user might experience are unlikely to show up with a suitability test. Moreover, the delay in inserting Norplant would also expose a woman on progestin-only pills to a period of time using a far less effective contraceptive. Use of several injections of Depo-Provera to test a woman's response to a long-acting progestin-only method makes no sense at all. The hormones are completely different, as are the fluctuations in hormone levels in the serum.

COMMON QUESTIONS ABOUT NORPLANT IMPLANTS

1. In what situations might Norplant implants be a better choice than the injectable contraceptive Depo-Provera?

In the following situations Norplant might be a better option for a woman than Depo-Provera:

- Weight gain is a major concern.
- Difficulty returning each 3 months for an injection.
- Fear of repeated shots.
- When method is discontinued, client will want to become pregnant right away. This consideration is particularly important for women late in their reproductive years who want contraception at the present time but will want to become pregnant right away after discontinuing contraception.
- Need for very effective reversible contraceptive for a long period of time. For example, use of Accutane for a year or more; long-term use of anticoagulants; chemotherapy for cancer to be followed by several years of not becoming pregnant before considering becoming pregnant.
- When a decrease in HDL cholesterol would be unacceptable.

2. Can anything be done for a woman who has persistent bleeding while using Norplant?

The problem is usually an atrophic endometrium. Stimulation of the endometrial lining followed by stopping hormonal stimulation usually controls the chronic spotting *temporarily*. Cycle your patient for several months. The additional hormones should not be a problem for most women if you use low-dose OCs; or a low dose of conjugated estrogens, ethinyl estradiol, or estradiol.

Explain to the woman experiencing this annoying side effect that repeating the use of these extra hormones would not be harmful, that the amount of blood loss is probably less not more, that she can have sexual intercourse in spite of the spotting, and that you would be happy to do an hematocrit to reassure her that she is not anemic. Keep in mind that she could have an unrelated problem such as a chlamydia infection, a fibroid, or a cervical infection.

D EPO-PROVERA (DMPA)

PROVIDING DEPO-PROVERA

The World Health Organization makes the reassuring statement: "In summary, DMPA and NET-EN appear to be acceptable methods of fertility regulation. Clinical evidence from more than 15 years of use as contraceptive agents shows no additional, and possibly fewer, adverse effects than are found with other hormonal methods of contraception...Studies thus far have not shown any serious short or long-term effects of DMPA or NET-EN."[52]

There are few precautions to the use of Norplant implants. These are noted in Table 11-6.

Toxicologic studies of DMPA in beagle dogs showed an increase in mammary gland tumors, some of which became malignant.[12] These studies have raised concern over the possibility of breast cancer in women using DMPA. Several studies in the United States and elsewhere have found no effect in humans (see Table 11-7). In a New Zealand study, 891 women with newly diagnosed breast cancer were compared with 1,864 women selected at random. Women were interviewed by telephone about their past use of contraceptives and any risk factors for breast cancer. Overall, the relative risk of breast cancer associated with any use of medroxyprogesterone acetate (Depo-Provera) was 1.0. In women aged 25-34 years, the relative risk was 2.0. The risk was greatest among women who used the drug for 6 years or longer. Despite the lack of an association overall, this study suggests that Depo-Provera may accelerate the presentation of breast cancer in young women, perhaps acting as a promoter in the late stages of carcinogenesis.[36] The WHO Collaborative Study failed to demonstrate a significantly increased risk for either breast cancer or cervical cancer among women using DMPA.[52,53]

Depo-Provera must always be provided to women on a completely voluntary basis. No hint of coercion should enter the picture. Even before DMPA was approved by the FDA, it was used in adolescent health care for mentally retarded adolescents, teenagers with emotional or behavioral problems, and adolescents characterized as having "out-of-control behavior" (delinquency, runaway, unstable social environment).[18] Attention to keeping DMPA completely voluntary is particularly important in these situations.

In the United States, DMPA is usually provided from vials each containing 150 mg of DMPA in each 1 cc. Depo-Provera produced in the United States has a 2-year shelf-life on the label; DMPA made in Belgium has a 5-year shelf-life. USAID hopes and expects that the FDA will approve a 3-year shelf-life labeling by the time that they start purchasing DMPA sometime in 1993.[38]

Table 11-6 Precautions in the provision of Depo-Provera injections

Refrain from providing Depo-Provera for women with the following diagnoses:

Precautions	Rationale/Discussion
Known or suspected pregnancy	Although current data do not show any increased risk for birth defects caused by taking hormones during pregnancy, it is best to avoid any exposure of the fetus to hormones.
Unexplained abnormal vaginal bleeding in past 3 months	Use of Depo-Provera usually leads to irregular menses, increased days of light bleeding or spotting, or amenorrhea. These Depo-Provera-induced changes may mask an underlying problem. Causes of bleeding may include pelvic inflammatory disease, cancer of the reproductive tract, pregnancy, hyper- or hypothyroidism, early or premenopause, or fibroids. Therefore until a diagnosis of unexplained vaginal bleeding is reached by the clinician, Depo-Provera injections should not be started.

Exercise caution if Depo-Provera injections are used or considered in the following situations and carefully monitor for adverse effects:

Precautions	Rationale/Discussion
Pregnancy planned in the fairly near future	Because of the prolonged delay in return of fertility a more readily reversible method may be advisable.
Concern over weight gain	Weight gain is predictable: 5.4 pounds (average) in the first year, 8.1 pounds after 2 years of use, and 13.8 pounds after 4 years of use (according to DMPA package insert); and 2.2 pounds per year (according to WHO)[52]

Active liver disease has been deleted from the above list as a reason to avoid Depo-Provera. Exercise special care when providing DMPA to women with severe, acute liver disease or liver tumors or to women with severe gallbladder disease.

Source: Angle and Murphy (1992).

   Deep intramuscular injections may be made into the deltoid or the gluteus maximus muscles. Injections into the deltoid may be less embarrassing, but may also be slightly more painful. The needle should be 2.5-4 cm in length and 21-23 gauge; both needle and syringe should be sterile.[52] *The area of the injection should NOT be massaged because this may lower the effectiveness of DMPA.* Injections usually are not painful.

Table 11-7 Risks of 5 types of cancers in DMPA users

Site of Cancer	No. of Cases Who Used DMPA/ All Cases (%)	No. of Controls Who Used DMPA/All Controls (%)	Relative Risk for Women Who Have Ever Used DMPA*
Breast	39/427 (9)	557/5,951 (9)	1.0
Cervix	126/920 (14)	545/5,833 (9)	1.2
Ovary	7/105 (7)	74/637 (12)	0.7
Endometrium	1/52 (2)	30/316 (9)	0.3
Liver	7/57 (12)	34/920 (12)	1.0

Sources: WHO (1986).
Liskin (1987).

Injections are scheduled every 3 months. In international circles, there has been some discussion of self-administered injections of DMPA. After a woman has received several injections, each 150 mg of DMPA has a contraceptive effect greater than 3 months. This means that the method is forgiving of the woman who returns late for her injection. Some programs will provide injections of DMPA up to 4 weeks late; women are informed that pregnancies are rare but may occur. When a woman does appear late for her shot, stress the importance of returning on time for injections in the future. Try to find out why women are late for injections. Reasons may be fear of cancer, changes in the pattern of menstrual bleeding, other side effects, cost of injections, time lost coming to the clinic, or partner or family disapproval of the method. Deal with these barriers sympathetically and try to help your client to overcome them.

Satisfaction with this method may increase if clients are told to anticipate menstrual irregularity during the first year and an increasing likelihood of amenorrhea in subsequent years.

MANAGING DEPO-PROVERA PROBLEMS AND FOLLOW-UP

At each 3-month follow-up visit, ask about weight gain and any problems or concerns a woman may have, date of last menstrual period, risk for HIV infection and other STDs (and counsel to use condoms consistently if at risk), and measurement of weight and blood pressure. In one of the largest studies of 3,875 DMPA users, headaches were noted in 17% of users, nervousness in 11%, decreased libido in 5%, breast discomfort in 3%, and depression in 2%.[40] Weight gain was greater among clinic patients than among private patients provided DMPA.[40] If annual examinations do not reveal any problems and the client is not gaining weight excessively or having any unacceptable symptoms, DMPA injections may be continued as long as desired. At the time of annual exams, in addition to the above evaluation, perform a complete examination and Pap smear, and order mammography and other procedures dictated in part by the age of the client.

Menstrual changes. Women need to be informed in advance of the changes that will occur in their menstrual cycles. Do not belittle the impact of bleeding changes. They are the major reason for discontinuation of this method. Spotting or breakthrough bleeding may be managed most easily in a family planning clinic by offering women a cycle or so of combined oral contraceptives. Five days of pills may be enough and may be repeated. Inform women that the irregular bleeding may return. Teenagers *can* manage the bleeding patterns occurring during DMPA use. Amenorrhea will increase over time. Amenorrhea is not harmful.

Allergic reactions. The *Physicians' Desk Reference* (PDR) notes that anaphylactic and anaphylactoid reactions may occur immediately following Depo-Provera injections. Fortunately, severe anaphylactic reactions to DMPA are rare. However, because DMPA is irretrievable once injected, emergency supportive measures such as epinephrine, steroids, and diphenhydramine should be available.

COMMON QUESTIONS ABOUT DEPO-PROVERA

1. In what situations might Depo-Provera injections be a better choice for a woman than Norplant implants?

Depo-Provera might be more acceptable or a wiser choice than Norplant implants for the woman who:

- Is very concerned by the thought of a minor surgical procedure.

- Has a history of sickle cell disease or of seizures, both of which may actually be improved by DMPA.[25]

- Is taking a medication that markedly increases production of liver enzymes which speed up the breakdown of levonorgestrel (the hormone elaborated by Norplant implants). This would include women on phenobarbital, phenytoin (Dilantin), primidone, carbamazepine, and phenylbutazone.

- Needs highly effective contraception for just a *few months*. For example, prior to tubal sterilization or a vasectomy; at the time of receiving rubella immunization; during use of a medication like Accutane (for acne), which is known to produce severe defects in babies if taken by a pregnant woman; or during use of anticoagulants or valproic acid.

- Needs *only a year* of extremely effective contraception: for example, a woman who has recently had a molar pregnancy and who must not become pregnant for 1 year.

- Has a preference for receiving medications by injection.
- Wants to keep all information about contraceptive use from her partner (for example, from an abusive husband who does not want her to use contraception).

2. Can a woman who is breastfeeding her baby receive Depo-Provera injections?

Yes, this is an excellent option for breastfeeding mothers. Postpartum bleeding may be somewhat less predictable if DMPA is given immediately postpartum.

3. Why is a method that was "bad" 10 years ago now a good method?

It has always been a good method. By the time Depo-Provera was approved in the United States, it was already being used by 8-9 million women throughout the world in over 90 countries that approved Depo-Provera before it was approved in the United States.

4. What is the most important difference between Depo-Provera (DMPA) and norethindrone enanthate (NET-EN) injections?

NET-EN injections are not available in the United States. They are injections of norethindrone in an oily base given at 2-month intervals for the first 6 months of use. Then NET-EN injections are given at intervals of 2–3 months.[17] DMPA is given every 3 months from the first 150 mg injection on. Other countries also have injections containing both an estrogen and a progestin.

   It is important that the woman using norethindrone enanthate (NET-EN) every 3 months *not be late* for her injection. That 3-month interval should not be exceeded or failure rates will increase. Depo-Provera is more forgiving of the woman who is late for her injection.

P ROGESTIN-ONLY PILLS (Minipills)

PROVIDING PROGESTIN-ONLY PILLS

Because of the small number of women who use minipills, large-scale studies that document benefits and side effects are unavailable. In general, progestin-only pills have lower effectiveness, more breakthrough bleeding, and fewer noncontraceptive benefits than combined OCs.

Table 11-8 Brand names of progestin-only pills

Progestin	Dose (mg)	Number of Tablets Per Package	Brand Names
Norethindrone (Norethisterone)	350	42/28	Micronor, NOR-OD Noriday, Norod
Norethindrone (Norethisterone)	75	35	Micro-Novum
Norgestrol	75	28	Ovrette, Neogest
Levonorgestrol	30	35	Microval, Noregeston, Microlut
Ethynodial diacetate	500	28	Femulen
Lynestrenol	500	35	Exluton

Most of the health benefits of progestin-only pills are probably similar to combined estrogen/progestin pills: decreased menstrual cramps or pain, less heavy bleeding, a shorter period, decreased premenstrual syndrome symptoms, and decreased breast tenderness. In theory, the thick, less penetrable cervical mucus in women on progestin-only pills should decrease the risk of pelvic inflammatory disease.

Progestin-only pills should theoretically be safer than combined pills. Progestin-only pills have not been shown to increase the risk of either cardiovascular complications or malignant disease and are less likely to cause headaches, blood pressure elevation, depression, and other side effects than are higher dose combined OCs.[49] However, the FDA-required class labeling in the package insert for progestin-only pills does not suggest different contraindications for minipills than for combined pills. The authors propose that these contraindications be replaced with the precautions noted in Table 11-9.

Progestin-only pills are not the best choice for women who are disorganized.[15]

MANAGING MINIPILL PROBLEMS AND FOLLOW-UP

The most important problems with progestin-only pills relate to the patterns of bleeding. Many of them may be managed much as they are for women using Norplant implants or Depo-Provera. The approaches for managing increased days of light or heavy bleeding, spotting, or amenorrhea are the same as would be considered for the woman using implants or injectable contraceptives: switch to a combined oral contraceptive, use supplemental estrogen (in the form of conjugated estrogens, 17-beta estradiol or ethinyl estradiol) use prostaglandin inhibitors, rule out pregnancy, and provide counseling.

Table 11-9 Precautions in the provision of progestin-only pills

Exercise caution if minipills are used or considered in the following situations and carefully monitor for adverse effects:

Precautions	Rationale/Discussion
Menstrual cycle changes	Irregularities in menstrual bleeding, including spotting, breakthrough bleeding, prolonged cycles, and amenorrhea are the major problems encountered by women on progestin-only pills. *Unexplained abnormal vaginal bleeding during the past 3 months is an important reason to avoid using progestin-only pills.*
Functional ovarian cysts	Functional ovarian cysts appear to occur at a slightly more frequent rate among progestin-only pill users. If the cysts are symptomatic, discontinuation of progestin-only pills is recommended, and the cysts will usually regress spontaneously in 1–2 months. Abdominal pain in a woman on progestin-only pills may be related to a functional ovarian cyst or an ectopic pregnancy.
Cardiovascular complications	There is no epidemiologic evidence that progestin-only pills increase a woman's risk for the cardiovascular complications that have been attributed to combined OCs.[14]
Breast cancer	The effect of progestins on breast cancer is not fully understood.
Medications	Medications such as rifampin/rifampicine and most antiseizure medications, which induce hepatic enzymes, reduce the effectiveness of very low-dose hormonal contraceptives. Recommend a back-up contraceptive.

As in the case with Norplant and IUD users, when a pregnancy occurs in a woman using progestin-only pills, it is more likely to be ectopic because of the contraceptive effect of progestin-only pills on the endometrial lining. In other words, POPs, Norplant, and IUDs are more effective at preventing intrauterine than ectopic gestations. Therefore, of the pregnancies that do occur, a higher percentage are ectopic than is true for women using no method of birth control.

COMMON QUESTIONS ABOUT MINIPILLS

1. What effect do minipills have on ovulation?

Women on the progestin-only pills now available in the United States will have one of the following three patterns:

- First, they may ovulate every month. Periods tend to be quite regular.
- Second, they may never ovulate, in which case periods tend to be very irregular; a woman may go months without any bleeding.
- Third, they may ovulate some months and not others, in which case periods are irregular.

2. Which women would benefit most by consistently using a back-up method?

Women with regular periods who are ovulating regularly.

3. During the first cycle of minipills are back-up contraceptives essential?

No, whether or not a woman ovulates the first month on minipills, the production of a thick cervical mucus starts immediately and continues as long as minipills are taken every day at about the same time.

4. During the first cycle of minipills are back-up contraceptives <u>wise</u>?

Perhaps. Minipills may be forgotten or taken late during that first cycle. Mistakes are more common the first month on any method of birth control.

5. Which women might benefit most by using a back-up contraceptive while on minipills?

Several groups of women might be encouraged to use a back-up contraceptive while taking minipills:

- In the first cycle (just to make sure pills are remembered and tolerated well)
- Late in taking a minipill (should use a back-up contraceptive until back on schedule)
- Very regular in their menstrual cycles (*e.g.,* every 28 days)—this is presumptive evidence that women are ovulating and this might make them lean in the direction of using a back-up contraceptive
- Anxious every time a period is late (there is less emotional wear and tear if a back-up method has been used)
- At any risk for HIV infection or sexually transmitted infections—use condoms consistently

INSTRUCTIONS FOR USING PROGESTIN-ONLY CONTRACEPTIVES

NORPLANT IMPLANTS

If inserted in the first 7 days of a menstrual cycle, Norplant is effective immediately. No back-up method is necessary. If Norplant has been inserted more than 7 days after your period starts, use a back-up method contraceptive if you have intercourse during the first 24 hours after Norplant insertion.

You are using a very effective contraceptive. Your six implants release levonorgestrel, a hormone like progesterone, which your ovaries produce. Levonorgestrel is the same hormone millions of women take each month in a number of different birth control pills. You are receiving very low amounts of levonorgestrel constantly. Your contraceptive is very safe and remains effective for 5 years, at which point it should be removed. You may want to get a new set of implants at that time.

You may have your implants removed at any time. The procedure for Norplant removal takes a bit longer than insertion and may require two visits. The contraceptive effects of Norplant end as soon as the implants are removed. Here is some additional information that might help you:

1. Norplant is one of the most effective contraceptives available. Only about 1 in 1,000 women who use the method will become pregnant in the first year. This failure rate is lower than that for the pill or IUD. In the first 2 years of use, Norplant is about as effective as female sterilization. Women who weigh more than 70 kg (154 pounds) may have higher failure rates than those who weigh less.

2. **Norplant becomes effective within 24 hours of insertion.**

3. **If you have pain after insertion,** return to see your clinician. You might need antibiotics for an infection. Try to avoid direct pressure on the insertion area for a few days. After the incision has healed, you may touch the skin over the implants. The soft, flexible implants cannot break inside your body, so you should not be concerned about putting pressure on the area.

4. **If you may be at risk for infection** with the virus that causes AIDS (human immunodeficiency virus or HIV) or any other sexually transmitted infection, continue to use condoms in addition.

5. **The Norplant implants may cause you to have irregular bleeding or more days of bleeding.** Despite an increased number of days of bleeding, the amount of blood lost is rarely enough to produce anemia. In fact, a woman tends to lose less menstrual

blood than she did before she started using Norplant. A follow-up visit is recommended if you experience heavy bleeding.

6. The hormone levels in Norplant are very low. They are so low that there is very little build up of the lining of your uterus. This means that there is very little lining to shed and you will notice very light periods or no periods at all. Your bleeding may be irregular. Generally the amount of blood loss is less than before Norplant implants are inserted. Some women become concerned when they have no bleeding at all while using Norplant. There is no harm to your health if you do not get your period. If you want to make sure you are not pregnant, you may return to the clinic for a pregnancy test, but you will probably not be pregnant. Menstrual bleeding does tend to become more regular after implants have been in place for 9–12 months, although you cannot count on this.

7. Most women do not have major problems with Norplant. Common side effects noted by women using implants include headaches, nervousness, nausea, dizziness, rash, acne, changes in appetite, weight gain, breast tenderness, hirsutism, and hair loss. Although ovarian cysts sometimes occur in Norplant users, they usually disappear on their own. Surgery is considered if a cyst remains beyond 10 weeks. Several other problems noted by women using Norplant may or may not be caused by the implant: breast discharge, inflammation of the mouth of the womb (cervicitis), mood change, depression, general malaise, weight loss, hypertension, and itching.

8. If you are seen by a clinician for a medical problem, mention that you are using Norplant implants.

9. **Replace the Norplant implants at the end of 5 years;** effectiveness decreases after this time. A new set of implants can be inserted when the old set is removed.

10. Return to your clinician if you have any questions. Watch for the following signs of potential problems:

Norplant Warning Signs

Caution

- Severe lower abdominal pain (ectopic pregnancy is rare but can occur)
- Heavy vaginal bleeding
- Arm pain
- Pus or bleeding at the insertion site (these may be signs of infection)
- Expulsion of an implant
- Delayed menstrual periods after a long interval of regular periods
- Migraine headaches, repeated very painful headaches, or blurred vision

Avoid bumping the area where your Norplant implants were inserted and keep this area dry for several days after insertion.

DEPO-PROVERA

You have chosen a very effective method of birth control: injections every 3 months of Depo-Provera. Birth control shots are used by more than 6 million women around the world, and Depo-Provera is the most commonly used injection. If you wish to get pregnant, discontinue birth control shots several months before you plan to conceive. The following information may help you use Depo-Provera:

1. **Use an additional contraceptive method for 2 weeks** after your first injection. This is not necessary if the first shot is given during the first 5 days after the beginning of a normal menstrual period.

2. **If you may be at risk for infection** with the virus that causes AIDS (human immunodeficiency virus or HIV) or any other sexually transmitted infection, continue to use condoms in addition.

3. **Return to the clinic every 3 months for another injection.**

4. Depo-Provera tends to make a woman's periods less regular, and spotting between periods is fairly common. Some women stop having periods completely. If your pattern of bleeding concerns you, return to the clinic to get a blood test for anemia, to rule out the possibility of a pregnancy, or to rule out the possibility of infection.

5. Weight gain is common in users of Depo-Provera. You will have to pay close attention to avoiding excessive calories if you want to avoid this side effect.

6. See your clinician if you develop any problems.

MINIPILL

1. **Have on hand a back-up birth control method such as foam, spermicidal tablets or suppositories, condoms, or a diaphragm. You will need to use your back-up method:**
   - While you are waiting to start progestin-only pills or minipills
   - During your first 7-28 days on minipills
   - If you miss a minipill, you should use a back-up method until you restart or until your next period.

   Progestin-only pills are very low-dose contraceptives. Your margin of error is not great. Do not count on this method unless you will be able to take pills every single day. Try hard to take your minipills at the same time every day. *Some women use a back-up method at all times to increase the effectiveness of this approach to birth control.*

2. **Swallow one pill each day until you finish your pill pack.** Then start your new pack the next day. Never miss a day. The evening meal may be the best time to take progestin-only pills.

3. **If you may be at risk for infection** with the virus that causes AIDS (human immunodeficiency virus or HIV) or any other sexually transmitted infection, continue to use condoms in addition.

4. **If you miss one minipill,** take it (yesterday's minipill) as soon as you remember. Also take today's minipill at the regular time even if that means taking two pills in 1 day. If you are more than 3 hours late taking a minipill, use your back-up birth control method for the next 48 hours (2 days).

5. **If you miss two or more minipills in a row,** there is an increased chance you could become pregnant. Immediately start using your back-up method. Restart your minipills right away and double up for 2 days. If your menstrual period does not begin within 4–6 weeks, see your clinician for an exam and a pregnancy test.

6. Keep track of your periods while you take minipills. If you have more than 45 days with no period, then you may want to see your clinician for an exam and pregnancy test.

7. **If you have spotting or bleeding between periods,** keep taking your minipills on schedule. If your bleeding is very heavy or if you have cramps, pain, or fever, see your clinician. Your bleeding may be caused by infection. In most cases, bleeding is not serious and will often stop after a few days. Bleeding is especially likely if you have missed one or more minipills. Bleeding is common during the first few months a woman takes minipills.

8. If you become ill with vomiting, severe diarrhea or both, use your back-up method of birth control along with your minipills until 48 hours (2 days) after your illness is over. Using your back-up method will give you extra protection in case your illness or the medication you are taking for that illness interferes with minipill effectiveness.

9. If you decide you want to become pregnant, plan to stop using minipills and change to another method of birth control, such as condoms, for 2 or 3 months. Once you are off minipills, your natural cycle should be reestablished. Your clinician will be able to determine your pregnancy due date more accurately if you have at least two natural menstrual periods before you become pregnant.

10. Stop minipills anytime you want, even in the middle of a pill pack. Remember, though, that protection from the minipill does not last after you stop. Begin using another method the very next day.

11. See your clinician regularly for routine checkups. Be sure to have a blood pressure check, Pap smear, breast exam, and pelvic exam.

12. **See your clinician right away if you have severe lower abdominal pain while using minipills.**

Progestin-Only Pills (Minipills) Warning Signals

Caution

- Abdominal pain—May be due to an ovarian cyst or an ectopic pregnancy.
  (Don't stop pills but contact us right away.)

- Pill taken late—Even if only 3 hours late use a back-up contraceptive for the next 2 days. Be careful to take minipill ON TIME.

REFERENCES

1. Affandi B, Karmadibrata S, Prihartono J, Lubis F, Samil RS. Effect of Norplant on mothers and infants in the postpartum period. Adv Contracept 1986;2(4): 371-380.
2. Affandi B, Santoso SS, Djajadilaga W, Hedispura W, Moelock FA, Prihartono J, Lubis F, Samil RS. Five-year experience with Norplant. Contraception 1987;36(4):417-428.
3. Angle M, Murphy C. Guidelines for clinical procedures in family planning. A reference for trainers. Program for International Training in Health (INTRAH); Chaper Hill NC; 1992.
4. Antal EG. Personal communication from Drug Information Clinical Pharmacist at the Upjohn Company to Robert A. Hatcher; March 18, 1993
5. Bertrabet SS, Shikary ZK, Toddywalla VS, Toddywalla SP, Patel D, Saxena BN. Transfer of norethisterone (NET) and levonorgestrel (LNG) from a single tablet into the infant's circulation through the mother's milk. Contraception 1987;35(6):517-522.
6. Broome M, Fotherby K. Clinical experience with the progestogen-only pill. Contraception 1990;42(5):489-495.
7. Cundy T, Evans M, Roberts H, Wattie D, Ames R, Reid IR. Bone density in women receiving depo medroxyprogesterone acetate for contraception. BMJ 1991;303(6793):13-16.
8. Darney PD, Atkinson E, Tanner ST, MacPherson S, Hellerstein S, Alvarado AM. Acceptance and perceptions of Norplant among users in San Francisco, USA. Stud Fam Plann 1990;21(3):152-160.
9. Diaz S, Herreros C, Juez G, Casado ME, Salvatierra AM, Miranda P, Peralta O, Croxatto HB. Fertility regulation in nursing women: VII. Influence of Norplant levonorgestrel implants upon lactation and infant growth. Contraception 1985;32(1):53-74.
10. Diaz S, Pavez M, Miranda P, Johannson EDB, Croxatto HB. Long-term follow-up of women treated with Norplant implants. Contraception 1987;35(6): 551-567.
11. Diaz J, Rubin J, Faundes A, Diaz M, Bahamondes L. Comparison of local signs and symptoms after the insertion of Norplant implants with and without a scalpel. Contraception 1991;44(3):217-221.
12. Finkel MJ, Berliner VR. The extrapolation of experimental findings (animal to man): the dilemma of the systemically administered contraceptives. Bulletin of the Society of Pharmacological and Environmental Pathologists, December 1973.
13. Fraser IS, Weisberg E. A comprehensive review of injectable contraception with special emphasis on depo medroxyprogesterone acetate. Med J Aust 1981;1(1):3-19.
14. Greenspan AR, Hatcher RA, Moore M, Rosenberg MJ, Ory HW. The association of depo-medroxyprogesterone acetate and breast cancer. Contraception 1980;21:563-569.
15. Guillebaud J. Contraception: your questions answered. New York NY: Pitman, 1985.

16. Haukkamaa M. Contraception by Norplant subdermal capsules is not reliable in epileptic patients on anticonvulsant treatment. Contraception 1986;33(6): 559-565.

17. Huezo CM, Briggs C. Medical and service delivery guidelines for family planning. London: International Planned Parenthood Federation Medical Department, 1992.

18. Isart F, Weber FT, Merrick CL, Rowe S. Use of injectable progestin (medroxy-progesterone acetate) in adolescent health care. Contraception 1992;46(1):41-48.

19. Jimenez J, Ochoa M, Soler MP, Portales P. Long-term follow-up of children breast-fed by mothers receiving depo-medroxyprogesterone acetate. Contraception 1984;30(6):523-533.

20. Klavon SL, Grubb G. Insertion site complications during the first year of Norplant use. Contraception 1990;41(1):27-37.

21. Koetsawang S. The effects of contraceptive methods on the quality and quantity of breast milk. Int J Gynaecol Obstet 1987;25(suppl):115-127.

22. Koetsawang S, Boonyaprakob V, Suvanichati S, Paipeekul S. Long term study of growth and development of children breast-fed by mothers receiving Depo-Provera (medroxyprogesterone acetate) during lactation. In: Zatuchni GI, Goldsmith A, Shelton JD, Sciarra JJ (eds). Long-acting contraceptive delivery systems: proceedings from an international workshop on long-acting contraceptive delivery systems, May 31-June 3, 1983, New Orleans LA. Philadelphia PA: Harper & Row, 1983:378-387.

23. Labbok MH. Contraception during lactation: considerations in advising the individual and in formulating programme guidelines. J Biosoc Sci 1985;9(Suppl):55-66.

24. Liskin L, Blackburn R. Hormonal contraception: new long-acting methods. Popul Rep 1987;Series K(3).

25. Mattson RH, Cramer JA, Caldwell BV, Siconolfi BC. Treatment of seizures with medroxyprogesterone acetate: preliminary report. Neurology 1984;34(9): 1255-1258.

26. Mattson RH, Cramer JA, Darney PD, Naftolin F. Use of oral contraceptives by women with epilepsy. JAMA 1986;256(2):238-40.

27. McCann MF, Liskin LS, Piotrow PT, Rinehart W, Fox G. Breastfeeding, fertility and family planning. Popul Reports 1984;12(2),Series J(24):525-575.

28. McCann MF, Moggia AV, Higgins JE, Potts M, Becker C. The effects of a progestin-only oral contraceptive (Levonorgestrel 0.03 mg) on breast-feeding. Contraception 1989;40(6):635-648.

29. McCauley AP, Geller JS. Decisions for Norplant programs. Popul Rep 1992;Series K(4).

30. Mishell DR, Kletzky OA, Brenner PF, Roy S, Nicoloff J. The effect of contraceptive steroids on hypothalamic-pituitary function. Am J Obstet Gynecol 1977;128(1):60-74.

31. Mishell DR. Long-acting contraceptive steroids. Postcoital contraceptives and antiprogestins. In: Mishell DR, Davajan V, Lobo RA (eds). Infertility, contraception, and reproductive endocrinology. Cambridge: Blackwell Scientific Publications, 1991.

32. Moggia AV, Harris GS, Dunson TR, Diaz R, Moggia MS, Ferrer MA, McMullen SL. A comparative study of a progestin-only oral contraceptive versus non-hormonal methods in lactating women in Buenos Aires, Argentina. Contraception 1991;44(1):31-43.

33. Odlind V, Olsson SE. Enhanced metabolism of levonorgestrel during phenytoin treatment in a woman with Norplant implants. Contraception 1986; 33(3):257-61.

34. Pardthaisong T. Return of fertility after use of the injectable contraceptive Depo-Provera: updated data analysis. J Biosoc Sci 1984;16(1):23-34.

35. Pardthaisong T, Yenchit C, Gray R. The long-term growth and development of children exposed to Depo-Provera during pregnancy or lactation. Contraception 1992;45(4):313-324.

36. Paul C, Skegg DCG, Spears GFS. Depot medroxyprogesterone (Depo-Provera) and risk of breast cancer. Br Med J 1989;299(6702):759-762.

37. Population Council. NORPLANT levonorgestrel implants: a summary of scientific data. Monograph. New York NY; 1990.

38. Rinehart W. Personal communication to Robert A. Hatcher, March 9, 1993.

39. Sarma SP, Hatcher RA. The Emory method for rapid removal of Norplant implants (in press).

40. Schwallie PC, Assenzo JR. Contraceptive use-efficacy study utilizing medroxy-progesterone acetate administered as an intramuscular injection once every 90 days. Fertil Steril 1973;24(5):331-339.

41. Sheth A, Jain U, Sharma S, Adatia A, Patankar S, Andolsek L, Pretnar-Darovec A, Blesey MA, Hall PE, Parker RA, Ayeni S, Pinol A, Li-Hoi-Foo C. A randomized, double-blind study of two combined and two progestogen-only oral contraceptives. Contraception 1982;25(3):243-252.

42. Shaaban MM. Contraception with progestogens and progesterone during lactation. J Steroid Biochem Mol Biol 1991;40(4-6):705-710.

43. Shaaban MM, Salem HT, Abdullah KA. Influence of levonorgestrel contraceptive implants, Norplant, initiated early postpartum upon lactation and infant growth. Contraception 1985;32(6):623-635.

44. Shikary ZK, Bertrabet S, Patel ZM, Patel S, Joshi JV, Toddywala VS, Toddywala SP, Patel DM, Jhaveri K, Saxena BN. ICMR task force study on hormonal contraception. Transfer of levonorgestrel (LNG) administered through different drug delivery systems from the maternal circulation into the newborn's circulation via breast milk. Contraception 1987;35(5):477-486.

45. Shoup D, Mishell DR, Bopp B, Fielding M. The significance of bleeding patterns in Norplant implant users. Obslet Gynecol 1993; 77:256-265.

46. Sivin I. Personal communication to James Trussell, August 13, 1992.

47. Sivin I. Internation experience with Norplant and Norplant II. Contraception 1988; 19(2): 81-94.

48. Speroff L, Darney P. A clinical guide for contraception. Baltimore MD: Williams & Wilkins, 1992.

49. Vessey MP, Lawless M, Yeates D, McPherson K. Progestin-only oral contraception: findings in a large prospective study with special reference to effectiveness. Br J Fam Plann 1985;10:117-121.

50. Virutamasen P, Wongsrichanalai C, Tangkeo P, Nitichai Y, Rienprayoon D. Metabolic effects of depo medroxyprogesterone acetate in long-term users: a cross-sectional study. Int J Gynecol Obstet;1986;24(4):291-296.

51. World Health Organization Collaborative Study of Neoplasia and Steroid Contraceptives. Depo-medroxyprogesterone acetate (DMPA) and cancer: memorandum from a WHO meeting. Bull WHO 1986; 64(3):375-382.

52. World Health Organization. Injectable contraceptives: their role in family planning, monograph. Geneva, 1990.
53. World Health Organization Collaborative Study of Neoplasia and Steroid Contraceptives. Breast cancer and depo-medroxyprogesterone acetate: a multinational study. Lancet 1991;338(8771):833-838.
54. World Health Organization Collaborative Study of Neoplasia and Steroid Contraceptives. Depo-medroxyprogesterone acetate (DMPA) and risk of invasive squamous cell cervical cancer. Contraception 1992;45(4):299-312.
55. Wyeth Laboratories. Norplant system prescribing information. Philadelphia PA: Wyeth Laboratories, December 10, 1990.
56. Mattson RH, Rebar RN. Contraceptive methods for women with neurologic disorders. Am J Obstet Gynecol 1993; 168: 2027-2032.

Fertility Awareness

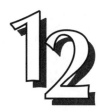

- Fertility awareness helps people understand how to become pregnant and how to avoid pregnancy.
- Fertility awareness is valuable for all men and women, regardless of which contraceptive they use.

- Among perfect users of the method, fertility awareness is effective for pregnancy prevention. Among imperfect users, however, it is very unforgiving.

Fertility awareness is the basic information on male and female reproduction that helps people understand how and when a woman can become pregnant. This information can help women plan or prevent pregnancies by identifying the fertile days of the menstrual cycle. A woman who knows when she is fertile can avoid pregnancy by abstaining from intercourse or by using other contraceptives (primarily barrier methods) during her fertile days.[6] Women who want to conceive can time intercourse accordingly.

Natural family planning methods are based on fertility awareness, with abstinence from intercourse during the fertile time. These methods include the calendar rhythm method, the basal body temperature (BBT) method, the ovulation or Billings method, and the sympto-thermal method. The term "natural" does not imply that other methods are unnatural, but that the natural signs and symptoms associated with the menstrual cycle are observed, recorded, and interpreted to identify the fertile time. The most commonly used signs and symptoms are menstrual bleeding, cervical mucus, and the basal body temperature.

Other fertility-awareness-based methods also require observation, recording, and interpretation of these signs and symptoms. However, rather than abstaining during the fertile time to avoid pregnancy, couples can use barrier methods.

MECHANISM OF ACTION

These methods are based on reproductive anatomy and physiology and are applied according to the signs and symptoms naturally occurring in the menstrual cycle. Calculations of the period of fertility take into account the sperm viability in the female reproductive tract, which is estimated to average 3 days (with a range from 2 to 7 days),[12] and the fertile period of the ovum, which is estimated to be 24 hours. Thus, the span of fertility may be from 7 days before ovulation to 3 days after.[20]

EFFECTIVENESS

Effective use of fertility-awareness-based methods requires that couples understand how to identify fertile days and then adapt their sexual behavior to accommodate their family planning intentions. Unintended pregnancies among women practicing these methods are primarily user-related. A sizable but unknown portion of the failures is attributable to improper teaching and poor use of the method.[8,17] Experts at the World Health Organization suspect that sexual risk taking during fertile days accounts for more accidental pregnancy than does inability to interpret chart records accurately.[19] In a German study,[4] users frequently took risks; most broke the rules at the beginning of the fertile phase, when they believed "nothing will happen this time." The concomitant use of barrier methods intended to be used during the fertile phase did not appear to reduce risk taking.

Among typical users, approximately 20% fail during the first year of use.[17,18] (See Table 12-1.) Among perfect users, the first-year failure rate would be substantially lower, ranging from 1%–9%. Some versions of the method are inherently more effective than others. The rate of accidental pregnancy among perfect users would be lowest if intercourse occurred after ovulation only (postovulation intercourse-only method). The sympto-thermal method and the ovulation method would be also be quite effective when used perfectly; however, the calendar method would be least likely to predict fertile days accurately.[17,18]

Perfect use of periodic abstinence implies that intercourse will not occur during the fertile period. Likewise, imperfect use implies that unprotected intercourse will occur during the period of peak fecundity. Thus, by definition, periodic abstinence is very unforgiving of imperfect use: failure rates during imperfect use will be approximately the same as pregnancy rates among women who are actually trying to become pregnant. On the other hand, failure rates during perfect use will be very low so long as the method can accurately identify the period of peak fecundity. Further discussion can be found in Chapter 27, with efficacy studies summarized in Table 27-4.

Table 12-1 First-year failure rates* for women using periodic abstinence, chance, and pills

Method (1)	% of Women Experiencing an Accidental Pregnancy Within the First Year of Use		% of Women Continuing Use at One Year (4)
	Typical Use (2)	Perfect Use (3)	
Chance	85	85	
Periodic Abstinence	20		67
Calendar		9	
Ovulation Method		3	
Sympto-Thermal		2	
Post-Ovulation		1	
Pill	3		72
Progestin Only		0.5	
Combined		0.1	

* See Table 5-2 for first-year failure rates of all methods.

Emergency Contraceptive Pills: Treatment initiated within 72 hours after unprotected intercourse reduces the risk of pregnancy by at least 75%.

COST

The cost of using a fertility-awareness-based method depends on whether users rely on periodic abstinence or a concurrent method of contraception such as a barrier. Periodic abstinence may require charts or special basal body temperature thermometers, which are relatively inexpensive. Clients who use concurrent methods instead of abstinence will obviously need to pay for the cost of the back-up contraceptive, although they would need a smaller supply of contraceptives such as spermicides because use would be confined to the fertile time. Clients who are trying to get pregnant may purchase ovulation predictor tests that cost about 30 dollars for a kit of five tests (good for 1 month of testing). In addition, the client will need to spend time with a counselor or instructor, who may charge a fee for service.

ADVANTAGES AND INDICATIONS

Fertility awareness increases the users' knowledge of reproductive physiology and enhances self-reliance. Some couples like the active involvement required of the male partner who must comply by abstaining or by using a condom or, possibly, withdrawal. Moreover, fertility-awareness-based methods produce no serious side effects.

Fertility awareness information can be used for the following purposes:

- **To conceive**—Couples have intercourse every day beginning about 5 days before the predicted day of ovulation until signs and symptoms show that ovulation has already occurred. (If the male partner has a low sperm count, intercourse every other day may be preferable.) Conception is more likely to occur with intercourse just before rather than just after ovulation.

- **To detect pregnancy**—A postovulatory temperature rise (see section on Basal Body Temperature Charting) that is sustained for 18 or more days is an excellent early indicator that pregnancy is under way.

- **To contracept**—For maximum contraceptive efficacy, couples should abstain from unprotected intercourse until 3 days after ovulation has been clearly documented, and chart as many cyclic patterns as they can.

- **To detect impaired fertility**—A series of cycle charts costs very little and can aid in diagnosing and treating fertility problems due to infrequent or absent ovulation. Women who do not ovulate tend to have a steady but meandering BBT pattern throughout the cycle, rather than the typical biphasic pattern.

- **To relieve premenstrual syndrome**—See Chapter 2 on The Menstrual Cycle.

Fertility awareness is important for all men and women, regardless of which family planning method they use or whether they choose to use family planning at all. In order to use a fertility-awareness-based method of family planning, women should be willing and able to observe, record, and interpret fertility signs and symptoms. Couples should be able to adjust their sexual behavior according to their fertility intentions. For users of natural family planning, this means that couples will need to abstain from vaginal intercourse for 10-14 days of the woman's menstrual cycle, depending on her cycle length and the method used. For users of fertility awareness plus another family planning method, this means that a barrier method will need to be used during intercourse on those days. Successful use of fertility-awareness-based methods also requires that a couple be able to communicate with each other about sexual matters.

DISADVANTAGES AND PRECAUTIONS

Periodic abstinence confers no protection against STDs or HIV. Lack of the male partner's cooperation will be a distinct obstacle for those women who wish to practice abstinence during the fertile days.[22]

Women for whom pregnancy would be highly undesirable or medically contraindicated should consider a more reliable method of contraception.

For other women, certain conditions may make fertility awareness methods more difficult to use:

- Irregular intervals between menses
- History of irregular menstrual cycles
- Irregular temperature charts
- Recent discontinuation of hormonal contraceptive methods
- Recent menarche
- Approaching menopause
- Discomfort with lack of sexual spontaneity during the preovulatory infertile and fertile days
- Inability to keep careful records

Fertility awareness methods are not recommended before regular menstruation has resumed postpartum. Fertility signs and symptoms are much more subtle during this period, and BBT is affected by the new mother's lack of sleep. Research is still under way to discover what instructions should be given to nursing women using these methods.[13]

COMPLICATIONS SHOULD PREGNANCY OCCUR

A number of studies have examined the question of whether aged ovum or sperm could adversely affect pregnancy outcome or the offspring. Although animal studies have shown some increase in fetal wastage and chromosomal abnormalities, human studies are not convincing.

Spontaneous abortion. Although a few studies have noted higher spontaneous abortion rates for conceptions occurring outside of the most fertile time zone, a number of other studies have rates in keeping with the clinically recognized pregnancy loss rate of 10%–15%.[15]

Birth defects. In a review of birth defects in couples using fertility awareness methods,[5] the data were not convincing one way or the other. If an increased risk of abnormal offspring exists when failures occur, this risk is of a low magnitude. In karyotyped spontaneous abortions, the prevalence of polyploidy was higher when conception occurred 15 or more days after the last menstrual period. No differences were observed in respect to monosomy X or autosomal trisomy.[15]

Birth size. Among liveborn infants, preliminary data from a study of more than 700 pregnancies suggests that birth length, weight, and head circumference are not correlated with timing of conception.[14]

PROVIDING GUIDANCE

During the first few cycles of charting, patients will probably need an instructor's help to interpret their records. Couples should be advised that the methods can be most effective when intercourse occurs only after ovulation. However, these methods are extremely unforgiving of imperfect use.[17]

Providers counseling couples should be aware that many couples who use fertility awareness methods engage in noncoital sexual activities. In a series of more than 400 couples, 84% of the men and 80% of the women achieved orgasm without intercourse with some regularity during periods of abstinence.[9,10]

CALENDAR CHARTING

Worldwide, the calendar rhythm method is the oldest and most widely practiced of the fertility awareness methods.[21] In the United States, three-fourths of women practicing periodic abstinence methods use the calendar method.[4]

Calendar charting allows women to calculate the onset and duration of their fertile period—the time during which a viable egg is available for fertilization by sperm. Calculation of the fertile period rests on three assumptions: (1) Ovulation occurs on day 14 (plus or minus 2 days) before the onset of the next menses; (2) sperm remain viable for 2-3 days; and (3) the ovum survives for 24 hours.

BASAL BODY (BBT) CHARTING (TEMPERATURE METHOD)

The basal body temperature is by definition the lowest body temperature of a healthy person taken upon wakening. A drop in BBT sometimes precedes ovulation by about 12–24 hours, and a sustained rise almost always follows for several days.[16] Body temperature rises under the influence of progesterone produced by the corpus luteum. The characteristic upward shift does not give any advance warning of ovulation; therefore, for many women, the BBT cannot be used to predict the exact day of ovulation. However, by recording the BBT for several days each menstrual cycle, a woman can identify when ovulation has passed and the infertile phase has started. By noting this temperature daily, a woman may determine her time of ovulation.

Figure 12-1 illustrates the BBT variations during a model menstrual cycle of 28 days. In reality, however, women exhibit striking variations from the model chart characteristics shown. One study found that six out of 30 women had no identifiable BBT pattern in a cycle when hormone tests clearly documented ovulation.[11] The typical biphasic pattern can be disrupted by illness, stress, travel, or interrupted sleep.

CERVICAL MUCUS CHARTING (OVULATION METHOD)

This approach is often referred to as the ovulation or Billings method of natural family planning. Cervical mucus changes appear in recognizable patterns among most ovulating women, even those whose cycles are otherwise

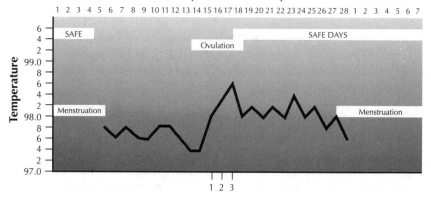

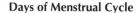

Figure 12-1 Basal body temperature variations during a model menstrual cycle

irregular. A woman obtains mucus directly from the vaginal opening, with either her finger(s) or toilet paper. Before checking her mucus, the woman first ascertains whether she feels a sensation of wetness or dryness. When checking the mucus, she focuses primarily on the quality (lubrication, elasticity, wetness, and tackiness) and only secondarily on the color and quantity. The general recommendation is to check the mucus before urinating.[3]

Mucus samples from fertile days also display ferning. Ferning means that a sample of mucus taken on a fertile day, smeared on a glass slide, and air dried will reveal a microscopic pattern resembling fern leaves. Ovulation most likely occurs within 1 day before, during, or 1 day after the last day of abundant, slippery discharge. To use the cervical mucus method most conservatively, the fertile period begins when any type of mucus is noted before ovulation.

Douching is not advised because it can wash out the mucus, making it practically impossible to notice discharge changes. Sometimes women secrete insufficient amounts of mucus for evaluating cyclic changes.

SYMPTO-THERMAL CHARTING

The various charting techniques may be used alone or in combination. The most common technique is for women to record changes in their mucus and cervix (symptoms) and in their basal body temperature (thermal). The external os of the cervix expands and the cervix becomes softer. Some women also notice and record ovulatory pain (mittelschmerz), which can include feelings of heaviness, abdominal swelling, rectal pain or discomfort, and lower abdominal pain or discomfort on either side. Pain can occur just before, during, or after ovulation.

The simultaneous dependence on these two indicators of the time of ovulation is called sympto-thermal charting or the sympto-thermal method when used for birth control. If couples use sympto-thermal charting for birth control, they must remember that intercourse can be safely resumed only on the fourth day following peak mucus and the third day following the thermal rise. If one occurs without the other, safety cannot be assumed and the second event must occur.

OVULATION DETECTION TESTS IN THE HOME

Home methods of ovulation detection can help the accuracy with which women determine their fertile days. Most research on ovulation prediction and detection instruments has focused on helping women with fertility problems. These instruments rely on either measuring the woman's temperature or detecting hormonal metabolites in the urine.[7]

Temperature based. Once a woman ovulates, her temperature rises (see section on Basal Body Temperature). Various devices for determining fertile time periods include The Rabbit, Rite Time, Fertil-A-Chron, and Ovudate.

Hormone based. Currently, assays to detect estrogen and pregnanediol glucuronides only confirm, not predict, ovulation. These include Qui del Q, Hi-Gonavis, Ovu-stick Self-Test, First Response, Ovutime-Ovulation Predictor, and Q Test Ovulation Test Kit. UNIPATH and Quidel are developing methods to predict ovulation. A test that could be used for periodic abstinence would need to predict ovulation about 5 days in advance. The Home Ovarian Monitor has been tested as a natural family planning device.[2] The urine test indicates the beginning fertile days when the estrone glucuronide levels are raised; the woman should abstain from intercourse. She then observes the pregnanediol glucuronide levels, and when they also rise, she can resume intercourse without further observation during the rest of the cycle.

Several other approaches are under study.[7] One kit measures the water content in cervical mucus. Others detect effects of preovulatory estrogen rises in cervical mucus or saliva. Breast milk changes are also under study, as are changes in electrical resistance of body fluids.

INSTRUCTIONS FOR USING MENSTRUAL CYCLE CHARTING

Menstrual cycle charting is a good method for couples who are committed to using their method correctly. Charting requires practice. For the first several cycles, abstain or use a back-up contraceptive method. If used to prevent pregnancy, these methods are most effective if the couple abstains or diligently uses an effective back-up contraceptive until after ovulation has occurred and the infertile days arrive. Although effective when used perfectly, natural family planning methods are unforgiving of imperfect use.

CALENDAR METHOD

1. To use this method, a menstrual calendar should first be maintained for several menstrual cycles.
2. Find the longest and shortest of the menstrual cycles. (A cycle begins on day 1 of menstrual bleeding and continues period through the day before the next period starts.)
3. Look at the fertile days chart (see Table 12-2) and apply the "minus 10, minus 20" rule.
   - Use the shortest cycle to find the first fertile day. The earliest day on which a woman is likely to be fertile is computed by subtracting 20 days from the length of her shortest cycle

Table 12-2 How to calculate your fertile period

If Your Shortest Cycle Has Been (# of Days)	Your First Fertile (Unsafe) Day is	If Your Longest Cycle Has Been (# of Days)	Your Last Fertile (Unsafe) Day is
21*	3rd Day	21*	10th Day
22	4th	22	11th
23	5th	23	12th
24	6th	24	13th
25	7th	25	14th
26	8th	26	15th
27	9th	27	16th
28	10th	28	17th
29	11th	29	18th
30	12th	30	19th
31	13th	31	20th
32	14th	32	21st
33	15th	33	22nd
34	16th	34	23rd
35	17th	35	24th

*Day 1 = First day of menstrual bleeding

- Use the longest cycle to find the last fertile day. The latest day on which she is likely to be fertile is calculated by subtracting 10 days from the length of her longest cycle. For example, if the shortest cycle has been 22 days, the first fertile day will be day 2. If the longest cycle has been 28 days, the last fertile day will be day 18.

4. Next find the dates of the first and last fertile days for the current menstrual period. For example, if the period starts September 6 and the chart says the first fertile day will be day 2, then the first fertile day will be September 7. If the last fertile day will be day 18, then the last fertile day this cycle will be September 23. In this example, the fertile days are September 7 through September 23.

5. **For conception:** Intercourse should begin a couple days before the predicted fertile days and continued throughout the fertile period.

6. **For contraception:** Abstinence from sexual intercourse or use of a back-up method of birth control (such as condoms, the sponge, spermicides, or a diaphragm) should be practiced during fertile days.

7. If the cycles begin to fluctuate wildly in length so that there are many more fertile days than safe days, another method of birth control may be needed.

BASAL BODY TEMPERATURE (BBT) CHARTING

1. Record daily BBT readings on a chart for 3–4 successive months. Most special BBT thermometers can be used orally, rectally, or vaginally, but the same site should be used consistently.

2. **Take and record BBT in the morning before getting out of bed** (after at least 3 hours of sleep).

3. **Record the temperature reading every day** on a special BBT chart (see Figure 12-1). Connect the dots for each day so a line connects dots from day 2 to day 3, etc.

4. The temperature will probably rise about 0.4°–0.8° F shortly before, during, or right after ovulation. This postovulatory temperature rise will stay elevated until the next period begins. The actual temperature and maximum temperature are not important, just the rise over the baseline.[1] If a sustained rise cannot be detected, then a woman may not have ovulated in that cycle. A true postovulatory BBT rise usually persists 10 days or longer.

5. Some women notice a temperature drop about 12–24 hours before it begins to rise after ovulation, whereas others have no drop in temperature at all. A drop in BBT probably means ovulation will occur the next day.

6. **For conception:** The temperature usually does not rise until after ovulation, so it is difficult to predict fertile days—you may miss the opportunity to become pregnant.

7. **For contraception:** Because ovulation may occur as early as day 7 of the menstrual cycle, a woman monitoring only her BBT should assume that she may be fertile from the beginning of her cycle or no later than day 4 (if she has cycles greater than 25 days long) until the temperature has remained elevated for 3 consecutive days. The safest way to use BBT charting for birth control is to avoid intercourse or use a back-up method of birth control all through the first half of the cycle.

CERVICAL MUCUS CHARTING

1. Record the mucus changes for at least two to three cycles to understand clearly the personal mucus signs. Many counselors advise complete sexual abstinence throughout the first cycle a woman charts her mucus changes to help her avoid confusing mucus with semen and normal sexual lubrication.

2. **Check the outside of the vagina every day** (whenever using the bathroom).

3. Wipe with toilet tissue. Notice whether any mucus can be collected; feel the mucus, particularly if it feels wet. Record the wettest mucus noted for each day.

Table 12-3 Summary of ovulation method of fertility regulation

Approximate Cycle Day: Phase	How Identified	Intercourse Allowed?
1-5: Menstruation*	Bleeding	No
6-9: Dry Days	Absence of cervical mucus	On alternate nights only
10: Fecund Period Begins	Onset of sticky mucus secretion	No
16: Peak Fecund Day	Last day on which slippery mucus (resembling raw egg white) is observed	No
20: Fecund Period Ends	Evening of the *4th* day after the peak day	After fecund period ends
20-29: Safe Period	From end of fecund period until onset of bleeding	Yes

*The cycle begins on the first day of menstruation.

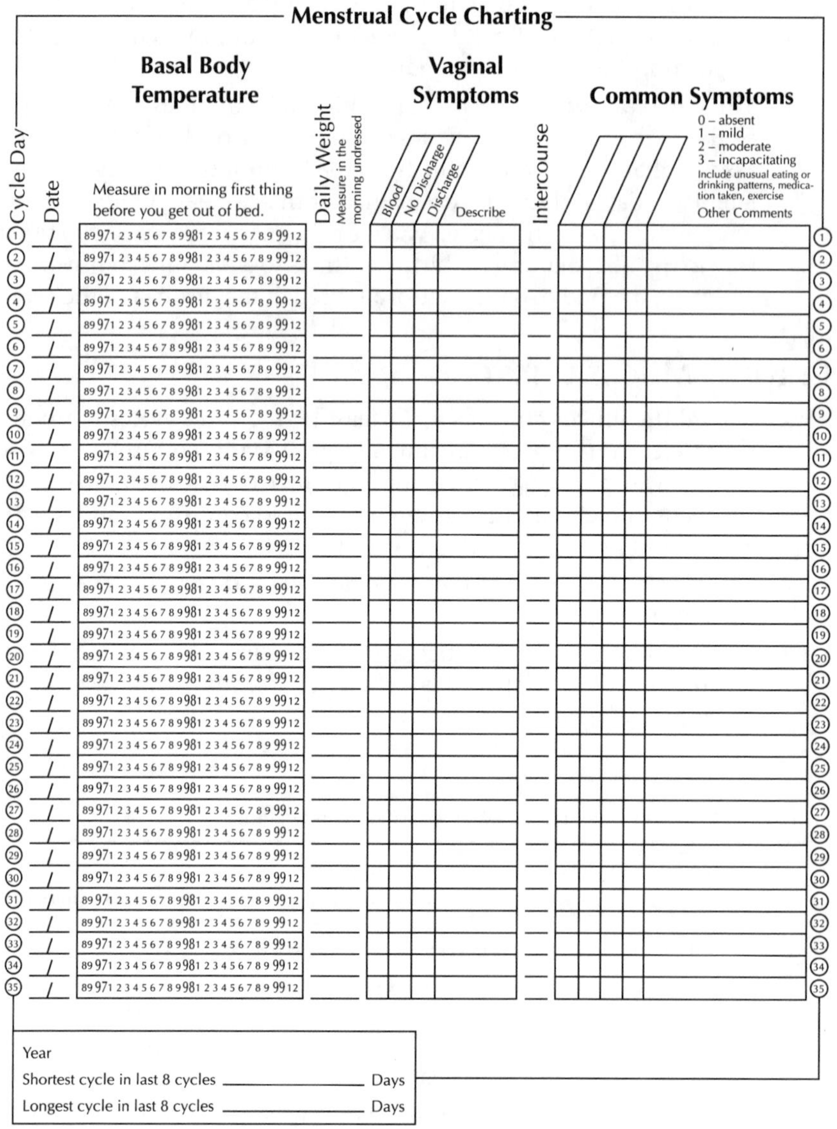

Figure 12-2 Menstrual cycle charting

4. **Note the pattern in the mucus changes during each cycle.** (See Table 12-3.)

   • During menstruation, blood covers up any other sensations of wetness or mucus.

   • After the menstrual period, the vagina may feel moist a few days, but not distinctly wet. There will be no mucus. (Some women do not have any of these dry days, especially if they have very short cycles.)

- Next may come mucus that is thick, cloudy, whitish or yellowish, and sticky. The vagina still does not feel distinctly wet. This phase can last for several days. Consider the sign of any mucus at all as indicative of fertile days.
- As ovulation nears, mucus usually becomes more abundant, and there is an increasingly wet sensation. Mucus becomes clear, slippery, and can stretch 2-3 or more inches between the thumb and forefinger. The peak or last day of wetness and abundant, clear, slippery mucus is assumed to be about the time of ovulation.
- After ovulation, the mucus becomes thick, cloudy, and sticky or is not present at all until the time of the next menstrual period.

5. Douching, vaginal infection, semen, foam, diaphragm jelly, lubricants, medications, and even the normal lubrication of sexual arousal may interfere with the ability to notice a clear-cut mucus pattern.

6. **For conception:** Begin having intercourse on the first day of wet sensations and mucus. The first day of mucus is best detected if intercourse occurs only every other day beforehand.

7. **For contraception:** Avoid intercourse or use another method of birth control during the first part of the cycle and up until the fourth day after a clear-cut peak mucus day. Remember that condoms are the only vaginal method of birth control that do not change mucus characteristics. Although the mucus signs are the best indicators of the beginning of the fertile time, mucus charting may not give enough advance warning of ovulation to prevent unplanned pregnancy. *Remember that sperm can survive several days, so avoid unprotected intercourse as soon as sticky mucus appears.*

8. Most women probably need help interpreting the records, especially during the first few cycles of charting.

REFERENCES

1. Albertson BD, Zinaman MJ. The prediction of ovulation and monitoring of the fertile period. Adv Contracept 1989;3(4):263-290.
2. Brown JB, Holmes J, Barker G. Use of the Home Ovarian Monitor in pregnancy avoidance. Am J Obstet Gynecol 1991;165(6-2):2008-2011.
3. Gulen D, Gillette N. The ovulation method: cycles of fertility. Portland OR: Ovulation Method Teachers Association, 1984.
4. Frank-Herrmann P, Freundl G, Baur S, Bremme M, Doring GK, Godehardt EAJ, Sottong U. Effectiveness and acceptability of the symptothermal method of natural family planning in Germany. Am J Obstet Gynecol 1991;165(6-2):2052-2054.
5. Hatcher RA, Stewart GK, Stewart FH, Guest F. Fertility awareness methods. In: Sciarra JW (ed). Gynecology and obstetrics. Philadelphia: Harper & Row, 1984.

6. Kass-Annesse B, Kennedy KI, Forrest K, Danzer H, Reading A, Hughes H. A study of the vaginal contraceptive sponge used with and without the fertility awareness method. Contraception 1989;40(6):701-714.
7. Labbok MH, Jennings VH. Advances in fertility regulation through ovulation prediction during lactation (lactational amenorrhea method) and during the menstrual cycle. Prepared under contract to the Institute for Reproductive Health (Contract No. DPE-3040-00-5064-00).
8. Labbok MH, Klaus H, Barker D. Factors related to ovulation method efficacy in three programs: Bangladesh, Kenya, and Korea. Contraception 1988;37(6): 577-589.
9. Marshall J, Rowe B. The effect of personal factors on the use of basal body temperature method of regulating births. Fertil Steril 1972;23(6):417-421.
10. Marshall J, Rowe B. Psychological aspects of the basal body temperature method of regulating births. Fertil Steril 1970;21(1):14-19.
11. Moghissi KS. Accuracy of basal body temperature for ovulation detection. Fertil Steril 1976;27(12):1415-1421.
12. Perloff WH, Steinberger E. In vivo survival of spermatozoa in cervical mucus. Am J Obstet Gynecol 1964;88(4):439-442.
13. Queenan JT, Moghissi KS. Natural family planning: looking ahead. Am J Obstet Gynecol 1991;165(6-2):1979-1980.
14. Simpson JL, Gray RH, Queenan JT, Kambic RT, Perez A, Mena P, Barbato M, Pardo F, Tagliabue G, Bitto A, Stevenson W. Fetal outcome among pregnancies in natural family planning acceptors: an international cohort study. Am J Obstet Gynecol 1991;165(6-2):1981-1982.
15. Simpson JL, Gray RH, Queenan JT, Mena P, Perez A, Kambic RT, Tagliabue G, Pardo F, Stevenson WS, Barbato M, Jennings VH, Zinaman MJ, Spieler JM. Pregnancy outcome associated with natural family planning (NFP): scientific basis and experimental design for an international cohort study. Adv Contracept 1988;4(4):247-264.
16. Stewart FH, Guest FJ, Stewart GK, Hatcher RA. Understanding your body. New York NY: Bantam Books, 1987.
17. Trussell J, Grummer-Strawn L. Contraceptive failure of the ovulation method of periodic abstinence. Fam Plann Perspect 1990;22(2):65-75.
18. Trussell J, Hatcher RA, Cates W, Stewart FH, Kost K. Contraceptive failure in the United States: an update. Stud Fam Plann 1990;21(1):51-54.

Coitus Interruptus (Withdrawal)

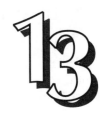

- Withdrawal is an important contraceptive choice for non-abstaining couples who have no other contraceptive method available at the time of intercourse.

- The method does not protect a couple against sexually transmitted diseases.
- The pre-ejaculate of HIV-infected men can contain HIV-infected cells.

Coitus interruptus, or the withdrawal method of birth control, was a natural response to the discovery that ejaculation into the vagina caused pregnancy. The method was probably widely practiced throughout history,[5] playing a predominant role in fertility declines occurring prior to the advent of the pill.

MECHANISM OF ACTION

Coitus interruptus prevents fertilization by preventing the contact between spermatozoa and the ovum. The male partner interrupts intercourse and withdraws his penis from his partner's vagina before he ejaculates.

EFFECTIVENESS

Although coitus interruptus has often been criticized as an ineffective method, it probably confers a level of contraceptive protection similar to that provided by vaginal barrier methods. Effectiveness depends largely on the male's ability to withdraw prior to ejaculation. How effective the method would be if used consistently and correctly is highly uncertain. Our best guest is that about 4% of perfect users would fail in the initial year.[6]

Among typical users, about 19% fail during the first year of use. See Table 13-1 (see also Tables 5-2 and 27-5).

A DVANTAGES AND INDICATIONS

As a method of birth control, withdrawal has several distinct advantages. It costs nothing, requires no devices, involves no chemicals, and is available in any situation. Practicing coitus interruptus causes no medical side effects. Couples who cannot or do not wish to use other contraceptive methods and who can accept the potential for unintended pregnancy would find withdrawal an acceptable alternative. It is a back-up contraceptive that is always available. Although only 2% of sexually active women report relying solely on withdrawal,[7] many men have probably used the method at sometime in their lives.

D ISADVANTAGES AND CAUTIONS

For some couples, interruption of the excitement or plateau phase of the sexual response cycle may diminish pleasure. Coitus interruptus has two other major disadvantages:

- First, the method is unforgiving of incorrect or inconsistent use, leading to a failure rate significantly higher than hormonal methods or IUDs in typical users. One reason for the contraceptive failure may be a lack of self-control that is demanded by the method. With impending orgasm, men (and women) experience a mild to extreme

Table 13-1 First-year failure rates* for withdrawal, chance, condoms, and pills

Method	Typical Use (%)	Perfect Use (%)	% of Women Continuing
Chance	85	85	
Condoms (male)	12	3	63
Pill	3		72
Combined		0.1	
Progestin Only		0.5	
Withdrawal	19	4	—

*See Table 5-2 for first-year failure rates for all methods.

Emergency Contraceptive Pills: Treatment initiated within 72 hours after unprotected intercourse reduces the risk of pregnancy by at least 75%.

clouding of consciousness during which coital movement becomes involuntary.[3] The man may feel the urge to achieve deeper penetration at the time of impending orgasm and may not withdraw in sufficient time to prevent semen from being deposited in his partner's vagina or on her external genitalia.

- Second, the couple is not protected from STDs, including HIV. Surface lesions, such as those from herpes genitalis (HSV) or human papilloma virus (HPV), may be actively infective. Not only does unintentional ejaculation pose a risk for infection, but so could the pre-ejaculate fluid released prior to ejaculation. In one prospective study, the condom failed to protect some users against gonorrhea because they were exposed to infectious secretions before the condom was used.[1] The fluid can contain HIV-infected cells,[2,4] although epidemiologic studies have not determined the infectious potential of the pre-ejaculate.

Some concern exists that the pre-ejaculate fluid may carry sperm into the vagina. In itself, the pre-ejaculate, a lubricating secretion produced by the Littre or Cowper's glands, contains no sperm. However, a previous ejaculation may have left some sperm hidden within the folds of the urethral lining. Examinations of the pre-ejaculate in a small study[4] indicated that the pre-ejaculate was free of spermatozoa in all of 11 HIV seronegative men and four of 12 seropositive men. Although the eight samples containing spermatozoa revealed only small clumps of a few hundred sperm, these could possibly pose a risk of fertilization. In all likelihood, the spermatozoa left from a previous ejaculation could be washed out with the force of a normal urination. However, this remains unstudied. Another study examining the pre-ejaculate for the presence of spermatozoa found none in the samples of 16 men.[2] These men were not azoospermic.

P ROVIDING THE METHOD

The couple may have penile-vaginal intercourse until ejaculation is impending, at which time the male partner withdraws his penis from the vagina and away from the external genitalia of the female partner. The man must rely on his own sensations to determine when he is about to ejaculate. The pre-ejaculate, which is usually released just prior to full ejaculation, goes unnoticed by both the man and the woman during the course of intercourse and so is not a sign that ejaculation is about to occur. The sexually inexperienced man may find it particularly difficult to achieve the self-control required for withdrawal.

Although the potential for the pre-ejaculate to lead to fertilization remains unstudied, it makes inherent sense for the man who has recently ejaculated to urinate, thereby voiding leftover semen prior to subsequent intercourse.

INSTRUCTIONS FOR USING COITUS INTERRUPTUS

1. Before intercourse, the man should urinate and wipe off the tip of the penis to remove any remaining sperm from a prior ejaculation.
2. When he feels he is about to ejaculate, the man should withdraw his penis from his partner's vagina, making sure that ejaculation occurs away from his partner's genitalia.
3. Withdrawal is not a good contraceptive method if
   - The man cannot predictably withdraw prior to ejaculation
   - The man intends to have repeated orgasms, which may cause the pre-ejaculate to contain spermatozoa.
4. **Withdrawal does not protect against HIV infection;** it may not protect against other STDs either, although the question remains to be studied. Abstinence or use of condoms provide far better protection.
5. Withdrawal is a considerably better method of contraception than no method at all.
6. The couple should **learn what options are available for post-coital protection** should any ejaculate come in contact with the vagina. The couple should try to have a supply of birth control foam or some type of spermicide available in case of unintentional ejaculation in or near the woman's vagina. Despite the seeming optimism of this suggestion, it is probably too late to stop some sperm from swimming up into the uterus.

REFERENCES

1. Darrow WW. Condom use and use-effectiveness in high-risk populations. Sex Transm Dis 1989;16(3):157-160.
2. Ilaria G, Jacobs JL, Polsky B, Koll B, Baron P, MacLow C, Armstrong D, Schlegel PN. Detection of HIV-1 DNA sequences in pre-ejaculatory fluid [Letter]. Lancet 1992;340(8833):1469.
3. Kinsey AC, Pomeroy WB, Martin CE, Gebhard PH. Sexual behavior in the human female. Philadelphia PA: W.B. Saunders Company, 1953.
4. Pudney J, Oneta M, Mayer K, Seage G, Anderson D. Pre-ejaculatory fluid as potential vector for sexual transmission of HIV-1 [Letter]. Lancet 1992;340(8833):1470.
5. Robertson W. An illustrated history of contraception. Park Ridge NJ: Parthenon Publishing Group, 1990.
6. Trussell J, Hatcher RA, Cates W, Stewart FH, Kost K. Contraceptive failure in the United States: an update. Stud Fam Plann 1990;21(1):51-54.

7. Trussell J, Vaughan B. Selected result concerning sexual behavior and contraceptive use from the 1988 National Survey of Family Growth and the 1988 National Survey of Adolescent Males. Princeton NJ: Princeton University, Office of Population Research Working Paper #91-12, 1991.

Intrauterine Devices (IUDS)

14

- The IUD is a single-decision method. It is easily inserted and removed.
- Ninety-eight percent of IUD users say they are happy with this method, and 60% of women with IUDs are repeat users.[28]
- The Cu T 380 A (ParaGuard) offers 8 years of very effective protection, with only about 2% of women becoming pregnant in the first year of use.

- In patients who are screened to assure that they are appropriate users for the method, IUDs are extremely safe.[18]
- Patients at risk of STDs, including HIV, should use another method (in place of or in addition to) such as the condom for protection.

In the 1970s, intrauterine devices (IUDs) were used by as many as 10% of contracepting women in the United States. A series of problems led to removal of most IUDs from the U.S. market and a negative perception among contraceptors and providers regarding IUD use.[9,14] Currently, fewer than 2% of women at risk of pregnancy in the United States use the IUD (see Table 5-1). Most IUD users are over the age of 35, and nearly 90% are in their 30s and 40s.[28] Client perceptions about the IUD come from many sources but principally arise from information given by family planning providers.[40]

MECHANISM OF ACTION

IUDs may affect sperm, ova, or the endometrium to prevent pregnancy. The exact mechanism of action of IUDs is not completely understood. Recent observations on processes that take place in the fallopian tube have indicated that IUDs exert effects that extend beyond the uterus.[33] In two studies, researchers recovered ova from 14 women using four types of IUDs and from 20 women not using any contraception. All women had recently had intercourse close to the time of ovulation. Clear signs of fertilization were apparent in half of the ova recovered from non-contraceptors but none of the ova recovered from IUD users.[2,29] Some process inactivates the ability of sperm or egg so that fertilization does not occur. The mechanism of action of the IUD in the prevention of fertilization appears to operate in one of two ways:

- *Sperm:* Immobilizes sperm; interferes with migration of sperm from vagina to the fallopian tubes.
- *Ovum:* Speeds transport of the ovum through the fallopian tubes.

Other enzymatic and biochemical processes, as well as local affects on the endometrium, have been identified; however, their role and contribution to the IUD function are unclear.[38]

IUD Options

Only two IUDs are available in the United States as this edition goes to press (see Figure 14-1). The Levonorgestrel IUD may be approved for use during the life of this edition.

The *CuT 380A* (Paragard), approved for 8 years of use, is provided through GynoPharma, Inc. In the United States, approximately 500,000 of these IUDs have been used through the end of 1992.[17] Throughout the world, more than 25 million Cu T 380A IUDs have been distributed in 70 countries.[24] The T shape is made with polyethylene, to which is added barium sulphate (to create x-ray visibility). Fine copper wire (314 mm^2) is wound around the vertical stem. Each of the two horizontal transverse arms has a sleeve of copper measuring 33 mm^2. The bottom of the T has a single filament polyethylene clear or whitish string that is knotted after passing through a hole in the T, creating a double string effect.

The *Progesterone T* (Progestasert System), approved for 1 year of contraceptive protection, is provided by Alza Corporation. Because the Progestasert System must be removed and replaced annually, we believe it should be used only in unusual circumstances such as allergies to copper. The T consists of ethylene vinyl acetate copolymer. The vertical stem contains a reservoir of 38 mg progesterone and barium sulphate (for visibility on x-rays) in a silicone oil base. It releases 65 mcg progesterone per day. The IUD is 36 mm long, 32 mm wide, and when placed in the inserter barrel, has a diameter of 8 mm. The blue-black double string attaches at a hole in the base of the T.

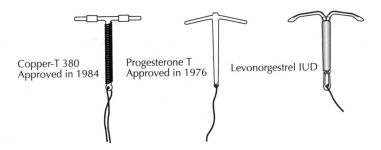

Figure 14-1 Two currently used IUDs in the USA and the Levonorgestrel-IUD (anticipated to be approved)

The *Levonorgestrel-IUD (LNg IUD)* was developed by Leiras. The active substance, levonorgestrel, is released directly into the uterus at a constant rate of 20 micrograms per day (thus the IUD is called LNg-20) for up to 5 years. This dosage decreases the hormonal systemic effects. The LNg-IUD is based on a NOVA T model polyethylene frame, with a cylinder of polydimethyl-siloxane/levonorgestrel mixture molded around its vertical arm. The cylinder is coated with a membrane that regulates the release of the hormone.

EFFECTIVENESS

IUD characteristics, such as size, shape, and presence of copper or progesterone, and user characteristics, such as age and parity, contribute to differences in effectiveness for different IUDs. The failure rate of IUDs also depends on a number of administrative, patient, and medical variables, including ease of insertion, clinician experience, patient detection of IUD expulsion, and the user's access to medical services. The failure rate tends to be lower if the IUD has the following characteristics:

- Medicated with copper, silver, progesterone, or another progestin
- Large surface area, especially for nonmedicated IUD
- Low expulsion rate
- Partial and complete expulsions detected quickly
- Inserted all the way to the top of the fundus of the uterus

The first-year failure rate in typical IUD users is 0.8% for the Cu T 380A and 2% for the Progestasert System. The lowest expected pregnancy rate (perfect use) is 1.5% with Progestasert System use and 0.6% with Cu T 380A use (one of the lowest failure rates of any contraceptive). See Table 14-1.

The estimate for perfect use of the Cu T 380A did not count pregnancies that resulted when the device was not known to be *in situ*. This was calculated based

Table 14-1 First-year failure rates* for women using IUDs, pills, Depo-Provera, Norplant, and sterilization

Method (1)	% of Women Experiencing an Accidental Pregnancy Within the First Year of Use		% of Women Continuing Use at One Year (4)
	Typical Use (2)	Perfect Use (3)	
Pill	3		72
Progestin Only		0.5	
Combined		0.1	
IUD			
Progesterone T	2.0	1.5	81
Copper T 380A	0.8	0.6	78
LNg 20	0.1	0.1	81
Depo-Provera	0.3	0.3	70
Norplant (6 Capsules)	0.09	0.09	85
Female Sterilization	0.4	0.4	100

*See Table 5-2 for first-year failure rates of all methods.

on the perhaps-questionable assumption that these failures should be classified as user failures and the empirically based assumption that expulsions are so uncommon that the denominator of the perfect-use failure rate is virtually the same as the denominator for the typical-use rate. The perfect-use estimate for the Progestasert System was derived analogously (see Chapter 27).

Over the long run, the LNg IUD is the single most effective method of reversible contraception available in the world today, followed closely by the Cu T 380A. The cumulative proportion of LNg IUDs failing in the first 7 years of use is only 1.1%,[34] compared with 1.7% for the Cu T 380A at the end of 7 years,[30] and 3.7% for Norplant at the end of 5 years (see Chapter 11 on Progestin-Only Contraceptives).

COST

The IUD costs less than or equal to any of the commonly used contraceptives. The total cost of an IUD insertion in a public family planning clinic would be between $200-$300. The costs would likely be higher in the private sector.

Table 14-2 Cost of IUDs

Clinic Visit (per year)	$ 60
IUD Insert	$ 30
IUD Cost (Cu T 380A)	$ 120
Lab (GC)	$ 9
TOTAL	$ 219

Source: Planned Parenthood of Sacramento Valley, CA (1993).

A DVANTAGES AND INDICATIONS

The IUD is a highly effective, safe, long-acting, single-decision method.

1. It is less expensive per year and easier to use than other methods.

2. Women who have contraindications to hormonal methods can use the IUD.

3. The progestin or progesterone-releasing IUDs decrease menstrual blood loss and the incidence and intensity of dysmenorrhea.

4. The LNg IUD appears to reduce the incidence of pelvic inflammatory disease[37] and is an effective treatment of menorrhagia.[3] Indeed, the LNg IUD combines the advantages of the Norplant and the IUD.

5. IUDs can prevent and treat Asherman's syndrome (adherence of the two walls of the uterus by synechiae) that occurs after some uterine surgery.

Ideal candidates for the IUD may include women who have medical contraindications to oral contraceptives, want a long-acting method, want a reversible method, are in a monogomous relationship, or are lactating or postpartum. However, voluntary contraception and informed consent, as discussed in Chapter 23 on Education and Counseling, must always form the basis for contraception decision making.

D ISADVANTAGES AND CAUTIONS

Certain complications from IUD use make screening critical for identifying women at risk. It is important to note that the IUD labeling may identify nulliparous women as a group that should not receive an IUD. We feel that an IUD is an option for women who have never had children but that the risks need to be discussed.

1. **PID.** The greatest risk of pelvic inflammatory disease (PID) associated with the use of the IUD occurs at its insertion.[13,22] (See Table 14-3.) This increased risk of infection may be associated with a microbiological contamination of the endometrial cavity at the time of insertion.[25] Strict asepsis at insertion and leaving the IUD in place for its life span can reduce the chance of developing PID. We recommend that the 1-year IUD (Progestasert System) be used only in unusual circumstances, such as allergies to copper. The LNg IUD has been shown to provide a protective effect against PID as compared with a copper-releasing IUD.[37] Women who have more than one sexual partner or whose partner has other sexual partners are at high risk for acquiring sexually transmitted diseases and, in turn, more likely to develop PID if they use an IUD.[22]

2. **HIV.** Whether IUDs increase the risk of acquiring an infection with the human immunodeficiency virus (HIV) is unknown. One study showed that among various contraceptors exposed to HIV, IUD users had higher risks as compared with nonusers and users of other contraceptive methods.[26] The effect of the IUD on the uterine lining may create an environment favorable to HIV transmission. The increased bleeding associated with IUD use may increase the transmission of the virus (for HIV-positive women); however, further study is required.

3. **Menstrual problems.** Increased dysmenorrhea may accompany IUD use. From 10%–15% of IUD users will have their IUD removed because of symptoms or signs associated with bleeding or spotting. However, the average IUD patient has an increase in blood loss that is usually minor and of little consequence.

4. **Expulsions.** Between 2%–10% of IUD users spontaneously expel their IUD within the first year. Young maternal age, abnormal amount of menstrual flow, and severe dysmenorrhea before IUD insertion are risk factors for Cu T 380A expulsion.[43]

5. **Pregnancy complications.** One-half (50%) of intrauterine pregnancies occurring with the IUD *in situ* end in spontaneous abortion.[23, 39] If the IUD is removed early in pregnancy, the abortion rate will

Table 14-3 PID risk after IUD insertion

Time After Insertion	PID Rate/1,000 Women-Years	Relative Risk
≤ 20 Days	9.66	6.36
≥ 20 Days	1.38	1.00

Source: Farley et al. (1992).

be approximately 25%.[23] Severe pelvic infections resulting in death are more likely to occur if the IUD is left in place in a pregnant woman.[7] Approximately 5% of women pregnant with an IUD in place will have an ectopic pregnancy.[39] Progestasert System users have a 6- to10-fold higher ectopic rate than copper IUD users.[1]

PRECAUTIONS

Table 14-4 lists the precautions for using the IUD. These are meant to encourage consideration of use of another contraceptive method, careful client assessment, informed medical consent, and infrequent use of an IUD among clients in those categories. Informed consent is required of any woman who will have an IUD inserted.

PROVIDING THE IUD

The apparent difference in performance between one IUD and another is often not as great as the difference between one clinic and another. The skill of the IUD inserter and the quality of counseling, selection, and follow-up are often more important than structural differences between IUDs.[6,38] With appropriate training, a broad range of trained personnel including nurses, nurse-midwives, physician assistants, and paramedical personnel can safely perform routine IUD insertions. Clinicians should practice first on a model, then counsel women and insert an adequate number of IUDs under supervision in order to demonstrate their competence. Rather than an absolute number requirement, a level of competence as determined by clinical supervision should be the criterion for certification.

INSERTION

Prior to insertion, obtain a medical history and advise the client of her suitability for use of available contraceptive methods. Assess and discuss the factors relating to safety and effectiveness.

An IUD can be inserted any time during the menstrual cycle as long as the woman is not pregnant:

- Immediately following childbirth, *i.e.*, within the first 10 minutes. If the IUD is inserted 1 or 2 days after childbirth, there is a greater risk of expulsion as the uterus contracts.[42] Post-placental insertions are infrequently performed in the United States.
- Six weeks postpartum and breastfeeding.
- Six weeks postpartum with no menses, not breastfeeding, and a negative sensitive pregnancy test.

Table 14-4 Precautions to the provisions of intrauterine devices

Refrain from providing an IUD for women with the following diagnoses:

Precautions	Rationale/Discussion
Active, recent, or recurrent pelvic infection (acute or sub acute): • postpartum endometriosis • infection following an abortion	Bacteria are introduced into the uterus at the time of IUD insertion. In addition, the IUD promotes a sterile inflammatory reaction inside the uterus that could, in theory, worsen existing PID. Finally, women with recent pelvic infection are likely to be at risk for future upper genital tract infections; the IUD is unique among all models of contraceptives in its failure to prevent upper genital tract infection.[4, 10, 13, 19, 31]
Known or suspected pregnancy	IUD insertion with a pregnancy in uterus has a high likelihood of leading to a spontaneous abortion with the possibility of septic abortion.[10, 19, 31]

Exercise caution if an IUD is used or considered in the following situations and carefully monitor for adverse effects:

Risk factors for PID: • purulent cervicitis, until treated • recent positive test for gonorrhea or chlamydia • recurrent history of gonorrhea or chlamydia	At the time an IUD is inserted through the cervical canal, bacteria from a STD in the canal can be introduced into the sterile uterine cavity, leading to PID. Most of the increased risk of PID actually attributable to the IUD comes in the initial 3 weeks following IUD insertion. Thereafter the increased attributable risk is minimal. If a vaginal infection is present, it should be treated, and should be resolved, before the IUD is inserted. The woman and her partner(s) must be treated for STDs before considering IUD insertion.
High risk for a sexually transmitted disease, including multiple sexual partners or a partner who has multiple sexual partners	IUDs fail to protect against STDs (in the vagina and cervix) ascending and causing upper genital tract infection.
Impaired response to infection: diabetes, steriod treatment, HIV disease	Women with impaired immune response may be at greater risk for severe PID.[4, 5, 8, 9, 10, 31]

(continued)

Table 14-4 Precautions to the provisions of intrauterine devices *(cont.)*

Exercise caution and carefully monitor for adverse affects:

Precautions	Rationale/Discussion
Risk factors for HIV infection and/or HIV disease	IUDs cause increased menstrual flow, and a sterile inflammatory reaction in the uterus with increased numbers of white blood cells. If the woman is HIV positive, the IUD may increase the risk of HIV transmission to her sexual partner(s); condoms should be recommended instead. In addition, the decreased immune response may increase the risk of pelvic infection.[4, 5, 8, 9, 10, 31]
Undiagnosed, irregular, heavy or abnormal vaginal bleeding; cervical or uterine malignancy (known or suspected), including unresolved Pap smear	For a woman with abnormal vaginal bleeding, gynecological problems should first be ruled out. Because IUDs may cause uterine bleeding between periods and may increase menstrual flow, bleeding abnormalities could be attributed to the IUD in error, and the woman's true problem of cervical or uterine malignancy may be missed.[4, 10, 19, 31]
History of ectopic pregnancy, particularly important consideration if future pregnancy is desired	Women with a past history of an ectopic pregnancy are more likely to have a history of pelvic infection. Although most IUDs are associated with a decreased risk, not an increased risk for ectopic pregnancy, other contraceptives have an even greater protective effect and also decrease a woman's risk for PID.[5, 8, 9, 31]
Previous problems with IUD: pregnancies, expulsion, perforation, pain, or heavy bleeding	Monitor patient carefully since a history of problems with the IUD exists.
Past history of severe vasovagal reactivity or fainting	IUD use can occasionally cause a vasovagal reaction. This is most likely to occur in a nulliparous woman with a small uterus. Use of paracervical anesthesia may decrease a woman's risk for severe pain or vasovagal reaction; 10 cc −20 cc of 1% lidocaine is recommended.[19]
Difficulty obtaining emergency follow-up care and treatment for pelvic infection	Infections from IUDs can be serious and, if untreated, can lead to hysterectomy or even death. Therefore, it is advisable to have a doctor nearby in case emergency care is needed.[19]

(continued)

Table 14-4 Precautions to the provisions of intrauterine devices *(cont.)*

Exercise caution and carefully monitor for adverse affects:

Precautions	Rationale/Discussion
Valvular heart disease such as aortic stenosis	Valvular lesions make women more susceptible to subacute bacterial endocarditis (SBE). Some clinicians recommend prophylactic antibiotics at time of IUD insertions. Others recommend avoiding IUD use in women at increased risk for SBE. Mitral valve prolapse is generally not considered a reason to avoid IUD use.[19]
Anatomical abnormalities of the uterus including: leiomyomata, endometrial polyps, cervical stenosis, bicornuate uterus, or a small uterus	Severe distortions of the uterine cavity could cause difficulties in insertion and increased chance of expulsion of the IUD.[5, 8, 9, 10, 31]
History of anemia	The increased menstrual blood loss from most IUDs can worsen anemia; however, the use of oral iron or nutritional counseling can reverse the effect.[5,8,9,10,31]
Women who have never had a child	While most of the increased risk of PID attributable to IUDs occurs in the 3 weeks immediately following insertion, other contraceptives have a protective effect against PID and are better options for the woman who has never had a child and wants children in the future. Nulliparous women tend not to tolerate an IUD as well as women who have carried a pregnancy to term. Some studies demonstrate a slightly increased risk of infertility in women with a history of IUD use. Return of fertility, however, is excellent for most women following IUD use.[5, 8, 9, 10, 15, 31]

- Six weeks or more postpartum, if the woman has had no menses, has not had sexual intercourse since delivery of her baby, or has used condoms or vaginal spermicides or another contraceptive method each time she has had intercourse.

- Immediately after or within 3 weeks of an uncomplicated first-trimester spontaneous or legally induced abortion.

- Any time in her menstrual cycle, if a woman has been consistently and reliably using birth control pills or another method or if she has a negative sensitive pregnancy test.

- Any time in her menstrual cycle, if the woman has not had intercourse since her last menses.
- Within 6 days of the unprotected coitus, if the woman desires a postcoital contraceptive device.

If there is any question of pregnancy, perform a pregnancy test or delay insertion until the next menstrual flow, which usually indicates that the woman is not pregnant. Inserting the IUD later in a woman's cycle (after day 18) may result in more pain and bleeding in the short term.[41] (See Table 14-5.)

The inconvenience to the patient caused by a policy that dictates when in the menstrual cycle IUDs may be inserted can impede an effective IUD program. In some settings, women may need to make special arrangements and may need to travel a long time to reach a family planning clinic. In addition, another clinic visit costs money—thus creating a barrier to services. As a rule, trust the history given by women in a family planning clinic. This basic principle contributes to thoughtful, dignified, and high quality family planning services. Reasons to support inserting the IUD at any time in the menstrual cycle include:

- Insertion during the entire menstrual cycle gives the patient (and provider) options for more convenient and flexible appointment times.
- The infection rate and the expulsion rate may be higher when inserted during menses (see Table 14-5).

Table 14-5 IUD termination rates (per 1,000 insertions) during the first and second postinsertion months, by menstrual cycle day of insertion

Reason for Termination	Menstrual Cycle Day of Insertion				
	1–5	6–10	11–17	18+	All Cycle Days
Expulsion	50.3	30.5	24.0	22.0	39.6
Pregnancy	3.0	4.1	4.8	6.1	3.7
Pain and Bleeding	20.9	20.6	27.2	36.7	22.7
Miscellaneous Medical	5.9	7.9	4.8	9.8	6.8
Personal	25.6	30.9	17.6	19.6	26.2
Pelvic Infection	3.0	3.1	3.2	1.2	2.9
Total	108.7	97.1	81.6	95.4	101.9

Source: White (1980).

- At midcycle the cervix is just as dilated as during menses and therefore the IUD can be inserted easily.[41]

Insertion Technique

To insert an IUD, move slowly and gently during all phases of the insertion. Because insertion methods differ slightly for the various IUDs, always read and follow the manufacturer's instructions on IUD insertion. Detailed course handbooks are available for trainers who wish to instruct clinicians in IUD insertion, withdrawal, and management techniques.[20] The methods differ depending on the size and shape of the IUD, inserter barrel, plunger, packaging, and strings. The following instructions for insertion generally apply to all IUDs but refer specifically to the Cu T 380A and Progestasert System IUDs.[1,16] Figure 14-2 describes the equipment required for IUD insertion.

1. Explain the IUD insertion procedure to the patient. Answer questions, eliminate myths about the method, and create a comfortable, confident atmosphere for the client.

2. Administer an analgesic agent or antiprostaglandin, which has been found helpful for some women.

3. Perform a careful bimanual exam to rule out pregnancy and active pelvic infection and to diagnose the position of the uterus. The track of IUD perforations is usually at 90 degrees to the axis of the fundus. An unrecognized retroflexed uterus increases the possibility of uterine perforation at the time of the IUD insertion.

4. After you have inserted a warm speculum and viewed the cervix, use a motion of concentric circles beginning at the os and spiraling outward on the cervix using an antiseptic solution such as a 1:2500 iodine solution. If the patient is allergic to iodine use a chlorhexidine (Hibiclens) solution.

5. In some instances, you may inject intracervical local anesthesia at this point (see Paracervical Block).

6. Grasp the anterior lip of the cervix with a tenaculum about 1.5cm to 2.0 cm from the os. Close the single-tooth tenaculum slowly, one notch at a time. (A small amount of local anesthesia may help decrease discomfort of tenaculum placement.)

7. Sound the uterus slowly and gently. Place a cotton swab at the cervix when the sound is all the way in. Hold the sound and the swab together and remove them at the same time. The distance between the tip of the sound and the tip of the swab gives a measure of the depth of the fundus to within 0.25 cm.

8. Load the IUD into the inserter barrel. Use sterile conditions. To minimize the chance of introducing contamination, do not remove the IUD from the insertion tube prior to placement in the uterus. Do

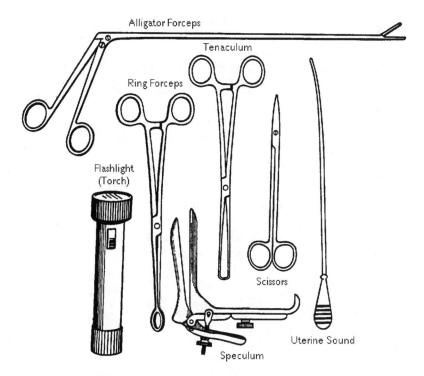

Figure 14-2 Minimal equipment for IUD insertion

not bend the arms of the "T" earlier than 5 minutes before it is to be introduced into the uterus. Strict aseptic technique can be maintained in the absence of sterile gloves by folding the arms in the partially opened package on a flat surface and pulling the solid rod partially from the package so it will not interfere with assembly.

9. Insert the IUD no further than is necessary to ensure the arms are retained in the tube. Introduce the solid rod into the insertion tube from the bottom alongside the threads until it touches the bottom of the Cu T 380A and Progestasert System. The insertion technique for the LNg IUD is similar to the Cu T 380A, but refer to manufacturer's instructions prior to use.

Progestasert System (Progestasert Intrauterine Progesterone Contraceptive System): Follow the directions on the package. The mechanism for folding the IUD is simple and requires only pushing on a firm surface to ready the device for insertion.

Cu T 380A (ParaGuard): Place your thumb and index finger on the ends of the horizontal arms while the IUD is still in the package. Push the insertion tube against the arms of the "T." Squeeze the arms down with thumb and index finger while using your other hand to maneuver the insertion tube to pick up the arms of the "T."

10. Adjust the movable flange on the tube so that it indicates the depth to which the IUD should be inserted and the direction in which the arms of the "T" will open. At this point, make certain that the horizontal arms of the "T" and the long axis of the flange lie in the same horizontal plane.

11. Introduce the inserter tube through the cervical canal into the fundus. Applying steady, gentle traction on the tenaculum that is grasping the anterior lip of the cervix. Insert the tube only up until the depth indicated by the flange. Do not force the insertion.

The Cardinal Rule for IUD Insertion:
Everything done at the time of IUD insertions and removal CAN and SHOULD be done slowly and gently.

12. Insert the IUD into the cavity of the uterus by retracting the outer barrel over the plunger (withdrawal technique). (See Figure 14-3.) Insert the IUD slowly and without much force. (This is the centerpiece of training: teaching clinicians the respect, feel, and confidence necessary to work with clients.)

13. Release the Cu T 380A or Progestasert System. Withdraw the insertion tube no more than 1/2 in.h while holding the solid rod completely still. This releases the arms of the "T."

14. To guarantee high fundal placement, the inserter tube is gently pushed up, until resistance is felt.

15. Withdraw the solid rod while holding the insertion tube stationary.

16. Withdraw the insertion tube from the cervix.

17. Clip the strings. Leave a sufficient length of the strings (1 in. or 2.5 cm) so that the woman can easily check for the presence of the IUD. In the patient's record, note the length of the visible strings.

18. Some clinicians have the patient feel for the strings of her IUD before she leaves the examining room. In any case, this procedure can be explained as part of the counseling process after the insertion.

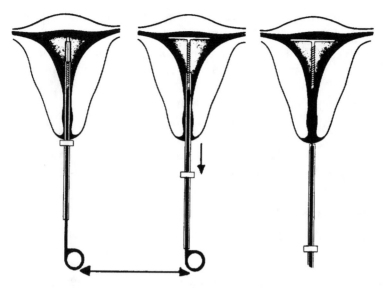

Source: Porter et al. (1983).

Figure 14-3 Withdrawal technique

IUDS in Nulliparous Women

Because of the increased risk of PID in IUD users, nulliparous women who wish to bear children in the future are generally poor candidates for IUDs. Exercise caution when inserting IUDs in nulliparous women, because they are more likely to experience vasovagal symptoms and postinsertion pain that would require immediate removal of the IUD. These problems are more common in a nulliparous woman who is anxious, has a narrow cervical canal, a small uterine cavity, an empty stomach, or a history of syncopal attacks. Gentleness, careful explanation, a warm and friendly environment, use of a small bivalve speculum, slow movement, and judicious use of paracervical anesthesia may help to avoid problems.

Prophylactic Antibiotics and IUD Insertion

No consensus exists on whether prophylactic antibiotics at the time of IUD insertion reduces postinsertion PID syndrome. The two published studies on this issue differed on the value of antibiotic prophylactics at the time of insertion.[21,32] If sexually transmitted infections are common in the population being served, some clinicians consider it wise to provide women with prophylactic antibiotics at the time of IUD insertion.

The following are guidelines that might be followed for prophylactic antibiotic use with IUD insertion:

- The patient must have no precautions to IUD insertion, no clinically acute infection, and no contraindications to taking antibiotics.
- Give the woman 200 mg of doxycycline orally at the time of insertion, followed by 100 mg 12 hours later.
- Breastfeeding women may be given 500 mg of erythromycin orally 1 hour before insertion or at the time of insertion, and 500 mg orally 6 hours after insertion. (Doxycycline is contraindicated during pregnancy and lactation because of potential affects on newborn bone.)

Immediate Postpartum Insertion of IUDs

If labor and delivery were normal, the uterus is firm, and bleeding has subsided, a Cu T 380A may be inserted immediately postpartum. (The authors recommend only the Paraguard because it has been shown to be the safest and most effective IUD model in postpartum women.) Manual post-placental IUD insertion, which occurs immediately following delivery of the placenta, and immediate postpartum insertion, which occurs during the first week after delivery, are safe and convenient approaches to birth control. They carry no increased risk of infection, perforation, or bleeding.[11,38] To minimize infection, use a sterile long-sleeved glove. Table 14-6 summarizes the major advantages and disadvantages of post-placental/immediate postpartum IUD Insertion.

High expulsion rates are a major drawback to immediate postpartum insertion. Rates of 9% in a study in China,[44] 22% in a Family Health International multicenter trial,[12] and 31%-41% in a WHO multicenter trial[42] have been reported. The expulsion rate for copper-bearing IUDs appears to be lower than the expulsion rate for Lippes Loops.[36] The chance

Table 14-6 Advantages and disadvantages of post-placental/immediate postpartum IUD insertion

Advantages	Disadvantages
• Patient already at health facility	• Expulsion rates higher
• Contraindication of pregnancy is not present	• Continuation rates slightly lower
• Fewer complaints of pain and bleeding	• Higher rates of missing strings
• Risk of perforation is same or lower	• Counseling postpartum is difficult
• Lower cost	• Special instructions needed about expulsions
• Insertion technique is easier to master	

Sources: O'Hanley et al. (1992); Stewart (1993).

of expulsion can be minimized with post-placental IUD insertion if the individual inserting the IUD is experienced, an ergot preparation enhances uterine contractility,[27] and the following techniques are used:

- Massage uterus until bleeding subsides
- Insert the IUD within 10 minutes of delivery of the placenta
- Administer Methergine (+/–) but no antibiotics or analgesia/anesthesia
- Grasp "Cu T" with ring forceps
- Grasp cervix with second pair of ring forceps
- Manually place the IUD in the uterine cavity
- Grasp abdomen/uterus with hand
- Place the IUD high in the fundus
- Release IUD and rotate ring forceps 45 degrees
- Move forceps laterally and remove
- Inspect vagina for string
- Replace string if it is visible

Because of the potential problem of expulsion, fully inform the client and encourage a postinsertion follow-up. In spite of higher expulsion rates, cumulative pregnancy rates for immediate postpartum IUD insertion are comparable to or lower than interval IUD insertions, perhaps because of the lower fertility of women in the postpartum period. With modern copper IUDs, proper insertion techniques, and adequate follow-up, rates for unplanned pregnancy with postpartum IUD insertion range from 2.0-2.8 per 100 users at 24 months.[27]

The string of the Cu T 380A may lie entirely within the uterine cavity after postplacental insertion. If a postpartum woman is examined 1 month after delivery and the string is not visible, determine the status of the Cu T 380A by sounding the uterine cavity (pregnancy at 4 weeks postpartum is very unlikely). Tease the string down to the cervical os. Otherwise, leave the string in the uterine cavity as long as the presence of the IUD was confirmed during sounding.

Paracervical Anesthesia or Paracervical Block

To prevent the pain from an IUD insertion or a difficult removal, place a paracervical block using no more than 10cc–20 cc of 1% lidocaine without epinephrine. Paracervical anesthesia is particularly beneficial at the time of insertion for a woman who has never been pregnant or for a woman who has a history of vasovagal reactions. The clinician should remember to ask the patient if she has any known allergies, especially to iodine or any local anesthetic. A suggested procedure for performing a paracervical block is as follows:

1. Perform a bimanual pelvic examination; insert a speculum into the vagina to obtain good visualization of the cervix.

2. Clean the cervix and vagina with antiseptic material.

3. Ask the patient to inform you if she experiences nausea, dizziness, ringing of the ears, or tingling of the lips from the procedure. It is not uncommon for these symptoms to occur, and they will pass quickly.

4. Inject 2 cc of lidocaine at the tenaculum site and then apply the tenaculum to the upper lip of the cervix.

5. Different clinicians use different placements of injections around the cervix. One technique is to inject 2cc–5 cc at sites corresponding to 4 o'clock to 5 o'clock and 7 o'clock to 8 o'clock on a clock face (a total of 10 cc).

6. Insert the needle just under the mucosa in the connective tissue. This method assures rapid and adequate distribution of the anesthetic because most of the smaller blood vessels and capillaries are in this region. Aspirate lightly with each injection to avoid direct intravenous injection.

7. Serious reaction will be extremely unlikely to occur by using less than a total of 20 cc lidocaine.

8. Anesthesia occurs in 2–5 minutes.

IUD Removal

When removing an IUD, always apply gentle, steady traction and remove the IUD slowly. If you cannot remove the IUD with gentle traction, use a tenaculum to steady the cervix and straighten the anteversion or retroversion. If this does not work, dilate the cervix with dilators. Dilators should always be available in a clinic managing IUD complications. For difficult removals, use a laminaria tent to dilate the cervix. A paracervical block may make the removal easier and less painful. Removing the IUD at the time of menses or at midcycle may be easier than at other times during the cycle.

If you do not see the strings, probe for them in the cervical canal with narrow forceps (or the alligator forceps). When the IUD (with or without its strings) is in the uterus, probe the endometrial cavity with alligator forceps (with which the strings or the IUD itself may be grasped), a hook, uterine packing forceps, or a Novak curette. Proficiency with one of these instruments for IUD removal when the strings are absent or entirely within the uterine cavity can prevent unnecessary hospitalizations.

Patient Counseling

A panel of experts at the Centers for Disease Control and Prevention has developed the following guidelines for informing women about IUDs:[10]

1. Foremost, allow the client to participate in choosing her method. She must be an informed user.

2. Make all presentations, counseling, and educational materials compatible with the language, culture, and education of the client.

3. Set aside a time for counseling as a routine part of the clinic visit. During the initial visit, a woman needs counseling to help her select a method, then additional counseling after the IUD insertion to learn about IUD use.

4. Be aware of the local myths and misconceptions about IUDs. Gaining this awareness may require background research. Address the misconceptions sensitively but directly.

5. Use a standard checklist outlining key information that the IUD user should know to help you remember important information to tell the user.

6. Ask the client to repeat important information.

7. Give each IUD user an identification card with the name and picture of the IUD. The card may note the date of insertion and recommended removal.

8. If a client is not accustomed to following a calendar, inform her about the recommended dates for checkups and IUD removal.

9. Sample IUDs should be available so that women can handle and examine them.

10. Provide flip charts, posters, and handouts describing key information about IUDs (and other available contraceptive methods).

M ANAGING PROBLEMS AND FOLLOW-UP

Serious complications from IUDs are usually preventable. When in doubt, take an IUD out. Seven potential complications from IUDs are listed in order of increasing severity.

SPOTTING, BLEEDING, HEMORRHAGE, AND ANEMIA

Abnormal bleeding may be either a sign of pregnancy or a sign of infection — two problems that must always be ruled out during the process of evaluating potential IUD clients.

CONDITION	ACTION
1. Patient has a Hgb of less than 11.5 gm at insertion:	• provide her with $FeSO_4$ (300 mg) to take 1 daily for 1–2 months (ferrous gluconate does not constipate patients as much as sulfate)

                    • instruct in proper nutrition, including iron rich foods

                    • repeat Hgb at 3-month followup

2. Within 3 months of the IUD insertion user complains of excess bleeding:

- reassure the patient that the bleeding will likely decline in subsequent cycles
- provide $FeSO_4$ (as in condition 1)
- provide ibuprofen 400 mg t.i.d. for first 3 days of cycle
- perform Hgb and treat (as in conditions 1, 4, and 7)
- examine for other pathology or symptoms such as:
  - cancer of the cervix and uterus
  - cervical and uterine polyps
  - leiomyomata
  - postcoital bleeding
  - chronic cervicitis
  - dysfunctional uterine bleeding

3. Excess bleeding is associated with pain:

- examine the patient to rule out a pelvic infection
- consider obtaining a sensitive pregnancy test to rule out pregnancy (including ectopic pregnancy)

4. Hgb is less than 9 gm:

- remove IUD
  - provide $FeSO_4$ (300 mg) daily × 2 months
  - repeat Hgb at 1 month
  - provide alternative method of contraception

5. Bleeding is thought to be associated with endometritis:

- remove IUD
  - culture for GC
  - treat presumptively with antibiotics (doxycycline × 10 days)
  - treat partner presumptively
  - provide alternative method of contraception

6. Patient desires IUD removal because bleeding is not tolerable:
- remove IUD
  - provide alternative method of contraception

7. Hgb falls >2 gm:
- remove IUD
- treat as in condition 4

8. Patient is over 40 and having prolonged menses:
- remove IUD
- if abnormal bleeding continues, refer for diagnosis and treatment with intermenstrual bleeding

CRAMPING AND PAIN

Slight pain may be felt at the time of IUD insertion and may be followed by cramping pain over the next 10–15 minutes. Cramping and abdominal pain may be signs of pregnancy or infection, two problems that must always be ruled out when evaluating clients with abdominal pain.

CONDITION	ACTION
1. Pain with sounding of the uterus during insertion:	• sound slowly and gently • consider smaller sound • if severe, desist and check alignment of uterine cavity; if OK, use a paracervical block
2. Cramping/pain immediately after insertion, for a day or so thereafter or with each menses:	
a. if severe:	– consider IUD removal
b. if mild:	– provide mild analgesia such as acetaminophen 1 gm every 4 hours as needed or ibuprofen 400 mg p.o. every 4 hours as needed
3. Pain at time of insertion, persistent and increasing, adding signs of abdominal tenderness:	
a. if strings are present:	– presume partial perforation has occurred; remove IUD and treat as pelvic infection
b. if strings are present and IUD is not:	– consider possibility of perforation (see IUD Removal section) – remove IUD

4. Partial expulsion of an IUD:
   a. if no infection of cervix or uterus:
      - may insert another IUD
      - provide 5-7 days of doxycycline 100 mg every 12 hours
   b. if infection of cervix or uterus or question of infection:
      - remove IUD
      - provide alternative contraception
      - treat with antibiotic as above and insert another IUD after 3 cycles

5. Pelvic inflammatory disease:
   • remove IUD, treat per section on PID

6. Severe postinsertion pain, reaction, syncope or seizure:
   • give spirits of ammonia per nasal inspiration
   a. if question of improper placement:
      - remove IUD, reevaluate uterus, resound, and reinsert another IUD
   b. if IUD felt to be properly positioned and pulse less than 60 beats/minute:
      - consider giving atropine 0.4-0.6 mg IM or IV
      - consider paracervical block
      - provide pain medication (*e.g.,* acetaminophen or ibuprofen)
      - remove IUD if necessary

7. Spontaneous abortion:
   • remove IUD
   • treat per section on pregnancy

8. Ectopic pregnancy:
   • treat per section on pregnancy

Expulsion of the IUD (Partial or Complete)

The symptoms of an IUD expulsion may include unusual vaginal discharge, cramping or pain, intermenstrual spotting, postcoital spotting, dyspareunia (for male or female), absence or lengthening of the IUD string, and presence of the hard plastic of the IUD at the cervical os or in the vagina.

   • If the IUD string is not felt, an expulsion may have occurred.

   • If menstrual period is delayed, check for IUD string. This may be the first indication of a "silent" expulsion.

CONDITION	ACTION
1. Partial expulsion:	• remove IUD
	• evaluate for pregnancy or infection —if present, treat as indicated
	• if neither pregnancy nor infection are present, reinsert another IUD and give 5-7 days of doxycycline 100 mg every 12 hours
2. Complete expulsion:	• insert another IUD per insertion guidelines

OTHER STRING PROBLEMS

CONDITION	ACTION
1. Partner is irritated by string:	
a. String has a short, sharp point coming from the cervix:	– counsel partner at time of insertion that he may feel string but it usually won't hurt him
	– cut string shorter and carefully record length
	– consider removing and replacing IUD, leaving string longer
b. String is long:	– try shortening the string
	– consider removing IUD
2. String is too long:	• rule out expulsion by exam and by sounding the cervix
a. IUD seems in place:	– trim string
b. Any doubt:	– remove IUD and replace with a new IUD
3. String is absent (either as determined by patient or examiner)	
a. Menses missed:	– rule out pregnancy by exam and pregnancy test. If both negative, evaluate as per 3b. If pregnancy detected, see next section on Pregnancy.
b. Menses not missed and no abdominal pain:	– advise use another method of contraception and wait until next menses; examine during next menses

i. IUD found:	– if IUD string not present, prepare cervix as per IUD insertion technique and explore uterus with alligator forceps
	– if string brought to appropriate place from cervical os and IUD not thought disrupted, treat with antibiotics and follow routinely
	– if any question of IUD dislodging or abnormal placement or position, remove IUD, treat with antibiotic and reinsert another IUD
ii. IUD not found:	– refer to physician
	– obtain ultrasound (or x-ray)
a. No IUD seen on ultrasound:	– obtain pregnancy test
	– insert another IUD per insertion guidelines
b. IUD seen on ultrasound:	– clarify location of IUD to determine whether or not perforated
	– may need to place another IUD; and take an x-ray or ultrasound of pelvis
	– if perforation, treat accordingly
	– if no perforation, then the x-ray should show two IUDs in the uterus (usually both will have to be removed and another inserted)

PREGNANCY

Approximately one-third or fewer of IUD-related pregnancies are attributable to undetected or partial expulsions. If the patient is pregnant with an IUD in place, the following is recommended.

- Inform the patient of the risk of spontaneous abortion.

- Determine whether the client wishes to continue the pregnancy. If the IUD has completely perforated the uterus and is in the abdominal cavity, it may not pose any risk to the pregnancy. Because the degree of perforation is usually not known, treat the condition as though the IUD were *in situ* and the string not seen.

CONDITION	ACTION
1. Patient is undergoing a spontaneous abortion:	• empty the uterus • remove the IUD • provide doxycycline or ampicillin for 7 days • rule out ectopic pregnancy
a. Severe pain:	– provide analgesic medication
b. Anemic:	– give $FeSO_4$
2. Patient requests to abort the pregnancy:	• refer for abortion
3. Patient wishes to continue the pregnancy and the IUD strings are visible:	• gently pull on the IUD string and remove the IUD • warn the patient that an ectopic pregnancy should be suspected • refer the patient for prenatal care
4. Patient wishes to continue the pregnancy and the IUD strings are not visible:	
a. Signs of an intrauterine infection exist:	– evacuate the uterus, and treat the patient with antibiotics – evacuate the tissue to rule out ectopic pregnancy – refer these patients for special care
b. Signs of infection do not exist:	– inform the patient to watch for signs of infection (such as pain, discharge, bleeding, fever, myalgia) and of ectopic pregnancy and instruct her where to go should those complications occur – refer for prenatal care – warn of possible perforation – recover the IUD at delivery

UTERINE PERFORATION, EMBEDDING, AND CERVICAL PERFORATION

The incidence of perforation is approximately 1 in 1,000. The IUD generally perforates the uterus at one of three sites: (1) uterine fundus, (2) body of the uterus and (3) cervical wall.

CONDITION	ACTION
1. IUD plastic device sticking through cervix:	• use alligator forceps to grasp IUD inside cervix in lower uterine cavity and push IUD back into uterus and then remove through cervical os • perform paracervical block, if needed, to perform procedure • provide analgesia • provide medication as needed • treat with antibiotics • provide alternative contraception • reinsert as per IUD insertion guidelines
2. IUD string does not allow IUD to be removed with significant pressure:	• try recommendations in section on lost strings • provide paracervical block
a. IUD found in uterus:	– use alligator forceps to grasp IUD in cervix or uterus and remove – if IUD not removable, refer for more specialized care
b. IUD not found in uterus or cervix (and string is seen):	– refer to gynecologist – use alternative methods of contraception – provide an antibiotic

If the IUD has perforated the uterus, it's possible that the IUD string could still be hanging outside of the cervix. In this case it would be difficult to detect that a perforation has occurred. This is one circumstance where expert help is truly required.

3. IUD perforation identified by x-ray or ultrasound and no string visible	
a. Pain, evidence of bowel obstruction, or pelvic infection	– refer to gynecologist or general surgery – treat with antibiotics; surgery may be required
b. No pain or evidence of obstruction, infection, or pregnancy	– provide patient with alternative contraception – inform patient of signs of

	obstruction or pelvic infection or where to go if those signs develop
c. Patient is pregnant and IUD is extrauterine	• provide information as per condition b and as per section on Pregnancy

PELVIC INFLAMMATORY DISEASE

PID is a serious complication, due either to the IUD itself or to STD exposure. PID due to the IUD itself occurs most commonly in the first few weeks following insertion. Pelvic infections need aggressive treatment and follow-up to be certain that the infection is adequately treated. An IUD should not be reinserted in someone who is at high risk for developing another pelvic infection or who has had PID in the past 3 months. The accurate diagnosis of PID is difficult. The following signs suggest PID:

- an oral temperature of 38° C, or above
- suprapubic tenderness and guarding
- tenderness/pain associated with moving the cervix during pelvic exam
- purulent discharge from the cervix
- tenderness of the uterus upon palpation
- adnexal tenderness or adnexal palpable mass or masses

CONDITION	ACTION
1. Patient is pregnant and has symptoms of PID	• see section on Pregnancy
2. Patient has mild pelvic infection defined as fever ≤ 38° C, no abdominal guarding, mild suprapubic, uterine, and/or adnexal tenderness and no adnexal masses	• remove IUD • provide alternative contraception • provide treatment (see Chapter 4) • reexamine in 1 week • inform patient to seek immediate care if symptoms worsen
3. Patient has moderate pelvic infection defined as fever <39° C, abdominal guarding and no rebound, and no adnexal masses, patient is not vomiting	• same as condition 2 • provide treatment (see Chapter 4) • consider hospitalization

4. Patient has severe pelvic infection with fever >39° C, guarding or rebound, pelvic masses or vomiting, or appears acutely ill

• refer to hospital care

PID is a serious, life-threatening problem that needs expert care.

INSTRUCTIONS FOR USING IUDs

BEFORE YOU HAVE YOUR IUD INSERTED:

Some women have a fair amount of pain or nausea immediately after IUD insertion. You may want to come to the clinic with your husband, partner, or friend in case you need someone to assist you home.

AFTER YOU HAVE YOUR IUD INSERTED:

1. **Check your strings.** Before you leave the office or clinic, learn how to feel the strings that protrude 2 inches or so into your vagina. If you cannot feel the strings or if you can feel the plastic part, your IUD may not protect you against pregnancy; use another method until you can return to the clinic to have your IUD checked. You can expel an IUD without knowing it. Check for the strings frequently during the first months you have the device, then after each period and any time you have abnormal cramping while menstruating.

2. **Beware of infection.** If at any time you have fever, pelvic pain or tenderness, severe cramping, or unusual vaginal bleeding, contact your clinician immediately because you may have an infection. Infections from IUDs can be serious and, if untreated, can lead to hysterectomy (removal of the uterus) or even death. When your IUD is inserted, find out where you can go to be treated for an infection. IUDs can occasionally cause internal pelvic infection (in contrast to vaginal infections) that can lead to chronic pain or infertility. Women in mutually faithful relationships appear to have little increased risk of infection.[22]

3. **Watch for your periods.** If you miss a menstrual period, contact your family planning provider immediately. The most commonly reported nuisance side effects of the IUD are increased menstrual flow, menstrual cramping and spotting, and increased mucous discharge. Remember that if you cannot tolerate the IUD, you can always have it removed. Heavier menstrual bleeding may be serious if you are

anemic. However, a small increase in the menstrual flow is normal with the IUD, especially during the first two to three periods.

4. Do not try to remove the IUD yourself. Do not let your partner pull on the strings. The clinician will have a better idea of the angle at which the IUD went in. It should come out the same way.

5. Learn and pay attention to the IUD Warning Signs.

Early IUD Warning Signs

Caution

P ■ Period late (pregnancy), abnormal spotting or bleeding

A ■ Abdominal pain, pain with intercourse

I ■ Infection exposure (any STD), abnormal discharge

N ■ Not feeling well, fever, chills

S ■ String missing, shorter or longer

REFERENCES

1. Alza Corporation. Progestasert intrauterine progesterone contraceptive system. Alza Product Information, 1986.
2. Alvarez R, Brache V, Fernandez E, Guerrero B, Guiloff E, Hess R, Salvatierra AM, Zacharios S. New insights on the mode of action of intrauterine devices in women. Fertil Steril 1988;49(5):768-773.
3. Andersson K, Rybo G. Levonorgestrel-releasing intrauterine device in the treatment of menorrhagia. Br J Obstet Gynaecol 1990;97(8):690-694.
4. Angle MA, Murphy C. Guidelines for clinical procedures in family planning. Chapel Hill NC: Program for International Training in Health, 1992.
5. Angle MA. Intrauterine devices: an evaluation of the epidemiologic evidence implicating IUDs in infertility, and a consideration of the policy implications for U.S.A.I.D., thesis. Chapel Hill, School of Public Health, University of North Carolina, 1987.
6. Arbab AAO, McNamara R, Lauro D, Aziz FA. Expanded services for intrauterine contraception in Sudan. East Afri Med J 1991;68(2):70-74.
7. Bernstine RL. Review and analysis of the scientific and clinical data on the safety, efficacy, adverse reactions, biologic action, utilization, and design of intrauterine devices. Final Report, Department of Health, Education, and Welfare/Food and Drug Administration, Technical Resources Development. Seattle WA: Batelle Memorial Institute, 1975.
8. Burnhill M. Intrauterine contraception. In: Corson SL, Derman RJ, Tyrer LB (eds). Fertility Control Boston: Little, Brown & Co., 1986:272.
9. Burnhill MS. The rise and fall and rise of the IUD. Am J Gynecol Health 1989;III(35):6-10.
10. Centers for Disease Control. IUDs: guidelines for informed decision making and uses. Atlanta GA: Centers for Disease Control, May 1, 1987.
11. Chi I-c, Farr G. Postpartum IUD contraception—a review of an international experience. Adv Contracep 1989;5(3):127-146.

12. Cole LD, Edelman DA, Potts DM, Wheeler RG, Laufe LE. Postpartum insertion of modified intrauterine devices. J Repro Med 1984;29(9):677-682.

13. Farley TM, Rosenberg MS, Rowe PJ, Chen SH, Meirik O. Intrauterine devices and pelvic inflammatory disease: an international perspective. Lancet 1992; 339(8796):785-78.

14. Forrest JD. Acceptability of IUD's in the United States. Presented at: A new look at IUD's – advancing contraceptive choices. New York, NY, March 27-28, 1992.

15. Guillebaud J. Contraception, your questions answered. New York NY: Churchill Livingstone, Inc., 1989.

16. GynoPharma. Prescribing information for the Copper T 380—an intrauterine copper contraceptive. Issued April 1988.

17. GynoPharma. Data on File. 1992.

18. Harlap S, Kost K, Forrest JD. Preventing pregnancy, protecting health: a new look at birth control choices in the United States. New York NY: The Allan Guttmacher Institute, 1991.

19. Hatcher RA, Stewart F, Trussell J, Kowal D, Guest F, Stewart G, Cates W. Contraceptive technology 1990-1992. New York NY: Irvington Publishers, Inc., 1990.

20. JHPIEGO Corporation, eds. JHPIEGO IUD Course Handbook. November 1992.

21. Ladipo OA, Farr G, Otolorin E, Konje JC, Sturgen K, Cox P, Champion CB. Prevention of IUD-related pelvic infection: the efficacy of prophylactic doxy-cycline at IUD insertion. Adv Contracept 1991;7(1):43-54.

22. Lee NC, Rubin GL, Borucki R. The intrauterine device and pelvic inflammatory disease revisited: new results from the Women's Health Study. Obstet Gynecol 1988;72(1):1-6.

23. Lewit S. Outcome of pregnancy with intrauterine device. Contraception 1970;2(1):47-57.

24. Mauldin WP, Segal SJ. IUD use throughout the world — past, present and future. In: Bardin CW, Mishell DR Jr. (eds). A new look at IUD's—advancing contraceptive choices. Stoneham MA: Butterworth-Heinemann, Publication forthcoming.

25. Mishell DR, Bell JH, Good RG, Moyer DL. The intrauterine device: a bacterio-logic study of the endometrial cavity. Am J Obstet Gynecol 1966;96:119-126.

26. Musicco M, Nicolosi A, Saracco A, Lazzarin A. IUD use and man to woman sexual transmission of HIV-1. In: Bardin CW, Mishell DR Jr. (eds). A new look at IUD's—advancing contraceptive choices. Stoneham: Butterworth-Heineman. Publication forthcoming.

27. O'Hanley K, Huber DH. Postpartum IUDs: keys for success. Contraception 1992;45(4):351-361.

28. Ortho Pharmaceutical Corporation. 1991 Ortho Annual Birth Control Survey. Raritan, New Jersey.

29. Ortiz ME and Croxatto HB. The mode of action of IUDs. Contraception 1987;36(1):37-53.

30. Rowe PJ. Research on intrauterine devices. Annual technical report 1991. Geneva, Switzerland: Special Programme of Research, Development and Research Training in Human Reproduction, World Health Organization, 1992:127-137.

31. Sample IUD training curriculum and protocol, unpublished manuscript. New York: Family Planning International Assistance, 1988;72(1):1-6.

32. Sinei SKA, Schulz KF, Lamptey PR, Grimes DA, Mati JKG, Rosenthal SM, Rosenberg MJ, Riara G, Njage PN, Bhullar VB, Ogembo HV. Preventing IUD-related pelvic infection: the efficacy of prophylactic doxycycline at insertion. Br J Obstet Gynaecol 1990;97(5):412-419.

33. Sivin I. IUDs are contraceptives, not abortifacients: a comment on research and belief. Stud Fam Plann 1989;20(6-1):355-359.

34. Sivin I, Stern J, Coutinho E, Mattos CER, Diaz SEMS, Pavez M, Alvarez F, Brache V, Thevenin F, Diaz J, Faundes A, Diaz MM, McCarthy T, Mishell DR, Shoupe D. Prolonged intrauterine contraception: a seven-year randomized study of the levonorgestrel 20 mcg/day (LNg20) and the Copper T380 A IUDs. Contraception 1991;44(5):473-480.

35. Stewart GK. Personal communication during Philippine Contraception Workshop, 1993.

36. Thiery M. Timing of IUD insertion. In: Zatuchni GI, Goldsmith A, Sciarra JJ, Osborn CK (eds). Intrauterine contraception: advances and future prospects. Philadelphia PA: Harper and Row, 1985; 365-374.

37. Toivonen J, Luukkainen T, Allonen H. Protective effect of intrauterine release of levonorgestrel on pelvic infections: three years' comparative experience of levonorgestrel and copper-releasing intrauterine devices. Obstet Gynecol 1991;77(2):261-264.

38. Treiman K, Liskin L. IUDs—a new look. Popul Rep 1988;Series B(5).

39. Vessey MP, Johnson B, Doll R, Peto R. Outcome of pregnancy in women using an intrauterine device. Lancet 1974;1:495-498.

40. Westhoff CL, Marks F, & Rosenfield A. Physician factors limiting IUD use in the US. Presented at: A new look at IUD's – advancing contraceptive choices; March 27-28, 1992; New York, NY.

41. White MK, Ory HW, Rooks JB, Rochat RW. Intrauterine device termination rates and the menstrual cycle day of insertion. Obstet Gynecol 1980;55(2):220-224.

42. World Health Organization. Special programs on research, development and research training in human reproduction. Task force on intrauterine devices for fertility regulation. Comparative multicenter trial of three IUDs inserted immediately following delivery of the placenta. Contraception 1980;22(1):9-18.

43. Zhang J, Chi I-c, Feldblum PJ, Farr MG. Risk factors for copper T IUD expulsion: an epidemiologic analysis. Contraception 1992;46(5):427-433.

44. Zhou SW, Chi I-c. Immediate postpartum IUD insertions in a Chinese hospital – a two year follow-up. Inter J Gynaecol Obstet 1991;35(2):157-164.

LATE REFERENCE

45. Porter CW, Waife RS, Holtrop HR. The health provider's guide to contraception. The international edition. Watertown MA: The Pathfinder Fund, 1983.

Voluntary Surgical Contraception (Sterilization)

- Healthy women are fertile until about age 50 to 51; healthy men are fertile essentially throughout life. Because most couples have all the children they want well before the end of their reproductive life span, couples will need effective contraception protection against unwanted pregnancies for many years.

- Voluntary surgical contraception (VSC), or contraceptive sterilization, has become one of the most widely used methods of family planning in the world for both developed and developing countries.

- VSC is one of the most effective methods—for men or women.

- A single decision and one surgical procedure provides a permanent long-term method. Reversal is expensive, not readily available, requires major surgery, and results are not guaranteed.

- VSC is one of the safest and most cost-effective contraceptive methods.

Since 1970, approximately 1 million sterilizations have been performed annually in the United States. In 1991, 490,958 vasectomies were performed[51] and in 1986, the year for which the latest figures are available, 640,000 tubectomies were performed in the United States.[6] Nearly 14 million women rely on sterilization as their contraceptive method: 9.6 million rely on female sterilization, and 4.1 million on vasectomy. (See Chapter 5.)

Better patient selection, improved anesthetic methods and patient monitoring, increased use of local anesthesia with light sedation, improved surgical techniques, better asepsis, and better trained personnel contributed to the improved safety of voluntary surgical contraception (VSC) over the past 20 years.

The ratio of male-to-female sterilizations varies widely from one part of the United States to another. Vasectomies are much more common in the West, while female sterilizations are preferred in the South. Those with higher incomes and higher levels of education seem to prefer sterilization: 12% of women with incomes under $6,000 compared with 33% for women with incomes greater than $30,000 are sterilized.[53]

Ideally, a couple should consider both vasectomy and female sterilization. They are comparable in effectiveness, and both are intended to be permanent. If both were equally acceptable, vasectomy would be the medically preferred procedure. The use of vasectomy depends upon the effort and emphasis of providers to make high quality vasectomy services available.

M ECHANISM OF ACTION

Sterilization for women involves mechanically blocking the fallopian tubes to prevent the sperm and egg from uniting.

Vasectomy is the male sterilization operation that blocks the vasa deferentia to prevent the passage of sperm into the seminal ejaculated fluid.

E FFECTIVENESS

FEMALE STERILIZATION

Failure rates associated with sterilization are lower than those associated with use of most temporary contraceptive methods during the first year. They are similar to rates given for some of the long-term methods, such as the levonorgestrel and T 380A IUDs and Norplant. Most studies of the common occlusion techniques—the Pomeroy and Pritchard techniques, Silastic ring, Filshie and spring clips, electrocoagulation, and the Irving technique—report first-year failure rates of less than 1%, usually 0.0%-0.8% (see Table 27-15). A recent analysis indicates a significantly higher risk of pregnancy with bipolar cautery than with unipolar cautery.[76] An overall failure rate of 0.4% for the first year is reasonable to expect. (See Table 15-1 and Tables 5-2 and 27-1.) Sterilization failures can be classified into five categories:[73]

1. Women who are pregnant at the time of sterilization (luteal phase pregnancy). These may or may not be reported as failures. Luteal phase pregnancies may be prevented when the sterilization is performed in the follicular phase, assuring the patient's use of effective contraceptive until after the sterilizing procedure, careful sexual history (and use of postcoital contraceptive when indicated), and selective use of the D&C procedure.

Table 15-1 First-year failure rates* for women using sterilization, condoms, pills, IUD, and Norplant

Method (1)	% of Women Experiencing an Accidental Pregnancy Within the First Year of Use		% of Women Continuing Use at One Year
	Typical Use (2)	Perfect Use (3)	(4)
Condom			
Male	12	3	63
Female (Reality)	21	5	56
Pill	3		72
Progestin Only		0.5	
Combined		0.1	
IUD			
Progesterone T	2.0	1.5	81
Copper T 380A	0.8	0.6	78
LNg 20	0.1	0.1	81
Norplant (6 Capsules)	0.09	0.09	85
Female Sterilization	0.4	0.4	100
Male Sterilization	0.15	0.10	100

*See Table 5-2 for first-year failure rates of all methods.

2. Surgical error, accounting for 30%-50% of failures.[47] Training of surgeons, good care of instruments, and routine accurate identification of tubes are key to limiting this problem.
3. Equipment failure when using any of the laparoscopic methods.
4. Fistula formation, most commonly with the electrocoagulation method.
5. Spontaneous reanastomosis, as in item 4, which is related to the method of occlusion. Carefully using accepted methods will minimize these problems.

Because surgical skill can seldom be separated from the inherent effectiveness of the occlusion technique, it is difficult to conclude that one technique will be superior. For surgeons well-trained in the techniques they perform, it is unlikely that important differences in effectiveness rates will occur among the recommended occlusion techniques described in this chapter. However, the literature does suggest guidance about which techniques will be more effective depending on pregnancy status and surgical approach. (See Occlusion Techniques under sections Postpartum and Postabortion Surgical Contraception and Interval Surgical Contraception.)

Vasectomy

Vasectomy is a very effective contraceptive method. Unfortunately, few studies of vasectomy clearly address the issue of pregnancy. Many studies report "failures," but these are failures to eliminate sperm from the ejaculate rather than to prevent pregnancies. Even the pregnancies that are reported may not always be due to the men undergoing vasectomy. True failure of the technique can result from spontaneous recanalization of the vas, division or occlusion of the wrong structure during surgery, and (rarely) a congenital duplication of the vas that went unnoticed during the procedure.

Studies that do report pregnancies are summarized in Table 27-16. These rates do not include pregnancies resulting from unprotected intercourse before the reproductive tract has been cleared of sperm, and thus are true method failures. One might expect a method failure rate of approximately 0.1% in the first year. (See Table 15-1 and Chapter 27.)

Cost

In the United States and throughout the world, the cost of sterilization procedures varies greatly. Unequivocally, however, female sterilization is much more expensive than male sterilization. Table 15-2 presents figures on the cost of sterilization in 1993 dollars.

Table 15-2 Cost of sterilization (US$)

	Female	Male
	Interval Laparoscopy or Minilaparotomy	Vasectomy
Public Sector*	± $1,200	$250–$400
Private Sector**	± $2,500	$500–$1,000

*Planned Parenthood of Sacramento Valley, CA, 1993
**Compilation of Sacramento County Physician and Surgery Center fees, 1993

Advantages and Indications

Female Sterilization

Voluntary surgical contraception (VSC) for women is a safe operative procedure. Reported fatality rates for the United States are in the range of 3 per 100,000.[67] By contrast, the maternal mortality rate is 7.9 deaths per 100,000 live births.[79] The risk of death from hysterectomy for benign disease is estimated to be 5/100,000–25/100,000[88] in women aged 35-44. Laparoscopy is associated with a lower mortality than is minilaparotomy, although this has been a debated topic in the past.[48]

Sterilization can be performed without increasing the health risks during the immediate postpartum period or in association with pregnancy termination, provided appropriate medical assessment is available. When immediate postpartum VSC is performed by trained personnel using local anesthesia, a small incision, and refined surgical technique, the normal postpartum stay (often 24 hours or less) is not prolonged. Suprapubic minilaparotomy (performed 4 weeks or more after delivery) can be performed on an outpatient basis with local anesthesia and light sedation, as can laparoscopy.

The method is ideal for those persons who are certain they wish no further children and need a reliable contraceptive method. Other advantages include the following:

- Permanent
- Highly effective
- Cost effective when cost is spread out over time
- Nothing to buy or remember
- No significant long-term side effects
- Partner compliance not required
- No interruption in lovemaking
- Very private/personal method

VASECTOMY

Vasectomy continues to be simpler, safer, and less expensive than female surgical contraception. It is a simple procedure that can be performed quickly, safely, and inexpensively. In the circumstances where the relationship is stable, the female has no other sexual partners, and the man has voluntary informed consent, vasectomy would be the preferred surgical contraceptive method.

The main advantages of vasectomy are:

- Highly effective
- Relieves the female of the contraceptive burden
- Inexpensive in the long run
- Permanent
- Highly acceptable procedure to most clients
- Very safe
- Quickly performed

DISADVANTAGES AND CAUTIONS

FEMALE STERILIZATION

Surgical contraception is not recommended for anyone who is not sure of their fertility desire. Other disadvantages include the following:

- Permanent
- Reversibility difficult and expensive
- Sterilization procedures technically difficult
- Requires surgeon, operating room (aseptic conditions), trained assistants, medications, surgical equipment
- Expensive at the time performed
- Morbidity and mortality high when considered for 1 year
- If failure, high probability of ectopic pregnancy
- No protection against STDs, including HIV

VASECTOMY

Vasectomy is not effective until sperm in the reproductive system are ejaculated. Complications such as bleeding or infection, although infrequent, do occur. As a contraceptive method, vasectomy provides only indirect protection from pregnancy for women. The major disadvantages of vasectomy are:

- Protection for the male (it is the female who is at risk for pregnancy)
- A surgical procedure requiring surgical training, aseptic conditions, medications, and technical assistance
- Expensive in the short term
- Serious long-term effects suggested (although currently unproved)
- Permanent (although reversal is possible, it is expensive, requires a highly technical and major surgery, and its results cannot be guaranteed.)
- Regret in 5%-10% of patients
- No protection against STDs, including HIV

Sperm antibodies. About one-half to two-thirds of men will develop sperm antibodies following vasectomy. However, no physiological evidence of any pathologic complication arising from the condition has been noted.[46,59] Although two studies performed on vasectomized monkeys suggested that the monkeys developed atherosclerotic plaques in the blood vessels at a greater rate than nonvasectomized monkeys,[1,12] extensive epidemiologic studies in men have found no adverse effects or increase in heart disease.[22,50,57,58,59,83] One study has found that vasectomy is not associated with an increase in mortality or morbidity from cardiovascular disease, but that there is a slightly increased risk of cancer in men who have been sterilized for 20 or more years.[23]

Prostate cancer. Recent studies have found a weak positive association between vasectomy and prostate cancer.[24,25] Past epidemiological studies on this relationship have been conflicting. Because much of prostate cancer is undetected and underreported, studies have a high chance of detection bias. A relationship between vasectomy and prostate cancer has no known biological plausibility.

The Final Statement from the Vasectomy and Prostate Cancer Conference held in March 1993 states that "Because the results of research to date on vasectomy and prostate cancer are inconsistent, and associations that have been found are weak, there is insufficient basis for recommending a change in clinical and public health practice at this time. In light of this:

- Providers should continue to offer vasectomy and to perform the procedure.
- Vasectomy reversal is not warranted to prevent prostate cancer.
- Screening for prostate cancer should not be any different for men who have had a vasectomy than for those who have not."[81]

PROVIDING SURGICAL CONTRACEPTION FOR FEMALES

Female sterilization involves ligation, mechanical occlusion with clips or rings, or electrocoagulation. Various surgical techniques are depicted in Figure 15-1. The choice of occlusion method depends upon the provider's training, personal experience, beliefs regarding effectiveness, and the availability of supplies. The differences in failure rates depend upon a number of factors, only one of which is the occlusion method.

The fallopian tubes are usually approached through the abdomen via a minilaparotomy incision and laparoscopy or via a laparotomy at the time of a caesarean section or other abdominal surgery. The surgical approach through the vagina via a colpotomy has been largely abandoned because of increased risks of infection and failure.

The timing of female sterilization, whether pregnancy-related or not, is very important for choosing the surgical approach, method of occlusion, presentation for counseling issues, use of staff and facilities, and organization of patient flow.

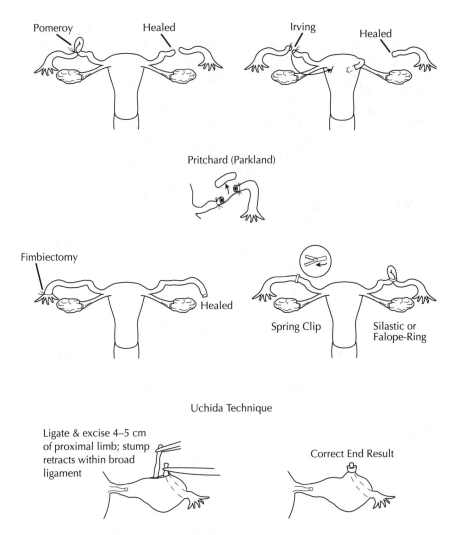

Figure 15-1 Tubal sterilization techniques

INTERVAL SURGICAL CONTRACEPTION

Suprapubic Minilaparotomy

Suprapubic minilaparotomy for "interval sterilization" (at 4 or more weeks after delivery) is performed when the uterus is fully involuted. The technique involves an abdominal incision 2cm–5 cm in length just above the pubic hairline. Through this incision the surgeon grasps the tubes and occludes them (see Figure 15-2.) For many women, the incision lies within the hairline and

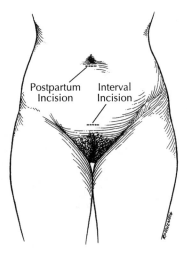

Source: Stewart et al. (1988).

Figure 15-2   Minilaparotomy incision site and size

so will not be visible. The minilaparotomy technique may be difficult if the woman is obese, the uterus immobile, or the tubes have adhesions from infection or previous surgery. This technique requires mobility of the pelvic structures so that by manipulation of the uterus the tubes can be moved into the incision site and thus be easily accessible.

In the preoperative assessment, assure that the patient has been appropriately counseled and provided an informed consent for surgical sterilization. Ask about pelvic disease, previous abdominal or pelvic surgery, diabetes mellitus, heart or lung disease, bleeding problems, allergies, and recent infections. Ascertain the date of last menstrual period and make certain that the woman is not pregnant. If the VSC procedure is done during a pregnancy termination procedure or postpartum, make certain the client has no pregnancy-related problems, particularly anemia. Examine the heart, lungs, abdomen, and general condition of the patient. Perform a pelvic exam, paying special attention to uterine position and mobility and presence of pelvic infection or masses. Laboratory evaluations usually include at least a hemoglobin measurement.

Procedure: The patient should empty her bladder by voiding or by catheterization immediately before the operation. Place the woman in the lithotomy position. If the uterus is not already anteverted, elevate the uterus manually or with a uterine manipulator (elevator) (see Figure 15-3.)

Correct placement of the incision is essential to avoid injury. If placed too high, the tubes will be difficult to reach; if placed too low, the bladder may be incised. Significant anatomical variation occurs among patients; thus, take great care in entering the abdomen. Light sedation can be given preoperatively

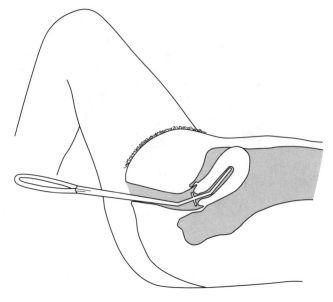

Source: Stewart et al. (1988)

Figure 15-3 A metal elevator raises the uterus and moves it from side to side so that the uterus and tubes will be closer to the incision.

and local anesthesia used to infiltrate layer by layer (see section on Anesthesia). When using local anesthesia, continue to communicate with the woman during the procedure to enhance the analgesic effect, reassure her and when necessary, elicit her cooperation. Surgical manipulation should be slow, gentle, and sensitive to the patient's complaints and response. Avoid unnecessary trauma or manipulation. Often a tubal hook or small Babcock forceps facilitates lifting the fallopian tube from the abdomen. Identify the fimbria to ensure that the structure is the tube and not the round ligament.

Use careful aseptic technique throughout. Achieve good hemostasis before closing the abdominal wound in layers. Growing evidence indicates that it is unnecessary to suture the peritoneal layer because small peritoneal defects will heal without adhesions.[89] This applies as well to subumbilical minilaparotomy.

Occlusion techniques. Occlusion options include the Pomeroy and Pritchard (Parkland) techniques, the Silastic or Falope-Rings, and the Spring clips (including the Filshie clip). The rings and clips require special applicators. Fimbriectomy and the Madlener procedures have been associated with higher failure rates and have no advantages over the Pomeroy and Pritchard techniques for routine cases. The Irving technique cannot be done through a minilaparotomy incision and is essentially useful only after a caesarean section.

Laparoscopy

The laparoscopy approach to sterilization (see Figure 15-4) involves making a small incision and inserting an instrument to visualize the tubes so that the surgeon can place rings (bands), apply clips, or electrocoagulate the oviducts. Use either a single- or double-puncture technique. The second puncture is used for manipulating the organs and occluding the tubes (see Figure 15-4). With single-puncture laparoscopy, pass the operating instrument through an opening beside the fiberoptic channel.

Principally because the incision is smaller, this method is less painful than minilaparotomy, has a low rate of complication, a short recovery time, and leaves only a small scar. The same equipment and skills can be used for endoscopic diagnostic procedures. The incision made for the laparoscope is small, and the patient and provider satisfaction with the method make it more attractive over time.

A recent report, however, indicates a decline in numbers of laparoscopic sterilizations as newer diagnostic and therapeutic endoscopic procedures are performed.[36] Disadvantages of laparoscopic sterilizations include the need for a specialist with expensive and intense training, equipment that is difficult to maintain, and a fully equipped operating room. Laparoscopic sterilization is not recommended for the immediate postpartum period, and complications may be serious.

Procedure: Laparoscopic sterilizations can be performed using local or general anesthesia. Local anesthesia with light sedation is usually adequate

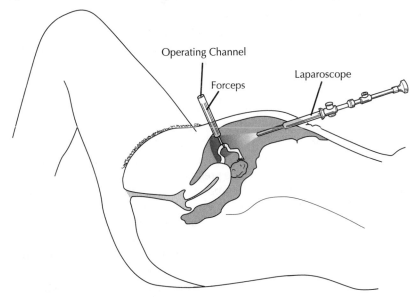

Figure 15-4 Laparoscopy

and offers safety advantages over general anesthesia, which can lead to compromised cardiorespiratory function.[37,55,56] With general anesthesia, control ventilation with endotracheal intubation. A higher level of training is required for administering general anesthesia than for administering local anesthesia.

Clean the perineal area, the vagina, and cervix. Scrub the abdominal site, with special emphasis on the naval. Stabilize the cervix with a tenaculum and a uterine manipulator. (See Figure 15-5.)

After making a small subumbilical incision, insert the Veress needle for insufflation. Apply upward traction on the abdomen. Advance the needle toward the pelvis, away from the great blood vessels. Place the patient in the Trendelenburg position and insufflate 1–3 liters of gas (the minimum needed for good visualization), nitrous oxide (N_2O), carbon dioxide (CO_2), or room air. Withdraw the needle and advance the trocar toward the pelvis, away from the great vessels, as the abdominal wall is firmly elevated. Remove the trocar from its sleeve (cannula) and insert the laparoscope. If double-puncture laparoscopy is used, make a second puncture under direct vision through the laparoscope in the abdomen. With single-puncture laparoscopy, insert the operating instruments through the operating channel of the laparoscope to grasp and occlude the oviducts. Variations from this description include "open laparoscopy," during which the peritoneal cavity is opened under visualization by the surgeon – similar to a subumbilical minilaparotomy. Then place a cannula for insertion of the laparoscope. This method avoids the blind entry of the sharp Veress needle and the trocar into the abdomen,[27,28,54] but has gained little support for general use.

If clips are used, place them on the isthmic portion of the tube at 1–2 cm from the uterus. Place Silastic rings 3 cm from the uterus. Perform electrocoagulation in the midportion of the tube away from other structures.[93] (See Figure 15-5.) After both tubes are occluded, inspect the pelvic organs to ensure that no injury or bleeding has occurred, the laparoscope is removed, all the gas is carefully expelled from the abdomen, the cannula is removed, and the incision is sutured closed.

Occlusion techniques. Silastic bands, unipolar electrocoagulation, and Filshie Clips appear to have similar short-term effectiveness rates when correctly applied, although the ectopic pregnancy rate appears to be higher with electrocoagulation (bipolar and unipolar) in the longer term (see section on Long-Term Complications).[80] A 10-year follow-up of unipolar and bipolar sterilization cases found higher failure rates with bipolar cautery than with unipolar cauter.[76] These high failure rates appear to be related to training and to technical problems with the instrumentation (*e.g.* incorrect wattage, etc.)[40,90] The spring clip has a lower force of compression than does the Filshie Clip and requires precise placement at a 90-degree angle across the tube with the isthmic portion of the tube positioned at the hinged part of the jaws in order to avoid failures.

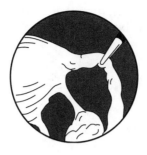

Source: Stewart et al. (1988).

Figure 15-5 A laparoscopy instrument grasps one tube in preparation for cautery or application of a ring or clip.

Vaginal Approach

The oviducts can be reached through an incision high in the vagina (called a colpotomy) posterior to the cervix. This allows direct visualization of the pelvic organs. The oviducts can also be reached through an endoscopic instrument called a culdoscope. In several countries, vaginal approaches have been found to be less safe and less effective than minilaparotomy and laparoscopic approaches. Infection has been more common, and the techniques are generally more difficult to learn and perform. Therefore, the vaginal approach should be used only for exceptional cases and performed in a well-equipped facility by a skilled surgeon.[89]

Transcervical Approach

Most of the hysteroscopic techniques to inject occlusive materials into the tubes are still experimental. Hysteroscopic techniques are difficult to learn, equipment is expensive, and the success rates for sterilization purposes have been generally disappointing.[66]

Also considered experimental are nonsurgical sterilization techniques using a chemical or other material to occlude the tubes through the cervix. Various agents, including quinacrine, methyl cyanoacrylate, and phenol have been used with varying success. The delivery systems are still being perfected to obtain higher levels of effectiveness and safety.[94]

The insertion of quinacrine pellets may hold potential as a method of nonsurgical sterilization. One study found that after two insertions of quinacrine pellets, 73% of women demonstrated bilateral tubal occlusion, and 94% did after a third insertion.[18] This method can be performed in any clinical setting capable of inserting an intrauterine device (IUD).[18]

Hysterectomy

Hysterectomy, whether performed through a vaginal or abdominal approach, carries a much higher risk of morbidity and mortality than other sterilization procedures. Therefore, it should not be performed for contraceptive purposes alone, but for a gynecologic disease or condition that justifies a hysterectomy.

POSTPARTUM AND POSTABORTION SURGICAL CONTRACEPTION

Subumbilical Minilaparotomy

The immediate postpartum period (within 48 hours of delivery) is the most common time for female sterilization in many countries and currently accounts for about 33% of female sterilizations in the United States.[68] This is largely explained by the greater convenience, lower costs, ease of surgery, and more efficient use of health resources. A hospital stay beyond that for a normal delivery (24 hours or less in many hospitals) is usually not required. (See also Suprapubic Minilaparotomy.)

Immediate postpartum VSC services should be an integral part of any maternity service. Many hospitals use a simple procedure room for postpartum VSC, although the delivery suite or operating theater is most commonly used. Following a procedure performed using local anesthesia and light sedation, the woman is often able to walk back to her bed with assistance. Preoperative assessment is facilitated because her health status can usually be assessed from the delivery and prenatal records. If minilaparotomy is performed at 10 or more hours after delivery, postpartum hemorrhage is unlikely to occur, and the status of the baby can be assessed more accurately.[62] (See Suprapubic Minilaparotomy for more on preoperative assessment.)

Procedure Immediately after delivery, the uterus and tubes are high in the abdomen. A small 1.5–3 cm incision just below the umbilicus is usually adequate to reach the tubes. Local anesthesia with light sedation and/or analgesia is frequently sufficient because several of the more painful aspects of minilaparotomy are reduced or eliminated:

- The incision is smaller
- Intra-abdominal manipulation of the tubes is less extensive
- The lithotomy position is not used
- The cervical tenaculum or uterine elevator are not required

The fallopian tubes are usually easier to reach if the incision is made over each tube by placing a hand on the side of the abdomen and moving the postpartum uterus.

When a minilaparotomy is not feasible, perform a laparotomy (defined as an incision larger than 5 cm), usually with use of general, spinal, or epidural anesthesia. Laparotomy incisions carry higher morbidity,[42] however, and the anesthesia methods also increase the risk and prolong recovery times. The laparoscope is not used in the immediate postpartum period because of the risk of injury to the large vascular uterus. In addition, the oviducts are edematous and vascular—thus larger. The laparoscopic occlusion methods are not appropriate.

Occlusion techniques. (See Figure 15-1.) The Pomeroy technique using plain catgut is an effective and safe approach and is the most widely employed method to occlude the tubes in the immediate postpartum period. A loop of tube in the midportion is ligated with plain catgut and is then excised. The Pritchard (Parkland) technique avoids the approximation of the cut ends and preserves more of the tube than the Pomeroy technique. The mesosalpinx is perforated in an avascular area; the tube is ligated in two places with one-zero chromic catgut; and the intervening segment is excised.[47,62]

A fimbriectomy has sometimes been performed since the ampullary and fimbrial portions of the tubes are more readily accessible than the isthmic and ampullary portions. However, the fimbriectomy method of sterilization has gained less favor because it is less reversible, removes more tissue, has been associated with high failure rates, and may cause more postoperative complications.

The Falope-Ring, the Fishie Clip, and the Spring Clip (Hulka, Rocket or Wolf Clip) are not suitable or recommended for immediate postpartum application. Electrocoagulation is also not recommended as a postpartum method. It is usually delivered via laparoscopy.

Cesarean Section

Tubal occlusion can be readily accomplished during cesarean section. However, because of the greater risks involved with cesarean section, it should not be performed solely to occlude the tubes.

High pregnancy rates following simple ligature by silk suture has resulted in methods that excise a portion of the tube. The use of the Pomeroy technique (a single plain catgut ligature at midportion of tube with excision of around 2 cm of ligature portion) at the time of a cesarean section has reported a slightly higher failure rate, but lack of surgical skill may be a factor.[38,39] The Pritchard (Parkland) procedure, shown in Figure 15-1, is the method now ideally favored. It involves two individual sutures, use of chronic catgut, and excision of a small central tubal portion. The Irving technique (which requires a wide surgical exposure for implanting the proximal end of the tube into the uterine wall and is thus possible with cesarean section) is one of the most effective methods and is unlikely to permit an ectopic pregnancy.[62]

Postabortion VSC

Tubal occlusion may be performed immediately after a first-trimester spontaneous or medically induced abortion as long as careful attention is given to counseling (clients have a higher risk of regret following postabortion sterilization[65]), informed choice, and medical contraindications. A minilaparotomy (incision somewhat higher than for a nonpregnant woman) or a laparoscopic approach may be used. The tubes will generally be less engorged and edematous than in the immediate postpartum period but will still require extra care during a minilaparotomy or a laparoscopy in which clips or Silastic rings are applied. (See sections on minilaparotomy and laparoscopy complications.)

Occlusion techniques may include the Pomeroy or Pritchard procedures with minilaparotomy. Failures with Silastic rings or spring clips used in the postabortion period are of less concern than in the immediate postpartum period.

ANESTHESIA

General anesthesia provided by trained personnel in appropriate settings can be safe and is the most frequently used method for female sterilization procedures in the United States. A discussion of general anesthesia is beyond the scope of this text. Local anesthesia with light sedation is generally sufficient to minimize the pain caused by sterilization procedures. By not compromising the normal physiological control of vital functions, a high level of safety can be maintained. It is important to avoid high doses of opioid (narcotic) analgesics and benzodiazepine (tranquilizer) sedatives that can compromise ventilation, sometimes dramatically, and may cause cardiovascular depression.

This therefore mandates that trained and competent personnel provide anesthesia support. A sample regimen for analgesia/local anesthesia follows for minilaparotomy, which is also suitable for laparoscopy with some modifications as noted. (Doses given are for an average adult body weight of 50 kg.)

Premedication

Sedate the woman with diazepam (Valium), 10 mg given with a sip of water 30–60 minutes before the operation. Midazolam (Versed), a new short-acting parenteral benzodiazepine, which is 3-4 times more potent than diazepam, may be substituted. (Give 2.5-3 mg intramuscularly 1 hour preoperatively, or 1-2.5 mg intravenously in the operating room.)

Given in the Operating Room

1. Atropine 0.4-06 mg intravenously.
2. Meperidine (Demerol) 50 mg intravenously. Other opioid analgesics or ketamine can be substituted for meperidine. The intravenous doses, each of which give analgesia approximately equivalent to 50 mg meperidine, are listed in Table 15-3.[89]

Table 15-3 Substititutes for meperedine anesthesia for female sterilization

Drug	Intravenous Dose	Analgesic Duration
Meperidine (Demerol)	50 mg	2–3 hours
Fentanyl (Sublimaze)	0.05–0.06 mg	30–60 minutes
Pentazocine (Talwin)	15–20 mg	2–3 hours
Butorphanol (Stadol)	1 mg	3–4 hours
Ketamine (Ketalar)	25–30 mg*	10–15 minutes

*Short acting – supplemental doses about one-third less than the initial ketamine dose may be given at 10-minute intervals as needed.

3. Promethazine (Phenergan) 25 mg intravenously.

4. Lidocaine local anesthesia. Infiltrate the skin and subcutaneous tissues with 1% lidocaine (=lignocaine) (Xylocaine) 10-15 ml (without epinephrine). After opening the peritoneal cavity, 5 ml of 1% lidocaine may be flowed onto each tube and the uterus. During laparoscopy, this step is optional if the instrument does not permit lidocaine application. During double-puncture laparoscopy, the second site will also be infiltrated. The maximum safe dose of 1% lidocaine (without epinephrine) is 5 mg/kg body weight; for a woman weighing 50 kg the maximum safe dose is 250 mg or 25 ml of 1% lidocaine. If only 2% lidocaine is available, dilute to 1% with 0.9% sodium chloride only in order to better obtain adequate volume for local infiltration and to avoid exceeding the safe dose. Some surgeons will use sodium bicarbonate (1 cc of 8.4% sodium bicarbonate (standard vile percentage) with 25 cc of 1% lidocaine) to decrease the burning sensation caused by the anesthesia infiltration in the subcutaneous space.

Monitor vital signs regularly during the operation and postoperatively until the woman is fully recovered and alert. The World Federation for the Advancement of Surgical Contraception publications describe anesthesia techniques in greater detail.[89]

PROVIDING VASECTOMY

Strictly adhere to the technical guidelines on providing vasectomy.[91] In a preoperative history, take an inventory of past illnesses and surgeries, bleeding disorders, allergies (particularly to local anesthetics and pain medications), heart disease, kidney and bladder infection, diabetes, anemia and sexually transmitted diseases. Evaluate the man's general health condition, including taking the pulse and blood pressure; assessing for local infections in the scrotal or inguinal area or inguinal hernia/previous surgery in the inguinal area; evaluating the scrotum for hydrocele or varicocele; and determining if the testicles are properly descended and/or are fixed in place. Assess the scrotal skin and subcutaneous tissues to see if there are factors that might affect a surgical procedure.

Laboratory examinations are not routinely performed, but should be available. If elements in the history or physical so indicate, obtain a lab test (*e.g.* liver function, bleeding and clotting time, etc.).

Procedure: Clip the man's hair from his scrotum and around his penis (if this was not already done at home). Wash the area with soap and water, just before surgery. Use an effective antiseptic (usually a water-based iodine or 4% chlorhexidine solution) to prep the scrotum, thighs, and perineum, and drape the area. Use sterile technique to perform the procedure. Anchor the vasa (two tubular structures, one in each side of the scrotum) with an atraumatic instrument or fingers. Infiltrate 1% lidocaine (lignocaine) without epinephrine into the area to be incised and then deeply into the perivasal tissue. Incise the skin and muscle overlying the vas, or open these with the no-scalpel method (see following section on No-Scalpel Vasectomy). Through this small incision, isolate the vas, occlude, and in most cases, resect a small portion (see Figure 15-6). Perform the same procedure for the vas on the other side. Close the incisions with absorbable suture. Some surgeons use only a single midline incision, and some do not suture small skin incisions.[2,33,89] If possible, the patient should rest 15 minutes to half an hour, or longer if needed, before he leaves.

Occlusion Techniques. Once the vas is isolated, divide it. The cut ends may be fulgurated to a depth of 1 cm in each direction by inserting a needle electrode or hot wire cautery into the lumen. Alternatively, some surgeons tie each end with a simple ligature using absorbable or nonabsorbable suture, being careful not to cut through the vas. Sperm granulomas occur more often at the cut ends after the ligature technique, possibly contributing to a somewhat higher failure rate than when fulguration is used. A segment of the vas may be removed to obtain greater separation, although this is not considered necessary. For either occlusion technique, create a fascial barrier between the ends by drawing the sheath over one end and suturing it.[2,89] This latter technique may decrease the failure rate.

A recent modification performed by a few surgeons is to leave the testicular end of the vas open ("open-ended vasectomy") and fulgurate the abdominal end to a depth of 1.5 cm. A fascial barrier may then be interposed. This method appears to reduce the frequency of postoperative congestive epididymitis without increasing the rate of painful sperm granulomas.[2,19,20,52] Some surgeons report increased failure rates, but open-ended vasectomy may reduce postoperative complaints. Success rates for reversal may also be higher than when both ends are fulgurated.

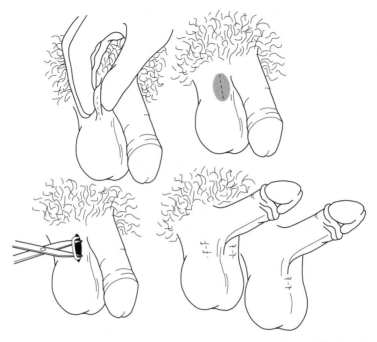

Source: Hatcher et al. (1983).

Figure 15-6 Sites of vasectomy incisions

NO-SCALPEL VASECTOMY

A new refined "no-scalpel" procedure is currently being used in many programs around the world, including in the United States. The no-scalpel vasectomy technique was developed in 1974 in China. It is the standard vasectomy technique in China, where more than 9 million men have had the procedure.[26] It is rapidly becoming the procedure of choice in Thailand, India, and Indonesia.[34,45] The surgical approach reaches the vas through a puncture in the scrotum rather than through a scalpel incision.[5] Thereafter, the surgical procedure is the same as the scalpel method. The no-scalpel method appears to have lower complication rates as compared with the scalpel method. This may especially help reduce anxieties about vasectomy for hematomas.[33]

This procedure employs two unique instruments. After local anesthetic is injected, a specially designed ring forceps encircles and firmly secures the vas without penetrating the skin. The second instrument, a sharp-tipped dissecting forceps, punctures and stretches a small opening in the skin and vas sheath. The vas is lifted out and occluded as with other vasectomy techniques. The same midline puncture site is used to deliver and occlude the other vas in an almost bloodless procedure. No sutures are needed to close the small wound (see Figure 15-7).

C OUNSELING FOR MALE AND FEMALE STERILIZATION

The goal of counseling is to provide the client with information and guidance that will result in their voluntary selection of a contraceptive method which they will use, which will be effective, and which will not have adverse effects. Sterilization methods have one characteristic that can offer an advantage or a disadvantage, depending upon how one looks at it. It is meant to be a permanent method of contraception. Reversals can be done in some people but are expensive, require major surgery, and the results are not guaranteed.

A number of circumstances can lead to a high degree of regret among users. Identifying these individuals prior to sterilization is helpful, but in most circumstances, unpredictable life changes are the cause of regret. Predictors of regret include the following:

- Loss of children
- Divorce or remarriage
- Desire for children/more children
- Sterilization used because of unhappiness with a reversible method

Two events correlate highly with requests for sterilization reversal: age of client and change in marital status.[10,31,85,86] Young clients need to be very carefully counseled to be certain their decision is based upon a sound assessment.

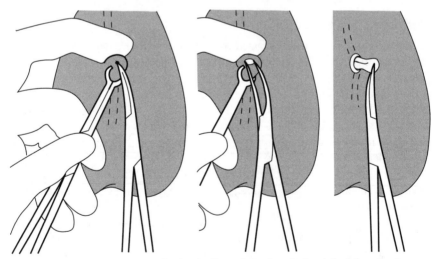

Reprinted with permission from the Population Information Program.

Figure 15-7 "No-scalpel vasectomy." The vas (dotted line) is grasped by special ring forceps and the skin and the vas sheath are pierced by sharp-tipped dissecting forceps (A). The forceps then stretch an opening (B) and the vas is lifted out (C).

VSC should be strongly discouraged in a man or woman whose marriage is unstable. The health and age of the youngest child may also be a factor in choosing this contraceptive method, particularly in areas of high infant mortality. Sterilization around the time of pregnancy is associated with an increased incidence of regret in many studies.[11,60,65,86] People who are poor,[31] (*e.g.* Medicaid clients), men and women of Hispanic origin,[31] and those who divorce[31,86] also make up a disproportionate group of those who would wish a reversal procedure.

The clear answer is to provide clients with choices. New and old long-term contraceptive methods (*e.g.* DMPA, TCu 380A IUDs, and Norplant) can be excellent methods for women who wish a permanent, single-decision method. In addition to choice, the availability of surgical reversal of sterilization seems ethically and programmatically justifiable.

In the United States, awareness of surgical contraception is widespread, and one of the interviewer's tasks is to assure that the individual correctly understands the procedure and has no misconceptions (see Table 15-4).

Give the client sufficient time to make a thoughtful, informed decision about a permanent method of contraception, especially women having immediate postpartum or postabortion (spontaneous or induced) sterilization. Whenever possible, the woman should have decided she wants a permanent method well before delivery or a pregnancy-related event or procedure. The concern is that her decision may be unduly influenced by the emotional and physical stress produced by the pregnancy and related events. Postpartum and postabortion sterilization clients have a higher rate of regret following sterilization.[85,86]

Women who come to the hospital for the first time during labor may be counseled after delivery when they are free of the immediate stresses related to labor and delivery and are not under the influence of sedatives. If the baby is healthy and the woman clearly desires no more children, she may be a suitable candidate for VSC. Husbands should also be brought into the discussion whenever possible; however, spousal consent should not be mandatory.

For postpartum clients, medical assessment after delivery is essential to assure the patient is a suitable surgical candidate. Medical problems such as eclampsia, postpartum hemorrhage, or endometritis might lead to postponing the VSC surgical procedure until a more optimal time.

Staff should be skilled in explaining and providing alternative postpartum methods, such as the intrauterine device (IUD) or Norplant, which may be inserted immediately postplacental or postpartum, if VSC is not the preferred choice. Women should feel no pressure to decide upon sterilization because of the unavailability of alternative methods or lack of clinical skill to provide them. Moreover, delayed VSC services should be available so that if uncertainty or any medical contraindication exists at the time, the procedure can be comfortably scheduled at 4 weeks or later after delivery.

Table 15-4 Counseling guidelines for surgical sterilization

The following guidelines may be helpful in any discussion of surgical contraception. We have developed the BRAIDED mnemonic for remembering them:

Benefits:	A single decision provides a permanent, highly effective, and "natural" method of birth control.
Risks:	Risks include infection, bleeding, complications of anesthesia, a slight chance of becoming pregnant in the future (but less than with other methods used over the years). Procedures to reverse the sterilization are expensive, involve major surgery and risk, are not available to everyone, and are often unsuccessful.
Alternatives:	Explain and make available reversible contraceptive methods.
Inquiries:	Encourage and answer questions; correct myths and misinformation.
Decision to Change:	Remind the client that he or she should feel free to decide against surgical contraception without loss of any medical or financial benefits.
Explanation:	Explain in detail the entire procedure and its possible side effects. Emphasize the permanence of the procedure. Be realistic about the chances of reversal. Explain what is known about effects on future health and sexual response (which should not be affected by the procedure). Inform clients of any costs they will bear. Make sure clients understand their obligations during the preoperative and postoperative periods.
Documentation:	The client's medical record should note the method and timing of surgical contraception, any complications that occurred during or after the procedure, and the management and outcome of any complications.

If the procedure is delayed beyond 4 weeks after delivery and she is not breastfeeding, the woman should be advised to use an effective contraceptive method until the sterilization procedure.

POLICY/LEGAL ISSUES

Laws and regulations regarding sterilization procedures have undergone many changes over the last number of years. Clinicians must be aware of certain rulings in counseling discussions with sterilization candidates.

1. Pragmatically, ethically, and legally, strict adherence to informed[72] choice and consent procedures is critical prior to sterilization.
2. Partner or spousal consent in the United States is not legally required.[13]
3. Clients using federal or state funds for sterilization must be age 21 or older, mentally competent, and must wait 30 days after signing a consent for performance of a VSC procedure.[21]

Arbitrary decisions by health professionals to restrict access to sterilization have been judged by courts in the United States to violate a woman's basic rights. Clear guidelines regarding eligibility for services, complying with law, and following the standards for informed choice and informed consent are most important in providing sterilization services.

The policy and legal status of providing sterilization to retarded women and men remains a problem. Clear guidelines that allow the procedures for deserving clients need to be established. Health care providers, policy makers, and the public should be informed of the ethical and legal issues involved in providing voluntary sterilization to those who may not be able to provide informed consent.

Informed Consent

Informed consent is the voluntary decision made by a person who has been fully informed regarding the surgical procedure and its consequences. Provide the information in a language that the client can understand. Most informed consent documents cover the following important points:

1. Type of operation, including risks and benefits
2. Availability of alternative methods of family planning
3. The fact that the operation, if successful, will prevent the client from having any more children
4. Intended permanence of sterilization
5. Possibility of reversal, but it is expensive, requires a highly technical and major surgery, and its results cannot be guaranteed
6. Possibility of failure (pregnancy) after the procedure
7. Option to decline surgical contraception without loss of medical or financial benefits

The client must always sign or mark the informed consent form. The surgeon or his or her authorized representative must also sign the form. The authorized representative may be the person with the primary responsibility for counseling the client.

Illiterate clients should mark the informed consent form with a thumbprint or "X"; a witness chosen by the client must also sign or mark the form. Preferably, the witness should be of the same sex as the client. The informed consent document should be readily understandable in the client's own language.

M ANAGING PROBLEMS AND FOLLOW-UP

FEMALE STERILIZATION

Complications occur in less than 1% of all sterilization cases. The types of complications vary by the type of surgical procedure and anesthesia. Most of these complications can be prevented by careful screening, local anesthesia with light sedation, close monitoring of vital signs, good asepsis, and careful surgical technique. Infection prevention in family planning programs must always be a high priority.[78] The seriousness of complications can often be minimized by early recognition and aggressive management.

Anesthesia complications can be severe; therefore, use local anesthesia, discussed in section on Anesthesia. Surgical complications require knowing that the abdominal wall is thin at the umbilicus and thus the dissection and entry into the peritoneal cavity must be cautious in order to avoid cutting the intestine.

- Brisk bleeding from the engorged postpartum vessels can be avoided by gentle handling of the tubes.
- Postoperative hemorrhage can be avoided if ligatures around the tubes are secure to prevent slipping.
- Infections are minimized by screening clients preoperatively and avoiding surgery on patients with prolonged ruptured membranes with evidence of current infections (with fever). Prophylactic antibiotics are usually given if the procedure is performed between the 3rd and 7th postpartum day. If the procedure cannot be performed within 7 days after delivery, it is often advisable to wait until 4–6 weeks postpartum, primarily because of the technical difficulty of reaching the oviducts.[62,89]

Laparoscopy Complications

Although complications from laparoscopy are not more common than from minilaparotomy, some are more severe.[56] The rate of laparoscopic complications is highly dependent on the level of surgical skill. To reduce complications, the operator should receive special training in laparoscopy. Surgeons performing fewer than 100 procedures per year have a much higher complication rate than more experienced surgeons.

The insufflation needle should have a blunt obturator (as does the Veress needle), and correct placement should be verified by aspiration, hanging drop, or pressure test.[89] Keep equipment in good working order; keep the trocar sharp. When removing the cannula after all gas has been expelled, reinsert the laparoscope to the end of the cannula to prevent omentum or bowel from herniating into the abdominal wall defects as the cannula is removed.[89]

Anesthesia. Anesthesia-related complications can be aggravated by the gas-filled abdomen and the Trendelenburg position, especially if general anesthesia is used.

Tears and transections. Complications such as mesosalpingeal tears and transection of the tube can occur with ring application, which may require laparotomy to control bleeding. Sometimes an additional ring can be placed on each severed end of the tube for hemostasis.

Instrumental trauma. Uterine perforation with the uterine elevator can usually be managed conservatively. Injuries to vessels, intestines, or other organs can occur with the insufflation needle or the trocar. General anesthesia back-up is necessary when doing laparoscopy sterilization procedures in order to manage rare complications of severe bleeding from a major vessel.

Burns. Bowel burns can occur from electrocoagulation, resulting in late perforation and peritonitis. Although the bipolar cautery may carry less risk of burns than unipolar electrocoagulation, most international agencies discontinued support for electrocoagulation in the early 1980s. Most laparoscopic injuries are not related to the cautery, but rather the trocar or other surgical instruments.[44] Bowel burns occur as a result of a direct insult to the bowel and not from indirect contact with a hot uterine tube or instrument.[16]

Minilaparotomy Complications

Wound infection. As with all surgical procedures, careful aseptic technique, proper skin preparation, sterilization of instruments, appropriate operating room technique, and diligent postoperative wound care decrease the likelihood of infection.

Uterine perforation with uterine elevator. Gentle use of *all* instruments on human tissues minimizes trauma. Determine uterine versing position prior to inserting the elevator.

Bladder injury. This common surgical complication occurs because of the proximity of the bladder at the lower incision. Careful dissection and attention to landmarks assist in prevention.

Intestinal injury. Recognition of tissue layers and careful entry into the abdominal cavity help in prevention. If injury is unrecognized, serious complications arise; therefore, prompt recognition is paramount.

Long-term Complications

Ectopic pregnancy. Rule out ectopic pregnancy any time a woman shows signs of pregnancy following tubal occlusion. Compared with an ectopic rate of 0.5%–1.0% among pregnancies of nonsterilized women, the rate of ectopic pregnancies among pregnancies in sterilized women ranges from 4%–73% of pregnancies, depending upon the procedure used.[47] One survey showed that 16% of clip pregnancies, 38% of ring pregnancies, 73% of unipolar pregnancies, 59% of bipolar pregnancies, and 44% of Pomeroy occlusion pregnancies were ectopic.[36]

A report from Korea of 4,361 ectopic pregnancies following sterilization suggests approximately a three-fold greater incidence of ectopic pregnancy associated with electrocoagulation than with the use of the Silastic ring. Ectopic pregnancies continued to occur at 6 and more years after sterilization. Ectopic pregnancy was most often related to the following:[41,84]

- Uteroperitoneal fistula after unipolar electrocoagulation
- Inadequate coagulation or recanalization after bipolar procedures
- Recanalization or fistula formation after the Pomeroy, clip, or ring procedure

Hormonal changes.   The effect of tubal occlusion on hormonal feedback between the pituitary and ovaries has been extensively studied.[3,14,77] While levels of LH, FSH, testosterone, and estrogen remain within the normal range, serum progesterone may decline;[17,49,63,64] other investigators have reached different conclusions.[3,14] No studies have evaluated presterilization and poststerilization levels.[35]

Menstrual patterns and other changes.   Abnormal menstrual patterns have been thought to occur following sterilization, and a "post-tubal-ligation syndrome" has been proposed. However, a specific and describable pattern of bleeding after sterilization has not been convincingly demonstrated.[4] Most studies find no changes, unpredictable changes, or that the changes could best be explained on the basis of discontinuing the pill or the IUD.[15,82] One study, however, found that increased menstrual flow and pain were significantly increased by the fifth year after sterilization.[87] Another study found that tubal sterilization is associated with a greater risk of hospitalization for menstrual disorders.[70] Further research needs to be conducted on this issue.

Psychological problems.   Psychological problems have been identified no more often in sterilized than in nonsterilized women.[9,82,87,90] A study on the impact of tubal sterilization and vasectomy on female marital sexuality found no detrimental long-term effects and, in fact, found an increase in coital frequency after 1 year in tubal sterilization women as compared with women not planning sterilization.[69]

Hysterectomy and other surgery.   Because of the questionable hormonal and menstrual changes following sterilization procedures, surgeries such as hysterectomies and D&Cs are sometimes performed. One study found an increased risk of hysterectomy among women who were sterilized while 20–29 years old but not among women sterilized over 30 years old.[74] No biological basis for these results, however, has been found. Consideration of these surgeries must be included in the long-term morbidity associated with sterilization.

VASECTOMY

Mortality is extremely rare (about one death in 300,000 procedures) when asepsis and surgical skills meet basic standards.[67] Bleeding complications with vasectomy can be minimized by careful surgical technique and assuring that men avoid strenuous activity for a day or two. Hematomas are also prevented by careful attention to hemostasis (controlling any bleeding) during the operation (see Table 15-5). Small noninfected hematomas may be managed with rest and analgesics; large, painful, or infected hematomas usually require surgical drainage. One of the main advantages claimed by the no-scalpel method is a decreased rate of bleeding complications.

Infections occurring with vasectomy procedures are prevented by strict aseptic practices, by sterilized equipment, and by having the patient keep the incision clean. If an infection does occur, it should be treated with antibiotics and frequently with wet heat to the area. Leakage of sperm from the occluded end of the vas can cause an inflammatory nodule (granuloma) that generally subsides spontaneously, although pain and medication may be required. The rare granuloma that increases in size, is painful, and does not recede may be treated surgically. Congestive epididymitis may occur due to back pressure in the occluded vas. With heat treatment and scrotal support, the condition usually subsides in a week.

REVERSAL OF FEMALE AND MALE STERILIZATION

VSC should be considered permanent, but even with careful counseling, some women and men will request reversal following a divorce or remarriage, a child's death, or the desire for more children.[30,71,85] The following points should be emphasized:

- Reversal requires major surgery and special skills.
- Some clients are not appropriate candidates because of the way the sterilization was performed, because of the client's or partner's advanced age, or because of the infertility of the spouse.
- Success cannot be guaranteed, even when the patient is a good candidate and the surgery is performed by an experienced microsurgeon.
- Reversal surgery is very expensive for both male and female procedures.

Table 15-5 Summary of medical complications of vasectomy

Complications	% of Procedures (N = 24,961)
Hematoma	1.6
Infection	1.5
Epididymitis	1.4
Granuloma	0.3
Failure	0.4

Source: Wortman (1975).

In addition, the candidate should understand that there are operative risks due to anesthesia and the usual risks of major abdominal or scrotal surgery. There is also a risk of ectopic pregnancy after reversal of female sterilization: The rate is about 5% for women who have an electrocoagulation procedure reversed and about 2% for women who have other occlusion techniques reversed.[47]

If the woman wishes to proceed after counseling, a laparoscopy is usually done to determine the condition of the tubes, and infertility tests may be performed for her and her husband. Most surgeons will not operate if less than 4 cm of healthy tube remains.

Success Rates for Reversal of Female Sterilization

Success rates based on intrauterine pregnancies after reversal surgery are highest for occlusion techniques that damage the smallest segment of oviduct (see Table 15-6).[47] If success rates were given as a percentage of all women requesting reversal, the differences would be further magnified, because many women are not accepted for surgery (as many as 70% in some studies) when the remaining length of healthy tube is inadequate.[30,71]

Higher success rates are generally achieved through the use of microsurgical techniques that require special training and combine several features including:

- Use of magnification (loupe, hood, or operating microscope)
- Accurate alignment of the fallopian tube segments and placement of sutures
- Constant irrigation of tissues to prevent drying
- Use of very fine suture and needles
- Microsurgical electrocautery to minimize bleeding
- Care to keep foreign materials from being left in the wound.

Table 15-6 Tubal damage and reversal pregnancy rate by tubal occlusion method

Technique	Tubal Damage cm	Reversal Pregnancy Rate %
Clip	1	88
Thermal Cautery	2	No Studies
Ring	3	75
Pomeroy	3–4	59
Electrocoagulation	3–6	43

Sources: Haber (1988), Liskin (1985).

Women must consider any sterilization technique as permanent, even clips, because reversal is not always successful and reversal surgery will not be available to all who want it. For women who are poor candidates for reversal surgery, *in vitro* fertilization (IVF) may be an option. (See Chapter 23 on Infertility.)

Success Rates for Reversal of Vasectomy

Microsurgical technique is important when restoring continuity of the vas, just as in female reversal. An operating microscope using higher magnification (25 power) is usually employed. Under these circumstances, reported pregnancy rates range from 16%–79%, with most rates approaching 50% or above. The success is determined in part by the time from vasectomy until reversal, with success rates being inversely related. (The greater the length, the less likely the pregnancy.)[7,8,43] The percentage of men with sperm in the ejaculate is higher, ranging from 81%–98%, which should not be presented to men as the measure of success, since pregnancy is the desired outcome, not presence of sperm.

The pregnancy success rate can depend on several factors, including the skill of the surgeon/microsurgeon. Factors that may reduce chances of success are (1) increased time since the vasectomy was performed, (2) presence of antisperm antibodies, (3) advanced age of the wife, and (4) the way the vasectomy was performed (long segment of vas removed, location near the epididymis, and use of cautery). Attempts to develop a plug, valve, or simple reversible vasectomy have not been successful.[46] Men must accept vasectomy as a permanent procedure even though improved microsurgical techniques have increased the chances of restoring fertility.

INSTRUCTIONS FOR VOLUNTARY SURGICAL CONTRACEPTION

FEMALE STERILIZATION

Preoperative Instructions

1. Be completely comfortable with your decision to use a surgical method for contraception. You must be certain that you understand and desire a permanent method of birth control. Be certain all of your questions have been asked and answered. You can change your mind at any time before the procedure or can postpone the operation if you need more time to think about it.

2. Shower or bathe just before surgery. Pay particular attention to the area around the umbilicus (navel) and the pubic hair.

3. **Do not eat or drink** in the 8 hours before surgery.

4. Have someone accompany you on the day of surgery, if at all possible. This person should accompany you when you go home. You should plan to have someone with you for the first 24 hours following surgery.

5. **Rest for at least 24 hours** after the procedure and avoid heavy lifting for 1 week.

6. Be prepared for pain over the incision and occasional pelvic aching or discomfort. The pain is usually not severe and can be relieved with mild pain medications provided to you.

7. Plan a flexible schedule for the week after the sterilization. Some women recover less quickly than others from the effects of anesthesia and surgery.

8. Be certain to ask questions if you have them.

Postoperative Instructions

1. **Rest for 24 hours following surgery.** Resume normal activities as you gradually become more comfortable.

2. **Avoid intercourse for 1 week** and stop if it is uncomfortable.

3. **Avoid strenuous lifting for 1 week** to allow the incisions to heal.

4. Return to the clinic or contact the clinic or doctor promptly if you develop:

Postoperative Warning Signs

Caution

■ Fever (greater than 100.4°F, 39°C)

■ Dizziness with fainting

■ Abdominal pain that is persistent or increasing

■ Bleeding or fluid coming from the incision

■ If you should ever get pregnant, you must be seen immediately

---

5. Take one or two analgesic tablets at 4- to 6-hour intervals if you need them for pain. (Do not use aspirin since it may promote bleeding.)

6. You may bathe 48 hours after surgery but avoid putting tension on the incision and do not rub or irritate the incision for 1 week. Dry the incision site after bathing.

7. Stitches will dissolve and do not require removal. (Note to provider: this instruction must be modified if nonabsorbable sutures such as silk are used.)

8. **Return to the clinic 1 week after the procedure** to make sure that the healing process is normal.

9. If you think you are pregnant at any time in the future, return to the clinic immediately. Although pregnancy after female surgical con-

traception is rare, when it does occur, chances are increased that it will be outside the uterus (an ectopic pregnancy). This is a dangerous life-threatening condition and must be treated immediately.

10. You should know that this method of birth control is permanent. Reversal surgery is possible under certain conditions, but it is expensive, requires highly technical and major surgery, and its results cannot be guaranteed.

VASECTOMY

Preoperative Instructions

1. Become completely sure of your decision to have a vasectomy. You must be certain that you understand and desire the permanence of vasectomy. You can change your mind at any time before the operation.

2. Before surgery while you are home, use scissors to cut all hair from around the penis and scrotum to approximately 1/4-in. in length.

3. Shower or bathe, washing the penis and scrotum thoroughly to remove all loose hairs.

4. If possible, have someone accompany you home when you have the procedure done. Do not ride a bicycle and avoid walking long distances or using other transportation that may rub or put pressure on the scrotum.

5. **Plan to remain quiet for approximately 48 hours** following the vasectomy. A 48-hour "rest" is important to decrease the risk of complications.

Postoperative Instructions

1. Following the surgery, return home and rest for about 2 days. If possible, **keep an ice pack on the scrotum for at least 4 hours** to reduce the chances of swelling, bleeding, and discomfort. Wear a scrotal support for 2 days. (Jockey shorts will be adequate.) You may be able to resume your normal activities after 2 or 3 days.

2. **Avoid strenuous physical exercise for 1 week.** Strenuous exercise means hard physical exertion or lifting or straining that could bring pressure to the groin or scrotum.

3. Do not shower or bathe for the first 2 days after the vasectomy.

4. The stitches will dissolve and do not have to be removed. (Note to provider: this instruction must be modified if nonabsorbable skin sutures, such as silk, are used or if are no skin sutures are used.)

5. **You may resume sexual intercourse after 2 or 3 days** if you feel that it would be comfortable; but remember, **you are not sterile immediately**. For many men, sperm will not be cleared from the tubes until after approximately 15 ejaculations. Until then, use

condoms or another method of birth control to prevent pregnancy. The best way of finding out if you are sterile is to have the doctor look at your semen under a microscope after you have 15 ejaculations.

6. If you have pain or discomfort, simple analgesics taken at intervals of 4–6 hours usually give adequate relief. (Note to provider: name and dose should be specified.)

7. It is important for you to know what is normal and what is abnormal following your surgery. You will probably have some pain and swelling in the scrotal region; the scrotum may be somewhat discolored. This is normal and should not worry you. Occasionally, blood from a tiny blood vessel may escape into the scrotum at the time of surgery, and bleeding may continue. Notify your doctor or health worker if you have any of the following danger signals or if you notice any other unusual body changes:

Postoperative Warning Signs

Caution

- Fever
- Bleeding or pus from the site of the incision
- Excessive pain or swelling

For any of these problems, you must return to the clinic for medical care without delay.

---

8. You should know that this method of birth control is permanent. Reversal surgery is possible under certain conditions, but it is expensive, requires highly technical and major surgery, and its results cannot be guaranteed.

REFERENCES

1. Alexander NJ, Clarkson TB. Vasectomy increases the severity of diet-induced atherosclerosis in Macaca fascicularis. Science 1978;201(4355):538-541.
2. Alderman P. The lurking sperm: a review of failures in 8879 vasectomies performed by one physician. JAMA 1988;259(21):3142-3144.
3. Alvarez-Sanchez F, Segal SJ, Brache V, Adejuwan CA, Leon P, Faundes A. Pituitary-ovarian function after tubal ligation. Fertil Steril 1981;36(5): 606-609.
4. Association for Voluntary Sterilization. Menstrual function following tubal sterilization. Biomed Bull 1981;2:1.
5. Association for Voluntary Sterilization. No-scalpel vasectomy: an illustrated guide for surgeons. New York NY: Association for Voluntary Surgical Contraception, 1992.
6. Association for Voluntary Surgical Contraception News 1989;27(July):1.
7. Bagshaw HA, Masters JRW, Pryor JP. Factors influencing the outcome of vasectomy reversal. Br J Urol 1990;52:57-60.
8. Belker AM, Konnak JW, Sharlip ID, Thomas AJ. Intraoperative observations during vasovasotomy in 334 patients. J Urol 1993;149(3):524-527.

9. Bledin KD, Cooper JE, Mackenzie S, Brice B. Psychological sequelae of female sterilization: short-term outcome in a prospective controlled study. Psychol Med 1984;14(2):379-390.
10. Boring CC, Rochat RW, Becerra J. Sterilization regret among Puerto Rican women. Fertil Steril 1988;49(6):973-981.
11. Chi IC, Gates D, Thapa S. Performing tubal sterilizations during a women's post-partum hospitalization: a review of the United States and international experiences. Obstet Gynecol Surv 1992;47(2):71-79.
12. Clarkson TB, Alexander NJ. Long-term vasectomy: effects on the occurrence and extent of atherosclerosis in rhesus monkeys. J Clin Invest 1980;65(1):15-25.
13. Coe vs. Bolton. United States District Court, Civil Action No. C-76-785-A. September 29, 1976 (N.D. Georgia).
14. Corson SL, Levinson CJ, Batzer FR, Otis C. Hormonal levels following sterilization and hysterectomy. J Repro Med 1981;26(7):363-370.
15. DeStefano F, Huezo CM, Peterson HB, Rubin GL, Layde PM, Ory HW. Menstrual changes after sterilization. Obstet Gynecol 1983;62(6):673-681.
16. DiGiovanni M, Vasilenko P, Belsky D. Laparascopic tubal sterilization. The potential for thermal bowel injury. J Repro Med 1990;35(10):951-4.
17. Donnez J, Wauters M, Thomas K. Luteal function after tubal sterilization. Obstet Gynecol 1981;57(1):65-68.
18. El Kady AA, Nagib HS, Kessel E. Efficacy and safety of repeated transcervical quinacrine pellet insertions for female sterilization. Fertil Steril 1993;59(2):301-304.
19. Errey BB. Follow-up of 6014 open-ended vasectomy cases. Personal communication with Gary Stewart, Sept. 4, 1987.
20. Errey BB, Edwards IS. Open-ended vasectomy: an assessment. Fertil Steril 1986; 45(6):843-846.
21. Federal Register 1978;43 Nov. 8:52146-52175.
22. Goldacre MJ, Holford TR, Vessey MP. Cardiovascular disease and vasectomy: findings from two epidemiologic studies. N Engl J Med 1983;308(14):805-808.
23. Giovannucci E, Tosteson TD, Speizer FE, Vessey MP, Colditz GA. A long-term study of mortality in men who have undergone vasectomy. N Engl J Med 1992;326(21):1392-1398.
24. Giovannucci E, Ascherio A, Rimm EB, Colditz GA, Stampfer MJ, Willett WC. A prospective study of vasectomy and prostate cancer in U.S. men. JAMA 1993;269(7):873-877.
25. Giovannucci E, Tosteson TD, Speizer FE, Ascherio A, Vessey MP, Colditz GA. A retrospective cohort study of vasectomy and prostate cancer in U.S. men. JAMA 1993;269(7):878-882.
26. Gonzales B, Barston-Ainley S, Vansintejan G, Li PS. No-scalpel vasectomy: an illustrated guide for surgeons. New York NY: Association for Voluntary Surgical Contraception, 1991.
27. Hasson HM. Open laparoscopy. Biomedical Bulletin, Association for Voluntary Surgical Contraception 1984;5(1).
28. Hasson HM. Open laparoscopy. In: Sciarra JJ (ed). Gynecology and obstetrics. Philadelphia PA: Harper & Row, 1982:44.
29. Hatcher RA, Dalmat ME, Delano GE, Fadhel SB, Kowal D, Mandara NA, Mati JK, Sai FT, Stewart FH, Stewart GK. Family planning methods and practice: Africa. DHHS, Center for Disease Control, 1983.
30. Henry A, Rinehart W, Piotrow PT. Reversing female sterilization. Popul Rep 1980;Series C(8):97-123.

31. Henshaw SK, Singh S. Sterilization regret among US couples. Fam Plann Perspect 1986:18(5):238-240.
32. Huber DH. Advances in voluntary surgical contraception. Outlook 1988;6(1).
33. Huber D. (Association for Voluntary Sterilization) Trip report, The People's Republic of China. June 19-30, 1985.
34. Huggins GR, Sondheimer SJ. Complications of female sterilization: immediate and delayed. Fertil Steril 1984;41(3):337-355.
35. Hulka JF, Peterson HB, Phillips JM. American Association of Gynecologic Laparoscopist's 1988 Membership Survey on Laparoscopic Sterilization. J Repro Med 1990;35(6):584-586.
36. Hulka JF. The spring clip: current clinical experience. In: Phillips JM. Endoscopic Female Sterilization. Downey CA: The American Association of Gynecologic Laparoscopists, 1983.
37. Husbands ME, Jr., Pritchard JA, Pritchard SA. Failure of tubal sterilization accompanying cesarean section. Am J Obstet Gynecol 1970:107(6):966-967.
38. Indian Council of Medical Research. Collaborative study on sequelae of tubal sterilization. New Delhi, 1982.
39. Kleppinger RK. An analysis of 7,000 laparoscopic sterilizations: unipolar, bipolar and mechanical occlusive. In: Phillips JM. Endoscopic female sterilization. Downey CA: The American Association of Gynecologic Laparoscopists, 1983.
40. Kwak Hyon-Mo. Laparoscopic sterilization: Korean experience, particularly ectopic pregnancy subsequent to female sterilization. Proceedings of the Pre-Congress Seminar of the XIth AUFOG Congress, Bangkok, Thailand, Dec. 1-4, 1987.
41. Layde PM, Peterson HB, Dicker RC, DeStefano F, Rubin GL. Risk factors for complications of interval tubal sterilization by laparotomy. Obstet Gynecol 1983;62(2):180-184.
42. Lee HY. Twenty-year experience with vasovasotomy. J Urol 1986;136(2):413-415.
43. Levy BS, Soderstrom RM, Dail DH. Bowel injuries during laparoscopy. Gross anatomy and histology. J Repro Med 1985;30(3):168-172.
44. Li S, Zhu J. Ligation of vas deferens with clamping method under direct vision. Unpublished, 1984.
45. Liskin L, Pile JM, Quillin WF. Vasectomy — safe and simple. Popul Rep 1983;Series D(4):61-100.
46. Liskin L, Rinehart W, Blackburn R, Rutledge AH. Minilaparotomy and laparoscopy: safe, effective and widely used. Popul Rep 1985;Series C(9):125-167.
47. Margolis A. Personal communication, to Gary K. Stewart 1992.
48. Mahgoub SE, Zeniny AE, Shourbagy ME, Tawil AE. Long-term luteal changes after tubal sterilization. Contraception 1984;30(2):125-134.
49. Massey FJ, Bernstein GS, O'Fallon WM, Schuman LM, Coulson AH, Crozier R, Mandel JS, Benjamin RB, Berendes HW, Chang PC. Vasectomy and health: results from a large cohort study. JAMA 1984;252:1023-1029.
50. Marquette C, Koonin L, Marston-Ainley S. Vasectomies in the United States: 1991. Presented at the American Public Health Association annual meeting, November 1992.
51. Moss WM. Vasectomy failure after use of an open-ended technique. Fertil Steril 1985;43(4):667-668.
52. Ortho Pharmaceutical Corporation. 1991 Ortho Annual Birth Control Survey. Raritan NJ.
53. Penfield AJ. Female sterilization by minilaparotomy or open laparoscopy. Baltimore MD: Urban and Schwarzenberg, 1980.

55. Peterson HB, Hulka JF, Spielman FJ, Lee S, Marchbanks PA. Local versus general anesthesia for laparoscopic sterilization: a randomized study. Obstet Gynecol 1987;70(6):903-908.

56. Peterson HB, DeStefano F, Rubin GL, Greenspan JR, Lee NC, Ory HW. Deaths attributed to tubal sterilization in the United States, 1977 to 1981. Am J Obstet Gynecol 1983;146(2):131-136.

57. Petitti DB. A review of epidemiologic studies of vasectomy. Biomedical Bulletin 1988;5(2). (Association for Voluntary Surgical Contraception, New York.)

58. Petitti DB, Klein R, Kipp H, Friedman GD. Vasectomy and the incidence of hospitalized illness. J Urol 1983;129(4):760-762.

59. Petitti DB, Klein R, Kipp H, Kahn W, Siegelaub AB, Friedman GD. A survey of personal habits, symptoms of illness, and histories of disease in men with and without vasectomies. Am J Public Health 1982;72(5):476-480.

60. Pitaktepsombati P, Janowitz B. Sterilization acceptance and regret in Thailand. Contraception 1991;44(6):623-637.

61. Planned Parenthood of Sacramento Valley, CA. Personal communication with Gary K. Stewart, 1993.

62. Pritchard JA, MacDonald PC Grant NF. Williams obstetrics, 17th ed. Norwalk CT: Appleton-Century-Crofts, 1985: Chapter 40.

63. Radwanska E, Headley SK, Dmowski P. Evaluation of ovarian function after tubal sterilization. J Repro Med 1982;27(7):376-384.

64. Radwanska E, Berger G, Hammond J. Luteal deficiency among women with normal menstrual cycles, requesting reversal of tubal sterilization. Obstet Gynecol 1979;54(2):189-192.

65. Ramsay IN, Russell SA. Who requests reversal of female sterilization? A retrospective study from a Scottish unit. Scott Med J 1991;36(2):44-46.

66. Reed TP, Erb RA. Hysteroscopic female sterilization with formed-in-place silicone rubber plugs. In: Phillips JM. Endoscopic female sterilization. Downey CA: The American Association of Gynecologic Laparoscopists, 1983.

67. Ross J, et al. Voluntary sterilization: an international fact book. Association for Voluntary Surgical Contraception, 1985.

68. Schwartz DB, Wingo PA, Antarsh L, Smith JC. Female sterilizations in the United States, 1987. Fam Plann Perspect 1989;21(5):209-212.

69. Shain RN, Miller WB, Holden AE, Rosenthal M. Impact of tubal sterilization and vasectomy on female marital sexuality: results of a controlled longitudinal study. Am J Obstet Gynecol 1991;164(3):763-771.

70. Shy KK, Stergachis A, Grothaus LG, Wagner EH, Hecht J, Anderson G. Tubal sterilization and risk of subsequent hospital admission for menstrual disorders. Am J Obstet Gynecol 1992;166(6-1):1698-1706.

71. Siegler AM, Hulka J, Peretz A. Reversibility of female sterilization. Fertil Steril 1985;43(4):499-510.

72. Soderstrom R. Clinical challenges: share warning information, court case teaches. Contra Technol Update 1981;2(1):8-9.

73. Soderstrom RM, Levy BS, Engel T. Reducing bipolar sterilization failures. Obstet Gynecol 1989;74(1):60-63.

74. Stergachis A, Shy KK, Grothaus LC, Wagner EH, Hecht JA, Anderson G, Normand EH, Raboud J. Tubal sterilization and the long-term risk of hysterectomy. JAMA 1990;264(22):2893-2898.

75. Stewart FH, Guest F, Stewart GK, Hatcher RA. Understanding your body. New York NY: Bantam, 1987.

76. Stewart GK. Personal communication with Herbert Peterson, 1993.
77. Stone SC, Dickey RP, Mickal A. The acute effect of hysterectomy (and laparoscopy) on ovarian function. Am J Obstet Gynecol 1975;121(2):193-197.
78. Tietjen L, Cronin W, McIntosh N. Infection prevention for family planning service programs: a problem-solving reference manual. Durant OK: Essential Medical Information Systems, Inc., 1992.
79. U.S. Bureau of the Census, Statistical Abstract of the United States: 1992 (112th ed.) Washington DC, 1992.
80. Uribe-Ramirez LC, Camarena R, Hernandez F, Diaz-Garcia M. A retrospective analysis of surgical complications of four tuboocclusive techniques. In: Phillips JM. Endoscopic female sterilization. Downey CA: The American Association of Gynecologic Laparoscopists, 1983.
81. Vasectomy and Prostate Cancer Conference. Department of Health and Human Services. The National Institute of Child Health and Human Development, The National Cancer Institute, The National Institute of Diabetes and Digestive and Kidney Diseases. March 2, 1993.
82. Vessey M, Huggins G, Lawless M, McPherson K, Yeates D. Tubal sterilization: findings in a large prospective study. Br J Obstet Gynaecol 1983;90(3): 203-209.
83. Walker AM, Jick H, Hunter JR, McEvoy J. Vasectomy and nonfatal myocardial infarction: continued observation indicates no elevation of risk. J Urol 1983;130(5):936-937.
84. Whong YW. Ectopic pregnancy subsequent to female sterilization. Korean Association of Voluntary Sterilization. December 1987.
85. Wilcox LS, Chu SV and Peterson HB. Characteristics of women who considered or obtained tubal reanatomosis: results from a prospective study of tubal sterilization. Obstet Gynecol 1990; 75(4):661-665.
86. Wilcox LS, Chu SY, Eaker ED, Zeger SL, Peterson HB. Risk factors for regret after tubal sterilization: 5 years of follow-up in a prospective study. Fertil Steril 1991;55(5):927-933.
87. Wilcox LS, Martinez-Schnell V, Peterson HB, Ware JH, Hughes JM. Menstrual function after tubal sterilization. Am J Epidemiol 1992;135(12): 1368-1381.
88. Wingo PA, Huezo CM, Rubin GL, Ory HW, Peterson HB. The mortality risk associated with hysterectomy. Am J Obstet Gynecol 1985;152(7-1):803-808.
89. World Federation of Health Agencies for the Advancement of Voluntary Surgical Contraception. Safe and voluntary surgical contraception. New York, 1988.
90. World Health Organization. Mental health and female sterilization: report of a WHO collaborative prospective study. J Biosoc Sci 1984;16(1):1-21.
91. World Health Organization. Technical and managerial guidelines for vasectomy services. Geneva: WHO, 1988.
92. Wortman J. Vasectomy — what are the problems? Popul Rep 1975;Series D(2): 25-39.
93. Yoon IB. The Yoon Ring as compared with other sterilization methods. In: Phillips JM. Endoscopic female sterilization. Downey CA: The American Association of Gynecologic Laparoscopists, 1983.
94. Zatuchni GI, Shelton JD, Goldsmith A, Sciarra JJ (eds). Female transcervical sterilization. Philadelphia PA: Harper & Row, 1983. (PARFR Series on Fertility Regulation).

Emergency Contraception: Postcoital Options

- Each year, 3.5 million women in the U.S. become pregnant unintentionally. More than half of these pregnancies occur because no contraceptive was used; some pregnancies occur because of contraceptive failure.

- Potentially, emergency treatment could reduce by 1.7 million the number of unintended pregnancies that occur in the U.S. each year. The number of abortions could be reduced by as much as 0.8 million.[15]

As long as condoms break, inclination and opportunity unexpectedly converge, men rape women, diaphragms and cervical caps are dislodged, people are so ambivalent about sex that they need to feel swept away, IUDs are expelled, and pills are lost or forgotten, we will need emergency, postcoital contraception. Our family planning technology is imperfect, and human situations are not always neat and tidy.

Widely available, accessible emergency contraception could have a tremendous impact. Simple, effective treatment options are available now; using them is legal. They are backed by two decades of research that demonstrates safety and efficacy. Unlike all other contraceptive methods, postcoital treatment does not require planning and implementation before it is needed, and it is the only possible way to reduce pregnancy risk in circumstances such as rape or mechanical failure of a barrier method. Emergency contraception brings family planning services to a whole new population of individuals at risk: those who have not been able to identify their risk in advance, or who have not recognized in advance their motivation to avoid pregnancy. Family planning services that do not provide postcoital treatment short-change their clients and miss the chance to reach many potential clients.

Mechanism of Action

MECHANISM OF ACTION

When a contraceptive emergency arises, there are several options. For most women who want treatment, emergency contraceptive pills will be the appropriate choice. Alternative hormonal regimens—danazol or progestin-only pills—may provide an option for women who need or want to avoid estrogen. Hormonal methods are effective because they temporarily disrupt ovarian hormone production and cause an absent or dysfunctional luteal phase hormone pattern.[9] An inadequate or absent luteal phase results in out-of-phase endometrial development, so the uterine lining is unsuitable for implantation. Also, hormone disruption may interfere with fertilization and cause disordered tubal transport.[10]

An IUD can be inserted up to 7 days after ovulation when unprotected intercourse has occurred earlier in the cycle. This is an excellent emergency option for a woman who otherwise is an appropriate IUD candidate, especially if she wants to continue with this method. IUD insertion alters the endometrium. An inflammatory response is triggered that makes the endometrium unsuitable for implantation and interferes with fertilization and transport.

For some women, early testing to detect pregnancy and use of very early abortion may be preferable to postcoital treatment. The chance of pregnancy with unprotected intercourse in one cycle is not high, and abortion is not a medically hazardous procedure.

Postcoital Options

Emergency contraceptive pills. Commonly available oral contraceptive pills that contain ethinyl estradiol and norgestrel can be used for postcoital treatment. This option, known as the "Yuzpe" regimen, requires two treatment doses, taken 12 hours apart, totalling 200 mcg of ethinyl estradiol and 2.0 mg norgestrel, *or* 1.0 mg levonorgestrel (see Table 16-1). The first dose should be given as soon as possible; there is no need to wait until the next morning, so use of the name "morning-after treatment" may not be desirable. Treatment is most effective if initiated within the first 12–24 hours after unprotected intercourse. Treatment is not likely to be effective if delayed longer than 72 hours. Evaluated in numerous studies, this regimen is the most widely used emergency treatment method.[3] A commercial product specifically for postcoital use is licensed and marketed in Europe. It is possible that additional oral contraceptive formulations, containing progestins other than norgestrel, also would be effective. Research on emergency contraception, however, has been reported only for norgestrel products.

Danazol treatment. This synthetic androgen has been used for emergency treatment with a schedule similar to the "Yuzpe" regimen. Two doses, 12 hours apart, totalling 800 mg and three doses, 12 hours apart, totalling 1,200 mg have been evaluated. Research on this method is limited,

Table 16-1 Emergency contraceptive pill options

Brand Name	Number of Tablets for Each Dose (Two Doses, 12 Hours Apart)
Ovral	2
Lo/Ovral, Nordette, or Levlen; Triphasil or Tri-Levlen (yellow pills only)	4

and efficacy results inconsistent. The danazol regimen was as effective as the "Yuzpe" regimen in one study,[23] but another study was stopped by its investigators because the efficacy was not acceptable.[19] Danazol emergency treatment, however, has a lower incidence of side effects such as nausea and vomiting than does use of emergency birth control pills.[13] Danazol may therefore be a reasonable option for women who are not able to tolerate oral contraceptives.

Progestin-only pill treatment. Short-term use of progestin-only pills has been evaluated as a method for women who have intercourse only intermittently (as in the Chinese "Visitors" pill) and for emergency use after unprotected intercourse. In the multiple-dose regimens studied, pills containing 0.75 mg of levonorgestrel have been used, with the first dose initiated no later than 8 hours after intercourse. The same dose is then repeated after 24 hours. If the woman has intercourse on subsequent days, she takes additional doses every 24 hours to a total of seven doses. Efficacy with this regimen appears to be similar to efficacy with emergency use of combined (estrogen and progestin) oral contraceptives, but abnormal bleeding patterns are common.[14] Another progestin-only regimen provides a single dose of 0.6 mg levonorgestrel taken within 12 hours of intercourse.[3] Unfortunately, no progestin-only oral tablets of appropriate dosage are available in the United States. An equivalent dose of levonorgestrel would require taking 16 Ovrette tablets to reach a total of 0.6 mg, or 20 tablets for each dose of 0.75 mg (Ovrette contains 0.075 mg of norgestrel; equivalent to 0.0375 mg of levonorgestrel). Also, initiating treatment within 8–12 hours would be problematic. This approach, however, might be helpful in providing care after rape for a woman who should not use estrogen.

Postcoital IUD insertion. Insertion of a copper IUD within 5–7 days after ovulation in a cycle when unprotected intercourse has occurred is extremely efficacious in preventing pregnancy.[4] This option, however, is used much less frequently than hormonal treatment;[20] women who need emergency treatment often are not appropriate IUD candidates. Insertion of an IUD is not wise if sexually transmitted disease is a possible risk, or if preserving fertility is a consideration for the woman. IUD product labeling specifies use only for parous women. IUD insertion is not likely to be a reasonable option after rape or when a woman is just beginning a new relationship; STD risk is high in these situations. Women who have multiple partners and women who have a history of pelvic infection or ectopic pregnancy are not appropriate IUD candidates.

Postcoital methods used in the past. High-dose estrogen treatment was used for emergency contraception in the 1960s. Postcoital use was an FDA-approved indication for DES (diethylstilbestrol); for this purpose, 25 mg–50 mg of DES were given twice daily for 5 days.[7] Other estrogen preparations also were used following the same regimen, with doses equivalent to DES 25 mg, such as ethinyl estradiol 2.5 mg, esterified estrogen 10 mg, conjugated estrogen 10 mg, and estrone 5 mg, for each dose. Efficacy using high-dose estrogen was as good or better than that for the emergency oral contraceptive method described above, but side effects were severe. The label indication for DES was discontinued, and DES postcoital treatment is no longer recommended.[8]

RU 486 and future prospects. Antiprogestogen drugs such as RU 486 may provide better postcoital treatment options in the future than those now available. RU 486 competes with the woman's ovarian progesterone for binding to progesterone receptors, thus blocking the action of progesterone. Without progesterone activity, the endometrium is unsuitable for implantation. Initial studies of RU 486, given in a single 600 mg dose within 72 hours after unprotected intercourse, have demonstrated excellent efficacy with a low incidence of side effects such as nausea and vomiting.[6,20] It is possible that a lower dose or wider time limits might also work. Optimal timing and dosage for this approach have yet to be established, but postcoital contraceptive use may turn out to be the most important role for antiprogestogen drugs.

Early pregnancy identification and early abortion. Vacuum aspiration, using a flexible 5-mm plastic cannula, can be performed very early in pregnancy. This procedure, sometimes called menstrual extraction or menstrual regulation, has been advocated in the past as an option for women who preferred not to know whether they were pregnant and as a way of avoiding the legal definition of abortion. It is a simple, low-risk procedure. Unfortunately, however, the likelihood of incomplete abortion, with continuing pregnancy requiring a second vacuum aspiration, is higher for vacuum aspiration performed before the end of the sixth week of pregnancy than it is for abortion performed at 7 weeks or later. Therefore, it is safer for the woman to wait until the sixth or seventh week, when placental tissue can be identified by the clinician performing the procedure, to assure that aspiration is complete (see Chapter 19). Also, widely available, inexpensive pregnancy test kits now permit accurate diagnosis of pregnancy as early as 7–10 days after fertilization, even before the woman's menstrual period is due. Consequently, there is no justification for performing any surgical procedure at all unless the woman definitely is pregnant.

EFFECTIVENESS

The risk of pregnancy with one act of intercourse ranges from approximately 0%–26%, depending on the cycle day of exposure in relation to ovulation. The risk of pregnancy is highest during the 3 days prior to ovulation and on the day of ovulation; during this interval, rates for pregnancy with one exposure range from 15%–26% (see Chapter 22 on Infertility, Table 22-5). To measure the efficacy of emergency contraceptive treatment, the number of pregnancies that occur despite treatment must be compared with the number that would have been expected if no treatment had been given.

Table 16-2 summarizes the results of the eight published studies of emergency contraceptive pill treatment that have included sufficient information to calculate an expected pregnancy rate. Analysis of these studies indicates that emergency contraceptive pill treatment reduces the risk of pregnancy by approximately 75%.[16]

Comparable efficacy rate calculations for alternative emergency options are not available

In one study that randomly assigned women to an 800-mg danazol regimen or to the Yuzpe regimen, danazol was somewhat more effective. In another study, a 1,200-mg danazol regimen (three doses of 400 mg given 12 hours apart) was found to be somewhat more effective than either an 800-mg danazol regimen or the Yuzpe regimen.[23] However, use of danazol

Table 16-2 Efficacy of emergency contraceptive pill treatment

Study	n	# Pregnancies
Yuzpe (1977)	152	1
Yuzpe (1982)	451	6
Tully (1983)	159	8
Van Stanten (1985)	461	5
Percival-Smith (1987)	610	12
Zuliani (1990)	407	9
Glasier (1992)	398	4
Webb (1992)	191	5

Total Cycles Studied: 2,829

Pregnancies Observed: 50 (1.8%)

Pregnancies Expected: 193 (6.8%)

Efficacy: Approximately 75%

was stopped on ethical grounds in one study because the interim analysis determined that the efficacy of the regimen was so slight.[19]

A Chinese multicenter study of 361 women who used 2–7 doses of progestin alone, as described above, found that pregnancy occurred in 1.4% of treated cycles.[1] With a single-dose progestin-only regimen, pregnancy occurred in 3% of treated cycles.[3]

Numerous studies have been reported for postcoital insertion of copper IUDs. A review of nine such studies, involving 879 women, found only one pregnancy and one possible spontaneous abortion.[4] IUD insertion was restricted to the first 5–7 days after unprotected intercourse in most of these studies; insertion as late as 10 days was allowed in the study that reported the pregnancies.

COST

One package of oral contraceptives (see Table 16-1) provides sufficient medication for emergency contraceptive pill treatment. If the woman already has a prescription, the cost of treatment would be about $20 for one pill pack. Otherwise the cost of a medical visit and additional laboratory tests that the clinician may perform, such as a pregnancy test, also would be required. Treatment with progestin-only pills would require one or two packages of Ovrette, and would cost $10–$20. Sufficient danazol to provide 800 mg–1200 mg (4–6 tablets) costs $14–$20. The cost for a copper IUD is $120 plus $40–$50 for insertion.

ADVANTAGES AND INDICATIONS

Emergency contraceptive treatment is the *only* option available to reduce pregnancy risk in circumstances such as rape or mechanical failure of a contraceptive device. It is also the only possible option when a couple realizes they do not want to risk pregnancy only after the risk has already been taken. All the other contraceptive possibilities require that motivation be recognized and acted upon in advance.

Available emergency options are simple, easy to use, and involve minimal medical risk. Drug exposure and side effects are of short duration.

INDICATIONS

Emergency options should be considered for any woman who has had unprotected intercourse within the last 72 hours, definitely does not want to be pregnant, and wants to consider treatment. It may be appropriate when:

1. A woman has had intercourse without using a contraceptive
2. A woman has missed multiple birth control pills in the 2 weeks preceding intercourse (more than three pills missed in midpack, or an interval of more than 7–9 days with no pills)[3]
3. A woman has missed one or more progestin-only pills, or had intercourse before completing at least 48 hours on a correct progestin-only pill schedule[3]
4. A woman's barrier method was inserted incorrectly, dislodged during intercourse, was removed too early, or was found to be torn
5. A condom slipped, broke, or leaked
6. Withdrawal or periodic abstinence has been unsuccessful
7. Ejaculation on the external genitalia has occurred
8. An IUD has been expelled or partially expelled
9. An IUD has been removed at midcycle (because removal was necessary)
10. A woman has been exposed to a possible teratogen (such as live vaccine, cytotoxic drug, extensive X-ray studies)
11. A woman has been sexually assaulted

Neither the total number of times unprotected intercourse has occurred nor the cycle day(s) of exposure are directly relevant to the decision. If multiple exposures have occurred, it is possible that fertilization and implantation have already taken place, in which case emergency treatment will not be effective. On the other hand, if pregnancy has not yet occurred, using emergency treatment can reduce the risk that pregnancy will result from unprotected intercourse within the last 72 hours. In either case, emergency contraceptive pill treatment would not be harmful. Reviewing the cycle time at which exposure occurred may enable the clinician to estimate whether pregnancy risk is high or low, but what determines whether emergency contraception is warranted is how the woman feels about reducing the risk, no matter whether the risk is high or low.

Some protocols for postcoital contraception have specified complex and limiting rules that withhold treatment in cases with more than one episode of unprotected sex, or with exposure on low-risk cycle days. Such limits may make sense in the context of research on efficacy, but are not necessary for routine clinical care. Instead, the issues to consider in deciding about treatment are:

1. Does the woman have any health problems that might make using short-term, high-dose estrogen and progestin unwise?
2. Would an alternative emergency option—danazol, progestin-only pill treatment, or insertion of an IUD—be better?
3. What would the woman do if pregnancy occurred despite emergency treatment?

A woman who would not plan to have an abortion needs to weigh the benefit of reducing the likelihood of pregnancy against the risk that the embryo could be exposed to hormones if emergency treatment fails or if she were already pregnant. Although no evidence indicates that taking oral contraceptive pills would be harmful during early pregnancy (see Chapter 10), it is prudent to avoid exposure to any unnecessary medication when planning optimal full-term pregnancy conditions.

D ISADVANTAGES AND CAUTIONS

Treatment with emergency contraceptive pills is not appropriate for a woman who has ever had any serious medical problems that would make use of oral contraceptives inadvisable. The same caution is applicable for use of progestin-only contraceptive pills, although fewer serious medical problems need to be considered in relation to use of progestin alone. Cautions for these products are described in detail in Chapters 10 and 11. Similarly, IUD insertion is reasonable only for a woman who otherwise is a good candidate for this method (see Chapter 14). Treatment with danazol is not wise for a woman who has any of the following conditions:

- Undiagnosed, abnormal vaginal bleeding
- Impaired liver, kidney, or heart function
- Porphyria

Because danazol could cause androgenic effects on an exposed female fetus, danazol should not be used if the woman does not plan to have an abortion if pregnancy occurs. It should not be used by a breastfeeding woman. Danazol can cause fluid retention, so may not be a wise choice for women with conditions that can be adversely affected by fluid gain, such as epilepsy, migraine, heart disease, or impaired kidney function.[11]

Side effects. Nausea and vomiting are very common during emergency contraceptive pill treatment. Nausea occurs in 50%–70% of those treated. As many as 22% experience vomiting as well.[19] Taking each dose with food may help prevent nausea. Some clinicians provide nonprescription antinausea medication such as dimenhydrinate (Dramamine) 50 mg to be taken 30 minutes before the second emergency pill dose if nausea occurs after the first dose.[20] Some clinicians also provide an additional dose of pills if the woman vomits within 1–3 hours after taking a dose.[3] Some women experience breast tenderness, abdominal pain, headache, or dizziness with emergency contraceptive pill treatment. Side effects subside within a day or two after treatment is completed.

Side effects are less common, but similar, after treatment with danazol or progestin-only pills. In the Chinese multicenter study of progestin-only treatment, 7% of women treated reported nausea, and 1% reported vomiting. Dizziness, abdominal pain, breast tenderness, sleepiness, vaginal discharge, and fatigue were reported by 1%–4% of subjects.[1] Rare but serious side effects have been reported in association with danazol treatment used for endometriosis or management of hereditary angioedema. Thrombophlebitis and thromboembolism, including stroke, have been reported, as have benign liver tumors, peliosis hepatis, and rare cases of hypertension related to pseudotumor cerebri.[11] Whether danazol is responsible for causing such effects, and whether they might occur with short-term treatment, is not known. Side effects after postcoital insertion of an IUD are the same as for insertion of an IUD under normal circumstances (see Chapter 14).

Menstrual cycle disturbance.   Emergency hormone contraception may alter the timing of the woman's next menstrual period. Menstrual bleeding may begin a few days earlier or a few days later than would have been expected. If menstrual bleeding does not commence within 3 weeks after treatment, however, evaluate to detect pregnancy.

PROVIDING EMERGENCY CONTRACEPTION

The authors believe that emergency contraceptive pills should be made available for over-the-counter sale (see Legal and Policy Issues). Since this is not now the case, however, the following guidelines are intended to meet current standards of care with respect to prescription drugs.

The first step in making emergency contraception a real option for patients is to make all patients aware that emergency treatment is possible. Include emergency postcoital pills on the list of contraceptive options in all educational materials and posters, and include it in routine contraceptive counseling. Remind patients that immediate action is needed if an emergency arises; treatment is most effective if started immediately; 72 hours after unprotected intercourse is the latest limit for initiating emergency pill use.

Providing emergency contraceptive pills in advance.   Women who are using barrier methods, condoms, withdrawal, or periodic abstinence are likely to be able to recognize when they are at risk: The method was not used or was used incorrectly, slipped out of place, or was damaged. Providing a prescription for emergency pills with written instructions, or an emergency kit containing a pill pack and instructions, may give them extra confidence in relying on their primary method. A routine family planning or health maintenance visit is an ideal opportunity to discuss emergency options, review medical history and exam findings to identify any risk factors for emergency use of oral contraceptives, and review instructions for deciding about and using emergency treatment. If the woman is able to understand the instruction sheet, has no serious medical problems, and is certain that she does not want to be pregnant, then providing an emergency prescription or an emergency kit is an excellent idea.

Providing emergency contraceptive pills after exposure. A request for emergency treatment demands an emergency response. Be sure that telephone protocols provide for an immediate response to any inquiry about emergency contraception; delay of even a few hours may make treatment less effective or inappropriate. Established patients can arrange to get emergency pills by telephone. A brief review of the patient's situation and medical history may be all that is needed. If the medical record is available to verify normal exam findings in the last year, the clinician will have extra confidence that pills can be prescribed safely. A visit for consultation or an exam is not necessary unless the patient needs help in deciding about treatment, has a medical condition or medical history risk factors that complicate decision making, or suspects that she may already be pregnant. It is not prudent, however, to prescribe any medication by telephone for an individual who is not an established patient.

If emergency contraception cannot be arranged by telephone, then arrange an emergency visit. If a same-day visit is not possible, refer the patient to an alternative resource for this service. At the time of the visit:

1. Review the patient's history, including past medical history, contraceptive history, and the date of last menstrual period, previous cycle length, estimated date of ovulation, date of unprotected intercourse(s), and number of hours since the first and the most recent unprotected episodes.

2. Estimate the date of ovulation and compare with intercourse timing. Discuss the likely risk of pregnancy with the patient, and the risk (if any) that pregnancy has already occurred.

3. Explore the patient's feelings about continuing pregnancy in the event that emergency treatment does not prevent pregnancy. There is no evidence that emergency hormone contraception would be harmful, but a normal outcome of any pregnancy cannot be guaranteed. Avoid any medication that is not necessary during pregnancy.

4. Identify any personal risk factors that warn against the use of oral contraceptives. Consider whether alternative hormone regimens or IUD insertion might be preferable.

5. Decide whether a physical examination and laboratory tests are needed.
   - If there is any doubt about exposure to unprotected intercourse in the previous cycle, obtain an ultrasensitive urine test to exclude pregnancy.
   - A blood pressure check is simple and reasonable, especially if normal blood pressure has not recently been documented.

- The indications for a pelvic examination are the same as they would be for any routine contraceptive consultation. Specifically, pelvic examination should be offered if pregnancy is suspected, if the woman has a history of pelvic pathology, if samples are needed for STD assessment, if IUD insertion is being considered, or if it is time for Pap screening. Otherwise, pelvic examination can be omitted, especially if the woman does not wish to have an exam.[3]

6. Discuss options with the patient, including possible risks and failure rates, necessary follow-up, alteration of menstrual period timing, and warning signs of possible pill complications that should prompt her to return for care (see Patient Instructions below). Help the patient decide whether she wishes to be treated.

7. Provide medication for treatment. If hormone treatment is used, administer the first dose immediately, as part of the visit if possible. Provide an extra dose of medication in case of vomiting, along with antinausea medication, or arrange for 24-hour availability in case vomiting occurs and additional medication is needed.

8. Plan for follow-up after treatment. A return visit and pregnancy test will be needed if the woman does not have a normal menstrual period within 3–4 weeks after emergency treatment. Document return of normal menses during a visit or at least by a follow-up over the telephone.

9. Plan for interim and ongoing contraception. The woman must avoid intercourse, or use a barrier method consistently and correctly, until the onset of her next menstrual period. If she has been taking oral contraceptives, she can either stop them and use a barrier method until her next menstrual period, or she can continue to take the remaining pills in her packet while using an additional barrier method for at least 7 days or until her next menstrual period.[2] When her menstrual period begins, she can resume taking oral contraceptives in the normal way or choose another ongoing contraceptive method best suited to her needs. Provide a prescription or supplies for future contraception as indicated. Often, when a woman needs an emergency contraceptive, she is also receptive to learning how to prevent having such a need in the future. Educators call this a "teachable moment."

MANAGING PROBLEMS AND FOLLOW-UP

A patient who experiences heavy bleeding or severe abdominal pain, or who is concerned or worried, needs an emergency follow-up visit. If severe gastrointestinal side effects occur after the first dose of emergency hormone treatment, the patient may need additional medication, or she may decide to discontinue treatment. Consider providing an extra hormone dose if the patient vomits soon after taking a treatment dose. Options for treating nausea include the following:

Nonprescription drugs

- Dimenhydrinate (Dramamine) 50 mg tablets, one or two tablets by mouth every 4–6 hours
- Cyclizine hydrochloride (Marezine) 50 mg tablets, one tablet by mouth every 4–6 hours

Prescription drugs (Warn patients not to drive or use dangerous equipment.)

- Trimethobenzamide hydrochloride (Tigan) 250 mg tablets, 1 tablet every 8 hours, or 200 mg rectal suppositories, 1 suppository every 8 hours
- Promethazine hydrochloride (Phenergan) 25 mg tablets, 1 tablet every 12 hours, or 25 mg rectal suppositories, 1 suppository every 12 hours.

Manage IUD problems, including bleeding, abdominal pain, cramping, or signs of possible infection such as fever or malaise, in the same way that they would be after IUD insertion at any other time (see Chapter 14). An emergency visit may be needed to identify infection or possible pregnancy or ectopic pregnancy.

Arrange for routine follow-up care within 3–4 weeks after treatment. Make sure that the patient is not pregnant and that she has whatever she needs for effective, ongoing contraception. If any uncertainty exists about the possibility of pregnancy, or if a normal menstrual period has not commenced within 3–4 weeks after treatment, perform a pelvic examination and an ultrasensitive urine pregnancy test.

Treatment failure resulting in pregnancy will require counseling, evaluation, and referral just as for any other patient diagnosed with unintended pregnancy. Guidelines for early pregnancy diagnosis and management are detailed in Chapter 2.

I NSTRUCTIONS FOR USING EMERGENCY CONTRACEPTIVES

Instructions for patients who have emergency insertion of an IUD are the same as for IUD insertion at any other time (see Chapter 14).

Patients provided with emergency hormone treatment should receive medication labeling that identifies the specific product prescribed, and the number of tablets needed for each dose (see Table 16-1). The following instructions can be used for emergency contraceptive pills provided in advance or for treatment provided after exposure. If emergency contraceptive pills are provided in advance, they also should be accompanied by additional information that enables the woman to determine whether taking them would be appropriate and safe (see example in Legal and Policy Issues).

INSTRUCTIONS FOR USING EMERGENCY CONTRACEPTIVE PILLS (ECPs)

1. **Swallow the first dose as soon as possible**—no later than 72 hours after having unprotected sex. Eating a snack or drinking a glass of milk reduces nausea.

   Swallow the second dose 12 hours after taking the first dose.

   Do not take any extra pills. More pills will probably not decrease the risk of pregnancy any further. More pills will increase the risk of nausea, possibly causing you to vomit.

2. Remember to eat or drink something to help prevent nausea. About one-third of women who use ECPs have temporary nausea. It is usually mild and should stop in a day or so. If you vomit within an hour after taking a dose, call your clinician. You may need to repeat a dose. You may need some antinausea medicine.

3. Watch for warning signs for the next couple of weeks. See your clinician at once if you have:
   - **severe pain in your leg (calf or thigh)**
   - **severe abdominal pain**
   - **chest pain or cough or shortness of breath**
   - **severe headaches, dizziness, weakness, or numbness**
   - **blurred vision, loss of vision, or trouble speaking**
   - **jaundice (yellowing of the skin)**

4. Your next period may start a few days earlier or later than usual. If your period doesn't start within 4 weeks, see your clinician for an exam and pregnancy test. If you think that you may be pregnant, see your clinician at once, whether or not you plan to continue the pregnancy. Emergency contraceptive pills may not prevent an ectopic pregnancy (in the tubes or abdomen). Ectopic pregnancy is a medical emergency.

5. As soon as you possibly can, begin using a method of birth control you will be able to use on an ongoing basis. Emergency contraceptive pills are meant for one-time, emergency protection. They are not as effective as other forms of birth control. If you want to resume use of birth control pills after taking ECPs, consult your clinician.

Protect yourself against AIDS and other sexually transmitted infections as well as against pregnancy—use condoms every time you have sex if you may be at risk.

The drugs used as ECPs are approved by the U.S. Food and Drug Administration (FDA) and are widely used for other purposes. These products have not been submitted to the FDA for approval for use as ECPs, but clinical research studies have shown that ECPs are safe and effective.

L EGAL ISSUES AND PUBLIC POLICY IMPLICATIONS

LEGAL STATUS OF EMERGENCY CONTRACEPTIVE TREATMENT

The emergency treatment options described in this chapter involve use of drugs or IUDs that have been approved by the U.S. Food and Drug Administration (FDA). However, no products have been approved specifically for emergency or postcoital use in the United States. FDA review and approval for drug and device indications normally is initiated at the request of the manufacturer, and no such application has been made. Because emergency use is not included as an indication in the FDA-approved product labeling, the manufacturers cannot recommend or market their products for this use. Use of approved drugs for unlabeled indications, however, is common, and is entirely legal. A 1982 FDA Drug Bulletin[5] provides clear guidance:

> **"Use of Approved Drugs for Unlabeled Indications:** The appropriateness or the legality of prescribing approved drugs for uses not included in their official labeling is sometimes a cause of concern and confusion among practitioners.
>
> Under the Federal Food, Drug, and Cosmetic (FD&C) Act, a drug approved for marketing may be labeled, promoted, and advertised by the manufacturer only for those uses for which the drug's safety and effectiveness have been established and which FDA has approved. These are commonly referred to as 'approved uses.' This means that adequate and well-controlled clinical trials have documented these uses, and the results of the trials have been reviewed and approved by FDA.
>
> The FD&C Act does not, however, limit the manner in which a physician may use an approved drug. Once a product has been approved for marketing, a physician may prescribe it for uses or in treatment regimens or patient populations that are not included in approved labeling. Such 'unapproved' or, more precisely, 'unlabeled' uses may be appropriate and rational in certain circumstances, and may, in fact, reflect approaches to drug therapy that have been extensively reported in medical literature.
>
> The term 'unapproved uses' is, to some extent, misleading. It includes a variety of situations ranging from unstudied to thoroughly investigated drug uses. Valid new uses for drugs already on the market are often first discovered through serendipitous observations and therapeutic innovations, subsequently confirmed by well-planned and executed clinical investigations. Before such advances can be

added to the approved labeling, however, data substantiating the effectiveness of a new use or regimen must be submitted by the manufacturer to FDA for evaluation. This may take time and, without the initiative of the drug manufacturer whose product is involved, may never occur. For that reason, accepted medical practice often includes drug use that is not reflected in approved drug labeling.

With respect to its role in medical practice, the package insert is informational only. FDA tries to assure that prescription drug information in the package insert accurately and fully reflects the data on safety and effectiveness on which drug approval is based."[FDA 82]

Family planning practice, including many clinic protocols, provides other precedents for using drugs for unlabeled indications. For example, oral contraceptive products have been used to manage hypothalamic amenorrhea, irregular or excessive menstrual bleeding, severe dysmenorrhea, and acne. There is no legal requirement for any special patient disclaimer or consent procedures in relation to unlabeled indications.

PUBLIC POLICY CHANGES NEEDED

Emergency contraceptive treatment should be available to everyone who needs it. Yet emergency options are not widely known, and many practical obstacles block the immediate access essential for success with this method. Emergency contraceptive pills would be an appropriate product for over-the-counter sale. Making emergency pill kits available without prescription or providing kits to all sexually active women when they visit a clinician for family planning services, gynecologic care, or sexually transmitted disease evaluation could greatly increase the potential role for this treatment. Medical problems that might make emergency pill use inadvisable are rare, and can be determined from medical history information. A physical examination or consultation with a clinician is not necessary unless the woman needs help in assessing medical risk factors or suspects that she may already be pregnant. With the help of clearly written guidelines (see following sample), a woman could herself determine whether it would be safe to use emergency contraceptive pills without professional consultation beforehand.

Current prescription requirements are intended to protect the small minority of women who might suffer harmful health effects that could be prevented by professional supervision. This benefit must be weighed against the risk and harm now suffered by women who experience unintended pregnancy that might have been prevented by wider availability of a simple treatment option. Current obstacles to access impose financial and human burdens, and medical risk as well; it is time to re-examine public policy, and begin removing obstacles.

EMERGENCY CONTRACEPTIVE PILLS (ECPs)
"Morning-after Treatment"

What if you need birth control after sex? What if—

- *You were forced to have sex.*
- *A condom broke or slipped off.*
- *You didn't use any birth control.*
- *Your diaphragm slipped out of place.*
- *You had sex when you didn't expect to.*
- *You stopped taking birth control pills for more than a week.*
- *You missed as many as half of your birth control pills in the past 2 weeks.*

If you have had unprotected intercourse, and are certain that you do not want to be pregnant, you may want to consider using emergency contraceptive pills (ECPs).

Are ECPs right for you? When you have sex without using birth control, your risk of becoming pregnant depends on *where you are in your menstrual cycle.* During your most fertile days—midway between two menstrual periods—the risk could be as high as 30%. By using ECPs, you decrease your chance of becoming pregnant by about 75%. For example, a 30% risk would be reduced to under 8%.

ECP treatment consists of two doses of hormone pills, with the first dose taken as soon as possible after unprotected intercourse. The hormones are estrogen and progestin, which are in regular birth control pills. ECPs provide a *short, strong burst* of hormones. This interferes with hormone patterns essential for pregnancy to continue. Hormone release from the ovary is reduced, and the development of the uterine lining is disturbed. These disruptions are temporary, lasting only a few days.

Timing is everything! ECPs must be taken as soon as possible—no later than 72 hours after unprotected sex.

- If you have had unprotected sex just once since your last normal period, and the unprotected sex was no more than 72 hours ago—ECPs make sense.
- If you have not had unprotected sex *more than once* since your last normal period, and the first unprotected sex was no more than 72 hours ago—ECPs make sense.
- But, if you have had unprotected sex more than once and at least one of these times was more than 72 hours ago, *you may already be pregnant.* If you are already pregnant, then ECPs will not work. On the other hand, if you are not already pregnant, your very recent unprotected time would be a reason to consider ECPs.
- If you would not have an abortion, you need to weigh the benefit of avoiding pregnancy against the risk of exposing the embryo to hormones if the ECPs fail or if you were already pregnant. In this case, talk to your clinician, who can help you weigh the pros and cons of using ECPs.
- If you are sure you would have an abortion—ECPs make sense.

Talk to your clinician *before* using ECPs if you think you might have become pregnant last month. Symptoms of early pregnancy can include:

- Breast tenderness
- Nausea
- Changes in your last menstrual period

Temporary side effects during ECP treatment are fairly common. About one-third of women experience nausea or vomiting. Less common temporary side effects are headache, breast tenderness, dizziness, and fluid retention. Many studies of ECPs have demonstrated that they work well. No serious health problems have been reported.

However, a woman using ECPs could have dangerous or even fatal complications that have been reported in very rare cases after normal, prolonged use of birth control pills. These include blood clots in the legs or lungs, heart attack, stroke, liver damage, liver tumor, gallbladder disease, and high blood pressure.

Talk to your clinician *before* using ECPs if you have ever had:

- Stroke
- Breast cancer
- Blood clots in your legs or lungs
- Any reason to think ECPs might pose a health risk for you
- Any serious medical disorder, such as diabetes, liver disease, heart disease, kidney disease, or high blood pressure

For some women, emergency insertion of an IUD (intrauterine device) may be a reasonable alternative to ECPs. To be effective, IUD insertion must be done within 5 days after unprotected intercourse. The IUD, however, is not a wise choice for a woman who intends to have a pregnancy in the future or has any current risk of exposure to sexually transmitted infections.

For most women, ECPs are a simple, safe option that can greatly reduce the chance of pregnancy after unprotected intercourse.

REFERENCES

1. He CH, Shi YE, Xu JQ, Van Look PF. A multicenter clinical study on two types of levonorgestrel tablets administered for postcoital contraception. Int J Gynecol Obstet 1991;36(1):43-48.
2. CSAC. Postcoital (emergency) contraception. Br J Fam Plann 1993;18(4):133-135.
3. CSAC. Emergency (postcoital) contraception guidelines for doctors. Br J Fam Plann 1992;18:3.
4. Fasoli M, Parazzini F, Cecchetti G, La Vecchia C. Post coital contraception: an overview of published studies. Contraception 1989;39(4):459-468.
5. FDA. Use of approved drugs for unlabeled indications. FDA Drug Bulletin 1982;12:1.
6. Glaiser A, Thong KJ, Dewar M, Mackie M, Baird DT. Mifepristone (RU 486) compared with high-dose estrogen and progestogen for emergency postcoital contraception. N Engl J Med 1992;327(15):1041-1044.
7. Johnson J. Contraception—the morning after. Fam Plann Perspect 1984;16(1): 266-270.
8. Kinch RAH. Diethylstilbestrol in pregnancy: an update. Can Med Assoc J 1982;127(9):812.
9. Landgren BM, Johannisson E, Aedo AR, Kumar A, Shi YE. The effect of levonorgestrel administered in large doses at different stages of the cycle on ovarian function and endometrial morphology. Contraception 1989;39(3):275-289.
10. Ling WY, Wrizon W, Zayid I, Acorn T, Popat R, Wilson E. Mode of action of dl-norgestrel and ethinylestradiol combination in postcoital contraception II. Effect of postovulatory administration on ovarian function and endometrium. Fertil Steril 1983;39(3):292-297.
11. Physicians' desk reference. 47th edition. Oradell NJ: Medical Economics Co., 1993.
12. Percival-Smith RKL, Abercrombie B. Postcoital contraception with dl-norgestrel/ethinyl estradiol combination: six years experience in a student medical clinic. Contraception 1987;36(3):287.

13. Rowlands S. Side effects of danazol compared with an ethinyloestradiol/norgestrel combination when used for postcoital contraception. Contraception 1983;27(1):39.
14. Task Force on Post-ovulatory Methods for Fertility Regulation. Postcoital contraception with levonorgestrel during the peri-ovulatory phase of the menstrual cycle. Contraception 1987;36(3):275-286.
15. Trussell J, Stewart F, Guest F, Hatcher R. Emergency contraceptive pills: a simple proposal to reduce unintended pregnancies. Fam Plann Perspect 1992;24(6):269-273.
16. Trussell J, Stewart F. The effectiveness of postcoital hormonal contraception. Fam Plann Perspect 1992;24(6):262-264.
17. Tully B. Postcoital contraception, a study. Br J Fam Plann 1983;119.
18. Van Stanten MR, Haspels AA. Interception II: postcoital low-dose estrogens and norgestrel combination in 633 women. Contraception 1985;31(3):275.
19. Webb AMC, Russell J, Elstein M. Comparison of Yuzpe regimen, danazol and mifepristone (RU 486) in oral postcoital contraception. Br Med J 1992;305(6859):927.
20. Webb A, Morris J. Practice of postcoital contraception—the results of a national survey. Br J Fam Plann 1993;18(4):113-118.
21. Yuzpe A, Lancee W. Ethinylestradiol and dl-norgestrel as a postcoital contraceptive. Fertil Steril 1977;28:932.
22. Yuzpe A, Percival-Smith RKL, Rademaker, AW. A multicenter clinical investigation employing ethinyl estradiol combined with dl-norgestrel as a postcoital contraceptive agent. Fertil Steril 1982;37(4):508.
23. Zuliani G, Columbo UF, Molla R. Hormonal postcoital contraception with an ethinylestradiol-norgestrel combination and two danazol regimens. Euro J Obstet Gynecol Reprod Biol 1990;37(3):253-260.

Postpartum Contraception and Lactation

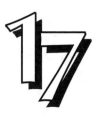

- Breastmilk is the ideal source of nutrition for infants and confers immunological protection against infection. Family planning clinic personnel can play an important role in promoting breastfeeding.

- The lactational amenorrhea method (LAM) is a highly effective, *temporary* method of contraception. However, to maintain effective protection against pregnancy, another method of contraception must be used as soon as menstruation resumes, the frequency or duration of breastfeeds is reduced, bottle feeds are introduced, or the baby reaches 6 months of age.

- Excellent contraceptive options for lactating women are (1) barrier methods such as the male and female condom, cervical cap, sponge and diaphragm—which also confer protection against STDs, (2) progestin-only methods such as the minipill, Norplant, and Depo-Provera, and (3) the Copper T 380A IUD and the LNg IUD.

- The combined pill is not a good contraceptive option for lactating women because estrogen decreases milk supply.

- HIV can be transmitted through breastmilk. Therefore, in the United States, where safe alternatives to breastmilk are available, HIV-infected mothers are advised to avoid breastfeeding.

A woman who delivers a child soon becomes capable of becoming pregnant again. Although the postpartum phase confers a period of infertility, that period may be brief, and the postpartum woman can regain her fertility before she can detect signs that her menstrual cycle will resume. The breastfeeding woman will have a longer period of infertility than will the non-breastfeeding woman; however, her return of fertility is also not predictable. Unfortunately, family planning clinicians sometimes discourage women from breastfeeding when promoting the use of those methods of contraception that clinicians provide. Clinicians can instead play an important role in promoting breastfeeding. Breastmilk is the ideal source of nutrition for infants and confers immunological protection against infection.

POSTPARTUM INFERTILITY

During pregnancy, cyclic ovarian function is suspended. The corpus luteum that arises from the ovulated follicle secretes steroids, including estrogen and progesterone, that are essential in maintaining pregnancy in the post-implantation stage. Later, steroids secreted by the placenta and conceptus emerge to play a more dominant role in hormonal support of the pregnancy. Luteal and placental steroids suppress circulating levels of follicle stimulating hormone (FSH) and luteinizing hormone (LH) but more importantly disrupt their pulsatile release from the pituitary.[20] When the placenta is delivered, the inhibiting effects of estrogen and progesterone are removed so that levels of FSH and LH gradually rise and pulsatile release by the pituitary of FSH and LH returns.[66]

Most nonlactating women resume menses within 4–6 weeks of delivery, but approximately one-third of first cycles are anovulatory, and a high proportion of first ovulatory cycles have luteal-phase defects. In the second and third menstrual cycles, 15% are anovulatory and a quarter of ovulatory cycles have luteal-phase defects. Among nonlactating women, the first ovulation occurs on average 45 days postpartum, although few first ovulations are followed by normal luteal phases.[16]

LACTATIONAL INFERTILITY

Lactation, or breastfeeding, further extends the period of inactive ovarian function and of infertility. Although plasma levels of FSH return to normal within 3 weeks postpartum in breastfeeding women, LH levels remain suppressed in the majority of lactating women throughout most of the period of lactational amenorrhea.[41]

Nipple and areola sensitivity increases at birth.[49] Infant suckling stimulates the sensory cells in the nipple and areola. Information is passed neurologically to the hypothalamus, stimulating the release of various hormones, including prolactin. Prolactin controls the rate of milk production but is not believed to play a major role in suppressing ovarian function. Instead, suckling appears to reduce directly the pulsatile release of gonadotropin releasing hormone (GnRH) by the hypothalamus,[41] perhaps by increasing hypothalamic ß-endorphin production.[14] The reduction in GnRH in turn suppresses the release of LH, which is required for follicle stimulation in the ovary. Small amounts of secreted estrogen are insufficient to produce normal follicular development and paradoxically appear to contribute to ovulatory suppression.[41]

Ovulation can occur even though the breastfeeding mother has not yet resumed menstruation. The probability that ovulation will precede first menses rises with postpartum duration, from 33%-45% during the first 3 months, to 64%-71% during months 4-12, to 87%-100% after 12 months.[4,34] In contrast, about 60% of ovulations have an adequate luteal phase among ovulations that precede first menses, a fraction that is constant with postpartum duration.[34] Consequently, lactational infertility decreases with time among amenorrheic women.

Fully or nearly fully unsupplemented breastfeeding is associated with longer periods of lactational amenorrhea and infertility than supplemented breastfeeding. Frequent, continuous stimulation of the breast by around-the-clock suckling strengthens the reflex that produces the contraceptive effect.[26] Both breastfeeding frequency per day and average suckling duration per breastfeeding episode contribute significantly to delaying the return of ovulation.[4,15] Breastfeeding frequency appears to be reduced far more by supplementary bottle feeds than by supplementary cup and spoon feeds.[4]

In summary:

- Breastfeeding delays the onset of ovulation and the return of menses;
- The longer a woman breastfeeds, the more likely menstruation will return while she continues to breastfeed; and
- The longer the return of menses is delayed, the more likely ovulation will precede the first menses.

CONTRACEPTIVE BENEFITS OF LACTATION

In developing nations, lactation plays a major role in prolonging birth intervals and thereby reducing fertility.[57,62] In developed nations, however, breastfeeding has a much smaller impact on reducing fertility because smaller fractions of infants are breastfed, and those who are breastfed receive food supplements and are weaned at earlier ages. For example, in Indonesia, 96% of infants are breastfed, and those who are breastfed are not weaned until they are 2 years old on average.[60] In contrast, only 52% of U.S. infants are breastfed and only 18% are breastfed for at least 6 months.[51] In the United States, there was a decline in the incidence of breastfeeding from the mid 1950s (about 30% of infants were breastfed) until the early 1970s (about 22% were breastfed), followed by a rapid rise until 1982 (about 60% were breastfed) and a slow decline thereafter (see Figure 17-1).[50]

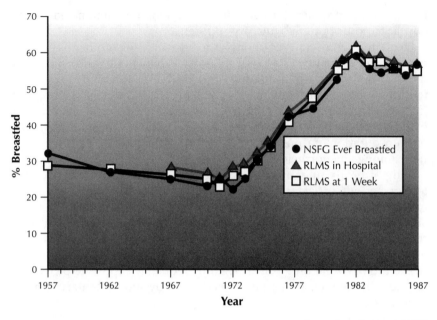

Figure 17-1 Incidence of breastfeeding, 1957-1987, National Surveys of Family Growth (NSFG) and Ross Laboratories Mothers Survey (RLMS)

THE LACTATIONAL AMENORRHEA METHOD (LAM) OF CONTRACEPTION

Breastfeeding *per se*, while an effective contraceptive at the population level in many developing countries, is an unreliable contraceptive for an individual woman because she can be at risk of pregnancy even though she is lactating. Because breastfeeding does suppress ovulation, it could be an effective temporary contraceptive as long as a woman could reliably recognize when she returns to the state of being at risk. The current consensus is that if the infant's diet is not supplemented (or supplemented only to a minor extent) and if the woman has not experienced her first postpartum menses, then "breastfeeding provides more than 98% protection from pregnancy in the first 6 months" following a birth.[26] One clinical study of this lactational amenorrhea method (LAM) demonstrated a cumulative 6-month life-table perfect-use failure rate of 0.5% among women who relied solely on LAM and used the method correctly.[46]

However, the precise extent of supplementation of an infant's diet can be difficult to determine. Furthermore, the 6-month criterion for LAM exists primarily because infant diets need to be supplemented after that time to ensure continued growth and development[38] and to avoid iron deficiency anemia.[3] Therefore, an important question is the degree to which the efficacy of LAM would be degraded if the supplementation criterion could be dropped. Combined data from several field trials revealed that cumulative pregnancy rates during lactational amenorrhea (regardless of whether the infant received supplementary food) at 6 and 12 months were 2.9% and 5.9%, respectively, compared with 0.7% at 6 months for LAM.[27]

These perfect-use failure rates during lactational amenorrhea compare favorably with those for some methods of contraception during perfect use (see Table 5-2). Clearly, however, even greater efficacy could be achieved by both breastfeeding and using another method of contraception, starting within 6 weeks postpartum. It is equally clear that LAM, and variants of LAM such as relying solely on lactational amenorrhea or relying on lactational amenorrhea for a maximum of 6 months regardless of supplementation, are very unforgiving of imperfect use.[2] If a woman wishes to rely on LAM, or any variant of LAM, and if she wishes to avoid becoming pregnant after the period when LAM affords contraceptive protection, then she must have another method of contraception available for use *before* LAM signals the return to the risk of pregnancy, and she must begin to use the method at that time.

POSTPARTUM SEXUALITY

Most American couples resume sexual intercourse within several weeks after delivery. Among lactating women, 66% are sexually active in the first month postpartum and 88% are sexually active in the second month postpartum.[13]

Contraception is only one counseling issue for postpartum women. Women—and men—may experience altered sexual feelings associated with bodily changes caused by pregnancy and delivery. Discussion of these bodily changes may help to alleviate a couple's anxiety. The following issues may be of particular concern:

- Tenderness in the perineum may cause intercourse to be painful.
- Vaginal lubrication may be diminished, particularly in the breastfeeding woman.
- Most women experience a heavy and bloody lochial discharge for a couple of weeks postpartum. This may interfere with a woman's feeling sexual and may also be a nidus for infection.
- Irrespective of whether the infant is breastfed, couples may find that the exhaustion caused by the responsibilities of being a new parent temporarily decreases sexual drive.
- Breasts are altered postpartum. Women may experience milk leakage. Couples may need to communicate feelings about whether touching the breasts is acceptable.

Depending on cultural and individual circumstances, the frequency of sexual intercourse may be altered during breastfeeding. Individual feelings about sexuality vary widely. The sexual desire of the male partner may be reduced by confusion about the role of the breasts in sexuality versus nursing the infant.[40] Breastfeeding causes a reduction in circulating estrogen. Hence, vaginal lubrication may be reduced. For some women, this vaginal dryness leads to a discomfort that is a strong disincentive for intercourse. Bonding between mother and child serves the important function of creating skills and commitment in the mother and trust and security in the infant but may interfere with the mother's emotional availability to her partner.[24] Breastfeeding mothers may be more vulnerable to exhaustion if frequent night feeding disturbs sleep. On the other hand, a birth (especially if planned) can be an exceedingly joyous experience that many couples find is enhanced by sexual intimacy. To some men and women, the shape or fullness of the lactating breast is particularly arousing. The breastfeeding woman may become more interested in sexual relations after a few months postpartum, when her perineum is less tender and she is experiencing some ovarian activity.[24]

I NITIATING CONTRACEPTIVE USE

Because postpartum infertility can be brief and lactational infertility unpredictable, contraceptive counseling should begin in the prenatal period. The first postpartum visit has traditionally been scheduled about 6 weeks after delivery, when involution of the uterus and healing have occurred. The authors, however, endorse the suggestion that the first postpartum visit be scheduled much earlier, 3 weeks after delivery.[54] The first postpartum visit is the focal point of many family planning programs and is a time when the individual woman is generally highly motivated to avoid another pregnancy. Such an opportunity should lead the clinician to educate the patient about her individual need for a contraceptive and to provide a method to the woman for immediate or later use.

The following considerations may prove useful when counseling and providing contraceptives to the postpartum woman, whether or not she is breastfeeding:

- Late pregnancy is a common time for a partner's infidelity.[37] Condoms are useful in preventing transmission of any STDs acquired during such encounters. Spermicides such as film, foams, foaming suppositories, creams, and jellies protect against some STDs. Spermicides and condoms may be used safely even in the immediate postpartum period.
- Withdrawal may be a good method for couples in the postpartum period. Its failure rate is comparable with that of the diaphragm and

spermicides (see Table 5-2). Moreover, if seminal fluid is not deposited in the vagina, the risk of sexually transmitting infections would be reduced.

- Postpartum endometritis is a serious complication. Clearly it is desirable to avoid the introduction of bacteria. The condom may be a particularly attractive option for some women.

- Avoid the diaphragm, cervical cap, and contraceptive sponge until 6 weeks after delivery. The diaphragm and cervical cap cannot be (re)fitted properly until that time. Moreover, the risk of toxic shock syndrome is increased when bleeding is present (see Chapter 9).

- Episiotomies may still be tender. Fitting a woman for cervical caps or diaphragms may cause discomfort.

- The sponge and the cervical cap (though not the diaphragm) have much higher failure rates among women who have delivered a child than among women who have not, *even during perfect use* (see Chapter 27). Information about this substantial decrease in efficacy for these two methods is essential if parous women are to make an informed choice of a contraceptive method.

- Postpartum abstinence, if practiced properly, is 100% effective in preventing pregnancy. Of course, it is extremely unforgiving of imperfect use. A woman should be counseled about other contraceptive methods should she desire to resume intercourse.

- IUDs can be inserted postpartum, either (1) immediately after the expulsion of the placenta (postplacental insertion), or (2) during the first week postpartum (immediate postpartum insertion), though preferably within 48 hours of delivery. Expulsion rates following postpartum insertion are higher than those following interval insertion, but they are lower for postplacental than for immediate postpartum insertion.[44] Discussion of this option before delivery will help to ensure that consent is fully informed (see Chapter 14). Some women experience mild uterine cramping when they breastfeed with an IUD in place, but the cramping does not usually interfere with lactation or with the effectiveness of the IUD. IUD insertion is less painful and pain and bleeding removal rates are lower for the lactating mother.[6,12] Although a few case reports and a small case-control study suggested that the risk of uterine perforation is higher among breastfeeding women, other studies find no evidence of increased risk and very low perforation rates in both breastfeeding and nonbreastfeeding women.[6,12,59] Nevertheless, it seems prudent to exercise special care, including careful sounding to determine uterine depth, when inserting an IUD postpartum.

CONTRACEPTION FOR THE NONBREASTFEEDING WOMAN

If she wishes to avoid becoming pregnant, the nonbreastfeeding woman should begin using a contraceptive method immediately postpartum or at least by the first postpartum examination (which would ideally occur 3 weeks rather than 6 weeks after delivery). Most nonbreastfeeding mothers have few restrictions placed on the method of contraceptive they can choose. Nonetheless, a few guidelines—in addition to those given above—are warranted:

- Combined oral contraceptives (OCs) may be prescribed immediately postpartum. However, caution women not to use them until at least 2 weeks after delivery. The risk of postpartum thrombophlebitis and thromboembolism is greatest just after delivery.[65] Delaying combined OC use for at least 2 weeks tends to bypass the period of peak risk for postpartum thrombotic complications.[40]
- Caution women that it is difficult to practice fertility awareness before their cycles are re-established and cyclic signs of fertility return.
- Suggest that lubricated condoms are a good option at least for the short period before the woman becomes better suited to her preferred method.
- Begin any discussion of immediate postpartum sterilization well before the delivery to help ensure that consent is fully informed.
- Norplant can be inserted and Depo-Provera can be safely injected immediately postpartum. Discussion of these options before delivery will help to ensure that consent is fully informed.

CONTRACEPTION FOR THE BREASTFEEDING WOMAN: NONHORMONAL METHODS

General comments regarding contraceptive use among postpartum women are given above. In addition, the following considerations are relevant for women who are breastfeeding.

Lactational amenorrhea method (LAM) provides effective protection against pregnancy for up to 6 months postpartum. Women who wish to use LAM need to know that if they wish to continue to avoid becoming pregnant, another method of contraception must be used as soon as LAM indicates a return to the risk of pregnancy. Those breastfeeding women who do not wish to use LAM could begin using contraceptives either immediately after delivery or at the first postpartum examination (which would ideally occur 3 weeks rather than 6 weeks after delivery). The ideal contraceptive would not interfere with the woman's ability to breastfeed.

Postpartum abstinence is practiced most widely in cultures that depend on breastfeeding for infant survival. In western cultures, however, the incentives for abstinence are fewer, making the method an unrealistic choice for many couples. Only 4% of lactating mothers in the United States have not resumed sexual activity by the third month postpartum.[13] Assure all women that intercourse will in no way harm milk production; pregnancy may cause changes in breast milk composition but does not prevent breastfeeding.

Spermicides and barrier methods have no effect on breastfeeding. The lubricated condom is especially useful in the postpartum period because of increased vaginal dryness. Spermicides such as film, foams, foaming suppositories, creams, and jellies also may help offset dryness due to estrogen deficiency. In the United States, barrier methods are the most widely used contraceptives among lactating mothers in the first 6 months postpartum.[13] In animal studies, nonoxynol-9 is absorbed through the skin and secreted in breastmilk.[7] The question of secretion in breastmilk has not been completely evaluated in humans.

Fertility awareness methods are not recommended before regular menstruation has resumed. These methods rely on detection of very minimal mucus changes. Some women can detect mucus changes during lactation, but research is still under way to discover what instructions should be given to nursing women using these methods.[48] For many women, however, the method may be more difficult to learn and practice during lactation because the mucus changes are more subtle than in nonlactating women. Basal body temperature (BBT) cannot be ascertained unless a woman has at least 6 hours of uninterrupted sleep; this requirement excludes those mothers who breastfeed during the night from using methods of periodic abstinence that involve recording BBT.[25]

The Copper T 380A IUD is also an excellent choice for the breastfeeding woman. The copper on the Copper T does not affect the quantity or quality of breastmilk.[63] (See the following section on Hormonal Methods for information on the IUDs containing progesterone.)

Tubal ligation is an excellent method for women who do not want to have more children. A tubal ligation can be performed immediately postpartum, although it can disrupt lactation if it requires general anesthesia or separation of mother and infant. Both problems can be minimized by performing the procedure with only regional or local anesthetic.[32] Discussion of this option before delivery will help to ensure that consent is fully informed.

Withdrawal in no way affects lactation.

CONTRACEPTION FOR THE BREASTFEEDING WOMAN: HORMONAL METHODS

The use of hormonal contraception by a lactating woman is an area of dispute among experts.[23] All steroids pass through the breastmilk to the infant. Estrogen decreases the volume of milk.

Progestin-only contraceptives (POCs)such as Norplant, the LNg IUD, the Progestasert IUD, Depo-Provera, and minipills do not have adverse effects on lactation, and some studies suggest they may even increase milk volume.[28,38] POCs do not have adverse effects on child growth and development.[1,9,22,28,39,43,45,52] Therefore, because their contraceptive efficacy is very high (see Table 5-2) and because they are simple to use, these methods are excellent options for lactating women who wish to postpone a subsequent pregnancy.

Studies of minipills have demonstrated no adverse effect on lactation or infant growth even when started in the first week postpartum.[39,43] Likewise, studies of Depo-Provera started 1–4 days postpartum or at 7 days postpartum[38] or within 6 weeks postpartum[29] have found no adverse effects.

In studies of the effects of Norplant on lactation and child development, this method has not been started until at least 30 days postpartum. In one Egyptian study, Norplant was inserted between days 30 and 42 postpartum in 50 lactating women. There was no difference in lactational performance between the Norplant group and two control groups. In all three groups, infant growth was above average for Egyptian infants. Among exclusively breastfed infants, weight gains in the early postpartum months were slightly but statistically significantly lower in the Norplant group.[53] In a second Egyptian study, Norplant was inserted between postpartum days 35 and 42 in 120 lactating women. There was no difference in breastfeeding performance between the women using Norplant and women in the control group. Moreover, there was no difference in infant growth or in psychomental development between the Norplant group and a control group.[52] In a Chilean study, Norplant was inserted between days 52 and 58 postpartum in 100 lactating women. There were no important differences in lactational performance between Norplant users and women in the control group. Among exclusively breastfed infants during the first year postpartum, average weights were slightly lower in the Norplant group than in the control group, but the difference was statistically significant only for the fourth through the sixth month. Average monthly weight gains did not statistically significantly differ between the two groups in the first 6 months postpartum among exclusively breastfed infants.[9] In an Indonesian study, Norplant was inserted 4–6 weeks after delivery in 60 lactating women. The weight and height growth curves were very similar among infants in the control and Norplant groups through the first 6 months postpartum.[1]

Although Norplant and Depo-Provera would probably have no adverse effects on lactation or infant health if used immediately postpartum, opinions about whether to do so vary. A prudent approach would be to share this information with the client, and, if the client consents, to wait until breastfeeding has been well established before inserting Norplant rods or giving the Depo-Provera injection. However, in those circumstances in which a breastfeeding woman is unlikely to return for a postpartum visit and requests Norplant before leaving the hospital after delivery (especially if she plans to supplement the infant's diet relatively soon after birth), the real long-term contraceptive benefit of using this method seems likely to exceed the theoretical risks. Because the contraceptive benefit to the lactating woman in obtaining Depo-Provera immediately postpartum is smaller and the theoretical risks might be higher (because the hormonal levels are relatively high in the immediate postinjection days), a case would be less compelling for injecting Depo-Provera before breastfeeding is well established. Discussion of these options before delivery will help to ensure that consent is fully informed.

Immediate postplacental or postpartum insertion of the LNg IUD and the Progestasert IUD has not been studied. High rates of expulsion of the Copper T 380A following postplacental and postpartum insertion raise concerns about expulsion rates for the LNg IUD and the Progestasert IUD (see Chapter 14). As with Norplant and Depo-Provera, discussion of these options before delivery will help to ensure that consent is fully informed.

Combined oral contraceptives are not the contraceptive of choice for breastfeeding mothers. There is clear evidence of a reduction in milk supply due to the estrogen component in combined pills, even those with low-dose preparations.[56,64] Use of combined pills may alter the composition of breastmilk, although results vary among studies; most studies report declines in mineral content. Nevertheless, the available evidence suggests that use of combined pills while nursing does not harm infants.[64] Just when combined pills can be provided to lactating women remains a subject of disagreement among experts. Although combined oral contraceptives can be prescribed immediately postpartum, it seems prudent to caution women not to use them until 6 weeks after delivery, for several reasons. First, low-dose combined oral contraceptives are less likely to interfere with breastfeeding when begun at this time than when begun earlier, because lactation will already be established. Nevertheless, milk volume will still be reduced.[56] This effect is of most concern to women who do not wish to supplement their infant's diet. Second, the risk of postpartum thrombotic complications is highest in the first few weeks after delivery.[65] Avoiding combined OC use during this period of highest risk is a sensible health precaution. Third, the lactating woman is likely to be at very low risk of becoming pregnant during the first 6 weeks postpartum, especially if she is not supplementing the infant's diet. Thus, combined OCs should not be needed in this period to protect against pregnancy. Some advise against using combined pills entirely when other alternatives such as the minipill are available.[17] In the United States, during the first month postpartum, 13% of lactating women who are sexually active rely on the pill; in the second, third and fourth to sixth months postpartum, 12%, 10%, and 7%, respectively, use the pill.[13]

Effects of Hormonal Contraception on the Breastfed Infant

Contraceptive steroids taken by the mother can be transferred to the nursing infant through breastmilk. The amounts, however, are small. The dose consumed by the infant (the equivalent of one pill for every 4 years of full lactation) is so low that no data and no biologic reasoning support the concern of a deleterious effect on the infant.[32] The concern is rather that estrogen suppresses the quantity of milk.

- The dose of contraceptive ethinyl estradiol (about 10 ng per day) reaching the infant of a mother taking combined oral contraceptives is comparable to the dose of the naturally occurring estradiol (from 6–12 ng per day depending on time of cycle) consumed by nursing infants of ovulatory mothers not taking oral contraceptives.[40]

- The quantity of progestin transferred to mother's milk varies with the type of progestin. The 17-hydroxy compounds (such as medroxyprogesterone acetate) enter the milk at approximately the same level as is found in the mother's blood, whereas the 19-nor compounds (such as norgestrel and norethisterone) enter the milk at only one-tenth the level in the blood.[58]

Combined oral contraceptive use during lactation is not the only possible source of estrogen and progestin exposure for the infant. When a mother becomes pregnant and continues to breastfeed a prior infant, that child is exposed to estrogen and progesterone in the mother's milk. Dairy cattle may also be pregnant at the time that they are milked, so that cow's milk and infant formula made from it may have relatively high levels of estrogen and progesterone.

Although early studies of high-dose oral contraceptives did demonstrate some effect of hormones on nursing babies,[8] most of those reports were anecdotal and have not been corroborated in women using low-dose pills. Although the short-term effects of absorbing contraceptive steroids through breastmilk appear minimal, the long-term consequences remain unstudied.[19,23,25]

B REASTFEEDING: ADVANTAGES TO THE INFANT

Mother's milk has both nutritional and anti-infective advantages for the infant. The particular mixtures of protein, fat, carbohydrate, and trace elements change to meet the infant's evolving needs as breastfeeding proceeds from month to month.[38] Furthermore, breastfeeding may help to cement the psychological bond between mother and infant. This bonding may lead to better psychological and intellectual development, though the evidence is inconclusive.[30] Finally, the infant ingests host-resistant, humoral, and allergy prophylaxis factors. These are particularly concentrated in the colostrum, the high-protein fluid secreted in the first few days postpartum.

Breastfed infants have lower risk of respiratory and gastrointestinal illness,[21,30,38] including neonatal necrotizing enterocolitis among preterm infants.[35] Breastfed infants are less likely to develop allergies, including eczema, cow's milk allergy, and allergic rhinitis.[38] Whether breastmilk is protective or alternative diets are allergenic cannot be determined from the available evidence.[30] Asthma may be less common and less severe among children who were breastfed.[30] Other benefits include a decreased incidence of otitis media[30,38] and dental caries.[31] Preterm infants who consume mother's milk in the early weeks of life have higher IQ scores,[36] although the association may not be causal.

B REASTFEEDING AND HIV

The human immunodeficiency virus (HIV), which causes AIDS, can be transmitted by an infected mother to her infant *in utero,* during childbirth, and through breastmilk. That HIV can be transmitted by breastfeeding has been conclusively demonstrated by prospective studies of mothers who were infected postnatally.[10,61] Rates of maternal-fetal transmission through all three routes combined average 25%-30%, with a high of 45% from Kenya and a low of 13% in Europe.[47] The majority of infants who are infected with HIV acquire the infection *in utero* or during childbirth. When the mother was infected prenatally, the additional risk of HIV transmission via breastfeeding is estimated to be 14%.[10]

All babies born to an HIV-infected mother carry passively acquired maternal antibodies to HIV. Those infants who are not infected will gradually lose maternal HIV antibodies, which may nevertheless persist in some cases until 15 months of age. Since standard tests for HIV detect HIV antibodies and not the virus itself, they cannot be used reliably to determine which infants born to HIV-positive mothers have been infected until the child has lost the maternal antibodies.[18] The problem, therefore, is that the HIV status of infants born to HIV-infected mothers cannot be ascertained until well after birth. Because of the risk to the (probably) uninfected infant, HIV-infected mothers in the United States, where safe alternatives to breastmilk are available, are advised to avoid breastfeeding.[5] It is possible that new inexpensive HIV tests will reliably yield positive results only if the infant is HIV-positive when cord blood is tested, even though a negative result would not conclusively mean that the infant was HIV-negative.[42] If such a test is developed, then HIV-positive mothers might be advised that an infant who tests positive could be breastfed.

In developing countries, breastfeeding has been shown to lower infant mortality significantly for three reasons. First, breastmilk is an uncontaminated source of nutrition. Second, the anti-infective agents in breastmilk guard the newborn against gastroenteritis and respiratory infections. Third, breastfeeding lengthens the intervals between births, thereby decreasing maternal depletion and competition between siblings for scarce resources, including parental attention.[57,62]

B REASTFEEDING: ADVANTAGES TO THE MOTHER

Breastfeeding is protective against ovarian and premenopausal breast cancer.[11,55] In addition, breastmilk has a zero price, whereas infant formula does not. Finally, breastfeeding promotes emotional bonding between mother and infant.

Lactation requires even more calories from the mother each day than does pregnancy. Women who do not breastfeed tend to retain the weight gained during pregnancy, whereas those who do breastfeed may return to normal weight more rapidly. This caloric demand is a potential benefit in Western countries where excess weight may be a health problem; where total calorie intake may be limited by economic and dietary resource deficits, it may be a problem for the mother's health. Another advantage to the breastfeeding mother is the rapid return of uterine tone. Oxytocin, which induces uterine contraction, is released from the posterior pituitary when the nipple is stimulated by suckling.

During lactation, the body's estrogen levels are very low, and vaginal lubrication may be less prolific than usual and begin later during sexual intercourse. This side effect disappears when cycling resumes or when the frequency of breastfeeding declines. Nursing mothers have added requirements for calories, protein, calcium, iron, and vitamins A, C, B_1, B_2, and B_3. The increased needs for specific nutrients can be provided by a well-balanced diet. Supplements are generally unnecessary unless the diet is deficient in one or more of these nutrients.[67]

I NSTRUCTIONS FOR BREASTFEEDING

1. Congratulations! Enjoy your baby, rest, and keep in touch with your clinician.

2. **If you are not breastfeeding, begin using a birth control method immediately.** You can become pregnant before your

first menstrual period after childbirth because ovulation can begin before menstruation.

3. **If you are breastfeeding and providing bottle supplements, begin using a birth control method as soon as your clinician advises,** but no later than the time of your first postpartum exam (which would ideally occur 3 weeks rather than 6 weeks after delivery).

4. **If you choose to rely on the lactational amenorrhea method (LAM) as a temporary method of contraception, you must feed your baby on demand, avoid any bottle feeds, and provide minimal supplements by cup or spoon.** Begin using another method of contraception when you resume menstruation, when you reduce the frequency or duration of breastfeeds, when you introduce bottle feeds, or when your baby turns 6 months old. See Figure 17-2.

5. **You can become pregnant while breastfeeding your baby, even before having your first menstrual period,** although the risk is greatly reduced if you feed your baby on demand, avoid any bottle feeds, and provide minimal supplements by cup or spoon. Most U.S. women do not follow breastfeeding patterns that confer maximum protection against pregnancy.

6. **Breastfeeding is a convenient, inexpensive, and nutritious way to feed your baby and it helps to protect the baby against infection and diarrhea.**

7. **Neither intercourse nor menstruation affect the quality and quantity of your breastmilk. You don't need to stop breastfeeding because you start having intercourse again or start your period.** You can continue breastfeeding when you start using another birth control method and even if you conceive another pregnancy. Pregnancy may cause changes in your breastmilk but does not prevent breastfeeding.

8. **Lubricants, such as K-Y jelly, birth control foam, or saliva, may make intercourse easier after childbirth** because decreased estrogen production during breastfeeding causes your vagina to lubricate itself more slowly.

9. **When you are nursing your child, your own nutrition is important.** Extra calcium, iron, and protein in addition to a regular well-balanced diet and sufficient fluid intake are helpful.

10. **Avoid smoking when nursing your baby.** Nursing women who smoke may transfer nicotine to their infant through their breastmilk. Nicotine is a poison that can harm the child. Babies should not

inhale smoke either. Smoking may also influence your ability to produce milk.

11. **Alcohol that you drink will be passed to your baby through breastmilk.** Your baby will have more difficulty metabolizing alcohol than you do, especially in the first few weeks after delivery. No good studies have been conducted to assess what level of alcohol consumption is safe. Thus it seems prudent to drink only modest amounts of alcohol.

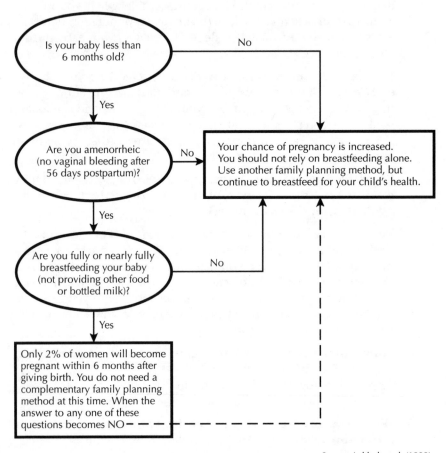

Source: Labbok et al. (1992).

Figure 17-2 Use of the lactational amenorrhea method (LAM) for child spacing during the first 6 months postpartum

12. **If you are using any medications while breastfeeding, be sure to tell your physician.** You will need advice concerning the best timing of medication ingestion to decrease infant exposure. Nevertheless, you can continue to breastfeed while using virtually all common drugs.

13. **If you are infected with HIV, the virus that causes AIDS, you could transmit the virus to your baby through breast-milk.** For this reason, most experts recommend that you not breastfeed your baby.

REFERENCES

1. Affandi B, Karmadibrata S, Prihartono J, Lubis F, Samil RS. Effect of Norplant on mothers and infants in the postpartum period. Adv Contracept 1986;2(4):371-380.

2. Bracher M. Breastfeeding, lactational infecundity, contraception and the spacing of births: implications of the Bellagio consensus statement. Health Transition Rev 1992;2(1):19-47.

3. Calvo EB, Galindo AC, Aspres NB. Iron status in exclusively breast-fed infants. Pediatrics 1992;90(3):375-379.

4. Campbell OMR, Gray RH. Characteristics and determinants of postpartum ovarian function in women in the United States. Am J Obstet Gynecol 1993;169(1):55-60.

5. Centers for Disease Control. Recommendations for assisting in the prevention of perinatal transmission of human T-lymphotropic virus type III/lymphadenopathy-associated virus and acquired immunodeficiency syndrome. MMWR 1985;34(48):721-726, 731-732.

6. Chi I, Potts M, Wilkens LR, Champion CB. Performance of the Copper T-380A intrauterine device in breastfeeding women. Contraception 1989;39(6):603-618.

7. Chvapil M, Eskelson CD, Stiffel V, Owen JA, Droegemueller W. Studies on nonoxynol-9. II. Intravaginal absorption, distribution, metabolism and excretion in rats and rabbits. Contraception 1980;22(3):325-339.

8. Curtis EM. Oral-contraceptive feminization of a normal male infant. Obstet Gynecol 1964;23(2):295-296.

9. Diaz S, Herreros C, Juez G, Casado ME, Salvatierra AM, Miranda P, Peralta O, Croxatto HB. Fertility regulation in nursing women. VII. Influence of Norplant levonorgestrel implants upon lactation and infant growth. Contraception 1985;32(1):53-74.

10. Dunn DT, Newell ML, Ades AE, Peckham CS. Risk of human immunodeficiency virus type 1 transmission through breastfeeding. Lancet 1992;340(8819): 585-588.

11. Eaton SB, Pike MC, Short RV, Lee NC, Trussell J, Hatcher RA, Wood JW, Worthman CM, Jones NB, Konner MJ, Hill K, Bailey R. Women's reproductive cancers in evolutionary context. Atlanta GA: Department of Radiology, Emory University, 1992.

12. Farr G, Rivera R. Interactions between intrauterine contraceptive device use and breast-feeding status at time of intrauterine contraceptive device insertion: analysis of TCu-380A acceptors in developing countries. Am J Obstet Gynecol 1992;167(1):144-151.

13. Ford K, Labbok M. Contraceptive usage during lactation in the United States: an update. Am J Public Health 1987;77(1):79-81.

14. Gordon K, Renfree MB, Short RV, Clarke IJ. Hypothalamo-pituitary portal blood concentrations of ß-endorphin during suckling in the ewe. J Reprod Fertil 1987;79(2):397-408.

15. Gray RH, Campbell OM, Apelo R, Eslami SS, Zacur H, Ramos RM, Gehret JC, Labbok MH. Risk of ovulation during lactation. Lancet 1990;335(8680):25-29.

16. Gray RH, Campbell OM, Zacur H, Labbok MH, MacRae SL. Postpartum return of ovarian activity in nonbreastfeeding women monitored by urinary assays. J Clin Endocrinol Metab 1987;64(4):645-650.

17. Guillebaud J. Contraception, your questions answered. New York NY: Churchill, 1985.

18. Hardy LM (ed). HIV screening of pregnant women and newborns. Washington DC: National Academy Press, 1991.

19. Harlap S. Exposure to contraceptive hormones through breast milk—are there long-term health and behavioral consequences? Intl J Gynaecol Obstet 1987;25(Suppl):47-55.

20. Hodgen GD, Itskovitz J. Recognition and maintenance of pregnancy. In: Knobil E, Neill JD, Ewing LL, Greenwald GS, Markert CL, Pfaff DW (eds). The physiology of reproduction. New York NY: Raven Press, 1988:1995-2021.

21. Howie PW, Forsyth JS, Ogston SA, Clark A, du V Florey C. Protective effect of breastfeeding against infection. Br Med J 1990;300(6716):11-16.

22. Jimenez J, Ochoa M, Soler MP, Portales P. Long-term follow-up of children breast-fed by mothers receiving depo-medroxyprogesterone acetate. Contraception 1984;30(6):523-533.

23. Johansson E, Odlind V. The passage of exogenous hormones into breast milk—possible effects. Intl J Gynaecol Obstet 1987;25(Suppl):111-114.

24. Kennedy KI. Fertility, sexuality and contraception during lactation. In: Riordan J, Auerbach KG (eds). Breastfeeding and human lactation. Boston MA: Jones and Bartlett Publishers, 1993:429-457.

25. Kennedy KI. Lactation and contraception. Ginecol Obstet Mex 1990;58(Suppl 1):25-34.

26. Kennedy KI, Rivera R, McNeilly AS. Consensus statement on the use of breast-feeding as a family planning method. Contraception 1989;39(5):477-496.

27. Kennedy KI, Visness CM. Contraceptive efficacy of lactational amenorrhoea. Lancet 1992;339(8787):227-230.

28. Koetsawang S. The effects of contraceptive methods on the quality and quantity of breast milk. Intl J Gynaecol Obstet 1987;25(Suppl):115-127.

29. Koetsawang S, Boonyaprakob V, Suvanichati S, Paipeekul S. Long-term study of growth and development of children breast-fed by mothers receiving Depo-Provera (medroxyprogesterone acetate) during lactation. In: Zatuchni GI, Goldsmith A, Shelton JD, Sciarra JJ (eds). Long-acting contraceptive delivery systems. Philadelphia PA: Harper & Row, 1983:378-387.

30. Kovar MG, Serdula MK, Marks JS, Fraser DW. Review of the epidemiologic evidence for an association between infant feeding and infant health. Pediatrics 1984;74(4-Suppl):615-638.

31. Labbok MH. Consequences of breastfeeding for mother and child. J Biosoc Sci 1985a;9(Suppl):43-54.

32. Labbok MH. Contraception during lactation: considerations in advising the individual and in formulating programme guidelines. J Biosoc Sci 1985b; 9(Suppl):55-66.

33. Labbok MH, Koniz-Booher P, Shelton J, Krasovec K. Guidelines for breastfeeding in family planning and child survival programs. Washington DC: Institute for Reproductive Health, Georgetown University, February 1992.

34. Lewis PR, Brown JB, Renfree MB, Short RV. The resumption of ovulation and menstruation in a well-nourished population of women breastfeeding for an extended period of time. Fertil Steril 1991;55(3):529-536.

35. Lucas A, Cole TJ. Breast milk and neonatal necrotising enterocolitis. Lancet 1990;336(8730):1519-1523.

36. Lucas A, Morley R, Cole TJ, Lister G, Leeson-Payne C. Breast milk and subsequent intelligence quotient in children born preterm. Lancet 1992;339(8788):261-264.

37. Masters WH, Johnson VE. Human sexual response. Boston MA: Little, Brown & Co., 1966.

38. McCann MF, Liskin LS, Piotrow PT, Rinehart W, Fox G. Breastfeeding, fertility and family planning. Popul Reports 1984;12(2), Series J(24).

39. McCann MF, Moggia AV, Higgins JE, Potts M, Becker C. The effects of a progestin-only oral contraceptive (Levonorgestrel 0.03 mg) on breastfeeding. Contraception 1989;40(6):635-648.

40. McGregor JA. Lactation and contraception. In: Neville MC, Neifert MR (eds). Lactation: physiology, nutrition, and breast-feeding. New York NY: Plenum Press, 1983:405-421.

41. McNeilly AS. Suckling and the control of gonadotropin secretion. In: Knobil E, Neill JD, Ewing LL, Greenwald GS, Markert CL, Pfaff DW (eds). The physiology of reproduction. New York NY: Raven Press, 1988:2323-2349.

42. Miles SA, Balden E, Magpantay L, Wei L, Leiblein A, Hofheinz D, Toedter G, Stiehm ER, Bryson Y, Southern California Pediatric AIDS Consortium. Rapid serologic testing with immune-complex-dissociated HIV p24 antigen for early detection of HIV infection in neonates. New Eng J Med 1993;328(5): 297-302.

43. Moggia AV, Harris GS, Dunson TR, Diaz R, Moggia MS, Ferrer MA, McMullen SL. A comparative study of a progestin-only oral contraceptive versus nonhormonal methods in lactating women in Buenos Aires, Argentina. Contraception 1991;44(1):31-43.

44. O'Hanley K, Huber DH. Postpartum IUDs: keys for success. Contraception 1992;45(4):351-361.

45. Pardthaisong T, Yenchit C, Gray R. The long-term growth and development of children exposed to Depo-Provera during pregnancy or lactation. Contraception 1992;45(4):313-324.

46. Pérez A, Labbok MH, Queenan JT. Clinical study of the lactational amenorrhoea method for family planning. Lancet 1992;339(8799):968-970.

47. Pizzo PA, Butler KM. In the vertical transmission of HIV, timing may be everything. New Eng J Med 1991;325(9):652-654.

48. Queenan JT, Jennings VH, Spieler JM, von Hertzen H (eds). Natural family planning: current knowledge and new strategies for the 1990s. Am J Obstet Gynecol 1991;165(6-Suppl):2013-2045.
49. Robinson JE, Short RV. Changes in breast sensitivity at puberty, during the menstrual cycle, and at parturition. Br Med J 1977;1(6070):1188-1191.
50. Ryan AS, Pratt WF, Wysong JL, Lewandowski G, McNally JW, Krieger FW. A comparison of breast-feeding data from the National Surveys of Family Growth and the Ross Laboratories Mothers Surveys. Am J Public Health 1991;81(8):1049-1052.
51. Ryan AS, Rush D, Krieger FW, Lewandowski GE. Recent declines in breast-feeding in the United States, 1984 through 1989. Pediatrics 1991;88(4):719-727.
52. Shaaban MM. Contraception with progestogens and progesterone during lactation. J Steroid Biochem Mol Biol 1991;40(4-6):705-710.
53. Shaaban MM, Salem HT, Abdullah KA. Influence of levonorgestrel contraceptive implants, Norplant®, initiated early postpartum upon lactation and infant growth. Contraception 1985;32(6):623-635.
54. Speroff L, Darney P. A clinical guide for contraception. Baltimore MD: Williams & Wilkins, 1992.
55. Speroff L, Glass RH, Kase NG. Clinical gynecologic endocrinology and infertility. Baltimore MD: Williams & Wilkins, 1989.
56. Tankeyoon M, Dusitsin N, Chalapati S, Koetsawang S, Saibiang S, Sas M, Gellen JJ, Ayeni O, Gray R, Pinol A, Zegers L. Effects of hormonal contraceptives on milk volume and infant growth. Contraception 1984;30(6):505-522.
57. Thapa S, Short RV, Potts M. Breastfeeding, birth spacing and their effects on child survival. Nature 1988;335(6192):679-682.
58. Toddywalla VS, Mehta S, Virkar KD, Saxena BN. Release of 19-nor-testosterone type of contraceptive steroids through different drug delivery systems into serum and breast milk of lactating women. Contraception 1980;21(3):217-223.
59. Treiman K, Liskin L. IUDs—a new look. Popul Rep 1988;16(1), Series B(5).
60. Trussell J, Grummer-Strawn L, Rodríguez G, VanLandingham M. Trends and differentials in breastfeeding behavior: evidence from the WFS and DHS. Popul Stud 1992;46(2):285-307.
61. Van de Perre P, Simonon A, Msellati P, Hitimana DG, Vaira D, Bazubagira A, Van Goethem C, Stevens AM, Karita E, Sondag-Thull D, Dabis F, Lepage P. Postnatal transmission of human immunodeficiency virus type I from mother to infant. New Eng J Med 1991;325(9):593-598.
62. VanLandingham M, Trussell J, Grummer-Strawn L. Contraceptive and health benefits of breastfeeding: a review of the recent evidence. Int Fam Plann Perspect 1991;17(4):131-136.
63. Wenof M, Aubert JM, Reyniak JV. Serum prolactin levels in short-term and long-term use of inert plastic and copper intrauterine devices. Contraception 1979;19(1):21-27.
64. Wharton C, Blackburn R. Lower-dose pills. Popul Rep 1988;16(3), Series A(7).
65. WHO Task Force on Oral Contraceptives. Contraception during the postpartum period and during lactation: the effects on women's health. Intl J Obstet Gynaecol 1987;25(Suppl):13-26.
66. Willson JR. The puerperium. In: Willson JR, Carrington ER, Ledger WJ, Laros RK, Mattox JH (eds). Obstetrics and gynecology. St. Louis MO: CV Mosby Company, 1987:598-607.
67. Worthington-Roberts BS, Williams SR. Nutrition in pregnancy and lactation. St. Louis MO: Times Mirror/Mosby College Publishing, 1989.

Pregnancy Testing and Management of Early Pregnancy

- With early pregnancy diagnosis, a woman planning to continue her pregnancy can begin prenatal precautions and medical care during the early, most vulnerable stages of fetal development.
- A woman considering abortion will have time for adequate counseling and decision making. Abortion can be performed when it is safest—early in pregnancy.

- Early pregnancy diagnosis helps ensure that ectopic pregnancy can be detected early. Early detection reduces the risk of life-threatening ectopic pregnancy complications. Early surgical management is more likely to preserve the affected fallopian tube.

Early pregnancy diagnosis is an essential part of every family planning program. Screening very early in pregnancy can avert serious complications and provide the pregnant woman with an opportunity to learn about precautions needed during pregnancy and prenatal care resources, or about options for abortion care. Early evaluation also provides an opportunity for HIV screening. Because HIV has such serious consequences, screen any woman who is pregnant or planning to become pregnant unless she and her partner have been mutually faithful for at least 10 years. Nonjudgmental, supportive counseling and information, including accurate and specific referral options for abortion, adoption services, and prenatal care, are essential services.

Inexpensive pregnancy test kits, sensitive enough to provide accurate results as early as 1 week after fertilization, are widely available and simple to use. Thus, there is no reason to impose an arbitrary delay in pregnancy evaluation based on the date of the woman's last menstrual period.

Clinical assessment and pregnancy testing should be offered as soon as the patient seeks these services.

PREGNANCY EVALUATION

Clinical evaluation for a woman who may be pregnant should include a review of pertinent history and symptoms, a laboratory test to detect human chorionic gonadotropin (HCG), and a pelvic exam. In most though not all cases, the last menstrual period date provides an accurate estimate of gestational age. A pelvic exam can confirm pregnancy test results and correlate uterine enlargement with menstrual dates. The pelvic exam is essential in identifying the possibility of abnormal pregnancy. Pregnancy diagnosis has several goals:

1. Determine whether or not the woman is pregnant.
2. Identify possible problems that require further evaluation and/or emergency intervention, such as ectopic gestation or threatened abortion.
3. Assess gestation length accurately (in weeks).
4. Help the patient make and implement her own plans for prenatal care or abortion.

History and symptoms. The most common sign that prompts a woman to seek pregnancy evaluation is an overdue menstrual period. Often the woman herself suspects pregnancy or has reason to believe that she could be pregnant. A particularly useful question to ask is simply: Do you think you are pregnant now? An unusually light or mistimed period may mean fertilization actually occurred before the last menstrual period (LMP), and for this reason, the date of the previous menstrual period (PMP) should be determined. The date when pregnancy symptoms began can help corroborate fertilization date. Breast tenderness and nipple sensitivity typically begin 1–2 weeks after fertilization; fatigue, nausea, and urinary frequency at about 2 weeks. Bleeding, spotting, or lower abdominal pain may signal ectopic gestation or threatened spontaneous abortion.

Physical examination. Cervical softening, blurring of the cervico-uterine angle, and uterine softening are early signs of pregnancy, appearing within the first 2–3 weeks after fertilization. If the uterine size does not correspond to the estimated length of gestation based on last menstrual period, consider possible reasons for the discrepancy (see Table 18-1) Ultrasound evaluation often is helpful in this situation.

PREGNANCY TEST BIOLOGY

Pregnancy tests detect HCG in a pregnant woman's urine or serum. Correctly interpreting pregnancy test results, however, is not entirely straightforward because:

Table 18-1 Possible reasons for discrepancy between uterine size and menstrual dates

Uterus Smaller Than Expected	Uterus Larger Than Expected
Fertilization later than dates suggest	Fertilization earlier than dates suggest
Ectopic pregnancy	Uterine leiomyomata (fibroids)
Incomplete or missed, spontaneous abortion	Twin gestation
Error in pregnancy test	Uterine anomaly
	Hydatidiform mole

  1. HCG levels change drastically over the course of pregnancy (see Figure 18-1).
  2. Test results, especially negative test results, must be interpreted in relation to the sensitivity, specificity, and characteristics of the particular test being used.

HCG Levels During Pregnancy

When the morula implants in the endometrium, the proliferation of trophoblastic cells initiates placental development and rapidly increasing HCG production. HCG can be detected in the woman's serum at low levels as early as 7–9 days after ovulation, very soon after implantation occurs. During the first 3–4 weeks after fertilization, the HCG level in normal

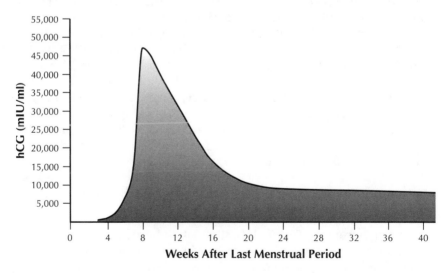

Source: Braunstein et al. (1976) with permission.

Figure 18-1 HCG levels during normal pregnancy

pregnancy doubles approximately every 2 days so that the serum level reaches 50–250 mIU/ml by the time of the first missed menstrual period (see Figure 18-2). HCG reaches a peak approximately 60–70 days after fertilization and then decreases.

In abnormal pregnancies, HCG levels often are abnormal. Elevated levels are normal with multiple gestation. Extremely high HCG production, with HCG levels as high as a million mIU/ml, can occur with molar pregnancy (hydatidiform mole). Such very high levels can be documented with a quantitative serum HCG test. Abnormally low HCG levels often occur before a spontaneous abortion or with an ectopic pregnancy. On the other hand, low levels may simply indicate that a normal pregnancy is earlier in gestation than menstrual dates suggest. For example, if ovulation was delayed slightly in the preceding cycle, fertilization will have actually occurred on cycle day 21 or later. Ovulation later than expected is not unusual, especially if the woman discontinued oral contraceptives in the previous menstrual cycle.

HCG Levels After Pregnancy

After a pregnancy is terminated by delivery or abortion, blood and urine HCG levels gradually decrease (see Figure 18-3). The initial decrease is quite rapid, so that an HCG level after 2 weeks should be less than 1% of the level at the time the pregnancy is terminated.[4] Following full-term delivery, the level will have dropped to less than 50 mIU within 2 weeks, and HCG will be undetectable after 3–4 weeks. In the case of first-trimester abortion, however, initial HCG levels may be much higher. If the abortion occurs at 8–10 weeks of gestation when HCG may be as high as 150,000 mIU, then 2 weeks after abortion the HCG levels may still be 1,500 mIU, high enough that all pregnancy tests will still be positive. HCG may be detectable by sensitive tests for as long as 40 days after first-trimester abortion.[20] If continuing intrauterine pregnancy, retained placenta fragments, or ectopic pregnancy are possibilities, consider obtaining serial quantitative HCG levels to track an upward or downward trend. If HCG is clearing normally from the bloodstream, the HCG level should decline steadily with a half-time of disappearance of no more than 24–48 hours.

Hormone Structure and Pregnancy Test Design

HCG is closely related in molecular structure to the pituitary hormones LH (luteinizing hormone), FSH (follicle stimulating hormone), and TSH (thyroid stimulating hormone). Each is composed of two subunits: an alpha and a beta subunit. The alpha subunits of LH, FSH, TSH, and HCG are virtually identical. Therefore, only a test that selectively identifies the beta subunit of HCG is specific for HCG.

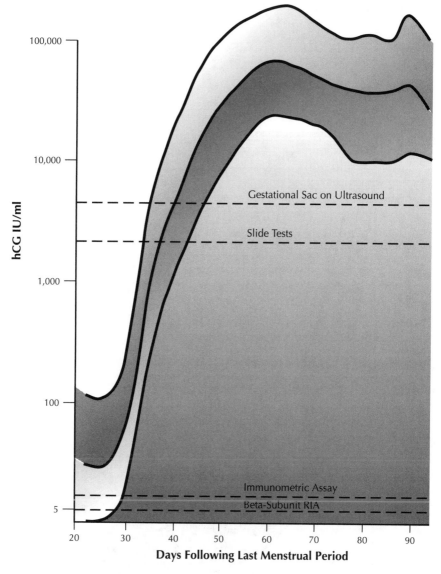

Source: Braunstein et al. (1978) with permission.

Figure 18-2 HCG levels in early pregnancy

Two-site, immunometric test kits appropriate for office or home use are specific for beta HCG, and so is the beta subunit radioimmunoassay used for quantitative serum HCG determination in the laboratory. Most agglutination inhibition slide tests, however, detect whole HCG rather than the beta subunit and therefore show at least some cross-reactivity with other

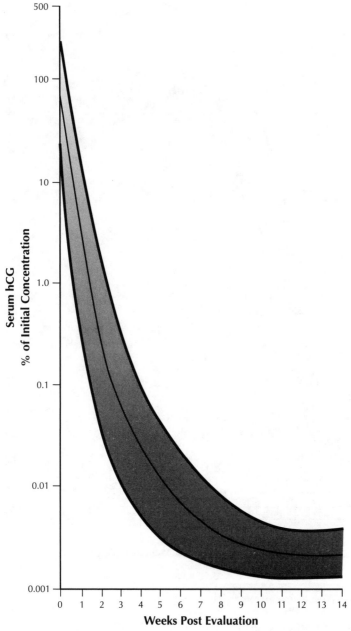

Source: Braunstein (1983) with permission.

Figure 18-3 HCG disappearance after pregnancy

hormones, especially LH. Because they are so inexpensive and simple to use, slide tests nevertheless may be an appropriate option in certain circumstances. Other, older test methods including tube tests and radioreceptor assays are no longer needed.

PREGNANCY TEST OPTIONS

Pregnancy testing has been revolutionized with the development of monoclonal antibody techniques. Many new test kits, as well as old familiar products, are available so that the array of options is bewildering and ever-changing. Test kits suitable for use in the family planning clinic or clinician's office are shown in Table 18-2.

IMMUNOMETRIC TESTS

Immunometric tests exploit technology that has made possible the inexpensive production of pure antibody in large quantities. Immunometric tests for pregnancy are based on the ELISA (enzyme-linked immunosorbent assay) assay design; they are sometimes called "two-site" or sandwich tests and require two different antibodies. One antibody captures the beta subunit of HCG; the other antibody is conjugated to an enzyme that provides a color change. Because immunometric tests are specific for the beta subunit of HCG, cross-reaction with other hormones is not a problem. Some test kits, which may also be suitable for clinic use, are available without prescription for home use.

Specificity.   Immunometric tests provide accurate qualitative (yes/no) results with HCG levels as low as 5–50 mIU/ml, depending on the specific test kit. With a urine test kit with a sensitivity of 25 mIU/ml, results are positive for some women as early as 3–4 days after implantation (10 days after fertilization); test results are positive for 98% of women within 7 days after implantation.[11]

Uses.   Immunometric tests can be used to confirm pregnancy, or to "rule out" the diagnosis of pregnancy. These tests are appropriate for screening prior to procedures such as biopsy or x-ray, or prior to prescribing a drug, that would be contraindicated during pregnancy. They are also appropriate in screening for possible ectopic pregnancy. Only 1% of patients with ectopic pregnancy would be missed (falsely negative) with a urine test sensitivity of 50 mIU/ml.[4]

QUANTITATIVE BETA HCG RADIOIMMUNOASSAY

Use of an RIA "blood test" as a qualitative (yes/no) pregnancy test does not have any advantage over immunometric urine tests. Immunometric kits

Table 18-2 Commonly used clinic and office pregnancy tests

Name (Manufacturer)	Sensitivity (mIU/ml)*	Time Required	# Steps/ Comments
Immunometric Tests: Specific for beta HCG, no LH, FSH, or TSH cross-reaction Reliably detect pregnancy 7–10 days after conception. Cost: $2.30–$7.00**			
CARDS (Pacific Biotech)	25	3 Min	1 Step/Urine
Clearview HCG (Wampole)	50	5 Min	1 Step/Urine
Icon II HCG (Hybritech)	20	5 Min	5 Steps/Serum
	25	4 Min	5 Steps/Urine
Nimbus (Biomerica)	10–25	5–15 Min	Serum or Urine Sensitivity depends on time
One Step (Wampole)	25	7 Min	1 Step/Serum
	25	5 Min	1 Step/Urine
PregnaGen (Biogenex)	40	4 Min	1 Step/Urine
Precise (Becton Dickinson)	25	4 Min	1 Step/Urine
Pro-Step HCG (Disease Detection Intl)	25	4 Min	1 Step, Dip/Serum
	25	3 Min	Urine
Quick Vue (Quidel)	25	3 Min	1Step/Urine
Surcell HCG (Kodak)	30	2 Min	2–3 Steps/Serum
	30	1 Min	2–3 Steps/Urine
	50	1 Min	2–3 Steps/Urine
Tandem Icon QSR (Hybritech)	<5	7 Min	Serum
Target (V-Tech)	50	4 Min	Urine
		5 Min	Serum
Testpack plus HCG (Abbott)	50	5 Min	1 Step/Urine
Testpack plus HCG combo (Abbott)	25	7 Min	1 Step/Serum
	50	4 Min	Urine
Agglutination Inhibition Slide Tests: Test antibody reacts to whole HCG, not specific for beta HCG; cross-reaction with LH, FSH, and TSH is possible. Reliably detect pregnancy 18 – 21 days after conception (32 – 36 days after last menstrual period). All require urine specimen. Cost $1.30–$2.30**			
Pregnosticon (Organon)	1,000–2,000	2 Min	
Pregnosis (Roche)	1,500–2,500	2 Min	
Wampole UCG (Wampole)	1,500–2,500	2 Min	

  * Sensitivity specified as the lower limit of reliable HCG detection in product literature. Test results may be positive at lower HCG levels in some cases.
** Bulk or nonprofit agency discount purchase may reduce costs significantly.

Source: Manufacturers' product literature (1993).

Note: Intermediate sensitivity slide tests that detect HCG levels of approximately 500 mIU/ml are also available, but cost as much as immunometric tests. Immunometric kits are more sensitive and easier to use.

are equally specific for HCG and provide sensitivity that is completely satisfactory for clinical evaluation, with immediate results, and at much lower cost.

Specificity. Because radioimmunoassay (RIA) provides accurate quantitative results with HCG levels as low as 5 mIU/ml, it can detect pregnancy reliably within 7 days after fertilization. The test may be positive a few days earlier. Because the RIA test procedure requires use of radioisotopes, it is appropriate for a laboratory associated with a hospital or large clinic. Tests are usually performed in batches because of expense; test processing requires 1-2 hours.

Uses. RIA can provide a quantitative result; serial test specimens can be used to check doubling time or disappearance time when ectopic pregnancy, impending spontaneous abortion, or possible retained placental fragments are being evaluated. Very high levels can be documented to confirm the diagnosis of molar pregnancy. Be sure to specify *quantitative beta* HCG when ordering this test. Also, serial tests should all be ordered from the same laboratory to avoid possible confusion about assay standardization differences between laboratories.

AGGLUTINATION INHIBITION SLIDE TESTS

Inexpensive agglutination inhibition slide tests, widely used for the last 15 years, depend on binding of HCG in the patient's urine with an anti-HCG antibody in the test solution. Binding of the test antibody prevents clumping (agglutination) of latex particles in the test solution.

Specificity. Because antibodies used in most slide tests are not specific for the beta subunit of HCG, cross-reactions are possible. To minimize problems of cross-reaction with LH, FSH, or TSH, slide-test sensitivity is set so that high levels of HCG are required to give a positive test result. A cross-reaction, therefore, is unlikely to be a source of clinical confusion. However, a test specimen obtained during the brief surge of LH just before ovulation or during the perimenopausal years may cause false positive results in a slide pregnancy test because of LH or FSH cross-reaction. Cross-reactivity with TSH is unlikely because its level is normally quite low.

Uses. Slide tests are inexpensive, easy to perform, and appropriate for confirming pregnancy when the gestation is between 6weeks and 16 weeks. HCG levels early in pregnancy (the first month after fertilization) and later in pregnancy (after 16–20 weeks' gestation) may be below the level detected by latex agglutination slide pregnancy tests. They are not appropriate to "rule out" pregnancy because early pregnancy, later pregnancy, ectopic pregnancy, and impending abortion may be missed. If the initial agglutination test is negative, a more sensitive test should be used (see Immunometric Tests), or the test should be repeated a few days later.

HOME PREGNANCY TESTING

Home pregnancy test kits offer the advantages of privacy, anonymity, and convenience. Moreover, they are popular. In a national survey, approximately 33% of pregnant women reported using them.[16] In another survey, 17% of college women reported that they had used a home test at least once. Most women chose home testing because results can be obtained quickly and confidentially.[12] Because home pregnancy test are easily accessible, a woman may identify pregnancy early and thus be more able to be an active manager of her own health care.

Specificity. Unfortunately, the accuracy of home tests in actual use may not be ideal. In one study of three commonly used home kits,[14] the predictive value was only 84% for positive home test results and 62% for negative results. Another researcher found that when test kits were used by non-technical personnel, results did not agree with standard laboratory test results in approximately 10% of 200 samples tested.[15] Test accuracy can be affected by the techniques and experience of the user, and by the user's ability to follow the test instructions precisely.[19] The most common error with home pregnancy tests is a negative result that occurs because the test was performed too early in pregnancy. An incorrect result could mislead a woman, causing her to delay in getting a clinical evaluation.

Uses. If a home test result is positive, clinical evaluation is needed to confirm the pregnancy, determine the length of gestation, and identify any possible risk for ectopic or abnormal pregnancy. If the home test result is negative, clinical evaluation also may be needed to determine the cause of menstrual delay or of the other symptoms that have prompted the test, especially if the woman does not resume normal menses soon. In either case, a second pregnancy test is likely to be indicated, so that the cost of the home kit may be an unnecessary expense. On the other hand, positive results may prompt a woman to change her lifestyle earlier than were she to wait for a clinical evaluation.

AVOIDING PREGNANCY TEST INTERPRETATION ERRORS

If pregnancy test results do not agree with other clinical signs, consider the possible reasons for the discrepancy. Plan appropriate follow-up or further evaluation to protect the patient against possible consequences of an incorrect test result:

1. **Any test result can be wrong.** Laboratory errors do occur, including specimen mix-up and incorrectly performed test procedures. For accurate results, instructions for the kit must be followed meticulously and timed with a stopwatch. Use control solutions to verify accuracy. Observe test-kit expiration dates.

2. **Know exactly what kind of pregnancy test was performed,** and what sensitivity the test has. Without this information, it is not possible to assess the clinical significance of a negative result or to evaluate the possibility of a false positive result.

3. **Send all serial specimens for quantitative beta HCG assays to the same laboratory.** Results of quantitative immunoassay performed by different laboratories may not be comparable because of differences between immunoassay kits and standards used by different manufacturers. Some laboratories record HCG levels in metric units; these can be roughly converted to mIU by multiplying the metric results by 5.2 (10 ng/ml = 52 mIU). Results should be multiplied by 1.5–2 for comparison to the first international standard and by 8–10 for the third international standard. Know what standard your laboratory uses.

4. **Do not base clinical management on the results of a home pregnancy test.** Although home kits have excellent theoretical accuracy, their use even by trained personnel may not reliably provide the sensitivity or specificity needed for optimal clinical management.[14,15,17] Be careful about accepting the results of a pregnancy test performed in another facility, especially if critical clinical situations such as ectopic pregnancy are possible.

5. **False negative results are common with agglutination inhibition tests.** False negative results frequently occur because the test is performed too early or too late in pregnancy. Abnormal pregnancy, urine that is too dilute, and medication that interferes with test result may all be responsible. Use an immunometric test (see Table 18-1) to "rule out" pregnancy.

6. **False negative results are rare with immunometric tests** but can occur if test procedures are performed incorrectly (such as excessive rinsing) or a test reader who has red-green color blindness.[3] Elevated lipids, high immunoglobulin levels, and low serum protein associated with severe kidney disease also can interfere with a test assay. If a false negative result is suspected, order a quantitative beta subunit radioimmunoassay.

7. **False positive pregnancy test results are not common,** but they can cause perplexing dilemmas:
   - False positive results with an *immunometric test* are very rare, but laboratory error is always possible. If a false positive result is suspected, obtain a quantitative beta subunit radioimmunoassay.

- If an agglutination inhibition *slide test* is positive, but the uterus is not enlarged, perform a confirmatory immunometric test. The positive result could be caused by *LH* or *FSH* cross-reaction, in which case the immunometric test will be negative because it is specific for beta *HCG*.

- Slide tests also can yield false positive results because of protein or blood in the urine specimen. Consider obtaining a confirmatory immunometric test if the urine specimen shows 1+ proteinuria or more. An immunometric test is likely to give an accurate (negative) result. When a positive pregnancy test is not confirmed by the presence of a pregnancy in the uterus, do not assume the test result is false. Seriously consider the possibility of an ectopic pregnancy.

8. In very rare cases, pregnancy test results are positive even though the patient is not pregnant because *HCG actually is present, originating from a source other than pregnancy.* HCG levels persist after a recent pregnancy or after HCG treatment. Low levels of HCG (5–30 mIU) may be associated with tumors of the pancreas, ovaries, breast, and many others.[2] Some normal postmenopausal women also have low levels of circulating HCG-like substance, whose origin is unknown.[4]

M ANAGING PROBLEMS IN EARLY PREGNANCY

Consider the possibility of spontaneous abortion or ectopic pregnancy whenever a woman in the reproductive years has symptoms such as abdominal pain, abnormal bleeding, or irregular or missed menstrual periods. The patient's history, as well as her own assessment of pregnancy risk, may be helpful. For example, in a study of women undergoing evaluation at a hospital emergency department, 63% of the women who thought they might be pregnant, were pregnant. A sensitive pregnancy test, however, is a prudent precaution to take, no matter what the woman's history indicates. In the previously cited study, 10% of women who reported a normal last menstrual period, and stated that there was no chance they could be pregnant, were nevertheless found to be pregnant.[21]

No matter what the cause or diagnosis, *Rh screening is indicated* for any woman with bleeding in pregnancy. The risk of Rh sensitization resulting from bleeding in early pregnancy is low, but treatment with Rh immune globulin is a wise precaution. *A blood count also is indicated at the time of initial evaluation.* The results may help assess the cumulative extent of bleeding and may provide an important baseline for later comparison if internal hemorrhage is suspected.

Abnormal bleeding, cramping, and abdominal pain can occur with threatened abortion, complete or incomplete spontaneous abortion, and ectopic pregnancy. However, these symptoms also can occur in an early pregnancy that subsequently progresses to a normal outcome. When these symptoms occur, perform an evaluation immediately: Exclude the presence of ectopic pregnancy and arrange appropriate care for possible spontaneous abortion.

POSSIBLE ECTOPIC PREGNANCY

A woman who has clinical evidence of possible ruptured ectopic pregnancy, such as hypotension and/or postural hypotension, severe abdominal pain, guarding, or rebound tenderness requires immediate referral for emergency surgery. An ultrasensitive pregnancy test is almost certain to be positive (false negative rate is less than 1%,[4] but agglutination inhibition tests are not sensitive enough to detect the lower HCG levels associated with ectopic gestation in about 50% of cases.[1] Because intervention should not be delayed, further nonsurgical evaluation is not prudent.

More commonly, the clinician considers the possibility of ectopic pregnancy because the woman has less serious and nonspecific symptoms such as bleeding in early pregnancy, uterine enlargement that does not correlate with dates (uterus is too small), or early vacuum abortion that has failed to recover identifiable placental tissue from the uterine cavity. Often the patient is completely asymptomatic. These situations allow time for further outpatient evaluation if the patient is willing and able to monitor her own symptoms carefully. While evaluation is pending, the patient must be warned to watch for ectopic pregnancy danger signs (see Table 18-3) and to return immediately for emergency care if danger signs occur. Further steps in evaluation might include the following:

1. **Quantitative beta HCG assay.** Although test results probably will not be available for at least 24 hours, an initial level can be compared with the beta HCG level 2 days later if diagnosis is still uncertain. A decline of 60% or more favors the diagnosis of normal HCG disappearance after spontaneous or induced abortion, or after spontaneous resolution of an ectopic pregnancy. A level of 1,000 mIU or less provides limited reassurance about the safety of outpatient management, because life-threatening intra-abdominal hemorrhage is rare with ectopic pregnancy at such an early stage of pregnancy.[18] However, clinically significant internal bleeding, while rare, has been reported even at levels below the 25 mIU/ml sensitivity of immunometric tests.

Table 18-3 Early pregnancy danger signs

Possible Ectopic Pregnancy
Sudden intense pain, or persistent pain, or cramping in the lower abdomen, usually localized to one side or the other
Irregular bleeding or spotting with abdominal pain when period is late or after an abnormally light period
Fainting or dizziness persisting more than a few seconds. These may be signs of internal bleeding. (Internal bleeding is not necessarily associated with vaginal bleeding.)

Possible Miscarriage
Late last period and bleeding is now heavy, possibly with clots or clumps of tissue; cramping more severe than usual
Period is prolonged and heavy—5 – 7 days of "heaviest" days
Abdominal pain or fever

Contact your clinician immediately or go to a hospital emergency room if you develop any of these signs.

Source: Stewart et al. (1987).

2. **Pathology phone report.** If an abortion has been performed, request a microscopic tissue evaluation and a report by phone. The pathologist may be able to identify placental villi and confirm intrauterine pregnancy, in which case the likelihood of simultaneous ectopic pregnancy is extremely remote.

3. **Ultrasound evaluation.** Pelvic ultrasound should be able to detect a fetus with cardiac activity inside the uterus by the 7th to 8th week of gestation dated from last menstrual period. The use of vaginal probe ultrasound moves this threshold forward by 7-10 days. With a vaginal probe, it is possible in some cases to detect a tiny gestational sac of 1 mm–3 mm in size in the uterus as early as 30 days after ovulation, when HCG is 900 mIU/ml or less.[8] With good abdominal ultrasound equipment and technique, a gestational sac should definitely be detected when the beta HCG is 1,800 mIU (by 5–6 weeks of gestation). A vaginal probe should detect a gestational sac when HCG is 1,000 mIU (by 4–5 weeks of gestation).[13]

Unfortunately, a sac-like ultrasound appearance, called a "pseudogestational sac," can occur in conjunction with ectopic pregnancy in as many as 10% of cases.[25] The other ultrasound signs of possible ectopic pregnancy, such as poorly defined adnexal mass and cul de sac fluid, are not specific enough for conclusive diagnosis. However, the diagnosis of ectopic pregnancy can be made conclusively if a gestational sac and fetal heartbeat are detected outside of the uterine cavity. The differential diagnosis usually includes intrauterine gestation earlier than menstrual dates would suggest, complete or incomplete spontaneous abortion, or pregnancy with a corpus luteum cyst. Unless intrauterine gestation can be identified with certainty or an extrauterine gestation is visible, ultrasound results do not provide a definite diagnosis.

If after completing these three diagnostic steps ectopic pregnancy cannot be excluded, arrange for surgical evaluation. Refer immediately if the patient becomes symptomatic during the process of evaluation. Laparoscopy will most likely be needed to ascertain the diagnosis.

In some cases, close observation alone may be an option: when beta HCG is low and declining, the patient remains asymptomatic, and the size of the ectopic pregnancy is small. Spontaneous abortion of an ectopic pregnancy followed by resorption occurs in as many as 83% of such cases in a reported series.[18] In this situation, the beta HCG will decline slowly to zero. Alternatively, some centers treat with methotrexate[24] or with etoposide[22] to induce dissolution of trophoblast tissue, thus causing a medical abortion. If gestation is early, it may be possible to evacuate the pregnancy through an incision in the fallopian tube wall during laparoscopic or abdominal surgery. When technically possible, this approach is preferred over salpingectomy or salpingo-oophorectomy for the patient who would like to preserve her future fertility.[1]

Early diagnosis is very important in ectopic pregnancy. Early diagnosis and intervention have helped to reduce ectopic pregnancy mortality from 35.5 deaths per 10,000 ectopic pregnancies in 1970 to 5.4/10,000 in 1988.[10] Also, early diagnosis allows more time for conservative management, which may help to preserve the woman's future fertility.

POSSIBLE SPONTANEOUS ABORTION

Approximately 15% of early pregnancies end in spontaneous abortion; the proportion is even higher if pregnancy losses are counted during the first 2 weeks of gestation, before the menstrual period is overdue and pregnancy is likely to be recognized. Missed abortion is also fairly common, but is unlikely to cause symptoms that would prompt the woman to seek care. Often the diagnosis is not suspected until prenatal exams reveal that uterine enlargement is not keeping pace with pregnancy dates, or an ultrasound evaluation fails to detect an expected fetal pole or cardiac activity at an appropriate time.

The diagnosis of spontaneous abortion may be made on the basis of a pelvic examination. If the cervix is dilated and products of conception are visible in the cervix or vagina, then abortion is inevitable. An ultrasound evaluation may help determine whether the uterine cavity is already empty. If the uterus appears to be empty and bleeding is not heavy, then uterine evacuation may not be necessary. Otherwise, vacuum aspiration can empty the uterus to resolve the woman's bleeding and cramping and to reduce the risk of infection. (See Chapter 19 for a description of vacuum aspiration procedures in early pregnancy termination.)

Vacuum aspiration is also indicated if bleeding is so heavy that it is life-threatening or if the woman does not want to continue the pregnancy. If the couple wants the pregnancy and the condition is not life-threatening, then intervention can be delayed while further evaluation is undertaken to determine whether the pregnancy may be viable. Serial quantitative beta HCG assays and an ultrasound evaluation are likely to document the diagnosis (see section on Possible Ectopic Pregnancy). When the pregnancy is desired by the couple, take time for a careful and thorough evaluation. Intervention on the basis of an initial exam or ultrasound will seem abrupt and shocking as the couple first begins to acknowledge the possibility of their loss and grief.

COUNSELING OBJECTIVES WITH PREGNANCY DIAGNOSIS

The issues surrounding personal fertility are complex, and a pregnancy diagnosis visit should provide the client an opportunity to clarify and articulate her feelings. Before beginning the physical exam and testing, find out what the woman hopes her result will be. When presenting the test results, elicit the client's reaction and allow time for her to express her feelings. Assess the woman's support system. Provide referrals if the patient feels counseling would be helpful. This is especially important if her own support system is not adequate. Emphasize that no decision based on the test results need be made that day. Encourage the woman to talk with her partner, family, or friends. Outline all the options available.

- If the client is pregnant and plans to continue her pregnancy, review precautions for optimal pregnancy (see Instructions for an Optimal Pregnancy) and be certain she has an appropriate resource for prenatal care. Remind her about danger signs of possible problems in pregnancy (see Table 18-3).
- If the client plans to continue her pregnancy, but does not want to parent the child, refer her to a resource that can help with adoption.
- If the client is pregnant but does not plan to continue her pregnancy, refer her for abortion services. In this case, the sooner the decision is made and acted upon, the safer the procedure will be.
- If the client is not pregnant and wishes she were, counsel her about her own fertility (see Chapter 23). If appropriate, refer her for fertility evaluation and help. Remind her about precautions for optimal pregnancy and about taking a daily vitamin that includes folic acid 0.4 mg before and during pregnancy.[9]

- If the client is not pregnant and is happy with the negative test result, then birth control counseling is appropriate. A pregnancy scare can be a good bridge from risk-taking to effective, ongoing contraceptive use.

- If the client is not clear how she feels about the test result, positive or negative, consider referral for counseling. Appropriate pregnancy counseling services are likely to be available through a local abortion facility. Be sure that pregnancy counseling referral resources you recommend have been carefully evaluated. Anti-abortion groups advertise pregnancy counseling services in some communities; these agencies do not provide the nonjudgmental environment that your clients are entitled to have in making a personal decision about pregnancy. A woman who is not pregnant, but who has ambivalent feelings about pregnancy, may want to consider working with a mental health professional to clarify her feelings.

INSTRUCTIONS FOR AN OPTIMAL PREGNANCY

Ideally, begin planning well before pregnancy occurs. For example, arrange for rubella testing at least 3 months beforehand. Stop taking oral contraceptives 3 months before trying to become pregnant.

1. **Review the medical and family history risk factors** for your own family and for your partner's family. Arrange genetic counseling or testing before pregnancy if Tay-Sachs disease is possible or if either family has had members with congenital abnormalities, Down's syndrome, hereditary anemia, or sickle cell anemia. Testing for AIDS is recommended for all women before they become pregnant.

2. **Plan ahead if you have a serious medical condition** such as diabetes or epilepsy, or if you take prescription medications for any reason. Talk to your clinician before stopping birth control. Your medications may need to be changed to avoid problems in pregnancy, and you will want to be sure your overall medical condition is under good control.

3. **Take a vitamin that includes folic acid 0.4 mg every day;** begin several months before you plan to be pregnant.

4. **Avoid exposure to potentially toxic agents** including:
   - Alcohol, smoking, excessive caffeine
   - X-ray of the abdominal area
   - Illegal drug use
   - Megadose vitamins (or mega-anything-else!)

5. **Do not take any medications** until you have discussed with your clinician the possible effects on pregnancy. This applies to prescription medications and to over-the-counter medications as well.

6. **Make healthy diet a top priority.** A restricted diet or weight loss can be dangerous for your fetus. Do not eat raw meat or fish. Avoid unpasteurized dairy products.

7. **Aim for fitness, but with moderation.** Daily exercise is a good idea. Although prolonged aerobic activities, such as long-distance running, and sports that may cause injuries such as horseback riding or skiing, may not be wise during pregnancy.

8. **Minimize your risk of STD exposure.** Avoid intercourse or use condoms if you have any doubts about possible exposure to sexually transmitted infection. STDs such as herpes, gonorrhea, or chlamydia can cause serious or lethal fetal complications.

9. **Avoid body temperature elevation.** Do not use a hot tub or sauna. Try to avoid exposure to contagious viral illnesses such as influenza.

10. **Avoid contact with cat fecal matter.** Toxoplasma infection during pregnancy can be dangerous for your fetus. Wear gloves if you do gardening. Put someone else in charge of emptying kitty litter.

11. **Have a pregnancy test and see your clinician as soon as possible** if you think you may be pregnant. Pregnancy dates will be most accurate if you have an exam within 2 weeks after missing your menstrual period. Early pregnancy diagnosis is especially important if you plan to have prenatal genetic testing.

12. **Watch for the danger signs of possible pregnancy complications.** Spontaneous abortion (miscarriage) and ectopic (tubal) pregnancy are most likely to cause symptoms within the first month or two of pregnancy. Contact your clinician immediately if you have danger signs.

REFERENCES

1. American College of Obstetricians and Gynecologists. Ectopic pregnancy. ACOG Technical Bulletin, Number 126. March 1989.
2. Bandi ZL, Schoen I, Waters M. An algorithm for testing and reporting serum choriogonadotropin at clinically significant decision levels with use of 'pregnancy test' reagents. Clin Chem 1989;35(4):545-551.
3. Bluestein D. Monoclonal antibody pregnancy tests. Am Fam Physician 1988;38(1):197-204.
4. Braunstein GD. HCG testing: a clinical guide for the testing of human chorionic gonadotropin. Monograph. Abbott Park IL: Abbott Diagnostics, 1992.
5. Braunstein GD. HCG expression in trophoblastic and nontrophoblastic tumors. In: Fishman WH (ed). Oncodevelopmental markers. Academic Press, 1983:351-371.

6. Braunstein GD, Karow WG, Gentry WC, Rasor J, Wade ME. First-trimester chorionic gonadotropin measurements as an aid in the diagnosis of early pregnancy disorders. Am J Obstet Gynecol 1978;131(1):25-32.
7. Braunstein GD, Rasor J, Danzer H, Adler D, Wade ME. Serum human chorionic gonadotropin levels throughout normal pregnancy. Am J Obstet Gynecol 1976;126(6):678-681.
8. Cacciatore B, Tiitinen A, Stenman UH, Ylostalo P. Normal early pregnancy: serum HCG levels and vaginal ultrasonography findings. Br J Obstet Gynecol 1990;97(10):899-903.
9. Centers for Disease Control. Recommendations for the use of folic acid to reduce the number of cases of spina bifida and other neural tube defects. 1992;41(RR-14):1-7.
10. Centers for Disease Control. Ectopic pregnancy—United States, 1988-1989. 1992;41(32):591-594.
11. Chard T. Pregnancy tests: a review. Hum Reprod 1992;7(5):701-710.
12. Coons SJ, Churchill L, Brinkman ML. The use of pregnancy test kits by college students. J Am Coll Health 1990;38(4):171-175.
13. Deutschman M. Advances in the diagnosis of first trimester pregnancy problems. Am Fam Phys 1991;44(suppl 5):15S-30S.
14. Doshi ML. Accuracy of consumer performed in-home tests for early pregnancy detection. Am J Publ Health 1986;76(5):512-514.
15. Hicks JM, Iosefsohn M. Reliability of home pregnancy-test kits in the hands of lay persons. [letters to the editor]. N Engl J Med 1989;320(5):320-321.
16. Jeng LL, Moore RM, Kaczmarek RG, Placek PJ, Bright RA. How frequently are home pregnancy tests used? Results from the 1988 National Maternal and Infant Health Survey. Birth 1991;18(1):11-13.
17. Latman NS, Burot BC. Evaluation of home pregnancy test kits. Biomedical Instrument and Technol 1989;144-149.
18. Leach RE, Ory SJ. Modern management of ectopic pregnancy. J Repro Med 1989;34(5):324-338.
19. Lee C, Hart LL. Accuracy of home pregnancy tests. DICP, Ann Pharmacotherapy 1990;24:712-713.
20. Marrs RP, Kletzky OA, Howard WF, et al. Disappearance of human chorionic gonadotropin and resumption of ovulation following abortion. Am J Obstet Gynecol 1979;135(7-8):731-736.
21. Ramoska EA, Sacchetti AD, Nepp M. Reliability of patient history in determining the possibility of pregnancy. Ann Emerg Med 1989;18(1):48-50.
22. Segna RA, Mitchell DR, Misas JE. Successful treatment of cervical pregnancy with oral etoposide. Obstet Gynecol 1990;76(5-2):945-947.
23. Stewart FH, Guest FJ, Stewart G, Hatcher RA. Understanding your body: every woman's guide to gynecology and health. New York NY: Bantam Books, 1987.
24. Stovall TG, Ling FW, Gray LA, Carson SA, Buster JE. Methotrexate treatment of unruptured ectopic pregnancy: a report of 100 cases. Obstet Gynecol 1991;77(5):749-753.
25. Thorsen MK, Lawson TL, Aiman EJ, Miller DP, McAsey ME, Erickson SJ, Quiroz F, Perret RS. Diagnosis of ectopic pregnancy: endovaginal vs. transabdominal sonography. AJR 1990;155:307-310.

Abortion

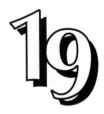

- Despite attempts to restrict the practice of legally induced abortion, it remains the most commonly performed surgical procedure in the United States.

- For a pregnant woman, legally induced abortion up to 20 weeks' gestational age is safer than continuing the pregnancy to term.

- Vacuum aspiration is the safest and most commonly used abortion method, accounting for over 90% of all procedures.

If all sexually active couples used a perfect contraceptive, and if all pregnancies carried no health risks to the woman, we would have no need for induced abortions. Unfortunately, we are far from this ideal world. Although we recognize the controversy surrounding the issue of induced abortion, the authors feel that it should be the right of each woman to make decisions regarding her own pregnancy, based upon accurate information. This brief review provides what we believe to be a factual basis for providing this important reproductive health service.

LEGAL STATUS OF ABORTION

Before 1970, legal abortion was generally unavailable in the United States. Beginning in that year, several large states on the East and West coasts passed legislation that allowed abortion under many circumstances. During the next 3 years, New York and California accounted for the majority of the legal abortions performed domestically.

In 1973, abortion became legal throughout the country. On January 22, 1973, the U.S. Supreme Court decided two landmark cases—*Roe v. Wade*[28] and *Doe v. Bolton*[29]—related to abortion. In brief, these decisions stated:

1. In the first trimester, the abortion decision and its performance must be left to the judgment of the pregnant women and her physician.

2. In the second trimester, the state, in promoting its interest in the health of the pregnant woman, may choose to regulate the abortion procedure in ways that are reasonably related to her health.

3. For pregnancy subsequent to viability, the state, in promoting its interest in the potentiality of human life, may, if it chooses, regulate and even proscribe abortion except when necessary, according to appropriate medical judgment, for the preservation of the life or health of the pregnant woman.

Legally induced abortion has become the most commonly performed surgical procedure in the United States. Over the past two decades, numerous and varied pieces of legislation attempting to regulate abortion services have been introduced at the local, state, and national levels.[2,7] Most recently, on June 29, 1992, the Supreme Court ruled that states could place restrictions interfering with provision of abortion services to include such possibilities as waiting periods, specific informed consent requirements, parental notification provision, and hospitalization requirements.[2] Over the next several years, the major confrontations are likely to occur at the state legislative level where both sides of the abortion issue will attempt to craft their agendas for the 1990s. Moreover, violence against abortion providers already has become epidemic during the past decade.[10] In addition, the majority opinion of the recent Supreme Court decision invited further judicial challenges to the constitutional basis of the original 1973 Roe decision.

WOMEN OBTAINING LEGAL ABORTIONS

Between 1972 and 1989, the number of reported abortions increased substantially (Table 19-1). Most of the increase occurred between 1972 and 1980, from approximately 600,000 to 1.3 million reported legal abortions.[19] During the decade of the 1980s, the number of reported legal abortions and the legal abortion rate (procedures per 1,000 women age 15-44) remained remarkably stable, varying each year by less than 5%. By 1989, nearly 1.4 million legal abortions were reported to the Centers for Disease Control and Prevention (CDC). This reported number of legal abortions is probably lower than the number actually performed. Totals provided by central health agencies are frequently lower than those obtained by direct surveys

Table 19-1 Characteristics of women who obtained legal abortions—United States, selected years, 1972-1989

Characteristics	Year			
	1972	**1978**	**1984**	**1989**
Reported Number of Legal Abortions	586,760	1,157,776	1,333,521	1,396,658
	% Distribution			
Residence				
In-State	56.2	89.3	92.0	91.0
Out-of-State	43.8	10.7	8.0	9.0
Age (Years)				
≤19	32.6	30.0	26.4	24.2
20–24	32.5	35.0	35.3	32.6
≥25	34.9	34.9	38.3	43.2
Race				
White	77.0	67.0	67.4	64.2
Black and Other	23.0	33.0	32.6	35.8
Marital Status				
Married	29.7	26.4	20.5	20.1
Unmarried	70.3	73.6	79.5	79.9
Weeks of Gestation				
≤8	34.0	52.2	50.5	49.8
9–10	30.7	26.9	26.4	25.8
11–12	17.5	12.3	12.6	12.6
13–15	8.4	4.0	5.8	6.6
16–20	8.2	3.7	3.9	4.2
≥21	1.3	0.9	0.8	1.0

Source: Koonin et al. (1992).

of abortion providers. Over the years, the number of legal abortions generated from surveys by the Alan Guttmacher Institute is 15% higher than the number reported to CDC.

Overall, women undergoing abortions tend to be young, white, and unmarried (Table 19-1). Most women have had no previous live births and are having the abortion procedure for the first time. Approximately half of all abortions are performed before the eighth week of gestation, and five out of six are performed before the thirteenth week of gestation. Younger women tend to obtain abortions later in pregnancy than do older women. Finally, with the widespread availability of abortion since 1973, more than 90 percent of women obtain the procedures in their states of residence.

THE DECISION-MAKING PROCESS

The decision-making process regarding abortion begins when the patient first suspects she is pregnant. Women need to be aware of both the timing of their menstrual cycle and also the symptoms of pregnancy. Delay in confirming pregnancy after the first 2 months increases the risks regardless of whether a woman chooses to terminate her pregnancy or to continue it. Complication rates increase the later in pregnancy either the abortion is performed or prenatal care is begun.[5]

Clinicians and pregnancy counseling staff should provide a supportive, non-judgmental setting in which the woman may explore her feelings concerning pregnancy once she finds that she is pregnant.[20] Women may need referrals to agencies providing services such as financial assistance, further counseling, first- and second-trimester abortions, prenatal care, and adoption.

Provide each woman with an opportunity to discuss whether or not to continue her pregnancy. Be empathetic and objective. In addition to providing basic information on family planning, the counselor should also be able to meet the counseling needs of most patients and identify high-risk patients who may need more extensive education, evaluation, or counseling. The criteria to ensure an informed choice/consent should be strictly followed (see Chapter 23).

Review the woman's feelings about the pregnancy, about abortion, about her partner, and about her future life plans. Some women desire and need extensive discussion about these subjects; others require minimal time. Ambivalence is common, since for many women the decision is complicated. If the patient is considering an abortion, the counselor should also explain the abortion procedure—how it is done, its discomforts, safety, risks, duration, and follow-up care instructions. Provide the patient with written information summarizing this discussion.

The patient may want her partner or other supportive persons to be involved in the process. The patient's wishes regarding third-party involvement must be honored.

ABORTION TECHNOLOGY AND CLINICAL MANAGEMENT

Several excellent overviews describe the clinical procedures in more detail.[9,15,27]

PRE-ABORTION PROCEDURES:

A medical history must be obtained before the abortion. This should cover these areas:

1. Recent menstrual history.
2. Prior obstetric and gynecologic history, including previous surgery on cervix or uterus, e.g., conization of cervix, cesarean delivery, and history of leiomyomata (fibroids). Inquire specifically about any complications of previous abortions.
3. Contraceptive history and future contraceptive plans/desires.
4. Allergies or intolerance to local anesthetics, analgesic agents, antibiotics, and other drugs.
5. Drugs (over-the-counter, prescription, and recreational) currently in use.
6. Acute or chronic illnesses, such as asthma or cardiac valvular disease, that might require more evaluation, adjunctive therapy, or special care regarding the performance of the abortion.

Perform a brief exam (vital signs, heart, lungs, and abdomen) and a thorough pelvic exam. During the pelvic exam, estimate (independent of the history) both the size of the pregnant uterus and the relationship of the cervix to the fundus (anteversion or retroversion). Determine the presence of any physical structure that might modify the procedure, such as uterine leiomyomata and adnexal masses. Ultrasound evaluation of the uterus is valuable in assessing length of pregnancy, pelvic architecture, and fetal position.

Recommended laboratory procedures include:

1. A pregnancy test (urine or serum).
2. A hemoglobin (or hematocrit). For those patients who are anemic, iron supplementation is recommended.
3. A D (Rh) antibody determination. Those patients who are D-negative should be advised to receive D immune globulin because of the risk of D to isoimmunization.
4. STD screening, where appropriate.

SURGICAL METHODS

In the United States, surgical methods are currently the most common abortion procedures:

Vacuum aspiration. Introduced to this country in 1967, this method is now the most widely used abortion procedure.[19] In 1989, 97% of the 1.4 million reported legal abortions were performed by suction curettage. This procedure offers the advantage of being a relatively simple technique for completely emptying the uterus in a short time through a small cervical dilation. The procedure may be performed using only local anesthesia, though many patients request general anesthesia.

Perform a bimanual examination to determine the uterine size and angle of the cervical-uterine junction. Insert the speculum and cleanse the cervix. Using a local anesthetic such as 0.5 % to 1 % lidocaine ester (limiting the amount to less than 2 mg/lb), place a paracervical block to reduce pain. Dilate the cervix using gently sloped Pratt or Denniston dilators. Laminaria or other osmotic dilators placed about 3-24 hours before the procedure can assist in dilating the cervix. After inserting a vacuum cannula and introducing negative pressure (usually from electrical vacuum pump), evacuate the products of conception. The cannula size generally used is 2 mm less than the number of weeks gestation (measured from LMP), although the next larger size may shorten the abortion procedure. After vacuum aspiration, use a sharp curettage to confirm complete evacuation. Finally, examine the tissue to document the pregnancy, to rule out the presence of an ectopic pregnancy or a hydatidiform mole, and to validate the complete uterine evacuation. To assist in confirming the pregnancy, suspend the chorionic villi in saline, tap water, or white vinegar and check the contents with backlighting.

The vacuum aspiration procedure can be done in an office through 14 weeks' gestation, provided that appropriate backup and preparation are available for dealing with potentially adverse situations, such as allergic reactions to medication, uterine atony, uterine perforation, seizure, or cardiac arrest. Surgical instruments are generally necessary to evacuate pregnancies later than 14 weeks' gestation.

Dilation and evacuation (D&E). D&E allows vacuum aspiration to be performed into the second trimester.[13] D&E is especially appropriate for procedures performed between 13 and 16 weeks' gestation, although many proponents use this method up through 20+ weeks.[16] An accurate estimate of the gestational age is crucial; intraoperative sonography may help. The cervix requires more dilation for a D&E than for a vacuum aspiration, since the products of conception in the second trimester are much larger. The surgeon may require crushing instruments along with a 140-mm vacuum cannula to remove the tissue and fluid. Osmotic dilators are often used to accommodate a gradual, less painful, and less traumatic dilation of the cervix. After administering a paracervical block or general anesthesia, remove the osmotic dilators and dilate the cervix as needed with mechanical dilators. The vacuum cannula, and other instruments as needed, can then evacuate the fetus and placenta from the uterus.

During this procedure, some clinicians use an intravenous infusion of oxytocin to encourage uterine contractions, thus limiting blood loss. However, others avoid using oxytocins until the procedure is completed for fear of "trapping" the fetal skull (often the last part removed) as the uterus contracts. Some clinicians use vasopressin with the paracervical or intracervical block to constrict uterine vessels and therefore decrease blood loss.

M EDICAL METHODS

FIRST TRIMESTER

Mifepristone (RU 486), together with prostaglandins, is being used to abort early pregnancies in European countries and China.[4] Despite success overseas, it is not currently available in the United States.[18]

Mifepristone is a progesterone antagonist that has been investigated both as an early abortifacient and as a once-a-month midcycle contraceptive. Combining mifepristone with a low-dose prostaglandin analogue appears to potentiate the effectiveness in terminating pregnancy without increasing the side effects.[4] This approach builds on the progesterone-blocking properties of mifepristone and the uterine stimulating activity of the prostaglandins. When the combination is administered within 3 weeks of the expected onset of the missed menstrual period, a complete abortion occurs in more than 95% of women. Mifepristone appears to be more effective the earlier in the pregnancy it is used. Complications are infrequent. About 1% of women with a successful abortion have uterine bleeding that requires curettage.

Depending on the availability of legal abortion in the United States over the next decade, medical methods for terminating early pregnancies may play an important role in expanding reproductive choices available to American women. However, these medical means have not been established to be as safe as first-trimester vacuum aspiration. Thus, clinicians must continue to compare these methods with the effective, safe, and widely available vacuum aspiration method for early abortion.

SECOND TRIMESTER

Agents

Currently, three main agents are being used for second-trimester abortion: hypertonic saline, hypertonic urea, and prostaglandin E2. However, in 1989, these methods accounted for only 1% of all abortions in the United States.[19] They have been replaced by D&E procedures that are safer, faster, and less expensive.

1. Hypertonic saline is probably the most widely used instillation agent. It has the advantages of being relatively inexpensive, readily available, and feticidal; in addition, considerable clinical experience with the procedure has been amassed. However, its disadvantages include higher rates of severe, disseminated intravascular clotting; myometrial necrosis if injected into the myometrium; and hypernatremia with convulsions and coma if infused directly into

the circulatory system. The hypertonic saline is usually made up in a 20%–25% solution.

2. Hypertonic urea is also used to terminate second-trimester pregnancies. The major advantages of this agent have been its relative safety, low cost, and feticidal effects. The major disadvantage has been the high failure rate when used as the sole abortifacient. Currently urea is primarily used in combination with prostaglandins to augment labor. Urea is used intra-amniotically by dissolving about 80 gm of urea in 200 cc of water.

3. Prostaglandin E2 is marketed as a vaginal suppository for evacuating a missed abortion. These 20 mg vaginal suppositories cause a high incidence of gastrointestinal side effects and often affect the thermoregulatory mechanism, causing a temperature elevation in some patients.[23]

Amniocentesis and Amnio-infusion

Amniocentesis (removal of fluid from the amniotic cavity) and amnio-infusion (infusion of medication into the amniotic cavity) are techniques central to the second-trimester instillation procedures.

After emptying her bladder, the patient lies in the supine position. Cleanse the amniocentesis site with an iodine disinfectant, and drape the site with sterile towels. No premedication is recommended. Infiltrate the skin over the injection site with a local anesthetic. Insert an 18-gauge spinal needle into the intrauterine cavity to obtain a flow of clear amniotic fluid.

Many clinicians will also insert osmotic dilators in the cervix either before or at the time of the amniocentesis to expedite the procedure and decrease the incidence of cervical lacerations. Prostaglandin suppositories can help soften the cervix.

Adjunctive Techniques

Laminaria.   This dried seaweed of the genus *Laminaria* is highly hygroscopic and can, over a period of time, dilate the cervix. Laminaria provide the advantage of being relatively painless and very effective. Use of laminaria can decrease the chance of cervical laceration or perforation. Place the laminaria so that they extend through the endocervical canal and dilate both the internal and external os. Usually, most of the cervical expansion occurs by 6 hours, but maximum dilation is not seen until 12-24 hours after placement of the laminaria.

Synthetic osmotic dilators.   Two synthetic hygroscopic dilators are used in the United States. Lamicel is a magnesium sulfate-impregnated sponge. Dilapan is an expanding polymer of polyacrilonitrile. Both produce faster cervical dilatation than laminaria. They have the advantages of uniform size (3 mm–5 mm diameter), assured sterility, and easy insertion and removal. Depending on cost, these synthetic dilators may eventually replace the natural products.

Oxytocin. Intravenous oxytocin (such as Syntocinon or Pitocin) may be used as an adjunct to vacuum aspiration to reduce the amount of bleeding. When used with second-trimester methods, oxytocin facilitates uterine contractions and hastens the abortion. When used with saline, oxytocin increases the risks of disseminated intravascular clotting, cervical laceration, and water intoxication, although it decreases the risks of infection and retained products of conception.

P REVENTING ABORTION COMPLICATIONS

Compared with childbirth (an alternative outcome for a pregnant woman), as well as other surgical procedures, legal abortion is remarkably safe.[5] In the two largest series of legally induced abortions reported to date, the rate of major complications is less than 1 in 200 cases.[10,14] The safety of the abortion procedure is helped by early diagnosis of pregnancy and prompt referral. When their complication rates are adjusted for gestational age, teenagers have lower complication rates than do older women.[6] The abortion method influences risks of complications: dilation and evacuation, for example, is significantly safer than that by instillation procedures in the 13- to 20-week (post-LMP) interval.[13]

Abortion-related problems are less likely under these conditions:

- The pregnancy is early.
- The patient is healthy.
- The patient is not ambivalent about having the abortion performed (or can cope with the feelings if she is ambivalent).
- The patient does not have gonorrhea or chlamydial infection of the cervix.
- The clinician is well-trained and experienced with abortion techniques.
- Osmotic dilators are used.
- Local anesthesia is used.
- The uterus is carefully and completely emptied.
- The clinician carefully examines the aspirated or curetted tissue to rule out the possibility of a molar or ectopic pregnancy.
- D-immune globulin is given to a D-negative woman.
- The patient understands the warning signs for potential postabortal problems.
- Prompt follow-up care is available on a 24-hour basis.

Prophylactic antibiotics can reduce complications from induced abortions.[12] A common dosage schedule is 100 mg of doxycycline, taken twice a day for 1–3 days. Many providers wait until after surgery to begin the antibiotics because of the problem of nausea and vomiting.

Table 19-2 Legal abortions, abortion-related deaths, and deaths per 100,000 procedures by selected characteristics, 1972-1987

Characteristic	Mortality Rate*	Relative Risk (95% CL)	
Age (Yr)			
≤19	1.0	1.0	Referent
20–24	1.3	1.3	(0.9, 1.8)
25–44	1.6	1.5	(1.1, 2.1)
Method			
Curettage	0.5	1.0	Referent
D&E	3.7	6.8	(4.9, 9.5)
Instillation	7.1	13.0	9.7, 17.5)
H/H	51.6	95.0	(69.6, 129.5)
Gestation (Wk)			
≤8	0.4	1.0	Referent
9–10	0.8	2.1	(1.3, 3.3)
11–12	1.4	3.7	(2.3, 5.8)
13–15	2.9	7.7	(5.0, 11.7)
16–20	9.3	24.5	(18.6, 32.3)
≥21	12.0	31.5	(22.2, 44.5)

*Rate per 100,000 procedures; CL = confidence limits; D&E = dilatation and evacuation; H/H = hysterectomy and hysterotomy.

Source: Lawson et al. (Manuscript submitted, 1992).

The risk of a woman's dying from a legal abortion is exceedingly rare.[22] The death-to-case rate for legal abortion is clearly related to the age of the woman, the type of procedure used, and the length of gestation (Table 19-2). Death is also associated with general health problems present at the time of abortion. In recent years, a disproportionate share of the percentage of deaths has been due to complications from general anesthesia or pulmonary embolism.[21]

SHORT-TERM POSTABORTION COMPLICATIONS

Legally induced abortion is, fortunately, an extremely safe procedure.[14] Because of this fact, any complaint by a woman after an abortion procedure should be taken seriously. The recognition and management of the potential serious postabortion problems is important:

Infection

Postabortal infections can be minimized by preabortal gonorrhea and chlamydia treatment, treatment of cervicitis, complete emptying of the uterus, and prophylactic antibiotics. Infections may be heralded by cramping, fever, discharge, and pelvic discomfort. Advise patients to seek help immediately if any suspicious symptoms develop after the procedure (See Warning Signs). If retained products of conception are suspected, remove them by a repeat vacuum aspiration after initiating a serum level of an antibiotic. If the infection has proceeded beyond the uterus, hospitalize the patient and administer parenteral antibiotics.

Intrauterine Blood Clots

The most common problem requiring a repeat aspiration is the presence of intrauterine blood clots.[24] These can occur either immediately or up to 5 days after the abortion; their presence is manifested by severe cramping and pain. The syndrome is diagnosed by a pelvic exam showing a large, tense, tender uterus without bleeding from the cervix. Simple vacuum aspiration remedies the problem. Use of oral ergotrate may help prevent this problem.

Continuing Pregnancy

On occasion (0.1%-0.3%), the attempt to terminate the pregnancy will not be successful. Carefully evaluating the products of conception after the procedure helps prevent such failures. A continuing pregnancy is recognized by ongoing symptoms of pregnancy and diagnosed by an enlarged uterus at the follow-up exam and a persistently positive pregnancy test. Thus, a careful history and physical examination are an important part of the postabortion exam. If the pregnancy has not been terminated, rule out an abnormal uterus (e.g., bicornuate), twin pregnancies, or an ectopic pregnancy.

Cervical or Uterine Trauma

Perforation of the uterus and laceration of the cervix are worrisome complications. Depending on their severity, treatment ranging from simple observation to hysterectomy may be required. Trauma may be prevented by using osmotic dilators for gentle cervical dilation and by applying gentle, firm, and steady traction when using the tenaculum on the cervix.[25] Women who have had a previous abortion have a reduced risk of cervical injury, whereas women under the age of 17 have an increased risk. Advanced gestational age and previous term delivery are risk factors for uterine perforation.[11] Use of local anesthesia, osmotic dilators, and clinician's experience in performing abortion procedures lower the risk of both cervical injury and uterine perforation considerably.

Bleeding

Bleeding during or after an abortion is common. Rates of hemorrhage range from 0.05 to 4.9 per 100 procedures depending on the definition used and the method of estimating blood loss. Local anesthetics, uterine-contracting agents (IV oxytocin or an ergotrate administered orally or intramuscularly), vascular constricting agents (intrauterine prostaglandins or oxytocin), and massaging the uterus minimize hemorrhage following a pregnancy termination. Severe, life-threatening disseminated intravascular coagulation can occur in advanced pregnancies and in those with intrauterine demise. This problem requires immediate expert care.

LONG-TERM POSTABORTION COMPLICATIONS

Increasing evidence indicates that first-trimester abortion performed by the vacuum aspiration technique has little effect on subsequent infertility, spontaneous abortions, premature delivery, and low birth weight babies.[3,8,17] If late somatic sequelae are eventually shown to be causally associated with prior induced abortion, they likely will be related to particular abortion techniques, such as the manner and caliber of dilation, the method of curettage used to evacuate the uterus, or the age of gestation at which the abortion was performed. Moreover, any risk of subsequent adverse reproductive outcomes would probably be increased for women who have already had one or more previous induced abortions.[17]

Much recent attention has been given to the alleged psychological and emotional harm occurring after an abortion. Major psychiatric sequelae after abortion are rare.[26] Moreover, the incidence of diagnosed psychiatric illness and hospitalization is considerably lower after legal abortion than after childbirth. Transient feelings of stress or sadness are common after the usually difficult decision to terminate a pregnancy.[1] Follow-up studies have shown no evidence of widespread long-term abortion psychologic trauma.

POSTABORTION CONTRACEPTION

A woman's decision to terminate an unplanned pregnancy represents an opportunity to discuss the contraceptive options available to prevent future unintended conceptions. Make sure she understands how to correctly use the method she chooses. If the unplanned pregnancy occurred while the woman was using a coitally dependent contraceptive (condom, spermicide, diaphragm), then consider suggesting a noncoitally dependent method.

REFERENCES

1. Adler NE, David HP, Major VN, Roth SH, Russo NF, Wyatt GE. Psychological response after abortion. Science 1990;248:41-43(4951).
2. Annas GJ. The Supreme Court, liberty, and abortion. N Engl J Med 1992;327(9): 651-654.
3. Atrash H, Hogue CR. The effect of pregnancy termination on future reproduction. Baillieres Clin Obstet Gynaecol 1990;4:(2)391-405.
4. Avrech OM, Golan A, Weinraub Z, Bukovsky I, Caspi E. Mifepristone (RU 486) alone or in combination with a prostaglandin analogue for termination of early pregnancy: a review. Fertil Steril 1991;56(5):385-393.
5. Cates W Jr. Legal abortion: the public health record. Science 1982;215(4540): (1)586-1590.
6. Cates W Jr, Schulz KF, Grimes DA. The risks associated with teenage abortion. N Engl J Med 1983;309(11):621-624.
7. Cates W Jr, Gold J, Selik RM. Regulation of abortion service: for better or worse? N Engl J Med 1979;301(13):720-723.
8. Frank PI, McNamee R, Hannaford PC, Kay CR, Hirsch S. The effect of induced abortion on subsequent pregnancy outcome. Br J Obstet Gynaecol 1991;98(10): 1015-1024.
9. Grimes DA. Surgical management of abortion. In: Mattingly R, Thompson JT (eds). TeLinde's operative gynecology. Philadelphia PA: J.B. Lippincott, 1991: 317-342.
10. Grimes DA, Forrest JD, Kirkman AL, Radford B. An epidemic of antiabortion violence in the United States. Am J Obstet Gynecol 1991;165(5):1263-1268.
11. Grimes DA, Schulz KF, Cates W Jr. Prevention of uterine perforation during curettage abortion. JAMA 1984;251(16):2108-2111.
12. Grimes DA, Schulz KF, Cates W Jr. Prophylactic antibiotics for curettage abortion. Am J Obstet Gynecol 1984;150(6):689-694.
13. Grimes DA, Schulz KF, Cates W Jr, Tyler CW. Midtrimester abortion by dilation and evacuation. N Engl J Med 1977;296(20):1141-1145.
14. Hakim-Elahi E, Tovell HM, Burnhill MS. Complications of first trimester abortion: a report of 170,000 cases. Obstet Gynecol 1990;76(1):129-135.
15. Hern WM. Abortion practice. Philadelphia PA: J.B. Lippincott, 1984.
16. Hern WM, Oaks AG. Multiple laminaria treatment in early midtrimester outpatient suction abortion. Adv Plann Parenthood 1977;7:(2)93-97.
17. Hogue CJ, Cates W Jr, Tietze C. Effects of induced abortion on subsequent reproduction. Epidemiol Rev 1982;4:66-94.
18. Klitsch M. Antiprogestins and the abortion controversy: a progress report. Fam Plann Perspect 1991;23(6):275-282.

19. Koonin LM, Smith JC, Ramick M. Lawson HOW. Abortion surveillance – United States, 1989. MMWR 1992;41(SS-5):1-33.
20. Landy U. Abortion counseling: a new component of medical care. Clin Obstet Gynecol 1986;13(1):33-41.
21. Lawson H, Atrash A, Franks A. Fatal pulmonary embolism during legal induced abortion, 1972-1985. Am J Obstet Gynecol 1990;162(4):986-990.
22. Lawson H, Frye A, Atrash A, Ramick M, Smith J. Legal abortion mortality in the United States, 1972-1987. Manuscript submitted, 1992.
23. Rakhshani R, Grimes DA. Prostaglandin E2 suppositories as a second-trimester abortifacient. J Reprod Med 1988;33(10):817-820.
24. Sands RX, Burnhill MS, Hakim-Elahi E. Postabortal uterine atony. Obstet Gynecol 1974;43(4):595-598.
25. Schulz KF, Grimes DA, Cates W Jr. Measures to prevent cervical injury during suction curettage abortion. Lancet 1983;1(i):1182-1184.
26. Stotland NL. The myth of the abortion trauma syndrome. JAMA 1992;268(15): 1078-2079.
27. Stubblefield PG. Pregnancy termination. In: Gabbe SG, Niebyl JR, Simpson JL (eds). Obstetrics: normal and problem pregnancies. New York NY: Churchill Livingstone, 1986:1051-1075.
28. Supreme Court of the United States. Jane Roe et al. vs. Henry Wade. Opinion No. 70-18, January 22, 1973.
29. Supreme Court of the United States. Doe et al. vs. Bolton. Attorney General of Georgia, et al. Opinion No. 70-40, January 22, 1973.

Menstrual Problems & Common Gynecologic Concerns

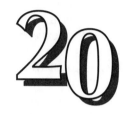

- Menstrual cycle events and reproductive hormones, whether they originate from inside the woman's own body or from hormone medication, have numerous effects. In many cases, the clinician's ability to identify and explain the symptom suffices, and no further evaluation or treatment is needed. Pain caused by ovulation, called mittelschmerz, is an example. If midcycle pain occurs exactly 14 days before a menstrual period, and lasts no longer than a day or two, a diagnosis of mittelschmerz can be made with confidence. Further testing is not necessary.

- In some situations, the potential for serious future consequences may make intervention wise even when the patient is not troubled by her symptoms. Amenorrhea evaluation, for example, is an important clinical priority. An amenorrheic woman may be at risk for osteoporosis if inadequate estrogen secretion is the reason her periods have stopped.

Initial management steps for common menstrual disturbances and for gynecological problems frequently encountered in the family planning clinic are presented in the following sections of this chapter. They include: dysmenorrhea, premenstrual syndrome, amenorrhea, menopause, adnexal masses, abnormal vaginal bleeding, toxic shock syndrome, and vaginal hygiene measures.

DYSMENORRHEA

Primary dysmenorrhea, or "normal" menstrual cramping, commonly begins during adolescence as soon as an ovulatory cycle pattern is first established. In a study of young women attending a family planning clinic, 80% experienced dysmenorrhea; for 18% it was severe enough to interfere with normal activities.[39] Primary dysmenorrhea is often accompanied by nausea, diarrhea, and vasomotor instability (episodes of weakness or fainting). This problem may persist throughout the reproductive years or may occur intermittently. Although dysmenorrhea may diminish with time, pregnancy is not a reliable cure, except for the 9 months of amenorrhea. Severe primary dysmenorrhea is unlikely to occur during anovulatory cycles.

Primary dysmenorrhea is caused by prostaglandins produced in the uterine lining and released into the woman's bloodstream as the lining is shed. Women with severe dysmenorrhea have greater production of these hormones than do women who do not experience cramps. Prostaglandins, which cause smooth muscle contraction, are responsible for excessive uterine muscle contractions, as well as for the other symptoms such as nausea and diarrhea that often accompany cramps.[47]

Dysmenorrhea can be a truly incapacitating problem. Pain usually begins coincident with menstrual shedding or just shortly before and is absent at other times in the cycle. If pain is not strictly limited to the menstrual phase, if its onset occurs after adolescence, or if its severity increases over time, then a more extensive evaluation is necessary. Consider the possibility of secondary dysmenorrhea.

Secondary dysmenorrhea means crampy pelvic pain caused by (secondary to) a disorder or disease. Gynecologic problems that can cause secondary dysmenorrhea include *pelvic inflammatory disease (acute or chronic), leiomyomata (fibroids), endometriosis, adenomyosis, endometrial hyperplasia, and endometrial cancer. Pregnancy problems, such as ectopic pregnancy, spontaneous abortion,* or retained products of conception also can cause pain similar to menstrual cramps. When evaluating crampy, pelvic pain, be sure to consider the possibility of infection or early pregnancy.

Contraception can affect primary dysmenorrhea markedly. Women using combined pills are unlikely to experience severe dysmenorrhea. Women using progestin-only pills and long-acting progestin injections also may have relief from dysmenorrhea. Approximately 30% of oral contraceptive users with previously severe dysmenorrhea, however, do not report improvement.[39] Progestin elaborated from the Progestasert intrauterine device may diminish menstrual cramps, whereas other IUDs are often associated with increased menstrual cramps and bleeding. Expulsion or partial expulsion of an IUD also may cause cramps. For some diaphragm users, dysmenorrhea is most severe when the device is in place.

Dysmenorrhea Treatment

For many women, simple measures such as taking aspirin (a mild prostaglandin inhibitor) or ibuprofen (a highly effective prostaglandin inhibitor available without prescription in 200 mg tablets), resting, and applying a heating pad are sufficient to relieve symptoms. Aspirin use can increase menstrual blood loss, while ibuprofen usually decreases the amount of flow.[14]

For women with severe dysmenorrhea, stronger measures are indicated. Severe dysmenorrhea may be an important, and entirely valid, reason to recommend hormonal contraception if the patient is able to use it. Prescription prostaglandin inhibitors (nonsteroidal anti-inflammatory drugs, NSAIDs) are also an appropriate choice (see Table 20-1). Contraindications to their use are limited:[35]

- History of allergy to aspirin, especially if a prior reaction involved the syndrome of nasal polyps, angioedema, and bronchospasm
- History of allergy to any NSAID (nonsteroidal anti-inflammatory drug)

Fatal reactions have been reported. Caution is also needed for patients who may have ulcer disease, kidney disease, or asthma. NSAIDs can cause gastric irritation, and significant gastrointestinal bleeding from NSAID-induced ulcers has been reported even in the absence of clinical ulcer symptoms. NSAIDs can affect renal blood flow and also can exacerbate asthma symptoms. Very rarely, cases of renal failure and of aseptic meningitis have been reported,[24] so warn patients to stop the medication and seek medical help if they develop hematuria or other possible signs of renal failure such as malaise or fatigue, vision problems, persistent headache, or fever.

Adverse reactions are quite uncommon, however, and side effects are unlikely to be a problem when these drugs are used for dysmenorrhea. Nausea and heartburn are the most common (see Table 20-2).

These drugs are effective because they inhibit prostaglandin synthesis. Be sure the patient understands that NSAIDs prevent cramps as well as treat pain. Relief of dysmenorrhea is more likely to be effective if treatment is initiated at the first onset of cramps or bleeding or even earlier, if possible.

If pain cannot be controlled with simple measures such as prostaglandin inhibitors or oral contraceptives, then evaluate further. Diagnostic laparoscopy may reveal an unsuspected gynecologic problem. For women who cannot use NSAIDs, or find them ineffective, a TENS unit (transcutaneous electrical nerve stimulation) may be an option.[45] In some cases, prescription diuretics are helpful, as are other prescription analgesics or narcotics. Surgical intervention such as presacral nerve ablation is a last resort in managing incapacitating, intractable dysmenorrhea.[26]

Table 20-1 Prostaglandin inhibitors

Drug Name, Tablet Strengths	Recommended Dose	Maximum Dose in 24 Hours
Approved for Treatment of Pain and of Primary Dysmenorrhea		
Ibuprofen* (IBU-TAB, Motrin, Rufen) 300, 400, 600, 800 mg	400 mg every 4 hours	3,200 mg
Meclofenamate Sodium (Meclomen) 50, 100 mg	100 mg every 8 hours	400 mg
Ketaprofen (Orudis) 25, 50, 75 mg	25–50 mg every 6–8 hours	300 mg
Mefenamic Acid (Ponstel) 250 mg	500 mg then 250 mg every 6 hours	
Naproxen (Naprosyn) 250, 375, 500 mg	500 mg then 250 mg every 6–8 hours	1,250 mg
Naproxen Sodium (Anaprox, Anaprox DS) 275, 550 mg	550 mg then 275 mg every 6–8 hours	1,375 mg
Approved for Treatment of Pain		
Diflunisal (Dolobid) 250, 500 mg	1,000 mg then 500 mg every 12 hours	1,500 mg
Etodolac (Lodine) 200, 300 mg	200–400 mg every 6–8 hours	1,200 mg
Fenoprofen Calcium (Nalfon) 200, 300, 600 mg	200 mg every 4–6 hours	3,200 mg
Ketorolac Tromethamine (Toradol) 10 mg	10 mg every 4–6 hours	120 mg

*Ibuprofen 200 mg is available without prescription (brand names include Aches 'N Pain, Advil, Medipren, Midol 200, Motrin, Nuprin).

Other nonsteroidal anti-inflammatory agents such as phenylbutazone (Butazolidin), sulindac (Clinoril), piroxicam (Feldene), indomethacin (Indocin), tolmetin sodium (Tolectin), and diclofenac sodium (Voltaren) are available for treatment of arthritis, and are effective prostaglandin inhibitors. They are not FDA-approved for treatment of dysmenorrhea because of more severe side effects. Zomepirac (Zomax) and suprofen (Suprol) were withdrawn from sale by their manufacturers because of adverse reactions.

PREMENSTRUAL SYNDROME

Most women who have normal ovulatory cyclic patterns are able to identify changes in mood or sense of well-being, energy level, propensity for fluid retention, and other personal signals that occur predictably in relationship to the menstrual cycle. For some women, cyclic symptoms are severely distressing

Table 20-2 Possible side effects of antiprostaglandin drugs

Severe

Allergic reaction. Do not prescribe these drugs for a patient who has had an allergic reaction to aspirin such as asthma, hives, runny nose, itching or rash, swelling or shock. Although these drugs do not contain aspirin, people who are allergic to aspirin are likely to be allergic to them as well.

Renal failure. Chronic, prolonged use of these drugs can cause azotemia, with malaise, fatigue, and loss of appetite, and overt renal failure, and may also cause nephritis with hematuria and proteinuria.

Meningitis. Severe persistent headaches, fever, muscle aches, and lab tests confirming aseptic meningitis have been reported. This is extremely rare. Patients recovered after stopping the drug.

Common (Experienced by at least 1% of users)*

Nausea and vomiting	Indigestion
Headache	Bloating and flatulence
Heartburn	Itching
Dizziness	Skin eruption, rash
Nervousness	Ringing ears
Abdominal or stomach pain	Loss of appetite
Constipation	Fluid retention and swelling
Diarrhea	

Rare (Experienced by less than 1% of users)*

Irritability, confusion	Palpitations
Depression, sleepiness	Visual disturbances
Kidney damage	Liver function changes
Mouth ulcers	Hepatitis, jaundice
Runny nose	Pancreatitis
Dry eyes and mouth	Heart failure
Bronchial spasm	Hair loss
Hearing loss	Dream abnormality, insomnia
Malaise	Elevated blood pressure
Abdominal pain with fever, chills, nausea, and vomiting	Change in anticoagulant drug effect
Allergic reaction, hives, blisters, red skin blotches, (see also "Severe" above)	Prolonged blood clotting time and other blood disorders
	Ulcer, stomach, or intestinal irritation or bleeding

*Reported for patients using medication continuously for arthritis.

Source: Physicians' Desk Reference (ed 47)
Adapted from: Stewart et al. (1987) with permission

or even disabling. The term premenstrual syndrome (PMS) encompasses a wide range of symptoms if the symptoms occur cyclically in the premenstrual (luteal) phase and are absent during the follicular phase. Dozens of possible PMS symptoms are described in the literature. Among the most common are:

- Dysphoria (depression, irritability, anxiety, nervousness, inability to concentrate, tension)
- Breast tenderness
- Fluid retention (bloating, edema, weight gain commonly 2–5 pounds, sometimes 10 pounds)
- Fatigue or exhaustion
- Headache
- Food cravings (especially for salt, sugar, or chocolate)

PMS complaints deserve compassionate attention. Some women with chronic problems such as asthma, epilepsy, or migraine, find that their symptoms are most severe during the premenstrual interval. When this is the case, oral contraceptives can suppress ovulation and provide a more uniform hormonal milieu throughout the cycle. Most women who suffer incapacitating PMS, however, are primarily troubled by their dysphoria symptoms. In some cases, intolerable symptoms just before menses reflect serious ongoing depression or psychiatric problems that are most obvious or incapacitating during the cyclic low point. Dealing with the PMS aspect of such problems is less crucial and less likely to be successful than efforts to restore better overall functioning; *when depression or psychiatric symptoms are severe, consider referral for psychiatric evaluation and treatment.*

The cause of PMS is not known, and numerous theories (with corresponding interventions) have been proposed, including nutritional deficiency, excess levels of prostaglandins, fluid balance abnormalities, progesterone deficiency, and central nervous system endorphin abnormalities.[27] Some researchers believe that PMS is not a single entity, but rather several separate entities, each with its own cluster of symptoms. Until PMS is better defined, and its etiology(ies) better understood, its management is strictly empirical.

No evidence exists that abnormal hormone patterns play a role in PMS,[42] so hormone testing is not indicated. There is evidence that hormone events during the luteal phase do not themselves directly trigger PMS symptoms. Researchers in one small study artificially terminated luteal phase hormone events and induced a follicular phase hormone environment during the premenstrual week. Women in the study who previously had reported severe PMS during "normal" cycles did not experience relief of their symptoms during the "artificial" cycle. Researchers concluded that events responsible for PMS symptoms must have occurred earlier in the cycle.[43] Prospective charting that demonstrates monthly recurrence of symptoms during the luteal phase is the only current diagnostic tool.

PMS Management

No single agent or regimen has been shown to be effective in treating the whole range of PMS symptoms.[47] Natural progesterone, strongly advocated by Dalton[99] has not proven to be more effective than placebo in six well-designed studies.[15,29] The possible health risks or long-term effects of progesterone are not known, and progesterone treatment regimens for PMS involve supraphysiologic doses (typically 400 mg to more than 3,000 mg daily). At high doses, progesterone may have a mildly sedative effect; or perhaps its believers are experiencing a placebo effect. In either case, alternative treatment approaches, which at least avoid incurring unknown drug risk, are a more prudent choice.

Vitamin and mineral supplements also have been extensively promoted for treatment of PMS symptoms. Like progesterone, their efficacy has not been validated in large-scale, double-blinded research, but they are probably safer. One small study, however, documented PMS symptom reduction with oral magnesium supplements (360 mg daily).[13] Evening primrose oil (Efamol 500 mg, 3 capsules b.i.d. from the 15th cycle day to menses) which provides gamma-linoleic acid and Vitamin E, also has been shown to alleviate PMS depression and mastalgia in placebo-controlled studies.[21,36,37] Use of high-dose vitamin B_6 is not wise. Peripheral neuropathy has been reported with use of vitamin B_6 supplements at doses as low as 500 mg daily.[4] L-tryptophan supplements can cause eosinophilia-myalgia syndrome with arthralgia, cough, dyspnea, fever, and edema.

Simple measures to improve overall well-being often greatly reduce PMS problems. Improved overall well-being is a desirable goal in any case, and is usually easier to achieve than is elimination of cyclic times that well-being is somewhat lower than average. Diet throughout the month, and especially during the premenstrual interval, should be high in complex carbohydrates and moderate in protein (emphasizing alternatives to red meat), but low in refined sugar and salt (sodium), with regular, small meals throughout the day. Women should reduce or eliminate their consumption of tea, coffee, caffeine-containing beverages, chocolate, and alcohol, and tobacco. They should follow scrupulously a regular program of aerobic exercise for at least 30 minutes three or four times weekly, especially during their premenstrual interval. Teaching relaxation response techniques also may be helpful. Women randomly assigned to learn relaxation from a 7-minute tape, and instructed to practice relaxation for 15 minutes twice daily, showed 58% improvement in PMS symptoms. In comparison, women instructed to sit quietly and read for the same amount of time had 27% improvement; women who simply charted symptoms had only 17% improvement.[17] Careful charting to correlate basal body temperature evidence of cyclic hormone events with symptoms, and the response to diet, exercise, and other interventions may help the patient to identify her own optimal regimen. Charting is described in Chapter 12.

Minimizing coffee, tea, and caffeine-containing beverages and products deserves special emphasis. The prevalence and severity of premenstrual symptomatology have a strong, dose-dependent, correlation with the amount of caffeine consumption.[41]

Additional steps to treat specific, individual symptoms also may be appropriate. Fluid retention problems may be treated with the diuretic spironolactone beginning a few days before symptoms are anticipated; other diuretics have not been better than placebo in controlled studies.[27] For most women, however, careful attention to sodium restriction is simpler and more effective in preventing cyclic fluid retention. Patients with PMS probably should avoid diuretics such as furosemide that can cause secondary aldosteronism and rebound edema.

Prostaglandin inhibitors (2–4 tablets daily beginning with the onset of symptoms, see Table 20-2) may be helpful, especially for women who have headaches or premenstrual cramping.[6]

Some women find that breast pain and tenderness improves with reduced caffeine consumption or with vitamin E (400 units twice daily) supplements, although neither of these interventions has effectiveness demonstrated in research. Evening primrose oil, described above, may be helpful in treating mastalgia. Bromocriptine efficacy also has been documented.[52] Premenstrual mastalgia, however, is not an FDA-approved indication for bromocriptine; it is an expensive drug, and side effects are common.

Intermittent treatment with alprazolam (Xanax), 0.25 mg three to four times daily for the last week of each cycle, is more effective than placebo in treating PMS symptoms.[31,46] Use of benzodiazepine tranquilizers, however, demands careful consideration and good clinical supervision because of the significant risk of drug dependence.[31] Efficacy for fluoxetine (Prozac 20 mg daily) also has been documented in a small, double-blind placebo-controlled study of women with severe PMS.[51]

Contraceptive choice may affect PMS symptoms. Low-dose, combined oral contraceptives suppress ovulation and provide a stable hormonal milieu throughout the month. Pills virtually eliminate cyclic symptoms for most women, although some pill users have problems all cycle long with symptoms similar to PMS. For many women, progestin-only minipills provide a similar benefit in reducing PMS-like cyclic symptoms.

A MENORRHEA

Because unsuspected pregnancy so often causes amenorrhea, an immediate evaluation is essential for any sexually active woman who reports amenorrhea. A pregnancy test is a wise precaution if the woman has any history of possible exposure to semen, even if true intercourse has not occurred, and even if the young woman has not yet begun having menstrual periods. Once pregnancy is excluded, evaluate further,[30] if:

- At age 15, the young woman has had no periods; secondary sexual characteristics are absent.

- At age 16 1/2, the young woman has had no periods (regardless of otherwise normal growth and development).

- A previously menstruating woman has missed three or more periods (whatever her previous cycle length), or has amenorrhea for 6 months or more.

In most cases, the cause of amenorrhea is benign. Aggressive evaluation is necessary, however, because treatment to restore a more normal hormone milieu may prevent serious problems in the future. If the woman has normal estrogen production, but absent periods because of anovulation, treatment with progestin may reduce her otherwise increased risks for endometrial hyperplasia and cancer. If she has inadequate estrogen production, treatment with estrogen and progestin can prevent osteoporosis.

If secondary amenorrhea occurs during use of hormonal contraceptives, and pregnancy is excluded, the problem may be resolved by changing to a different pill, changing to a different method of contraception, or by adding supplementary estrogen (such as conjugated estrogen 0.625 mg daily) for the last 5–7 days of the pill cycle. If amenorrhea persists for 6 months despite these measures, then evaluate the woman for secondary amenorrhea. It is possible that some other problem is responsible for amenorrhea.

EVALUATION OF AMENORRHEA

Speroff, Glass, and Kase[47] recommend the following steps for evaluating and treating amenorrhea. This simple scheme for initial evaluation can be managed appropriately in a family planning clinic. The first three steps can all be completed at the first visit.

Step 1. Medical history and exam. *Obtain an appropriate medical history* including previous menstrual history, drug or medication use, changes in weight or eating habits, and recent physical exercise patterns. Determine whether other symptoms are present, especially galactorrhea, headache, visual problems, and possible signs of androgen excess such as body or facial hair growth. Perform a physical exam and a pelvic exam. Verify specifically that the patient has a patent vaginal orifice and canal, a normal-appearing cervix, and that the uterus is present. Unless these findings suggest that referral for more extensive evaluation is needed, proceed with the following steps.

Step 2. Exclude the possibility of pregnancy.

Step 3. Laboratory studies and progestin challenge test. *Order blood tests* for prolactin and thyroid stimulating hormone (TSH). If galactorrhea is present, order also an x-ray evaluation of the sella turcica (coneddown view, lateral projection). If the patient has headaches or visual problems, order sella evaluation as in step 6. Administer a progestin challenge test (medroxyprogesterone acetate 10 mg daily for 5 days, or progesterone in oil 200 mg, IM).

- If bleeding does not occur, proceed to step 4.
- If bleeding occurs (spotting is sufficient), galactorrhea is not present, and prolactin and TSH are normal, no further evaluation is necessary. The diagnosis is anovulation, and treatment with progestin can be initiated (described in the next section).
- If TSH is elevated, the diagnosis is hypothyroidism (very rare) and treatment with thyroid will be effective in restoring normal cyclic patterns and will resolve galactorrhea, if present. If prolactin is elevated (greater than 100 ng/ml), then further evaluation of the pituitary (see step 6) is necessary. If this evaluation proves normal, continue surveillance with prolactin testing and coned-down x-ray view studies every 12 months as long as spontaneous menses are absent. Bromocriptine treatment is indicated if the patient wishes to ovulate so that she can become pregnant, or if she finds the galactorrhea troublesome or uncomfortable.
- If the coned-down sella view is abnormal, order further sella evaluation tests, as in step 6.

Step 4. Estrogen and progestin challenge. *Administer an estrogen and a progestin in a cyclic pattern* such as conjugated estrogen 2.5 mg daily for 21 days with medroxyprogesterone acetate 10 mg daily for the last 5 days.

- If bleeding occurs, proceed to step 5.
- If bleeding does not occur, repeat the estrogen/progestin stimulation for one additional month. If amenorrhea persists, the uterus is responsible for amenorrhea. Further evaluation, such as by hysteroscopy, will be necessary to identify and treat Asherman's syndrome, and referral to a gynecologist will probably be necessary.

Step 5. Pituitary function studies. *Order blood tests for FSH and LH* (follicle stimulating hormone and luteinizing hormone). Allow an interval of 2 weeks following step 4 so that the FSH and LH levels will not be influenced by the estrogen and progestin you have prescribed in step 4. Also, remember that the transient LH surge just prior to ovulation normally produces LH levels that are three times the baseline level. If the patient's LH test result is high, but menstrual bleeding occurs exactly 2 weeks later, repeat the LH determination.

- If FSH and LH are low or normal, proceed to step 6.
- If FSH is high, LH is normal, and the woman is of perimenopausal age (46-52 years), then further evaluation is not necessary. The diagnosis is menopause. As menopause approaches FSH often begins to rise before LH rises. In very rare cases, a tumor may secrete FSH or LH. Lung cancers and pituitary tumors can do so, but are so infrequent that further evaluation is not necessary unless other symptoms or signs of malignancy are present.
- If both FSH and LH are high, menopause (ovarian failure) is the cause of amenorrhea. If the woman is in the normal menopausal age range, 45-55, no further evaluation is necessary. If the woman is younger than 45, then the diagnosis may be premature menopause or other less common disorders such as gonadotropin-producing tumor, single gonadotropin deficiency, resistant ovary syndrome, premature ovarian failure secondary to autoimmune disease, or chromosomal mosaicism. Refer the patient to a gynecologist for further evaluation. Treatment to replace the premature loss of hormones for any woman aged 45 years or younger (see treatment following) should be strongly encouraged.

Step 6. Pituitary tumor studies. *Order CT scan or MRI* (magnetic resonance imaging) evaluation of the sella turcica (thin section coronal CT with intravenous contrast enhancement, or sella MRI).

- If the sella is abnormal, refer the patient for further evaluation. Treatment with bromocriptine is likely to be recommended if the tumor is large or shows rapid growth.
- If the sella is normal, hypothalamic suppression is responsible for amenorrhea. Initiate treatment with estrogen and progestin.

TREATMENT OF ANEMORRHEA

Once the cause of amenorrhea is established, initiate treatment. In some cases, hypothalamic suppression can be corrected by altering its cause: reducing excessive athletic training, for example, or modifying a medication regimen. Otherwise treatment should simply replace the missing estrogen and progesterone until normal cyclic function resumes. Combined oral contraceptives are an appropriate choice, especially if the woman needs contraceptive protection. Inform the woman, however, that similar amenorrhea problems are likely to recur when she stops using pills and that a delay in achieving pregnancy is likely. She should anticipate the need for intervention to induce ovulation and allow for extra time to conceive. Alternatively, conjugated estrogen and medroxyprogesterone acetate, prescribed as for postmenopausal hormone treatment (see following section) are appropriate.

If chronic anovulation with development of multiple ovarian follicles (often called polycystic ovary syndrome) is the cause of amenorrhea, then endogenous estrogen production is adequate or high, and replacement with progestin alone is sufficient. Medroxyprogesterone acetate 10 mg daily for 10 days every month is appropriate unless spontaneous ovulatory cycles resume.

Combined oral contraceptives are also an appropriate choice for a woman with anovulation, especially if the woman needs contraceptive protection. Oral contraceptives supply the needed progestin replacement and also suppress the woman's excessive ovarian hormone production which may help reduce symptoms caused by androgen excess. Symptoms of excess androgen are common with polycystic ovary syndrome, and may include acne and growth of dark facial and body hair.

Withdrawal bleeding should occur after each cycle of oral contraceptives or after each progestin batch. If withdrawal bleeding does not occur, then complete the remaining steps in the evaluation of amenorrhea (steps 4 through 8).

M ENOPAUSE

During the climacteric (a transition that usually occurs in women between the ages of 45 and 55), the number of maturing ovarian follicles gradually decreases. The ovaries are no longer able to respond to the pituitary stimulating hormones, so estrogen levels are low and production of FSH and LH increases dramatically. During this interval, fertility declines, and menstrual cycles may be erratic, with diminished menstrual flow. *Menopause, cessation of menstrual periods, occurs at a median age of 51,* but it can occur as early as 45 or as late as 55. Menopause before age 45 is defined as premature menopause. In some cases, the diagnosis of menopause is straightforward: cessation of menses at an appropriate age accompanied by typical hot flushes. Hot flushes usually begin with a spreading wave of warmth extending from the trunk to the face. During a flush, the skin may appear reddened, and sweating may be evident. Flushes typically last just a few minutes and occur several times daily or awaken the woman at night.

If there is any doubt about the diagnosis of menopause, blood tests for FSH and LH can resolve the issue. Cessation of menstrual periods for 12 months, at an appropriate age, or elevated FSH and LH levels in the menopause range, are good evidence that fertility has ended and that a woman can safely stop using contraception.

Many women have unpredictable, irregular cycles preceding menopause, with intermittent menopause symptoms. If bleeding occurs more frequently than once a month, then evaluate as abnormal bleeding (see the "Abnormal Bleeding" section in this chapter). During this interval, FSH levels may be elevated, but LH is still in the normal range and occasional ovulatory cycles may occur. Contraception is still needed.

CONTRACEPTION IN THE PERIMENOPAUSAL YEARS

Perimenopausal women who are healthy non-smokers with no risk factors for heart disease may want to continue oral contraceptives until menopause. Progestin-only minipills also are an option, and can be used by some women who are not good candidates for combined oral contraceptives (see Chapters 10 and 11). Long-acting progestin contraceptives such as Norplant or Depo-Provera can be continued through menopause. Irregular bleeding patterns, however, are problematic for perimenopausal women because abnormal bleeding that is persistent will need to be evaluated even if contraceptive hormone exposure is its most likely cause. Other contraceptive options for women in this age group include condoms, vaginal barriers, and IUDs.

Surgical sterilization is the most prevalent contraceptive method among women in the perimenopausal age range. *A decision to undergo tubal ligation during perimenopause, however, deserves thoughtful risk/benefit/cost analysis.* Because fertility is low, a woman can expect highly effective protection with any of the temporary methods, including vaginal barriers. So for her, the advantages of sterilization surgery are less compelling than they are for women who make the decision earlier in their reproductive years.

Women using oral contraceptives are unlikely to have signs that indicate when menopause is occurring. Beginning when the woman is age 50, *check serum FSH and LH annually to identify menopause* so that contraception can be discontinued. Perform the blood test at the end of the pill-free week.

MEDICAL MANAGEMENT ISSUES AT MENOPAUSE

Except for hot flushes, which are extremely common, most women are able to make the climacteric transition without serious difficulty. Problems associated with reduced estrogen levels such as vaginal dryness and diminished bladder control tend to begin later, months or years after menopause, and may persist or worsen, whereas hot flush problems usually subside in intensity within the first few years. When a woman reaches menopause, review the personal pros and cons of postmenopausal hormone treatment, information on calcium balance, and routine health screening measures such as mammography and lipid surveillance. The minimum daily calcium requirement increases from 1,000 mg daily for perimenopausal adult women to 1,500 mg after menopause for women who do not take estrogen. Dietary sources provide 400 mg–600 mg of calcium for the average woman, so supplements are likely to be necessary regardless of the decision about hormone treatment.

Estrogen treatment overview. Hormone treatment is a reasonable option for many women. Reviewing research available, the American College of Obstetrics and Gynecologists (ACOG) concluded that epidemiologic studies "strongly suggest" that estrogen treatment reduces the risk of cardiovascular disease for postmenopausal women.[1] There are no large prospective studies to provide cause-and-effect proof, however, and heart disease prevention is not an FDA-approved indication for estrogen use. The magnitude of benefit with estrogen suggested by the retrospective studies is very large: meta-analysis of 21 studies found a 50% reduction in the risk of a coronary event.[3] Hormone treatment also reduces osteoporosis risk and ameliorates symptoms such as hot flushes, vaginal dryness, and sleep disturbance; these are the FDA-approved indications for its use. There is some evidence also that estrogen can favorably affect mood and memory, and skin thickness and collagen content.[1] Overall well-being also is likely to be enhanced for women who experience severe flushing problems or menopause symptoms such as fatigue, irritability, or depression that may be related to chronic sleep disturbance caused by flushes at night.

Osteoporosis prevention. Protection against bone loss is a significant medical concern because fractures, especially hip fractures, cause substantial morbidity and mortality in the elderly. Adequate calcium intake and weight bearing exercise are helpful, but cannot alone prevent bone loss, especially for women who have one or more *osteoporosis risk factors, such as a family history of osteoporosis, medical problems or medications that adversely affect bone, slenderness and short stature, and nonblack ethnicity.* Women who do not want to use estrogen, or cannot, should have bone density assessment at menopause. If bone density is more than one standard deviation below the median for age, consider treatment.[38] Estrogen, if not contraindicated, is the simplest approach. Otherwise, consider alternative treatment options such as calcitonin or biphosphonate (etidronate).

Uterine cancer risk. The most clearly documented adverse consequence of estrogen treatment after menopause is a four-fold to eight-fold increase in risk for endometrial cancer. This consequence can be avoided by providing progestin for 12 days each month along with estrogen.[30] Women who use a combined estrogen and progestin regimen after menopause have a lower risk for endometrial cancer than do untreated women. Even if progestin is not provided, overall life-expectancy is greater for estrogen-users than it is for untreated women; this is true even for users who actually develop endometrial cancer.[19]

Breast cancer risk. The possibility that postmenopausal hormone treatment could affect breast cancer risk is of special concern. Research results are in conflict and because the pathophysiology of breast cancer is not known, it is not possible to speculate with confidence about the role that exogenous hormones might play. Because breast cancer ranks second only to lung cancer among women, this is a very significant issue. Several carefully-executed, large epidemiologic studies have shown no excess breast cancer risk for menopausal hormone users.[23,50] Several other studies, however, have found increased risk, at least for some users. Analysis based on 16 studies concluded that breast cancer risk may be increased by 30% after 15 years of estrogen use; no increased risk was apparent until 5 years of use. The risk was greatest for women who had a family history of breast cancer.[48] A possible protective effect of concomitant progestin administration has been suggested,[16,47] but a 1989 study of Swedish women[5] found the excess breast cancer risk to be highest for women who took progestin along with estradiol. Women using conjugated estrogen or estriol in the Swedish study did not incur increased risk, whether or not progestin was used concomitantly. *Until the cause(s) of breast cancer are understood, continuing concern and awareness are the watchwords.* Breast surveillance with conscientious clinical exams and annual mammography are important for all women in this age group.

Medical issues in hormone treatment. Contraindications to menopausal estrogen treatment include:[1]

- Unexplained vaginal bleeding
- Active liver disease
- Chronic, impaired liver function
- Recent vascular thrombosis (with or without emboli)
- Carcinoma of the breast
- Endometrial carcinoma, except in certain circumstances

What risk, if any, estrogen poses for a woman with a past history of thrombosis is unknown. The decision to use estrogen should be approached cautiously, with careful surveillance, for any woman who has had thrombophlebitis in the past. Other relative contraindications include seizure disorder, hypertension, familial hyperlipidemia, migraine headache, and gallbladder disease.[1] The risk of breast cancer recurrence with estrogen treatment is unknown. The risk of ovarian cancer and cervical carcinoma recurrence, however, is believed to be unaffected by hormone treatment.[1] Hormone treatment could aggravate endometriosis symptoms or cause growth of uterine leiomyomata, but in practice, these effects are not common.

Hormone treatment side effects. Breast tenderness, a common initial side effect of treatment, subsides after the first few weeks of treatment in many cases. Some women have nausea; taking estrogen at meal time may help. Fluid retention and uterine cramps occasionally are a problem during progestin administration, and may be reasons to reduce the progestin dose. Some women tolerate better the continuous, moderate blood levels of estrogen that occur with use of estradiol patches than they do the daily hormone peaks that occur with oral administration. A night-time peak, however, may be helpful for a woman with sleep disturbance; taking hormone pills in the evening may maximize her symptom relief.

Providing hormone treatment. A typical treatment regimen provides conjugated estrogen 0.625 mg daily for 25 days each month, with medroxyprogesterone acetate 10 mg daily for the last 10–13 days of estrogen treatment in each cycle.[30] Several other treatment schedules are fairly common. Estrogen given continuously, with progestin on the first 10–13 days of each month, may be helpful for women who experience menopause symptoms during the non-hormone interval in interrupted schedules. Estrogen and progestin given together for 5 days each week, or continuously without interruption, are used in an attempt to avoid bleeding.

Research to clarify optimal regimens, doses, and choice of drugs for menopause treatment is surprisingly limited. Available products are shown in Table 20-3. *Long-term research that documents cardiovascular benefit for estrogen users is entirely based on data for women who took estrogen (primarily conjugated estrogen) alone,* with no progestin. Because of the increased risk of endometrial cancer, women who have a uterus, and choose to use estrogen alone, need annual endometrial biopsy surveillance.

Whether regimens that provide progestin along with estrogen confer cardiovascular benefit similar to treatment with estrogen alone is not known. Protection against endometrial cancer risk is documented for cyclic progestin treatment, but studies of continuous progestin and estrogen treatment are very limited.[30] Research on endometrial hormone receptors, and histologic response to hormone exposure, suggests that for protection against endometrial cancer, the duration of progestin treatment is important. So if progestin-related side effects, such as fluid retention, are a problem, reducing the dose of progestin (to 5 mg or 2.5 mg of medroxyprogesterone acetate) is preferable to reducing its duration.[30] A woman who has had a hysterectomy does not need progestin.

Reliable protection against osteoporosis requires a dose of at least 0.625 mg conjugated estrogen or its equivalent, although some evidence suggests that a dose of 0.3 mg accompanied by an aggressive intake of calcium (1,500 mg– 2,500 mg daily total) can provide a similar benefit.[12]

Testosterone treatment has been suggested for women who have problems with diminished libido. Available hormone products include fixed estrogen/testosterone combinations. Little information, however, is available about long-term effects of testosterone treatment in women, and problems such as acne and increased facial hair have been reported. Intermittent use is possible; the increased libido effect is likely to occur within a few days after starting oral treatment.

Cyclic hormone treatment is likely to be associated with monthly bleeding after each progestin batch. *Bleeding at any other time, or any postmenopausal bleeding in a woman not receiving progestin, requires prompt evaluation.* Irregular bleeding is not uncommon during the first 3–6 months of treatment with a continuous progestin/estrogen regimen. If this occurs, perform an endometrial biopsy. Uterine cancer has been reported among women using a continuous regimen.[25]

Table 20-3 Menopausal treatment products

Hormone	Brand Name/Doses
Estrogens	
Conjugated Estrogens	Premarin 0.3 mg (green), 0.625 mg (maroon) 0.9 mg (white), 1.25 mg (yellow), 2.5 mg (purple)
Estropipate (Estrone)	Ogen 0.625 mg, 1.25 mg, 2.5 mg, 5.0 mg Ortho-est "0.625" (0.75 mg), "1.25" (1.5 mg)
Estradiol	Estrace 1 mg, 2 mg–scored
Estradiol	Estraderm 0.05 mg, 0.1 mg–patches (8 in pack) change patch 2x weekly
Ethinyl Estradiol	Estinyl 0.02 mg, 0.05 mg, 0.05 mg
Estrogen with Methyl Testosterone (MeT)*	
Conjugated Estrogen	Premarin 1.25 with MeT 10 mg Premarin 0.625 with MeT 5 mg
Esterified Estrogen	Estratest 1.25 estrogen with MeT 2.5 mg Estratest H.S. 0.625 estrogen with MeT 1.25 mg
Estrogen Vaginal Creams*	
Conjugated Estrogen	Premarin Vag Cream 0.625 mg/g 42.5 g tube; 1–4 g applicator
Estropipate	Ogen Vag Cream 1.5 mg/g 42.5 g tube; 1–4 g applictor
Dienestrol	Ortho Dienestrol Cream 0.01% (estrogenic potency unknown) 78 g tube
Estradiol	Estrace Vag Cream 0.01% (0.01 mg/g) 42.5 g tube; 1–4 g applicator
Progestins	
Medroxprogestrone Acetate	Amen 10 mg–scored Cycrin 10 mg–scored Provera 2.5 mg, 5 mg, 10 mg–scored
Norethindrone***	Norlutin 5 mg–scored
Norethindrone Acetate***	Norlutate 5 mg–scored Aygestin 5 mg–scored
Methyltestosterone*	
Methyltestosterone	Android 10 mg, 25 mg–scored Metandren 10 mg, 25 mg–scored Testred 10 mg–capsules Virilon 10 mg–capsules

(continued)

Table 20-3 Menopausal treatment products *(cont.)*

Hormone	Brand Name/Doses
Nonhormonal Products	
Clonidine	Catapres-TTS-1 (0.1 mg/day)–Transdermal -TTS-2 (0.2 mg/day)–1 patch/week -TTS-3 (0.3 mg/day) Clonidine 0.1 mg tablets
Belladonna 0.2 mg Phenobarbital 40 mg Ergotamine 0.6 mg	Bellergal-S–scored One tab b.i.d.
Bioflavinoids	Hy-C tablets Mevanin-C capsules Peridin-C tablets

Source: Adapted from Stewart et al. (1987) with permission.

*Methyltestosterone can cause masculine changes such as growth of coarse, dark body hair, scalp hair loss (balding), deepened voice, and increased sex drive; risks for developing liver tumor may also be increased.

**Vaginal estrogen absorption results in somewhat lower blood estrogen levels than the same dose given orally. Notice that Estrace and Dienestrol cream contain a smaller amount of estrogen than do the other products available. To use a low vaginal estrogen dose (equivalent to 0.3 mg conjugated estrogen vaginally), measure 1/8 of an applicator of Premarin, or 1/16 of an applicator of Ogen, or a whole applicator of Estrace or Dienestrol.

***These synthetic progestrins may be less desirable than medroxyprogesterone acetate because of blood lipid effects.

Alternatives to estrogen. When estrogen is contraindicated, treatment with progestin such as medroxyprogesterone acetate 10–20 mg daily or Depo-Provera 150 mg every 3 months, may reduce hot flushes. Progestin also provides some protection against bone loss.[47] Estrogen-containing vaginal cream is an option for treating vaginal dryness. Vaginal symptoms respond to local treatment at a much lower dose than is needed systemically. The use of this cream may not be associated with an increased risk of endometrial cancer.[10] Alternatives to hormone treatment for hot flushes include bioflavinoids, Bellergal, and clonidine (see Table 20-3). Women who must avoid hormones need to be aware that commonly recommended herbal preparations such as ginseng may not be a wise choice since they, too, have estrogenic effects.[20]

MANAGEMENT ISSUES AT MENOPAUSE

Many women experience changes in menstrual patterns beginning months or even years before menopause. Typically, cycle length is shortened. The ovaries become less responsive to pituitary hormones. Pituitary sensitivity to estrogen and progesterone also is altered.[22] Shortened follicular phase duration and inadequate luteal phase patterns can result in cycles as short as 18–21 days. Anovulatory episodes are common and can result in skipped menses or long cycle intervals. Overall, menstrual timing, as well as the duration, amount, and character of menstrual bleeding, are more variable during this time than earlier in the reproductive years.

At the same time in a woman's life, uterine cancer risk becomes a serious concern. Uterine cancer is rare before the age of 40, but its incidence increases in the perimenopausal years. *Abnormal bleeding is the most common early sign of uterine cancer* and of precursor abnormalities such as atypical endometrial hyperplasia. Women who have one or more risk factors for uterine cancer, especially, deserve careful surveillance. Risk factors include: obesity, hypertension, diabetes mellitus, previous breast or ovary or colon cancer, previous uterine hyperplasia or polyps, history of polycystic ovary disease, anovulatory cycle patterns, infertility, family history of uterine cancer, and previous radiation treatment involving the pelvis. *Evaluate to detect hyperplasia or cancer whenever a woman in this age range experiences abnormal bleeding,* including:

- Bleeding episodes with less than 18–21 day intervals
- Prolonged or unpredictable, intermittent bleeding
- Bleeding during cyclic hormone treatment that does not coincide with the conclusion of a progestin treatment interval (bleeding beginning earlier than the 11th day of progestin treatment)
- Any bleeding at all during continuous hormone treatment
- Any bleeding at all after menopause in a woman not taking hormones

The first steps in evaluation of bleeding are to *verify the origin of bleeding and to exclude pregnancy and pelvic infection* as possible causes. Perform an ultrasensitive pregnancy test if pregnancy is possible; ectopic pregnancy incidence is higher for women in the late reproductive years than is the case for younger women. If the woman has uterine tenderness, a past history of, or current risk factors for, pelvic infection, obtain blood tests such as white blood cell count, differential, sedimentation rate, and C-reactive protein. Prescribe a treatment trial with antibiotics.

Perform a pelvic examination during a bleeding episode to verify its source. Bleeding from vaginal or cervical lesions such as cervical cancer are uncommon possibilities that need to be remembered. For this reason, *the initial evaluation should include a Pap smear.* Abrasion or laceration in a severely atrophic vagina sometimes causes bloody vaginal discharge.

In most cases, endometrial biopsy or office hysteroscopy with biopsy is appropriate for initial evaluation of abnormal bleeding.[22] These procedures usually can be performed with local anesthesia, and should be scheduled at a time that the patient is not actively bleeding if this is possible without incurring undue delay. Pelvic ultrasound, to measure the thickness of the endometrial lining, also may be helpful in identifying women with possible hyperplasia or cancer.

If endometrial biopsy results are benign, prescribe cyclic progestin, or cyclic progestin and estrogen. If bleeding resolves promptly, then further evaluation is not necessary. *Bleeding that persists despite hormone treatment, however, mandates further evaluation* with hysteroscopy and more extensive biopsy or D&C (dilation and curettage). In some cases, the cause of bleeding can be corrected at the time of evaluation, especially when hysteroscopy is utilized. Both benign polyps and submucus leiomyomata are common and often can be removed with hysteroscopic surgery.

MANAGEMENT OF AN ADNEXAL MASS

Adnexal masses are extremely common. In some cases, the patient may seek evaluation because of lower abdominal pain (usually unilateral), tenderness, dyspareunia, or a sense of fullness in the lower abdomen. Often, ovarian enlargement is an incidental finding during a pelvic exam, and the patient is entirely asymptomatic.

Evaluation and management depend on the age of the patient, the size of the mass, and the accompanying symptoms, if any. *Be sure that the problem is not an ectopic pregnancy or an ovarian neoplasm.* Pelvic infection and endometriosis can present with similar symptoms.

Malignant ovarian tumors are uncommon in women under 30 years of age.[11] If the ovary is not massively enlarged (5 cm or less in size), the possibility of pregnancy has been excluded, and clinical evidence does not suggest infection or endometriosis, it is reasonable to defer further evaluation for 2–4 weeks for a woman 30 years of age or younger. The most likely diagnosis is a functional ovarian cyst, which is likely to shrink in size or disappear within one cycle. Follow-up pelvic exam will be normal. Treatment with oral contraceptives for one or two cycles can be used to suppress ovarian activity, but there is no evidence that this approach expedites resolution.

Functional cysts occur when follicular development is unusually exuberant, so that the normal ovulatory follicle or corpus luteum is unusually large. Functional cysts can be as large as 8 cm–10 cm in diameter, dwarfing the ovary. In some cases, the presence of a functional cyst disrupts cyclic hormone events temporarily, so that the expected menstrual period is delayed or the character and timing of menstrual flow is altered.

In rare cases, functional cysts can cause severe pain associated with leakage from the ruptured cyst or torsion of the involved adnexa. Cyst rupture can also be associated with intra-abdominal hemorrhage significant enough to require surgical intervention. In most cases, however, the cyst and its accompanying symptoms will resolve spontaneously within a few weeks.

Women who are using oral contraceptives are less likely than other women to develop functional cysts. This noncontraceptive benefit prevents approximately 35 hospitalizations annually for every 100,000 pill users who otherwise would have undergone surgery because of functional cysts.[32] The protection is not absolute, however, so functional cysts do occasionally occur despite oral contraceptive use. A 1987 report of seven cases suggested a possible link between use of triphasic oral contraceptives and the occurrence of large functional ovarian cysts.[8] A follow-up study, however, found no evidence of an increase in such cysts between 1979 and 1986 during which time the use of multiphasic oral contraceptives grew from zero to 3 million users.[18]

If ovarian enlargement persists, or if the woman is over age 30 or has a very large cyst, then evaluate further. Pelvic ultrasound may be helpful in documenting the size and character of a cyst. Ultrasound should help differentiate between a fluid-filled, simple cyst and a solid tumor or a complex cyst that would be consistent with ovarian neoplasm. Abdominal x-ray (flat plate) or MRI (magnetic resonance imaging) also may help identify calcifications or fatty deposits characteristic of dermoid or other ovarian tumors.

Even if these studies are reassuring, however, surgery is likely to be necessary to secure a definitive diagnosis. Among postmenopausal women, ultrasound characteristics were able to distinguish between benign and malignant masses for most women, but failure to undertake surgery would have missed the diagnosis of cancer in 6% of cases in one series.[28]

M ENSTRUAL HYGIENE AND TOXIC SHOCK SYNDROME

Toxic shock syndrome (TSS) is a rare but serious illness. It causes high fever (102° F or higher), vomiting, diarrhea, dizziness, weakness, myalgia, sunburn-like rash followed by desquamation, and in severe cases, hypotension, shock, coma, and death. The reported mortality rate associated with admission to the hospital for TSS was about 10% before 1980 but had declined to 2.6% by 1983[7] as less severe cases were recognized and treated earlier in the course of the disease. TSS is caused by a toxin (or possibly by more than one toxin) produced by *Staphylococcus aureus* bacteria. TSS may occur in the wake of staphylococcal infection anywhere in the body, but most reported cases are associated with using tampons during a menstrual period. In 99% of menstrual cases, TSS is associated with use of tampons. No tampon product is exempt, including natural sea sponges.[7] The risk of TSS increases during the postpartum period and after an initial TSS episode. Recurrence of TSS during subsequent menstrual periods is common.

The incidence of TSS increased significantly beginning in 1977 when super-absorbent tampon materials were first introduced. Because of concerns about TSS, products such as the Rely tampon that utilized these materials were withdrawn from sale, polyacrylate rayon was removed from all tampon products, and new standards for describing tampon absorbency were adopted. All tampon products carry a warning and a description of TSS symptoms. Even with tampon use, however, the risk of TSS is low. TSS incidence has been estimated at 1–3 cases per 100,000 menstruating women per year.[33]

An association between TSS and use of vaginal barrier contraceptives including the contraceptive sponge, the diaphragm, and the cervical cap, has also been documented.[44] The magnitude of this risk, however, is low. Schwartz estimates that 2.25 cases of nonmenstrual TSS may occur annually for every 100,000 women using barrier methods.[44] These cases would result in 0.18 death per 100,000, a mortality that is one-tenth the mortality caused by pregnancies due to method failure in the same number of barrier users. Because TSS can be life-threatening, however, women who use vaginal barrier contraceptives need to know about TSS and be familiar with TSS precautions and danger signs (see Table 20-4). FDA-approved product labeling for these products includes a warning about TSS. *Use of oral contraceptives reduces TSS risk.*[49] The risk of TSS is higher for young women (age 15–24) than for older women.

V AGINAL HYGIENE

Douching is a common practice that may cause adverse health consequences. Data from the National Survey of Family Growth, 1988, showed that 37% of U.S. women, ages 14–44, had douched regularly. Rates were surprisingly similar in all age groups and geographic areas. More educated, wealthier women were the least likely to report douching (17% and 28% respectively); black women were the most likely to douche (66%). Women in this nationally representative survey who reported a history of STD (gonorrhea, chlamydia, herpes, or genital warts) were less likely to have douched regularly than were women with no STD history. Conversely, women with a history of pelvic inflammatory disease were more likely to report having douched regularly than were women who did not report pelvic inflammatory disease.[2] Several other studies have documented a *statistical association between frequent douching and an increased risk for pelvic inflammatory disease and also for ectopic pregnancy.*[34,40]

These associations do not prove that douching causes the increased risk, although it may. Possibly, women who choose to douche do so because of exposure to a larger number of partners or because of vaginal discharge problems. The studies provide no reassurance that douching is safe or desirable. Discuss douching practices with patients. A discussion of the reasons a woman douches may be an opportunity to *teach her about possible risks of sexually transmitted disease and about how to identify early infection signs, such as abnormal vaginal discharge, that mandate evaluation.*

Table 20-4 Patient instructions: minimizing toxic shock syndrome (TSS) risks

1. Using sanitary pads instead of tampons almost entirely eliminates your risk for TSS, but even if you do use tampons the risk is low.

2. If you use tampons, choose the lowest absorbency that meets your menstrual flow needs, and be sure to change them at least every 8 hours. If possible, allow a tampon-free interval every day. For example, you may want to use sanitary pads at night.

3. Wash your hands with soap before inserting anything into your vagina (for example, a tampon, your diaphragm, a contraceptive sponge, or vaginal medication).

4. Follow instructions for vaginal contraceptive products carefully. Do not leave a sponge or your diaphragm or cervical cap in place in your vagina longer than the recommended time, and do not use these products during a menstrual period.

5. During the first 12 weeks after childbirth, you should not use tampons or contraceptive sponges or a cervical cap. It may be best to avoid using a diaphragm as well.

6. Watch for the danger signs of TSS, especially during menstrual periods. If you think you may have mild TSS, remove your tampon and see your clinician. Early TSS symptoms can seem like flu.

7. If you have had TSS, it is safest to stop using tampons entirely, and to avoid contraceptive sponges as well. It also may be prudent to avoid using a diaphragm or cervical cap.

8. TSS danger signs are:
   Fever (temperature of 101°F or more)
   Vomiting
   Diarrhea
   Dizziness
   Feeling faint or weak
   Muscle aches
   Rash-like sunburn
   In severe cases, TSS can cause shock, and even death.

REFERENCES

1. American College of Obstetricians and Gynecologists. Hormone replacement therapy. ACOG Technical Bulletin No. 166. Washington DC: ACOG, 1992.

2. Aral SO, Mosher WD, Cates W Jr. Vaginal douching among women of reproductive age in the United States: 1988. Am J Publ Health 1992;82(2):210-214.

3. Barrett-Connor E, Bush TL. Estrogen and coronary heart disease in women. JAMA 1991;265(14):1861-1867.

4. Berger A, Schaumberg HH. More on neuropathy from pyridoxine abuse. N Eng J Med 1984;311(15):986-987.

5. Bergkvist L, Adami HO, Persoon I, Hoover R, Schaiver C. The risk of breast cancer after estrogen and estrogen-progestin replacement. N Engl J Med 1989;321(5):293-7.

6. Budoff PW. Use of prostaglandin inhibitors in the treatment of premenstrual syndrome. Clin Obstet Gynecol 1987;30(2):453-464.

7. Centers for Disease Control. CDC Surveillance Summaries. Epidemiology of toxic shock syndrome, United States, 1960-1984. 1984;33(3SS):19SS-22SS.
8. Caillouette JC, Koehler AL. Phasic contraceptive pills and functional ovarian cysts. Am J Obstet Gynecol 1987;156(6):1538-1542.
9. Dalton K. The premenstrual syndrome and progesterone therapy. 2nd ed. London: William Heinemann Medical Books, 1984.
10. Deutsch S, Ossowski R, Benjamin I. Comparison between degree of systemic absorption of vaginally and orally administered estrogens at different dose levels in postmenopausal women. Am J Obstet Gynecol 1981;139(8):967-968.
11. Eriksson L, Kjellgren O, von Schoultz B. Functional cyst or ovarian cancer: histopathological findings during 1 year of surgery. Gynecol Obstet Invest 1985;19:155-159.
12. Ettinger B, Genant HK, Cann CE. Postmenopausal bone loss is prevented by treatment with low-dosage estrogen with calcium. Ann Int Med 1987:106:40-45.
13. Facchinetti F, Borella P, Sances G, Fioroni L, Nappi RE, Genazzani AR. Oral magnesium successfully relieves premenstrual mood changes. Obstet Gynecol 1991;78(2):177-178.
14. Fraser IS, McCarron G. Randomized trial of 2 hormonal and 2 prostaglandid-inhibiting agents in women with a complaint of menorrhagia. Aust NZ J Obstet Gynaecol 1991;31(1):66-70.
15. Freeman E, Rickels K, Sondheimer SJ, Polansky M. Ineffectiveness of progesterone suppository treatment for premenstrual syndrome. JAMA 1990;264(3):349-353.
16. Gambrell RD Jr. Proposal to decrease the risk and improve the prognosis of breast cancer. Am J Obstet Gynecol 1984;150(2):119-132.
17. Goodale IL, Domar AD, Benson H. Alleviation of premenstrual syndrome symptoms with the relaxation response. Obstet Gynecol 1990;75(4):649-655.
18. Grimes DA, Hughes JM. Use of multiphasic oral contraceptives and hospitalizations of women with functional ovarian cysts in the United States. Obstet Gynecol 1989;736:1037-1039.
19. Henderson BE, Paganini-Hill A, Ross RK. Decreased mortality in users of estrogen replacement therapy. Arch Intern Med 1991;1511:75-78.
20. Hopkins MP, Androff L, Benninghoff AS. Ginseng face cream and unexplained vaginal bleeding. Am J Obstet Gynecol 1988;159(5):1121-1122.
21. Horrobin DF, Phil D. The role of essential fatty acids and prostaglandins in the premenstrual syndrome. J Repro Med 1983;28(7):465-468.
22. Jutras ML, Cowan BD. Abnormal bleeding in the climacteric. In: Chihal HJ, London SN (eds). Menstrual cycle disorders. Obstetrics and Gynecology Clinics of North America. Philadelphia PA: WB Saunders Co. 1990;17(2).
23. Kaufman DW, Miller DR, Rosenberg L, Helmrich SP, Stolley P, Schottenfeld D, Shapiro S. Noncontraceptive estrogen use and the risk of breast cancer. JAMA 1984;252(1):63-67.
24. Lawson JM, Grady MJ. Ibuprofen-induced aseptic meningitis in a previously healthy patient. West J Med 1985;143(3):386-387.
25. Leather AT, Savvas M, Studd JW. Endometrial histology and bleeding patterns after 8 years of continuous combined estrogen and progestogen therapy in postmenopausal women. Obstet Gynecol 1991;78(6):1008.
26. Lichten EM, Bombard J. Surgical treatment of primary dysmenorrhea with laparoscopic uterine nerve ablation. J Repro Med 1987;323(1):37-41.

27. Lurie S, Borenstein R. The premenstrual syndrome. Obstetrical and Gynecological Survey 1990;45(4):220-228.

28. Luxman D, Bergman A, Sagi J, David MP. The postmenopausal adnexal mass: correlation between ultrasonic and pathologic findings. Obstet Gynecol 1991;77(5):726-728.

29. Maxson WS. The use of progesterone in the treatment of PMS. Clin Obstet Gynecol 1987;30(2):465-477.

30. Mishell DR Jr, Davajan V, Lobo RA. Infertility, contraception and reproductive endocrinology. 3rd ed. Oradell NJ: Medical Economics Co., 1991.

31. Mortola JL. Premenstrual syndrome. Western J Medi 1992;156(6):651.

32. Ory HW. The noncontraceptive health benefits from oral contraceptive use. Fam Plann Perspect 1982;14(4):182-184.

33. Petitti DB, Reingold AL. Recent trends in the incidence of toxic shock syndrome in Northern California. Public Health Briefs 1991;81(9):1209-1211.

34. Phillips RS, Tuomala RE, Feldblum PJ, Schachter J, Rosenberg MJ, Aronson MD. The effect of cigarette smoking, *Chlamydia trachomatis* infection and vaginal douching in ectopic pregnancy. Obstet Gynecol 1992;79(1):85-90.

35. Physicians' desk reference. 47th ed. Oradell NJ: Medical Economics Co, 1993.

36. Puolakka J, Makarainen L, Viinikka L, Ylikorkala O. Biochemical and clinical effects of treating the premenstrual syndrome with prostaglandin synthesis precursors. J Repro Med 1985;30(3):149-150.

37. Pye JK, Mansel RE, Hughes LE. Clinical experience of drug treatments for mastalgia. Lancet 1985;8451:373-376.

38. Riggs BL, Melton LJ. The prevention and treatment of osteoporosis. N Engl J Med 1992;327(9):620-627.

39. Robinson JC, Plichta BA, Weisman CS, Nathanson CA, Ensminger M. Dysmenorrhea and use of oral contraceptives in adolescent women attending a family planning clinic. Am J Obstet Gynecol 1992;166(2):578-583.

40. Rosenberg MJ, Phillips RS. Does douching promote ascending infection? J Repro Med 1992;37(11):930-938.

41. Rossignol AM, Bonnlander H. Caffeine containing beverages, total fluid consumption, and premenstrual syndrome. Am J Public Health 1990;80(9):1106-1110.

42. Rubinow DR, Hoban MC, Grover GN, Galloway DS, Roy-Byrne P, Anderson R, Merriam GR. Changes in plasma hormones across the menstrual cycle in patients with menstrually related mood disorder and in control subjects. Am J Obstet Gynecol 1988;158(1):5-11.

43. Schmidt PJ, Nieman LK, Grover GN, Muller KL, Merriam GR, Rubinow DR. Lack of effect of induced menses on symptoms in women with premenstrual syndrome. N Engl J Med 1991;324(17):1174-1179.

44. Schwartz B, Gaventa S, Broome CV, Reingold AL, Hightower AW, Perlman JA, Wolf PH. Nonmenstrual toxic shock syndrome associated with barrier contraceptives: report of a case-control study. Rev Infect Dis 1989;2(1):S43-S49.

45. Smith RP, Heltzel JA. Interrelation of analgesia and uterine activity in women with primary dysmenorrhea. J Repro Med 1991;36(4):260-264.

46. Smith S, Rinehard VS, Ruddock VE, Schiff I. Treatment of premenstrual syndrome with alprazolam: results of a double-blind, placebo-controlled randomized crossover clinical trial. Obstet Gynecol 1987;70(1):37-43.

47. Speroff L, Glass RH, Kase NG. Clinical gynecologic endocrinology and infertility. 4th ed. Baltimore MD: Williams & Wilkins Co., 1989.

48. Steinberg KK, Thacker SB, Smith SJ, Stroup DF, Zack MM, Flanders WD, Berkelman RL. A meta-analysis of the effect of estrogen replacement therapy on the risk of breast cancer. JAMA 1991;265(15):1985-1992.
49. Wager GP. Toxic shock syndrome: a review. Am J Obstet Gynecol 1983;146(1): 93-102.
50. Wingo PA, Layde PM, Lee NC, Rubin G, Ory HW. The risk of breast cancer in postmenopausal women who have used estrogen replacement therapy. JAMA 1987;257(18):209-215.
51. Wood SH, Mortola JF, Chan YF, Moossazadeh F, Yen SSC. Treatment of premenstrual syndrome with fluoxetine: a double-blind, placebo controlled, crossover study. Obstet Gynecol 1992;80(3):339-344.
52. Ylostalo P. Cyclic or continous treatment of the premenstrual syndrome (PMS) with bromocriptine. Europ J Obstet Gynecol Repro Biol 1984;17(5):337-343.

Cervical Cytological Screening

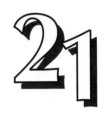

- The Pap smear is a cost-effective approach to substantially decrease cervical cancer.
- The risk factors for squamous cancers of the cervix follow an epidemiologic pattern similar to many sexually transmitted infections.

- HIV-infected women should receive Pap smears at least annually and their positive Pap smear findings managed aggressively.
- Optimal treatment of low-grade SIL lesions remains controversial. High-grade SIL should be followed by colposcopic evaluation.

A reproductive health care visit represents an ideal opportunity to offer cancer screening tests. The Pap smear, more than many other screening tests, has proven its cost effectiveness over the years.[28] Although negative press reports in the mid-1980s shed doubts upon Pap smear quality, early detection of premalignant lesions by Pap smears prevent at least 70% of potential cervical cancers.[27]

Of the remaining 30%—those women who actually develop cervical cancer—

- 8% elude cytological detection because of imperfections in cytological technology or the biologic behavior of malignant lesions.
- 22% represent women who develop cervical cancer because of failure to regularly seek Pap smears; women whose cancers could have been prevented with early detection and treatment.

Consequently, the most effective use of health care resources in the prevention of cervical cancer is to ensure that *all* women have receive Pap smears at indicated intervals, and to properly manage women found to have abnormalities on cytological screening.

Over the years, there has been a tendency to "link" cervical cytological screening with the use of prescription contraceptives, especially oral contraceptives (OCs). In many cases, a woman could get a prescription for OCs only when she underwent an annual examination, which necessarily included a Pap smear. In this way, women have been compelled to receive desirable public health screening tests as a by-product of their need for contraception. More recently, some experts have proposed unlinking Pap smears from OC prescriptions, based on the philosophy that while beneficial screening tests must be supported upon their own merits, interventions unrelated to cervical cancer screening (*e.g.*, OC prescription, abortion) should not be used as an opportunity to predicate Pap smear performance.[8,26] Regardless of one's attitude on this issue, the message that clinicians must promote is that periodic Pap smears are desirable, and in some cases, lifesaving screening tests, irrespective of a woman's contraceptive method. Furthermore, OCs should never be restricted or withheld from a woman solely because she has an abnormal Pap smear. There is no reason to believe that OC use will hasten the progression of an existing cervical lesion. All too often, the tragic result of withholding OCs is an unintended pregnancy in a woman with cervical dysplasia, making diagnosis more difficult and often delaying treatment.

PATHOPHYSIOLOGY

The cervix consists of two types of epithelium:

- Squamous epithelium, which covers the vagina and the portio vaginalis of the cervix
- Columnar epithelium, which covers the endocervical canal, and in younger women, the area around the external cervical os.

At menarche, when estrogen levels rise and *Lactobacillus sp.* consequently colonize the vagina, the vaginal pH drops into an acidic range. This environment changes the exposed fragile columnar epithelial cells around the cervical os, leading to their replacement by squamous epithelium, a process referred to as squamous metaplasia. As this process proceeds over decades, the advancing edge of the squamous epithelium (referred to as the squamocolumnar junction, or SCJ) migrates centrally toward the cervical os, and ultimately, into the endocervical canal. Squamous metaplasia is most rapid during adolescence and accelerates further during pregnancy.

In colposcopic terminology, the field of squamous metaplasia is referred to as the transformation zone (TFZ), and its inner border is defined as the active squamocolumnar junction. Because squamous cell cancers and their precursors virtually always develop within the transformation zone, both cytological and colposcopic evaluation focus upon the TFZ.[21]

The immature metaplastic cell is uniquely vulnerable to events that can modify the DNA component of the cell nucleus, consequently developing into a premalignant or frankly malignant cervical lesion. There is now widespread agreement that the cause of cervical dysplasia is point mutation in metaplastic cells resulting from human papilloma virus (HPV) infection and other carcinogenic co-factors.[22] Although more than 60 DNA-types of HPV have been identified, only a limited number are associated with premalignant and malignant epithelial lesions of the lower genital tract:

- HPV types 6 and 11 frequently are isolated from cervical condylomata and low-grade lesions and are felt to exhibit low malignant potential.
- HPV types 16 and 18, 31, 33, and 35, and a few others, considered to be "high risk" HPV types, also may be found in low-grade lesions, but more commonly are present in high-grade lesions and cervical squamous and adenocarcinomas.[9]

RISK FACTORS FOR CERVICAL CANCER

HPV infection alone is insufficient to initiate the development and proliferation of a premalignant lesion. A facilitating agent, or co-factor, appears to be necessary to act in concert with HPV to initiate these premalignant changes. For example, cigarette smoking has been identified as a powerful co-factor, doubling a smoker's risk of cervical cancer in comparison with a nonsmoker.[2,29]

Epidemiologic data are consistent with the biological mechanism cited above. Two decades ago, studies in Canada demonstrated the primary epidemiologic risk factors for the development of cervical cancer:

- **Early onset of intercourse** (defined as a sexual debut before 20 years old)—metaplasia is most active during adolescence, making a young woman more vulnerable to cell changes.
- **Three or more sexual partners** in one's lifetime—the greater the number of sexual partners, the greater the risk of acquiring a high risk type of HPV.[7]
- **Male sexual partner who has had other partners,** especially if a previous partner had cervical cancer.
- **Clinical history of condyloma acuminata.**

It is clear that the risk factors for squamous cancers of the cervix follow an epidemiologic pattern similar to many sexually transmitted infections. These cancers are often referred to as being a sexually transmitted disease.

Protective factors include:

- Virginity
- Long-term celibacy
- Life-long mutual monogamy
- Long-term use of condoms

Factors that seem to have no effect on cervical cancer risk include history of herpes simplex virus infection, circumcision status of the male partner, religious background, or number of pregnancies.[25] The effect of race and socioeconomic status are controversial, because while studies show higher rates of cervical cancer among African-American women and women of lower socio-economic status, it is unclear whether this is related to access to Pap smears and other medical care or to other undetected confounding variables.[4]

HIV INFECTION AND CERVICAL CANCER RISK

Recent studies of cohorts of women with HIV infection have demonstrated disturbing findings regarding cervical neoplasia. Although most studies are small and are not well controlled, HIV-infected women do appear to have higher rates of HPV infection, premalignant cervical lesions, and cervical cancer.[6,16] When cervical cancer occurs in HIV infected women, the lesion may progress more rapidly, probably due to the underlying immunodeficiency.[15] In 1992, the CDC changed its surveillance definition of AIDS to include cervical cancer in an HIV-positive woman as an AIDS indicator disease.[5] Although an early uncontrolled study suggested that HIV-infected women had substantially higher rates of falsely negative Pap smears,[17] more recent studies have yielded inconsistent results.[1] While much needs to be learned regarding the natural history of cervical neoplasia in HIV infected women, three clinical recommendations can be made at this time.

1. HIV-infected women should receive Pap smears at least annually. Many, though not all, experts recommend that HIV-infected women undergo a baseline colposcopic evaluation at the time of initial diagnosis of HIV infection.

2. There is no role for expectant management when an HIV-infected woman has abnormal Pap smear result. Perform colposcopy after a single reading of atypical squamous cell of undetermined significance (ASCUS) or squamous intraepithelial lesion (SIL).

3. Do not assume that treatment is futile for the woman who has both HIV and premalignant or malignant cervical disease. Because women with both conditions are more likely to die of cervical cancer, the aggressive treatment of cervical disease will prolong life in most cases.

TECHNICAL ASPECTS OF CYTOLOGICAL SCREENING

High accuracy in cytological screening is dependent upon a good quality cervical sample, appropriately performed slide preparation, and competent cytopathologic interpretation.

Timing. A Pap smear may be performed at any time that heavy menstrual bleeding is not present. However, optimal timing is midcycle in a woman who has not has intercourse for 24 hours and has not placed any substances in her vagina for at least 48 hours.

Sampling. Moisten the speculum with warm water. Never use other lubricants because they may cause cell clumping on the slide and interfere with cytological interpretation. Using a large cotton-tipped applicator in a gentle wiping motion, remove excess cervical mucus. The order of specimens sampled is critical: Those samples most easily contaminated by blood should be obtained earlier in the sampling sequence. Sampling of the vaginal pool is not helpful in premenopausal women and may actually decrease the quality of the sample by adding degenerating cells and other debris. If additional cervical sampling is necessary for evaluation of infection, collect the samples *after* completing the Pap smear. A sample for gonorrhea testing should be followed by a sample for chlamydia testing.

Slide preparation. First sample the exocervix, using a wooden or plastic spatula rotated 360 degrees around the exocervix. Immediately place the sample on a glass slide, creating a monolayer covering most of the slide's surface. Second, sample the endocervical canal, preferably using a brush sampling device, or if not available, a saline-moistened cotton-tipped applicator. Plate this sample directly over the first sample by gently rolling the brush or swab over the surface of the slide, again attempting to achieve a monolayer of material. Unless specifically requested by the cytopathology laboratory, there is no need to use separate slides for each sample or to segment the exocervical sample in one section of the slide and the endocervical sample in another section. Fix the sample immediately in order to avoid airdrying.

C YTOLOGICAL SCREENING INTERVALS

The issue of Pap smear screening intervals has been a contentious one, mainly because of disagreements over the basic assumptions utilized in cost-effectiveness analyses. In August 1987, a Pap Smear Consensus Statement was issued by a number of medical organizations:[27]

> All women who are, or who have been sexually active, or who have reached 18 years old, (should) have an annual Pap test and pelvic exam. After a woman has had three or more consecutive, satisfactory, normal annual exams, the Pap test may be performed less frequently at the discretion of her physician.

Many clinicians find that this statement provides minimal guidance, because the term "physician discretion" is rather nebulous. More useful are guidelines that account for epidemiological risk factors in the design of Pap smear sampling intervals for individual women.

A central concern in determining screening intervals is the risk of a falsely negative Pap smear. A false-negative smear is one that has been interpreted as normal in a woman who has an actual cervical abnormality. The longer the sampling interval, the greater risk that a falsely negative Pap smear will delay the diagnosis of a cervical lesion. For example, if a woman chooses a 3-year sampling interval, a single false negative smear could result in a delay of up to 6 years in the detection of her lesion.

The rate of false negative Pap smears averages about 20%, ranging from as low as 5% to as high as 70%.[12,30] If two Pap smears are performed in a short interval, the rate of falsely negative smears is reduced to 4% (20% x 20%). If three smears are performed, the rate of false-negative smears falls to 0.8%. Table 21-1 contains the recommendations for Pap smear screening intervals used by Title X Family Planning programs.[27]

PAP SMEAR REPORTING SYSTEMS

The original Pap smear reporting system, as devised by Papanicolaou and Traut in 1942, was designed for the purpose of diagnosing cervical and uterine cancer.

In older terminology, premalignant squamous epithelial changes were referred to as *dysplasia,* and lesions with increasing degrees of involvement of the cervical epithelium were graded in severity as mild, moderate, and severe dysplasia, with full-thickness epithelial lesions referred to as carcinoma-in-situ (CIS). In general, dysplasia was considered of lesser importance than CIS, which in the 1950s was considered equivalent of an early cervical cancer.[24]

Since the 1970s, this terminology has been replaced with the term *cervical intraepithelial neoplasia* (CIN), in which CIN I is considered equivalent to mild dysplasia, CIN II is equal to moderate dysplasia, and CIN III encompasses both severe dysplasia and CIS. The CIN classification system was devised to stress the fact the premalignant squamous lesions of the lower genital tract represent a continuum of the same process, and that the severity of the CIN lesion is irrelevant as long as it is detected and treated before invasion occurs.

Currently, The Bethesda Classification System (TBS) for cervical cytological screening is rapidly replacing the Papanicolaou reporting system as an *international* cervical cytopathology reporting standard.[20] (See Table 21-2.) The Bethesda System differs from the Papanicolaou reporting system in three important ways:

1. It abandons the "class" approach to diagnosis and provides a narrative descriptive diagnosis only.
2. It accounts for new information regarding the pathophysiology of premalignant genital tract lesions by including the diagnosis of HPV

Table 21-1 Pap smear screening intervals

Risk level	Characteristics	Interval

Extremely low-risk	• Virginal
	• Never an abnormal Pap *and*
	  – ≥5 benign Pap smears and hysterectomy for benign disease
	  – ≥10 benign Pap smears, including 1 at older than 60 years; presently over 65 years old
		Pap smear not necessary

Low-risk	• Onset of sexual activity at >20 years old • < 3 sexual partners (ever) • User of barrier contraception • No history of HPV or STDs • Non-smoker • Previously normal Pap smear	Yearly for 3 years, then every 2-3 years
High-risk	• Onset of sexual activity at <20 years old • 3 or more sexual partners • History of HPV or STDs • Previously abnormal Pap Smear • Cigarette smoker	Yearly
Post-hysterectomy	• Cervical or uterine malignancy • Premalignant cervical lesion • Benign cervix and uterus	• Every 3 months for 2 years, every 6 months for 3 years, then yearly • Every 6 months for 2-3 years, then yearly • Every 3-5 years
DES-exposed daughters		• First Pap at onset of menstruation, 14 years old, or onset of intercourse • Baseline colposcopy after onset of intercourse • Vaginal and cervical Pap smears every 6-12 months until 30 years old Thereafter, yearly cervical and vaginal Pap smears

Table 21-2 Comparison of The Bethesda Classification, CIN classification, and Papanicolaou reporting

Bethesda System	CIN Classification	Papanicolaou
Low-grade SIL	HPV change	Atypia: koilocytotic, warty, condylomatous
	CIN I	Mild dysplasia
High-grade SIL	CIN II	Moderate dysplasia
	CIN III	Severe dysplasia, carcinoma-in-situ

infection and limiting use of the term "atypia." Also added is the term *squamous intraepithelial lesion* (SIL): low-grade SIL refers to findings previously referred to as HPV change and CIN I, while high-grade SIL includes CIN II and CIN III lesions.

3. It more clearly defines the relationship between the cytopathologist and the referring provider by defining cervical cytological screening as a consultation with a cytopathologist, rather than the simple submission of an analyte to a laboratory.

One of the most profound changes in TBS is the effort to modify deeply entrenched management patterns based in the Papanicolaou reporting system: women with "atypical" Pap smears often were not managed aggressively and could be followed with a repeat smear, while those with Pap smears showing CIN I were managed aggressively with immediate colposcopic evaluation.

Conversely, the critics of TBS claimed[10] that lumping these conditions together was inappropriate, since women previously requiring different evaluation schema now would have to be managed in the same manner. The critics feared that mandating colposcopic evaluation for women with low-grade SIL on Pap smear, but who in fact had a benign HPV infection, could result in over utilization of resources and over treatment. Alternatively, if women with low-grade SIL were to be managed conservatively with repeat Pap smears, unacceptable delays in the diagnosis of CIN lesions might occur.

Convincing evidence, however, shows that HPV changes and CIN I represent *the same entity:*[14]

- Virologically, both HPV change and CIN I are in most cases associated with the presence of HPV types 6 and 11, although either lesion may demonstrate the presence of high-risk HPV types 16 and 18.

- Morphologically, the two lesions appear colposcopically as acetowhite epithelium with few or no vascular changes.

- Histologically, the nuclear and cytoplasmic characteristics of the lesions are very similar and commonly are indistinguishable under the microscope.

Finally, and most importantly, the natural histories of the two lesions appear to be the same, in that 15%-20% of untreated lesions progress, while the remainder either regress or remain unchanged for long periods of time. CIN II and CIN III were combined into the category of high-grade SIL for similar reasons: that the lesions are difficult to differentiate histopathologically, and if they are comparable in size, treatment is the same for the two lesions.

M ANAGEMENT OF ABNORMAL PAP SMEAR RESULTS

Cervical cytological reports conforming with The Bethesda System format will always include a statement of sample adequacy and a general categorization of the sample being normal or abnormal. Abnormalities are grouped into four broad categories: infection, reactive and reparative changes, squamous cell abnormalities, and gland cell abnormalities (Table 21-3).

Table 21-3 The Bethesda System reporting categories

Category	Reading
Infection	• Fungus consistent with *Candida sp.* • *Trichomonas vaginalis* • Predominance of coccobacilli consistent with a shift in vaginal flora • Bacteria morphologically consistent with *Actinomyces sp.* • Cellular changes associated with herpes simplex virus
Reactive and reparative changes	• Cellular changes associated with inflammation • Atrophy with inflammation • Miscellaneous: radiation, IUD, DES, etc.
Squamous cell abnormalities	• Atypical squamous cells of undetermined significance (ASCUS) • Low-grade SIL • High-grade SIL • Squamous cell cancer
Gland cell abnormalities	• Endometrial cells, cytologically benign, in a post-menopausal woman • Atypical glandular cells of undetermined significance (AGCUS) • Adenocarcinoma

NORMAL, PROBLEMS WITH THE
ADEQUACY OF THE SPECIMEN

Satisfactory, but limited by... The condition that most often limits the interpretation is an inadequate sampling of endocervical cells. Their presence indicates that in the process of sampling the transformation zone, the active squamocolumnar junction was included. If a normal or benign result is reported, take the next Pap smear at a routine interval. A result that describes inadequate or absent endocervical cells, but provides no other categorization or diagnosis, must be managed as an unsatisfactory smear (below).

Even with the best of sampling efforts, however, endocervical cells are absent in as many as 10% of Pap smears obtained from premenopausal women and as many as 50% from postmenopausal women. These cells are also more likely to be absent from smears from OC users and pregnant women. Thus, a 1988 CDC Consensus Statement declared that the presence of endocervical cells *per se* is not necessary in a Pap smear.[27] The proportion of Pap smears with this reading provides an important opportunity to monitor Pap smear technique. If the percentage of Pap smears with no endocervical cells present exceeds 10%-15%, remedial action is necessary. If clinician education regarding Pap smear technique and a switch to brush sampling devices does not result in improvement, the laboratory's cytopathologist must be consulted in order to determine whether the problem lies with the laboratory or the provider and to define further steps necessary to rectify the problem.

Unsatisfactory for evaluation... Inadequate sampling, air drying, excessive red or white blood cells, or other factors make interpretation of the smear impossible. Repeat the smear, preferably when the woman is at midcycle and has not had intercourse or used vaginal products for at least 24 hours. Do not repeat the Pap smear earlier than 6 weeks from the previous smear; repetitive sampling over short periods of time may increase the risk of falsely negative smears due to decreased exfoliation of abnormal cells and a greater likelihood of reparative changes. Postmenopausal women with one or more unsatisfactory Pap smears due to vaginal atrophy should apply topical vaginal estrogen cream for 4-6 weeks, then receive a repeat Pap smear no earlier than 1 week after completing the medication in order to avoid sampling interference caused by the vehicle of the topical medication. Unless a woman has a history of endometrial hyperplasia, progestin withdrawal is not necessary after this short course of estrogen exposure. If the proportion of unsatisfactory smears within a practice is greater than 10%, remedial action in consultation with the cytopathologist is indicated.

ABNORMAL DESCRIPTIVE DIAGNOSES

Infection

Fungus consistent with Candida sp. In most cases, *Candida* reported on Pap smear is due to normal vaginal colonization with low levels of *Candida*, rather than frank vaginal candidiasis. *Candida* colonization is not dangerous to the affected woman or her sexual partner. Review the woman's medical record. If she received treatment for vaginal candidiasis at the time the Pap smear was taken or since then, she does not need to be notified. However, if she was not treated for vaginal candidiasis, notify her that *Candida* were present. If she is symptomatic, ask her to return for evaluation and treatment. Repeat the Pap only if the inflammation due to the candidiasis is of sufficient severity that the cytopathologist recommends that the Pap smear be repeated after treatment is complete.

Trichomonas vaginalis. While the Pap smear is a relatively insensitive test for the detection of trichomonas—it detects trichomonads in only about one-half of infected women—its specificity is as high as 98%.[13] When the Pap report indicates presence of trichomonas, review the woman's medical record to determine whether the infection was recently treated. If it has been, no further action is required. If it has not been treated, offer treatment to avoid horizontal transmission to a new sexual partner and to prevent conversion of asymptomatic trichomonas colonization into an uncomfortable case of symptomatic vaginal trichomoniasis. The practice of requiring microscopic saline suspension confirmation of trichomonads is illogical because such a relatively insensitive test (about 60%) should not be used to confirm a test of high specificity. Repeat the Pap smear after the next routine screening interval, unless the narrative report mentions obscuring inflammation and indicates the need to repeat the Pap smear after treatment.

Predominance of* Coccobacilli *consistent with shift in vaginal flora. This reading refers to changes detected in the bacterial flora of the vagina in which the normal *Lactobacillus* are not abundant but *Coccobacilli* are seen in numbers greater than normal. While this description was devised to *suggest* the possibility of bacterial vaginosis (BV), it is both an insensitive and nonspecific indicator of BV. The clinical diagnosis of BV is made solely on clinical findings (see Chapter 4 on Sexually Transmitted Disease), and neither vaginal culture nor Pap smear findings have any role in the diagnosis of this condition. Management is controversial: Many clinicians feel that no further evaluation is necessary and that the next Pap smear should be performed at the routine interval, while others feel that the woman should be informed of this result and offered clinical evaluation for BV.

***Bacteria morphologically consistent with* Actinomyces spp.** *Actinomyces israelii* is an anaerobic bacteria capable of causing a severe pelvic infection, especially in women over 35 years old with current long-term IUD use. A large majority of IUD wearers with *Actinomyces* on Pap smear have asymptomatic cervical colonization (not infection) that does not require antibiotic therapy. IUD users with *Actinomyces* on their Pap smear must be examined in order to determine whether there is evidence of pelvic infection. If symptoms or physical findings suggest pelvic actinomycosis, remove the IUD and initiate intensive antibiotic therapy. Advise the woman to use another method of contraception and not have an IUD reinserted. While no definitive data support a particular course of action for patients with asymptomatic *Actinomyces* colonization, it is prudent to remove the IUD and insert a replacement IUD only after a repeat Pap smear performed 3 months later shows the absence of *Actinomyces*.

Cellular changes associated with herpes simplex virus (HSV). Although an insensitive indicator of cervical herpes simplex shedding, the Pap smear is a specific indicator. Although many women insist on culture verification of HSV infection it is likely that cervical shedding will have ceased in the 1-2 weeks since the Pap smear was taken, so a confirmatory HSV culture will be futile and wasteful of resources. Advise the infected woman to provide this information to her obstetrical care provider so that precautions may be taken to minimize the risk of vertical transmission of HSV to a newborn. Unless inflammation interferes with the interpretation of the Pap smear, the next Pap smear should be performed at the routine interval.

Reactive and Reparative

Reactive cellular changes associated with inflammation. Nonspecific reactive inflammatory changes may be associated with the following: benign metaplasia, mechanical or chemical irritation, post-traumatic repair, chlamydial or gonococcal endocervicitis, viral infection, invasive cervical cancer, or other unknown factors. Of these possibilities, the only infectious conditions amenable to antibiotic therapy are gonococcal and chlamydial endocervicitis. Women who have been recently evaluated for these organisms and found to be uninfected do not require further evaluation or antibiotic therapy. Women who have not been evaluated recently should be examined. Either provide empirical antibiotic treatment for women diagnosed with mucopurulent cervicitis or perform gonorrhea and chlamydia tests and treat women who test positive. Empirically treating women with inflammatory Pap smears with topical antibiotic sulfa creams *is of no value* in either the treatment of cervical infection or the resolution of abnormal Pap smears and is to be condemned.[23]

Rarely, the only Pap smear finding in a woman with a preinvasive or an invasive cervical carcinoma is the persistent finding of inflammation or inflammatory atypia. For this reason, many gynecologic oncologists recommend that women with persistent, unexplained inflammation on Pap smear receive colposcopic evaluation. If this regimen is accepted, women who have been treated for a cervical infection or those evaluated and found not to be infected should receive their next two Pap smears at 3- to 6-month intervals. If unexplained inflammation again is found during this surveillance period, colposcopic evaluation is recommended.

Atrophy with inflammation. Atrophy with inflammation is most common in postmenopausal women or those with estrogen-deficiency states. Treatment of the vaginal atrophy is indicated only if the woman has symptomatic atrophic vaginitis; it is not necessary for the asymptomatic woman. Pap smear screening intervals should not be modified and notification of the woman is unnecessary. However, because atrophy may cause a cytological picture similar to dysplasia, a postmenopausal woman with a Pap smear showing ASCUS or low-grade SIL should be treated with a vaginal estrogen cream for 4-6 weeks, followed by a repeat Pap smear.

Intrauterine contraceptive device. Cytological changes associated with the use of an IUD detected on Pap smear are of a benign nature and do not require further investigation.

Squamous Cell Abnormalities

Atypical squamous cell of undetermined significance (ASCUS). The ASCUS reading refers to the finding of cells with nuclear atypia that are not normal yet not consistent with a diagnosis of low-grade SIL. Findings suggestive of HPV effect (koilocytotic atypia, condylomatous atypia) are explicitly excluded from this category and classified as low-grade SIL. While intended to be an unusual reading, ASCUS accounts for as much as 10% of Pap smear results in some laboratories. Because of confusion regarding the meaning of the ASCUS finding, the updated 1991 Bethesda System[3] requires the cytopathologist to further qualify the diagnosis by stating that either "reactive changes" are present or that "a premalignant/malignant process is favored." This differentiation is critical for clinical management. If ASCUS results are not reported in this manner by your laboratory, consult with the cytopathologist and request clarification.

Management of ASCUS Pap smears is controversial because few studies assessed the natural history of these lesions or their optimal management. Until more is known, an ASCUS/premalignant change reading should be considered to be equivalent to a reading of low-grade SIL. Alternatively, ASCUS/reactive Pap smears probably represent a benign process and no further evaluation is necessary.

Low-grade SIL. This category encompasses HPV effects (koilocytotic atypia, condylomatous atypia) and CIN I. Because few data are available to validate management of low-grade SIL, clinicians must make an "educated guess" until optimal management patterns are further defined by large epidemiological studies. Only 15%-20% of low-grade SIL lesions will progress to a higher-grade lesion.[18,19] Efforts must focus upon identifying and treating those women with lesions destined to progress. In light of the relatively slow temporal progression of SIL lesions, expectant management of women with low-grade SIL on a single Pap smear is acceptable, *assuming that the woman is a good follow-up candidate.* In this situation, Pap smears should be done every 4–6 months for three intervals, and if any subsequent Pap smear report over the next 12–18 months shows ASCUS/premalignant change or SIL, the woman must be referred for colposcopic evaluation. Conversely, if all Pap smears are reported as normal during this period of increased surveillance, the woman may return to a routine screening pattern afterward. Women who are *not good follow-up risks,* or those who request immediate evaluation, should be advised to receive colposcopic evaluation after a single low-grade SIL Pap smear reading.

High-grade SIL. Refer women with high-grade SIL for colposcopic evaluation, even if the Pap smear was obtained during pregnancy, if a benign Pap smear has been obtained since the SIL reading, or if no visible cervical lesion is present. A comprehensive list of indications for colposcopy is included in Table 21-4.

Gland Cell Abnormalities

Endometrial cells, cytologically benign, in a postmenopausal woman. Endometrial cells found on Pap smear are an insignificant finding in premenopausal women with normal ovulatory cycling. However, because the endometrium normally is atrophic in postmenopausal women, the finding of endometrial cells may be the result of exfoliation from a focus

Table 21-4 Indications for colposcopy

- Pap smear showing high-grade SIL
- Persistent finding of "atypical squamous cells of undetermined significance (ASCUS)-premalignant process favored" or of low-grade SIL on Pap smear (any two abnormal Pap smears performed at 4- to 6-month intervals within a 12- to 18-month observation period), in a patient who will reliably return for repeat smear
- Persistent inflammation after treatment of proven infection or if persistent Pap smear finding with no infection documented
- Pap smear showing atypical glandular cells of undetermined significance
- Cervical leukoplakia (white lesion visible to the naked eye without the application of acetic acid) or other unexplained cervical lesion, regardless of Pap smear result
- Baseline examination of a woman with a history of in-utero DES exposure
- Baseline examination of a woman known to be infected with the human immunodeficiency virus (HIV)
- Unexplained or persistent cervical bleeding, regardless of Pap smear result

Women with Pap smear results reporting squamous cell or adenocarcinoma of the cervix must be referred immediately for expert consultation with a physician experienced in the management of gynecologic cancers.

---

of endometrial hyperplasia or adenocarcinoma. For this reason, consider the finding of endometrial cells in a postmenopausal woman as a danger sign and sample the endometrium. Because a premenopausal woman with chronic anovulation also is at risk for endometrial hyperplasia, manage the finding of endometrial cells in the same way.

Atypical glandular cells of undetermined significance (AGCUS). AGCUS may result from bacterial or HPV infection of glandular cells, adenocarcinoma-in-situ (adenoCIS), or adenocarcinoma. However, because adenocarcinomas of the cervix are associated with a rate of false-negative Pap smears as high as 40%,[11] women with AGCUS Pap smears require aggressive evaluation in order to exclude a cancer diagnosis. There is no role for observation (repeat Pap) in this situation. Management consists of a thorough endocervical curettage (ECC), optimally done within the context of a colposcopic evaluation. Even if this test reveals only benign columnar epithelium, many experts suggest more frequent Pap smear screening intervals for at least 12 months.

Squamous cell carcinoma, endocervical adenocarcinoma. Immediately refer women with Pap smear results showing squamous or adenocarcinoma of the cervix for expert consultation with a physician experienced in the management of gynecological cancers.

TREATMENT OF SQUAMOUS INTRAEPITHELIAL LESIONS

Over the past 5 years, management protocols have become much more conservative, due to the recognition that most low-grade SIL lesions will not progress to higher-grade lesions. While this trend is likely to continue, it will require greater diligence to follow-up on the part of both providers and patients.

Typical papillary condyloma acuminata of the cervix, once histologically proven by cervical biopsy, should be treated rather than observed. This aggressive approach decreases the amount of friable cervical tissue, which may increase receptivity to HIV infection and may decrease the risk of viral transmission to a partner. Cryotherapy will be the least invasive and most inexpensive treatment modality in most cases, although some situations may require the use of LEEP or laser. The use of trichloroacetic acid and topical 5-FU for the treatment of cervical condyloma and SIL is considered to be investigational and is not recommended.

The optimal treatment of low-grade SIL (flat condyloma and CIN I) remains a major focus of controversy. Because the lesion has indeterminate malignant potential, many clinicians assume that progression is a possibility and treat (ablate) the entire "at risk" transformation zone. Alternatively, because risk of progression is only about 20% and the lesion is not dangerous until it does progress, other clinicians follow the patient until there is evidence of high-grade SIL or documented persistence of low-grade SIL. There is universal agreement that high-grade SIL must be treated, because the risk of progression to cervical cancer is both more likely and more immediate.

REFERENCES

1. Adachi A, Fleming I, Burk RD, Ho GY, Klein RS. Women with human immunodeficiency virus infection and abnormal Papanicolaou smears: a prospective study of colposcopy and clinical outcome. Obstet Gynecol 1993;81(3):372-377.
2. Brinton LA, Schairer C, Haenszel W, Stolley P, Lehman HF, Levine R, Savitz DA. Cigarette smoking and invasive cervical cancer. JAMA 1986;255(23):3265-3269.
3. Broder S. Rapid communication — The Bethesda system for reporting cervical/vaginal cytologic diagnoses — report of the 1991 Bethesda workshop. JAMA 1992;267(14):1892.
4. Centers for Disease Control. Black-white differences in cervical cancer mortality — United States, 1980-1987. MMWR 1990;39(15):245-248.
5. Centers for Disease Control. 1993 revised classification system for HIV infection and expanded surveillance case definition for AIDS among adolescents and adults. MMWR 1992;41(RR-17):1-19.
6. Centers for Disease Control. Risk for cervical disease in HIV infected women— New York City. MMWR 1990;39(47):846-849.
7. Fidler HK, Boyes DA, Worth AJ. Cervical cancer detection in British Columbia: a progress report. J Obstet Gynaecol Br Commonw 1968;75(4):392-404.
8. Grimes DA. Over-the-counter oral contraceptives — an immodest proposal? [editorial]: Am J Public Health 1993;83(8):1092-1094.
9. Gross G, Ikenberg H, Gissman L, Hagedorn M. Papillomavirus infection of the anogenital region: correlation between histology, clinical picture, and virus type: proposal of a new nomenclature. J Invest Dermatol 1985;85(2):147-152.
10. Herbst AL. The Bethesda System for cervical/vaginal cytologic diagnoses: a note of caution. Obstet Gynecol 1990;76(3-1):449-450.
11. Hurt WG, Silverberg SG, Frable WJ, Belgrad R, Crooks LD. Adenocarcinoma of the cervix: histopathologic and clinical features. Am J Obstet Gynecol 1977;129(3):304-315.
12. Koss LG. The Papanicolaou test for cervical cancer detection: a triumph and a tragedy. JAMA 1989;261(5):737-743.
13. Kreiger JN, Tam MR, Stevens CE, Nielsen IO, Hale J, Kiviat NB, Holmes KK. Diagnosis of trichomoniasis: comparison of conventional wet-mount examination with cytologic studies, cultures and monoclonal antibody staining of direct specimens. JAMA 1988;259(8):1223-1227.
14. Kurman RJ, Malkasian GD, Sedlis A, Solomon D. From Papanicolaou to Bethesda: the rational for a new cervical cytologic classification. Obstet Gynecol 1991;77(5):779-782.
15. Maiman M, Fruchter RG, Guy L, Cuthill S, Levine P, Serur E. Human immunodeficiency virus infection and invasive cervical carcinoma. Cancer 1993;71(2):402-406.

16. Maiman M, Fruchter RG, Serur E, Remy JC, Feuer G, Boyce J. Human immunodeficiency virus infection and cervical neoplasia. Gynecol Oncol 1990;38(3): 377-382.
17. Maiman M, Tarricone N, Vieira J, Suarez J, Serur E, Boyce JG. Colposcopic evaluation of human immunodeficiency virus-seropositive women. Obstet Gynecol 1991;78(1):84-88.
18. Montz FJ, Monk BJ, Fowler JM, Nguyen L. Natural history of the minimally abnormal Papanicolaou smear. Obstet Gynecol 1992;80(3-1):385-388.
19. Nasiell K, Roger V, Nasiell M. Behavior of mild cervical dysplasia during long-term follow-up. Obstet Gynecol 1986;67(5):665-669.
20. National Cancer Institute Workshop. The 1988 Bethesda System for reporting cervical/vaginal cytological diagnoses. JAMA 1989;262(7):931-934.
21. Reid R. Preinvasive disease. In: Berek JS, Hacker NF (eds). Practical gynecologic oncology. Baltimore MD: Williams & Wilkins, 1989:195-239.
22. Reid R, Greenberg M, Jenson AB, Husain M, Willett J, Daoud Y, Temple G, Stanhope CR, Sherman AI, Phibbs GD, Lorincz AT. Sexually transmitted papillomaviral infections. I. The anatomic distribution and pathologic grade of neoplastic lesions associated with different viral types. Am J Obstet Gynecol 1987;156(1):212-222.
23. Reiter RC. Management of initial atypical cervical cytology: a randomized, prospective study. Obstet Gynecol 1986;68(2):237-240.
24. Richart RM. A modified terminology for cervical intraepithelial neoplasia. Obstet Gynecol 1990;75(1):131-133.
25. Schiffman MH. Recent progress in defining the epidemiology of human papillomavirus infection and cervical neoplasia. J Natl Cancer Inst 1992;84(6): 394-398.
26. Trussell J, Stewart F, Potts M, Guest F, Ellertson C. Should oral contraceptives be available without prescription? Am J Public Health 1993;83(8):1094-1099.
27. U.S. Department of Health and Human Services. Improving the quality of clinician Pap smear technique and management, client Pap smear education, and the evaluation of Pap smear laboratory testing: a resource guide for Title X family planning projects. Washington DC: U.S. Department of Health and Human Services, Public Health Service, Office of Population Affairs, Office of Family Planning, 1989:3-4, 59.
28. U.S. Preventive Services Task Force. Screening for cervical cancer. In: Guide to clinical preventive services: an assessment of the effectiveness of 169 interventions. Baltimore MD: Williams & Wilkins, 1989:57-62.
29. Winkelstein W. Smoking and cervical cancer — current status: a review. Am J Epidemiol 1990;131(6):945-957.
30. Yobs AR, Swanson RA, Lamotte LC. Laboratory reliability of the Papanicolaou smear. Obstet Gynecol 1985;65(2):235-244.

Infertility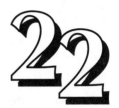

- Maintaining the ability to become pregnant until desired family size is completed is a principle goal of primary care and of family planning.
- Prevention of STDs must be a principle goal of reproductive health care and primary care.
- A reproductive life plan should be established by the family planning clinic.
- A basic level of fertility assessment can take place in the family planning clinic, after which specialty help should be sought.

The availability of infertility services might be seen as a litmus test for the definition of voluntary family planning versus population control. Given the cultural demands of most societies, and the scope of need, the problem requires the attention of family planning and health providers.

The problem of infertility provides several opportunities and responsibilities for family planning health care providers. At the minimum, providers must dispense or recommend only safe, effective means of delaying or spacing children that will not impair future fertility. The family planner's responsibility for prevention should exceed the "do no harm" approach to include the seeking and distributing of information about infertility prevention. Sexually transmitted diseases (STDs) are the leading cause of preventable infertility. (See Chapter 4 for more information about STD prevention, diagnosis, and treatment.) In addition, if family planners are to serve the needs of general reproductive health care in their community, they should provide some degree of initial evaluation and counseling for infertility. Infertility is a problem not only for the woman but for the couple, thus a family planning center may need to expand its philosophy and its services to include men. This fits within the framework of family planning as the responsibility of both men and women.

The extent of infertility varies among countries and among different populations within countries. Levels of infertility may be influenced by differences in prevalence of sexually transmitted diseases; access to adequate health care for sexually transmitted diseases, abortion, and childbirth; environmental factors affecting levels of disease transmission; occupations of reproductive age men and women; chemical toxins; nutrition; and genetically determined factors. Secondary infertility is especially decreased by access to adequate obstetric health care and may be two to three times as prevalent as primary infertility in some developing regions. It seems that our methods and ability to assist couples overcome some cause of infertility are increasing faster than methods of prevention.

A technical distinction exists between infertility and subfecundity: fertility refers to the actual production of children whereas fecundity refers to the capacity to reproduce. In the medical literature, infertility is used synonymously with subfecundity.

The following definitions are adapted from the World Health Organization's definitions of infertility in a couple:

Primary infertility: The couple has never conceived despite unprotected intercourse for at least 12 months.

Secondary infertility: The couple has previously conceived but is subsequently unable to conceive within 12 months despite exposure to unprotected intercourse.

Pregnancy wastage: The woman is able to conceive but unable to produce a live birth (unable to carry the fetus to a viable age).

Subfertility: The couple has difficulty in conceiving jointly because both partners may have reduced fecundity. In this sense, "subfertility" is used interchangeably with the term "subfecundity."

In this chapter, the term "infertility" is used to mean either a woman's inability to conceive and bear a living child or a man's inability to impregnate a woman.

PROBABILITY OF PREGNANCY

The chance of getting pregnant is the subject of discussion at nearly every interaction with infertile couples. The need to be knowledgeable and clear about this issue is a major responsibility of the family planning provider.

By using the criteria of a 20% chance of pregnancy each cycle among the normal fertile population, the cumulative pregnancy rates might be plotted as per Figure 22-1. These numbers show that 95% of couples are pregnant by the 13th cycle. On the other hand, if the chance of pregnancy is smaller, as for clients who are having donor insemination (DI) using frozen sperm or for patients who are undergoing ovulation induction, this possibility of pregnancy would follow a similar life-table curve—albeit with a more prolonged, lower slope.[16,19,36] The various probabilities cumulate, and these "cumulations" rise even more quickly when the probabilities are higher.

In actual populations, neither curve in Figure 22-1 is likely to be obtained. While the probabilities of conception may remain roughly constant over time for an individual couple (assuming that behavior does not change), they will decline for a group because the most fecund will become pregnant first. As time passes, those who have not conceived constitute a less fecund group. This consideration again points to the danger of diagnosing infertility on the basis of failure to conceive within 12 months (or even 24 months). Stated another way, those who conceive within 12 months and those who fail to conceive within 12 months do not constitute two radically different groups with respect to their underlying fecundity. Those in the first group have on average higher fecundity than those in the second group. But the second group contains only a minority (perhaps about a quarter) who will never conceive. The remainder simply take a little longer to become pregnant.

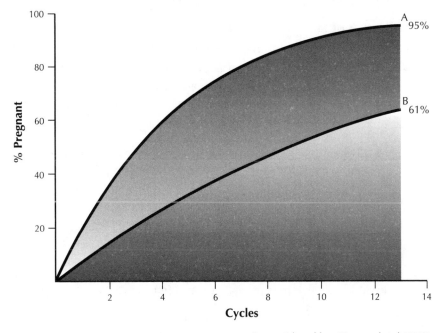

Source: Adapted from Hammond et al. (1983).

[A] Cumulative pregnancy curve assuming cyclic fecundability of 20%.

[B] Cumulative pregnancy curve assuming cyclic fecundability of 7%.

Figure 22-1 Cumulative pregnancy curves assuming two levels of fecundability

Cumulative pregnancy rates for surgical patients, *i.e.,* those treated for endometriosis or tuboplasty, tend to rise quite steeply until 12 months and then gradually stabilize until 36 months, after which pregnancies rarely occur.[15,20]

REQUIREMENTS FOR FERTILITY

For a couple to produce a child unassisted by the new fertility technology, both partners must be fecund. The properties of the fecund male include:

1. Normal spermatogenesis and ductal system (normal count, motility, and biologic structure/function)
2. Ability to transmit the spermatozoa to the female vagina, through
   - Adequate sexual drive
   - Ability to maintain an erection
   - Ability to achieve a normal ejaculation
   - Placement of ejaculate in the vaginal vault

The properties of the fecund female include:

1. Adequate sexual drive and sexual function to permit coitus
2. Functioning reproductive anatomy and physiology which include:
   - A vagina capable of receiving spermatozoa
   - Normal cervical mucus to allow passage of spermatozoa to the upper genital tract
   - Ovulatory cycles
   - Fallopian tubes which will function to permit the sperm and ovum to meet and allow migration of the conceptus to the uterus
   - A uterus capable of developing and sustaining the conceptus to maturity
   - Adequate hormonal status to maintain pregnancy
3. Normal immunologic responses to accommodate sperm, conceptus, and fetal survival
4. Adequate nutritional, chemical, and health status to maintain nutrition and oxygenation of placenta and fetus

Psychological, anatomical, or physiological alterations can interfere with the occurrence of pregnancy. In the United States, the male is principally responsible in 40% of infertile couples and the female in 40%, while in 20% the cause is unknown or problems exist with both partners.[19,43]

The categories of infertility are shown in Table 22-1. The diagnoses of infertility are noted in Table 22-2.

Table 22-1 General categories of infertility in developed countries

Category	% of Couples
Type of Infertility	
Primary	71
Secondary	29
No cause found in either	14
Female causes only	31
Male cause only	22
Causes found in both	21
Became pregnant	12

Source: WHO (1986).

In most developed countries, sexually transmitted diseases leading to pelvic inflammatory diseases (PID) are the leading preventable causes of infertility. In most developing countries, the major preventable causes are sexually transmitted diseases, postpartum infection, and postabortion infection.

FACTORS AFFECTING REPRODUCTIVE PERFORMANCE

A frequently made statement concerning infertility is that 10%–15% of couples are not able to conceive within 1 year if they are using no

Table 22-2 Male and female diagnoses of infertility in developed countries

Diagnosis	% of Couples
Female Diagnosis	
No demonstrable cause	40
Bilateral tubal occlusion	11
Acquired tubal abnormalities	12
Anovulatory regular cycle	10
Anovulatory oligomenorrhea	9
Ovulatory oligomenorrhea	7
Hyperprolactinemia	7
Male Diagnosis	
No demonstrable cause	49
Accessory gland infection	7
Idiopathic low motility	3
Primary testicular failure	10
Varicocele	11

Source: WHO (1986).

contraception and attempting to achieve a pregnancy. This percentage merely represents an aggregate summary statistic and usually will be of little value when counseling an individual or couple regarding the "chance" of conception. Several factors, discussed below, are known or are strongly suspected to affect the probability of conception. Figures 22-2 and 22-3 schematize the relationship, between various direct and indirect causes of infertility.

Age of woman. The effects of age on fertility are moderate, and do not begin until the late 30s.[26] Older women take longer to conceive, but both clinicians and patients must carefully distinguish "waiting longer" from "never being able to conceive." Table 22-3 demonstrates the effects of age from three separate studies. The primary point is that the standard measure of infertility (failure to conceive in 12 months) is very misleading because it confuses total inability to conceive with a delay in conception. In fact, the majority of "infertile" couples do conceive, whether or not they are treated.

The age issue is complicated by a host of other factors, including frequency of intercourse, age of the male partner, and the cumulative effect of medical and gynecologic problems.

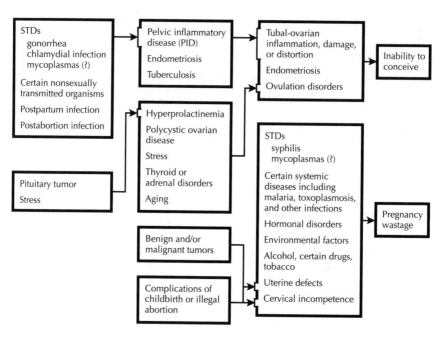

Source: Sherris (1985).

Figure 22-2 Relationships between selected direct and indirect causes of female infertility

Age of man. The age of the male has a significant effect on coital frequency and problems with sexual function, which are directly related to the chance of a pregnancy. Age of the male appears to have little impact on capability of the sperm and thus on reproductive performance.

Lack of understanding of reproductive biology. Another barrier to optimal fertility is a lack of understanding of vital information such as timing and frequency of intercourse. For example, the menstrual taboos of some groups that delay coitus until after menses may prevent conception in some women with short cycles and long menstrual periods. Patient education is therefore of primary importance in fertility counseling and family planning.

Coital frequency. Infrequent coitus is a common cause of infertility.[24] Coital frequency is positively correlated with pregnancy rates (see Table 22-4).[22] Other data and models based upon various biologic probabilities give similar projections.[35] Although the sperm count may be slightly decreased by an intercourse frequency of once per day or once every other day, the motility and number of sperm in the normal male would be sufficient to achieve a pregnancy.[31]

Timing of intercourse. Intercourse prior to ovulation is key in maximizing the chance of pregnancy (see Table 22-5). Sperm cells can survive over 72 hours in the female genital tract. The ovum has a much shorter life expectancy of only 12 hours if it is not fertilized. In fact, the "window of time" for fertilization is thought to last only a few hours, thus requiring sperm availability in the genital tract at or shortly after ovulation.

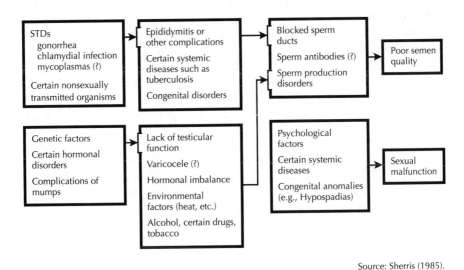

Source: Sherris (1985).

Figure 22-3 Relationships between selected direct and indirect causes of male infertility

Table 22-3 % of women with impaired fecundity, by age and parity.*

	Parity		
Age	Nulliparous	Multiparous	All Parities
15–24	8.4	7.1	7.6
25–34	20.0	8.3	10.9
35–44	36.4	8.8	11.4
15–24	20.5	8.4	10.7

*Data are from the 1988 National Survey of Family Growth.

Source: Mosher (1990).

Coital technique. Optimally the cervix should be maximally exposed to the semen deposited in the vagina. If a woman's uterus is anteflexed (tipped slightly forward, as 70% of uteri are), the best position for pregnancy-inducing intercourse may be with the woman on her back, with hips supported and elevated by a pillow, and to remain in the supine position for 20 minutes or so after intercourse. This position would tilt the vagina to allow the semen to pool near the cervix. Having the woman remain in the supine position for 20 minutes or so after intercourse may give sperm more contact time with the cervix, allowing more sperm to ascend to the fallopian tubes.

Lubricants. Some lubricants such as Surgilube and K-Y Jelly may have some spermicidal properties. Because of their lubricating quality, some spermicidal preparations may mistakenly be used by some couples trying to conceive.

Douching. Routine douching after intercourse or as part of "normal" hygiene should be discouraged. Although an unreliable method of birth control for couples of average fertility, douching may kill the very sperm that might have united with an egg in couples of marginal fertility.

Multiple sexual partners. Exposure to multiple partners increases the risks for sexually transmitted disease and PID, with potential sequelae of

Table 22-4 Frequency of intercourse and probability of conception within 6 months

Frequency of Intercourse	% Achieving Pregnancy Within 6 Months
<1 per week	17
1 per week	32
2 per week	46
3 per week	51

Source: MacLeod (1953).

Table 22-5 Probability of conception in the absence of contraception by day of coitus with respect to estimated time of ovulation

Coital Day	Average Likelihood of Conception
-5	0.00
-4	0.11
-3	0.20
-2	0.15
-1	0.26
0 (ovulation)	0.15
1	0.09
2	0.05
3	0.00

Source: Trussell and Kost (1987).

irreversible tubal damage and ectopic pregnancy. Having multiple sexual partners also increases the risk of cervical intraepithelial neoplasia (CIN) and other conditions that may require treatment such as freezing the cervix, laser treatment, conization and, possibly, hysterectomy. Some women develop antibodies to sperm, a condition that some clinicians believe is more likely to occur in women exposed to multiple partners. Regular use of condoms (except when pregnancy is desired) may help to prevent STDs, CIN, and the development of antisperm antibodies.

Sexually transmitted diseases. The relationship of sexually transmitted diseases and pelvic inflammatory disease is discussed in Chapter 4.

1. *Gonorrhea and chlamydia* are major causes of cervicitis and PID in the female (associated with tubal disease and pelvic adhesions). In the male, these organisms cause urethritis, epididymitis, and, possibly, accessory gland infection. These traditional infectious diseases may account for between 10% and 90% of all infertility, dependent upon geographic region and particular group studied. Although pelvic inflammatory disease is the major etiology of tubal infertility, chronic cervicitis may produce subfertility in some women. Chlamydia apparently causes more severe subclinical tubal inflammation than gonorrhea, with subsequent tubal damage, despite its more benign course of signs and symptoms.[12,45] Inadequately treated chlamydial salpingitis may appear to improve despite progressive tubal damage caused by the inflammatory response. Pelvic inflammatory disease of any etiology produces tubal scarring with resolution of the infection/inflammation. Infertility occurs when

bilateral intratubal adhesions interfere with the movement of sperm and ova either by completely occluding the tube or by damaging the delicate mucosa and cilia necessary for proper tubal functioning. Other pelvic adhesions (scars) may limit tubal mobility, motility, or contact with the ovary, thus interfering with capture of ova. Many of the same factors of pelvic damage that impair fertility also increase the likelihood of ectopic pregnancy, which may further damage the reproductive system.[5]

2. *T-Mycoplasma* (ureaplasma) is a sexually transmitted infection that contributes to the infertility of some males and females. Mycoplasma are frequently found in patients with other STDs, but conclusive proof of independent damage caused by these common organisms has been elusive.[40]

3. *Human papillomavirus* (HPV) is a sexually transmitted agent that frequently is a precursor to cervical dysplasia. The impact upon fertility is therefore dependent upon treatment, which may range from a required hysterectomy (should cervical cancer be diagnosed) to cryosurgery, cone biopsy, or similar treatment of the cervix for simple dysplasia. Cervical treatment may reduce fertility because of cervical transport problems subsequent to scarring and/or damage to the cervical mucous-producing cells. This damage to the cervix can be serious enough to cause "cervical incompetence" and thus contribute to preterm deliveries and possible pregnancy loss.

Parasitic and other infectious diseases.   Some parasitic and other infectious diseases can lead to infertility and fetal wastage.

1. *Toxoplasmosis, malaria, filariasis, schistosomiasis, leprosy (Hansen's Disease), and tuberculosis* are causes of infertility not likely to be encountered in the United States.

3. *Mumps,* leading to orchitis (testicular inflammation), may cause secondary testicular atrophy in the small number of men infected after puberty. Bilateral orchitis occurs in perhaps 1% of adult males with mumps; most will recover without impaired fertility.[40]

Previous pregnancy.   Problems which can occur around the time of delivery can cause very serious difficulties for future conception. Aside from mortality, the morbidities of infection, lacerations, uterine injury, rare hemorrhagic events requiring transfusions and even necessitating hysterectomy, as well as the emotional trauma of a difficult pregnancy all may inhibit future successful pregnancies. Indeed the stress of raising a child, while difficult to measure, is likely a very major contributor to future pregnancy problems.

Postpartum infections and postabortion infections caused by common nonsexually transmitted organisms and by sexually transmitted diseases can be a major cause of infertility. Postabortion infections are most common where safe, legal abortions are not available.

Sickle cell disease. Sickle cell disease has been documented as a cause of recurring priapism in some afflicted men, with possible impotence due to tissue and nerve damage, leading to male infertility. In women, sickling crises or alterations in placental blood flow or oxygenation have been clearly associated with an increased rate of fetal wastage.[30]

Nutrition. A drop of 10%-15% below normal weight can interfere with fertility in women. Percentage body fat should be greater than 22% to permit regular, ovulatory cycles.[11] Women with eating disorders such as anorexia nervosa or bulimia may be at increased risk of menstrual dysfunction, and may be overrepresented in infertility clinics.[44] Obesity may also lead to less frequent ovulation or to less frequent intercourse, thereby contributing to fertility problems.[41]

Toxic agents. The role of toxic agents in infertility is increasingly apparent and may well emerge as one of the principle causes of infertility with no demonstrable anatomic cause. Exposure to these agents can occur from occupational hazards (*e.g.*, farming, factory work, semiconductor industry, or mining); contaminated air, water, or food supply; drug ingestion; or other exposures.

Lead, toxic fumes, and exposure to pesticides are suspected causes of or contributors to infertility.[50,52] In women, lead poisoning reduces conceptions and is associated with fetal wastage. Individual case reports of spontaneous abortion in agricultural workers illustrate the need for further study. In men, exposure to lead can reduce both sex drive and sperm count. Pesticide exposure can also reduce sperm count.[50]

Smoking/alcohol. Smoking and alcohol use may cause poor sperm quality, and marijuana use has also been implicated in lower sperm motility and count. In women, both smoking and heavy alcohol use are associated with lower the conception rates[2] and increased rates of spontaneous abortion. Smoking also appears to increase slightly the risk of placenta previa. Smoking and alcohol use also negatively affect the developing fetus and may result in low birth weight babies.[43]

Medications. Some medications may affect male fertility by causing impotence, retrograde ejaculation, or temporarily impaired spermatogenesis. Narcotics, tranquilizers (such as phenothiazines), monoamine oxidase inhibitors (antidepressants), some antihypertensives, and drugs such as guanethidine and methyldopa may cause impotence. Amoebicides, antimalarial drugs, nitrofurantoin, sulfasalazine, cimetidine, certain antihypertensives, and methotrexate may affect sperm production.[4,34,39] In women, habitual use of narcotics or barbiturates apparently decreases regularity and effectiveness of ovulation. Systemic, powerful anticancer drugs exert many tissue effects that may include testicular or ovarian failure. These drugs may thus abolish spermatogenesis or ovulation temporarily or permanently after only one cycle of chemotherapy for some individuals. An increased number of cycles or higher doses generally decreases the chance of future fertility. *In utero* exposure to DES may diminish the fertility for both women and men.[3] Rates for testicular cancer, sperm abnormalities, and undescended testicles may be higher than usual for males exposed to DES.[4] Many other prescription medications, including tetracycline, retinoic acid derivatives (Accutane), several antiseizure medications, some antidepressants, some tranquilizers, and coumadin are examples of drugs which are clearly associated with an increased risk of fetal defects. Many of these drugs may also be associated with fetal wastage, although they more commonly cause increased rates of malformation rather than spontaneous abortion.[43] Avoidance of all medications while attempting to conceive and during pregnancy is advised whenever possible.

Surgery. Many types of surgery in men and women have a negative impact on fertility. If surgery is necessary, the potential impact on fertility should be discussed and options outlined. Any surgery that removes a vital reproductive structure, such as the uterus, tubes, or both gonads, will cause infertility. In men, sexual function may be reversibly or irreversibly impaired by surgery involving the penis, scrotum, prostate, and pelvis (which may cause nerve damage). In women, ovarian, cervical, or uterine surgery for benign processes may cause subsequent difficulties with conception, ovulation, or fetal wastage. Adhesions from any pelvic or abdominal surgery may interfere with conception.

It is imperative that all surgery be discussed in detail preoperatively, and that specific instructions be given to the surgeon by the client regarding future fertility intentions. Ask the surgeon to report on findings of the pelvic organs and obtain a copy of the operative report for the personal files of the client.

Radiation. Exposure to radiation may be occupational, accidental, iatrogenic, or as a therapeutic component of cancer treatment. Dosage and type of irradiation, as well as the site or focus of energy, may produce different results. Therapeutic radiation treatments in men or women can sometimes be tailored to minimize gonadal exposure to optimize future fertility and gonadal function. In men, the testicular germinal epithelium enclosing the seminiferous tubules may be reversibly incapacitated by irradiation, and chromosomal aberrations may occur.[33] Also, testicular cancer risks may be increased by irradiation.[4] In women, irradiation may cause ovarian failure, fetal wastage, or fetal damage.[43]

Physical exertion/heat. Some highly trained women athletes such as long-distance runners and professional dancers may experience reversible amenorrhea without any apparent long-term detrimental effects upon their fertility.[11] However, they may be at increased risk for bone loss.[17] Men who take frequent hot showers or whirlpool treatments, and men whose occupations involve subjecting the body to high temperature (*e.g.*, furnace workers) may subject the scrotum to temperatures high enough to reduce sperm production temporarily.[46] There is no evidence that endurance training leads to male infertility.[1]

Tight clothing. Jockey shorts and tight pants have been postulated to have the same suppressive effect on sperm production as do hot showers, because of high temperatures in the scrotal region; however, there is no evidence which supports this hypothesis.

Life plans. Patients who have set future goals and fertility objectives may find it easier to take preventive or active steps to preserve their fertility. Although many people have trouble planning for the future, health providers should realize that counseling about sexually transmitted diseases, contraception, and sexual behavior will be more meaningful for patients who have identified fertility objectives. Clearly, efforts to have children during the most fertile age is an issue to stress in the reproductive life plan.

PREVENTING INFERTILITY

The family planning or primary care clinic should give healthy individuals access to preventive fertility counseling and medical examination for early diagnosis and treatment of sexually transmitted diseases. Routine screening of sexually active individuals for STDs prevalent in the population may also prevent adverse consequences for those who do not know about the infections to which they may be exposed. Barrier contraceptives and spermicides reduce the risk of infections, such as gonorrhea and chlamydia, and consequently reduce PID.[6] On the other hand, IUDs can increase the risk of pelvic inflammatory disease with consequent reduction in fertility (see Chapter 14).[8,9] Pills appear to decrease the likelihood of acute gonococcal pelvic infection,[37] while they may increase the risk of acquiring cervical chlamydia.[7] Furthermore, pills may protect against tubal damage.[7] (See Chapter 10.)

Family planners who desire to prevent infertility should:

1. Be up to date in knowledge regarding the prevention, diagnosis and treatment of STDs and of PID.

2. Be aware that contraceptive choice influences the risk of PID.

3. Begin or continue public health education efforts so that the consequences of untreated sexual infection may be fully understood by your clients and particularly by all young people.

4. Work within the community to ensure that all individuals including minors have access to early and confidential diagnosis and treatment of STDs.

5. Encourage sexually active young people to use condoms, diaphragms, and spermicides, and to avoid IUDs.

6. Assist young persons in identifying risk factors and hence persons who will transmit infections to them. (From a public health perspective primary prevention would include avoiding exposure as well as avoiding infection if exposed.)

INTRAUTERINE DEVICES (IUDS)

The IUD is associated with an increased risk of contracting PID.[7,10,21] The risk of pelvic infection is apparently small for noninfected couples in mutually faithful relationships. In addition, the incidence of PID with the use of the Levonorgestrel IUD may be less than with other IUDs.[47] Recent studies suggest that previous risk estimates of PID among IUD users may have been overestimated.[7]

Family planning workers should take the following actions:

1. Be extremely conservative in using IUDs for nulliparous women who plan future childbearing. Many clinicians will not insert IUDs into nulliparous women.

2. Avoid recommending the IUD to women who may not understand about risk to future fertility, but who are at greater risk for sexually transmitted diseases and pelvic inflammatory disease (especially true of adolescents).

3. Urge further refinements in current IUDs (specifically, tailless types need to be evaluated and considered for use in areas where the incidence of sexually transmitted disease is high).

4. Screen for STDs in all patients in whom an IUD is inserted.

5. Never insert an IUD into a woman with an untreated STD.

6. Consider giving antibiotic prophylaxis for 1 week after IUD insertion in areas where the incidence of sexually transmitted disease is high.

7. Assume that a vaginal discharge in the presence of an IUD signals an infection until proven otherwise. (See Chapter 14 for more information about IUDs.)

8. Be certain that clients are aware of the danger signs of a pelvic infection and know where to go and what to do if these signs occur.

THE PILL

Oral contraceptive users have a lower risk of symptomatic pelvic inflammatory disease than IUD users or those who use no contraceptive method.[7] Decreased menstrual flow and myometrial activity, along with a less penetrable cervical mucus, may exert a protective effect against certain types of pelvic inflammatory disease in pill users.[7] (See Chapter 10.)

Amenorrhea and temporary infertility following pill use linked to the much publicized oversuppression syndrome (post-pill amenorrhea) do not appear to threaten female fertility seriously. The above symptoms are most commonly found in women who have irregular menses before beginning oral contraceptive therapy. This temporary condition is usually amenable to treatment by using standard ovulation induction drugs such as clomiphene citrate. It is now accepted that the risk of cervical infection with chlamydia is enhanced among oral contraceptive (OC) users (as compared with non-users).[7,49] The risk of ascending infection is currently unknown, but oral contraceptive use may lessen the damaging effects of inflammation.[7]

The question of an increased risk of CIN among OC users has not been settled. Because an increased risk of CIN occurrence among pill users appears likely, early diagnosis and treatment is important.

Family planning workers should take the following actions:

1. Educate patients about the relationship between the pill and pelvic inflammatory disease.
2. Urge pill users at high risk for sexually transmitted disease to use barrier contraception as well and to limit their number of sexual partners.
3. Assure Pap smears are done annually.

BARRIER METHODS

The use of condoms and other barrier methods can reduce the risk of acquiring a sexually transmitted disease such as chlamydia and gonorrhea, both of which are associated with pelvic inflammatory disease and tubal infertility. (See Chapter 4.) Because the risk of infertility increases with each episode of PID, clients who have had a previous episode of PID should be counseled about barrier methods to avoid infection.

Unprotected intercourse can lead to the development of sperm antibodies in women, although it is unclear whether immunity to sperm causes infertility. The use of condoms has been widely encouraged to reduce the risk of developing immunologic reactions to sperm.[42]

STERILIZATION

In the United States, 14 million women rely on female or male sterilization as their contraceptive method. These rates are highest among married women between 35 and 50 years old, 50%-60% of whom rely on sterilization.[32] (See Chapter 15.)

Family planners have expressed concern over the number of requests for sterilization reversal, an expensive procedure with uncertain prognosis. In a survey of 100 female patients, the reasons for requesting reversal were:[13]

Table 22-6 Reason for sterilization reversal

Change of marital status	63%
Death of child	17%
More children wanted (marital status same)	10%
Psychological reasons	6%
Other tragedy	4%

Family planning workers should take the following actions:

1. Emphasize the permanence of the procedure.
2. Avoid using the term "tying the tubes" to describe sterilization procedures; to some patients, such reference might imply that "untying the tubes" is feasible.[13] (See Chapter 15 for more information about sterilization procedures.)
3. Make efforts to assure clients have access to reversal procedures. This may require changes in laws relating to health insurance and in public funding of health systems.

ABORTION

No epidemiologic evidence supports a fertility risk to women experiencing first-trimester vacuum abortions. A slightly increased risk to reproductive performance exists when larger cervical dilation is used for some D&C abortion procedures and when the abortion is performed in the second trimester.[18] Abortions resulting in severe complications (*e.g.*, hysterectomy) are so rare that they are not readily apparent in statistical evaluations of fertility risk. The most obvious way to prevent these rare occurrences is to prevent the pregnancy (and thus the abortion). A full-term pregnancy still has a greater negative impact on long-term fertility than does safe, legal abortion.

Family planning workers should take the following actions:

1. Advise patients of the potential for complications.
2. Avoid using sharp curettes for first-trimester abortions if a vacuum aspiration may be used instead.
3. Use gradual dilation with laminaria (to not more than 11 cm if possible).
4. Prescribe prophylactic antibiotics whenever interference or illegal abortion is suspected (some clinicians recommend routine antibiotic prophylaxis for all abortions).

5. Vigorously treat septic abortions.
6. Provide contraceptive counseling to all abortion patients.
7. Screen for and treat STDs (gonorrhea and chlamydia) prior to surgery, or treat all patients with prophylactic antibiotics effective against resistant strains of disease-causing organisms.
8. Follow up for early signs of infection (see Chapter 19).
9. Have abortion complications treated by knowledgeable providers.

INFERTILITY (FERTILITY) EVALUATION

Triaging (sorting by urgency) is the important task of the first counselor to see the infertile client or couple. Discussion, investigation or referral, rather than advice to "wait and see," should be the general response to the inquiring couple who has tried unsuccessfully to conceive. Although typically one may wish the couple to have had sufficient exposure (e.g., 12 months) before beginning a work-up, a client discussion should occur if requested. Expediting an infertility evaluation is especially important if:

- The woman is in her late 30s. Because a steep decline in fertility occurs after age 40, women over age 35 should receive priority for early assessment. The assessment should be concise, complete, and accomplished quickly.
- The woman reports irregular menses. This symptom could signal sporadic ovulation, a condition unlikely to improve spontaneously unless the woman is a teenager, and may in fact be a sign of premature ovarian senescence or failure (early menopause). Irregular or abnormal bleeding may be a symptom of pelvic infection or other gynecologic disease, making evaluation necessary. Many of these problems are easily and successfully treated.
- The medical history for the couple includes mumps in the man; repeated miscarriages, ectopic pregnancy, or pelvic inflammatory disease in the woman; or previous pelvic surgery or other serious medical problems in either partner. Because time is not likely to improve such problems, but rather will allow the couple's fecundity to steadily diminish, a diagnosis and remedy should be sought promptly.
- The woman has severe progressive dysmenorrhea or dyspareunia. These symptoms may suggest endometriosis or other pelvic disease.
- The woman used an IUD in the past; had a pelvic infection; had surgery on an ovary, a tube, or uterus; or has any reason to suspect damage to her pelvic organs (e.g., endometriosis, ovarian cyst, fibroid). An early assessment, including a laparoscopy, may be in

order, which can then lead to an early diagnosis and treatment, or to reassurance that "more time" is needed.

- The couple lives in an area with a high endemic incidence of STDs.
- An early assessment of men or women with DES exposure *in utero* may be in order because of the known risk of reproductive system effects.
- Neither partner has ever produced a pregnancy, despite unprotected intercourse.

While economic, personnel, and laboratory resources may be limited, some basic initial services should be provided by most family planning programs. The following basic services may help some couples improve fertility and may expedite further evaluation and treatment for others who need more. The goals of the clinician or health care team initiating the evaluation process for a couple begin with the first four items listed and, where resources and training permit, include all of the following:

- Educating the patients.
- Gathering pertinent historical information.
- Providing a thorough physical exam.
- Providing a resource for reassurance, counseling, and emotional stability including referral as needed. Referral sources may be found by consulting with the American Fertility Society or the local Resolve group. (See resources at end of chapter.)
- Systematically evaluating the possible defective areas. Basic infertility services include:[39]
  - Counseling couples about fertility awareness techniques (described in Chapter 12) and optimizing coital timing
  - Checking couples for asymptomatic STD infections that could cause subfertility
  - Determining whether ovulation takes place, as indicated by basal body temperature and/or cervical mucus records (or urine LH test kits where available)
  - Performing semen analyses
- Making a plan and initiating treatment based upon information gathered and counseling couples with potentially serious fertility problems or undetected reasons for infertility about their options for further evaluation and treatment.
- Reassessing progress at predetermined intervals.
- Referring couples to other infertility specialists and/or adoption agencies as needed. Explain the anticipated short- and long-term costs and chances for success with further treatment, and discuss the options of adoption or remaining childless.

HISTORY AND PHYSICAL ASSESSMENT

After interviewing the couple together, the counselor should interview the man and woman separately to obtain confidential information. Having both partners present for the physical exams may ensure that both partners understand the anatomy and related issues discussed. This idealized scenario may not be comfortable or possible for some patients (and many clinicians as well).

Before beginning the evaluation process, explain the main steps that will be needed for diagnostic evaluation and the capacity of your facility. If referral becomes necessary, try to assure that procedures are not duplicated unnecessarily and that an orderly, agreed upon evaluation can be continued. Following a standard set of guidelines, such as the WHO flow sheet of the standardized approach to the infertile couple,[52] will enhance the effectiveness of referral prognosis.

Physical examination of the woman. Visual evaluation of hair distribution and of body and breast development can indicate endocrinopathy or developmental deficiencies such as hypogonadism, adrenal hyperplasia, hypothyroidism, ovarian dysfunction, and hyperprolactinemia. A complete pelvic exam (palpation of uterus and adnexae, speculum exam of vagina and cervix) should reveal any uterine hypoplasia, adnexal tumors, or cervical lesions and should indicate whether dyspareunia may be a problem.

Physical exam of the man. Again, visual inspection of sexual characteristics can identify such endocrinopathies as hypogonadism or Klinefelter's syndrome (the genetic XXY anomaly often associated with infertility). A penile exam can reveal hypospadias (displacement of the urethral opening) or phimosis (constriction of the foreskin). The testicular exam detects atrophy, tumors, epididymal cysts, cryptorchidism (undescended testicles), vas thickening or absence, hydrocele (fluid accumulation in testes or along spermatic cord), or varicocele (dilation of the veins of the spermatic cord in the scrotum).

The history and physical exam may indicate the need for further evaluation. Our approach is only one of many potential testing options. A recommended schedule of evaluation is described in Table 22-7.

Semen evaluation. Usually, arrangements must be made with the laboratory prior to bringing in a specimen for a semen evaluation. (Table 22-8 gives directions for obtaining a semen specimen.) The technician will look for a volume of 2 cc-5 cc, directional motility in over 60% of sperm present, 60% normal morphology, and a count of at least 20 million sperm/ml. If the sperm count is at least 15-20 million, the absolute number of sperm is probably less critical than their motility and their morphology. The presence of bacteria or white blood cells, as well as semen viscosity, should also be recorded. More than one evaluation may be necessary to assess accurately

Table 22-7 A fertility assessment visit schedule

The initial assessment of the couple should proceed in a systematic manner, with the objective of completing the first line of infertility evaluation within approximately 2–3 cycles. A suggested schedule for visits is as follows:

Visit 1:
Family planning clinic visit (ideally day 5–10 of menstrual cycle)
Ideally previous medical records obtained
Male and female complete medical history
Male and female physical examination
Develop investigation plan

Between Visits:
Male obtain physical exam if not already completed
Male semen evaluation
Male and female laboratory tests (although the blood tests might ideally be done later
Male and female be certain that all past and pertinent records are obtained
Begin BBTs and fertility awareness record keeping

Visit 2:
Clinic visit (pre-ovulatory day 13 of 28-day cycle or time by LH kit)
Intercourse 12 hours prior to clinic visit
Postcoital test

Between Visits:
Day 22 of 28-day cycle
Serum progesterone
Other blood tests as indicated

Visit 3:
Clinic visit (day 26 of 28-day cycle)
Endometrial biopsy

Between Visits:
Radiologist office (day 5–10 of menstrual cycle when not bleeding)
Hysterosalpingogram

Visit 4:
Clinic visit
Consultation
Review all records and information to date

Depending upon the above findings (after discussing with the patient), we would then proceed with some other investigations which might include:

- Diagnostic Laparoscopy and Hysteroscopy
- Hormonal Studies
- Immunologic Studies
- Tests of Sperm Function
- Other Tests as Indicated

the sperm/semen status, particularly if the results are borderline. The WHO recommends two samples taken at least 2 weeks apart.[51] (Table 22-9 provides the WHO criteria for semen evaluation.)

Table 22-8 Directions for collecting semen for evaluation

1. Abstain from intercourse (no ejaculation) for at least 3 and no more than 5 days. Do not drink any alcohol or take a hot shower or hot bath immediately prior to producing the specimen.

2. Produce a semen specimen by masturbation into a small, sterile, dry, wide-mouthed jar. Be sure the entire specimen is captured in the container. We can provide the container if you wish. You may use the restroom in the office building or obtain the specimen elsewhere.

3. Take the specimen to the laboratory as soon as possible after obtaining the specimen. Note the exact time the specimen was obtained and write it and your name on the container. The specimen must arrive in the laboratory within 1 hour of collection.

4. Try to keep the specimen close to body temperature during transit.

Following the initial history, physical exam, and basic diagnostic laboratory procedures, inform the patient about the further tests that may need to be performed and about initial recommendations.

INTERMEDIATE ASSESSMENTS AND TESTS

Patients should be instructed in recording basal body temperatures and charting mucus changes, as described in Chapter 12. This documentation often is helpful in verifying ovulation, determining timing and frequency of intercourse, and educating the client about the physiology of the menstrual cycle. The timing of various tests can also be recorded and guided by this documentation.

A postcoital (Sims-Huhner) test is obtained +/- 12 hours after intercourse approximately 1 day prior to ovulation. A small amount of cervical

Table 22-9 Criteria for a normal semen sample

A semen sample was considered normal if all of the following conditions were met:

Spermatozoa

Concentration	$>20 \times 10^6$/ml
Motility	>40% progressively motile
Morphology	>50% normal (ideal) forms
Viability	>60% live
Agglutination	no

Seminal Fluid

Normal Appearance
Normal Viscosity
Less Than 10^6 WBCs/ml

mucus is drawn into a thin catheter from the endocervical canal and evaluated. Ideally, there is an abundance of acellular, watery cervical mucus that ferns, has a spinnbarkeit of greater than 8 cm, and has greater than 10 motile sperm/HPF. The sperm should swim with good motility and in one direction.[28]

MORE SPECIALIZED TESTS (NOT AVAILABLE AT MOST FAMILY PLANNING CLINICS)

Endometrial biopsy is obtained using a paracervical block on cycle day 26 of a 28-day cycle (or post-ovulation day 12) to see whether the changes in the endometrium are uniform with the expected secretory effect. Occasionally, a dysynchrony can occur, producing a luteal phase problem that would require treatment with either ovulation inducers or supplemental progesterone (Clomid or progesterone suppositories). These biopsies are most useful (1) when read by an experienced histologist or pathologist who evaluates endometrial biopsies frequently enough to discriminate phases of secretory maturity and (2) when read in conjunction with patient information about the day of the menstrual cycle and serum progesterone levels.

Tubal patency should be confirmed either by laparoscopy or hysterosalpingogram (HSG). The HSG is typically performed early in the menstrual cycle after bleeding has stopped but prior to ovulation. A laparoscopy can be performed on day 26 of a 28-day cycle when an endometrial biopsy is performed (and thus reduce pain).

Laparoscopy usually requires general anesthesia and is classified as a major surgical procedure. However, this approach should be strongly considered when pelvic pathology is suspected, *e.g.*, the patient has a history of PID, a long history of IUD usage, or is older and just beginning her work-up. These procedures are somewhat uncomfortable for the woman, but they provide considerable information about anatomical abnormalities or damage or obstruction of the tubes. It may be combined with a hysteroscopy to rule out uterine anomalies, adhesions, or submucous fibroids.

During HSG, radiopaque dye is inserted into the uterus and x-ray photographs document its spread through the uterus and tubes. Because a hysterosalpingogram can cause serious recurrence of pelvic inflammatory disease, prophylactic antibiotics are recommended for patients with a history of pelvic inflammatory disease.

This initial evaluation will identify the basic causes of infertility in up to 80% of couples. The next level of evaluation is, in general, well beyond the scope of most family planning clinics, but might involve immunologic studies, test of sperm function, and other tests as indicated.

Costs

Economic considerations are critical if these services are introduced. The costs of the more technology-driven evaluations and treatment far exceed the resources of most people, and most health programs. Careful consideration must be given to determine the extent of service to be covered in the family planning clinic.

B ASIC TREATMENT POSSIBILITIES

Frequently, the role of the provider in infertility is to reassure (intelligently) and intervene at the right time. A principal responsibility is to tell the patient when the time has come to consider adoption, to discontinue therapy, or to proceed in some other course.

The treatment of identified problems is well outlined in general references, so it will not be described in great detail here. Instead, a highly simplified summary of the general strategies for counseling patients will be discussed. Infertility therapy, like any other medical therapy, is generally directed toward curing or improving diagnosed anatomic and physiologic problems. In addition, comprehensive infertility treatment seeks to maximize the chance of pregnancy by optimizing all conditions for conception (for example, by instructing patients about optimal timing of intercourse and by eliminating any factors that potentially diminish fertility, such as those discussed in the preceding sections of this chapter). For a significant portion of patients who have no identifiable cause of infertility, the comprehensive approach is the only therapeutic option, provided that all possible diagnostic tests have been adequately completed. Although specific treatments require experienced practitioners, specialized equipment, precise timing, or great expense, they are still not perfect.

Male infertility may be treated with insemination from donor sperm to overcome male factor infertility problems including azoospermia or impotence. Particular attention must be paid to guaranteeing that the semen does not carry any organisms that produce sexually transmitted diseases, including acquired immunodeficiency syndrome (AIDS). (Criteria for preparation, storage, and screening are set by the American Fertility Society. Their current recommendation is to use sperm that has been frozen and quarantined for 6 months. If the donor is still HIV-antibody negative after 6 months, the sperm may be released.[14])

Female infertility may be treated with a much wider range of approaches:

1. *Cervical mucus problems* impairing conception may be treated with insemination or uterine instillation of a small amount of specially prepared sperm.

2. *Cervical incompetence* interfering with continuing pregnancy may be treated with cerclage, bed rest, or both. Cerclage is the passage of strong suture material around the cervix, like a purse string, to prevent premature dilation.

3. *Ovulation disorders* can be treated with drugs to induce ovulation, such as clomiphene citrate which suppresses estrogen's ovulation-suppressive effect. In women whose ovulation is suppressed by hyperprolactinemia (high blood levels of the pituitary hormone prolactin), ovulation may be induced with prolactin-suppressing drugs such as bromocriptine.

4. *Damage to ovaries,* such as torsion, surgical removal, hemorrhagic cyst, or premature menopause that has eliminated primordial follicle tissue required to produce new ova, can only be overcome by some use of high-technology fertility medicine with an ova donated from another woman.

5. *Uterine/tubal abnormalities* may be addressed by appropriate specific corrective surgical procedures (in some cases microsurgery). Some congenital uterine/tubal anomalies, such as true bicornuate uterus, may not be amenable to surgical repair. In the case of tubal damage caused by endometriosis, hormonal suppression of the displaced endometrial tissue may be prescribed before or instead of surgery. Tubal or pelvic scarring due to pelvic inflammatory disease may be improved with microsurgery of the tube or laparotomy to allow lysis of pelvic adhesions. Currently, the delicate cilia and mucosa of the tubal lining cannot be surgically regenerated, and the variable effects of the body's capacity to repair itself produce a low rate of tubal "cure." In vitro fertilization (see following discussion) may be the only way to bypass damaged fallopian tubes.

High technology approaches to overcoming infertility have had some remarkable developments in the past 15 years. These expensive methods require expert practitioners and procedures and result in successful pregnancies at rates near the normal fecundity rates. The following are two of the major high technology approaches:

- *Gamete intrafallopian tube transfer (GIFT)* involves placing a mixture of ova and sperm into the fallopian tube. It is used primarily for unexplained infertility, where the fallopian tubes appear normal. The sperm is collected, washed, incubated, and prepared prior to laparoscopic harvesting of the oocytes. At the time of laparoscopy, both the sperm and oocytes are placed into the fallopian tube. (National surveys indicate a pregnancy rate of 29% per treatment cycle.)[25]

- *In vitro fertilization (IVF)* involves placing mature ova (harvested either at laparoscopy or transvaginally using an ultrasound-directed needle to aspirate the oocyte) with specially prepared sperm in a laboratory tissue culture medium and incubating them to allow fertilization. Fertilized ova that have successfully attained a certain maturity (generally between two and eight cell divisions) are placed in the uterus via a transcervical catheter. (National surveys indicate a pregnancy rate of 19% per treatment cycle.[25])

GIFT and IVF frequently utilize ovulation stimulation drugs to increase the number of ova ready for harvest.

ADOPTION

Many couples faced with infertility who desire children choose adoption. Open adoptions involving cooperation of the adopting parents and birthparents in all phases of the process are becoming more widespread. Licensed adoption agencies may or may not allow communication between the birthparents and adopting parents, and tend to involve a longer wait than independent adoptions. Couples may seek the help of providers who have contact with women with unwanted pregnancies. Attorneys, clergy, friends, and independent adoption centers can also aid in matching couples with birthparents. Adopting children from other countries, older children, or children with special needs may minimize the waiting period. The family planning provider should present these options to infertile clients, along with referrals to adoption resources.

THE COPING PHASE

Many couples who seek help for infertility eventually do achieve pregnancy, often in the course of preliminary investigation.[38,52] Their risk, however, for ectopic pregnancy, miscarriage, and perinatal mortality are higher than average, and some will eventually confront the reality of childlessness.

The impact of permanent infertility, coupled with the stresses of fertility evaluation and treatment, may damage a couple's relationship or an individual's self-concept. Normal reactions to the diagnosis of infertility include processes similar to other grieving processes: surprise, denial, isolation, anger, guilt, sorrow and, finally, resolution.[27] Depression and prolonged stress can follow diagnosis and treatment. In addition, couples may experience a great strain on their relationship. Clinicians need to recognize how disruptive infertility diagnosis and treatment can be for couples.[23]

Family planning agencies can take an active and complementary role in helping infertile couples to cope:

- Provide full information on adoption and fostering, with names and addresses of local agencies.

- Refer couples for psychological counseling if depression appears serious.
- Refer couples to infertility networks and support groups specifically designed to help people with infertility problems. (See the Resources at the end of the chapter.)
- Remain sensitive to the special vulnerability of infertility patients.

RESOURCES

1. Resolve, Inc. National Office
   P.O. Box 474
   Belmont, MA 02178

2. American Fertility Society
   2131 Magnolia Ave. #201
   Birmingham, AL 35256

3. Adoptive Families of America
   3333 Highway 100 North
   Minneapolis, MN 55422
   (612) 535-4829

REFERENCES

1. Arce JC, De Souza MJ. Exercise and male factor infertility. Sports Med 1993;15(3):146-69.
2. Baird DD, Wilcox AJ. Cigarette smoking associated with delayed conception. JAMA 1985;253(20):2979-83.
3. Barnes AB, Colton T, Gunderson J, Noller KL, Tilley BC, Strama T, Townsend DE, Hatab P, O'Brien PC. Fertility and outcome of pregnancy in women exposed in utero to diethylstilbestrol. New Eng J Med 1980;302(11):609-613.
4. Castleman M. Sperm crisis. Medical Self-Care 1980;Spring:26.
5. Cates W, Rolfs RT, Aral SO. Pathophysiology and epidemiology of sexually transmitted diseases in relation to pelvic inflammatory disease and infertility. Proceedings of the Seminar on Biomedical and Demographic Determinants of Human Reproduction. Liege, Belgium: International Union for the Scientific Study of Population, 1988.
6. Cates W, Stone KM. Family planning, sexually transmitted diseases and contraceptive choice: a literature update—Part I. Fam Plann Perspect 1992;24(2):75-84.
7. Cates W, Stone KM. Family planning, sexually transmitted diseases and contraceptive choice: a literature update—Part II. Fam Plann Perspect 1992;24(3):122-128.
8. Cramer DW, Schiff I, Schoenbaum SC, Gibson M, Belisle S, Albrecht B, Stillman RJ, Berger MJ, Wilson E, Stadel BV. Tubal infertility and the intrauterine device. N Engl J Med 1985;312(15):941-947.
9. Daling JR, Weiss NS, Metch BJ, Chow WH, Soderstrom RM, Moore DE, Spadoni, LR, Stadel BV. Primary tubal infertility in relation to the use of an intrauterine device. N Engl J Med 1985;312(15):937-941.

10. Farley TM, Rosenberg MS, Rowe PJ, Chen JH, Meirik O. Intrauterine devices and pelvic inflammatory disease: an international perspective. Lancet 1992;339(8796):785-788.
11. Frisch RE. Fatness and fertility. Sci Am 1988;258(3):88-95.
12. Gjonnaess H, Dalaker K, Anestad G, Mardh PA, Kuile G, Bergan T. Pelvic inflammatory disease: etiologic studies with emphasis on chlamydial infection. Obstet Gynecol 1982;59(5):550-555.
13. Gomel V. Microsurgical reversal of female sterilization: a reappraisal. Fertil Steril 1980;33(6):587-597.
14. Guidelines for gamete donation: 1993. The American Fertility Society. Fertil Steril 1993;59(2 Suppl 1):1S-9S.
15. Guzick DS, Rock JA. Estimation of a model of cumulative pregnancy following infertility therapy. Am J Obstet Gynecol 1981:140(5):573-578.
16. Hammond MG, Halme JK, Talbert LM. Factors affecting the pregnancy rate in clomiphene citrate induction of ovulation. Obstet Gynecol 1983;62(2):196-202.
17. Highet R. Athletic amenorrhoea: an update on aetiology, complications and management. Sports Med 1989;7(2):82-108.
18. Hogue CJ, Cates W, Tietze C. Effects of induced abortion on subsequent reproduction. Epidemiol Rev 1982;4:66-94.
19. Keller DW, Strickler RC, Warren JC. Clinical infertility. Norwalk CT: Appleton-Century-Crofts, 1984.
20. Lauritsen JG, Pagel JD, Vangsted P, Starup J. Results of repeated tuboplasties. Fertil Steril 1982;37(1):68-72.
21. Lee NC, Rubin GL, Ory HW, Burkman RT. Type of intrauterine device and the risk of pelvic inflammatory disease. Obstet Gynecol 1983;62(1):1-6.
22. MacLeod J, Gold RZ. The male factor in fertility and infertility: VI. Semen quality and certain other factors in relation to ease of conception. Fertil Steril 1953;4(1):10-33.
23. Mahlstedt PP. The psychological component of infertility. Fertil Steril 1985;43(3):335-46.
24. Masters WH, Johnson VE. Advice for women who want to have a baby. Redbook Magazine 1975;(3):70-74.
25. Medical Research International, Society for Assisted Reproductive Technology, The American Fertility Society. In vitro fertilization-embryo transfer (IVF-ET) in the United States: 1990 results from the IVF-ET Registry. Fertil Steril 1992;57(1):15-24.
26. Menken J, Trussell J, Larsen U. Age and infertility. Science1986;233(4771):1389-1394.
27. Menning BE. Counselling infertile patients. Contemp Ob/Gyn 1979; February.
28. Moghissi KS. The cervix in infertility. In: Hammond MG, Talbert LM (eds). Infertility: a practical guide for the physician. 2nd ed. Oradell NJ: Medical Economics Books, 1985:84-101.
29. Mosher WD, Pratt WF. Fecundity and infertility in the United States, 1965-88. Advance Data From Vital and Health Statistics of the National Center for Health Statistics. Number 192, December 1990.
30. Pernoll ML, Benson MC (eds). Current obstetric and gynecologic diagnosis and treatment. 6th ed. Norwalk, CT: Appleton-Lange, 1987.
31. Pfeffer WH. An approach to the diagnosis and treatment of the infertile female. Med Aspects Hum Sex 1980;14(4)121-122.
32. Report on the 1991 Ortho Annual Birth Control Study. Raritan NJ.Ortho Pharmaceutical Corporation.

33. Roland M. Infertility therapy: effects of innovations and increasing experience. J Repro Med 1980;25(1):41-46.
34. Schlegel PN, Chang TS, Marshall FF. Antibiotics: potential hazards to male fertility. Fertil Steril 1991;55(2):235-42.
35. Schwartz D, MacDonald PDM, Heuchel V. Fecundability, coital frequency and the viability of ova. Pop Stud 1980;34(2):397-400.
36. Schwartz D, Mayaux MJ. Female fecundity as a function of age: results of artificial insemination of 2,193 nulliparous women with azoospermic husbands. N Engl J Med 1982;306(7):404-406.
37. Senanayake P, Kramer DG. Contraception and the etiology of pelvic inflammatory disease: new perspectives. Am J Obstet Gynecol 1980;138(7-2):852-860.
38. Shane JM, Schiff I, Wilson EA. The infertile couple: evaluation and treatment. In: CIBA Clinical Symposia 1976;28:2-40.
39. Shane JM. Ambulatory evaluation of the infertile patient. In: Ryan GM (ed). Ambulatory care in obstetrics and gynecology. Grune & Stratton, 1980:303-316.
40. Sherris JD, Fox G. Infertility and sexually transmitted disease: a public challenge. Popul Rep 1983 (reprinted 1985);Series L(4):113-115.
41. Shoupe D. Effect of body weight on reproductive function. In: Mishell DR, Davajan V, Lobo RA. Infertility, contraception & reproductive endocrinology, 3rd ed. Cambridge: Blackwell Scientific Publications, 1991.
42. Shushan A, Schenker JG. Immunological factors in infertility. Am J Repro Immunol 1992;28(3-4):285-287.
43. Speroff L, Glass RH, Kase NG. Clinical gynecologic endocrinology and infertility, 4th ed. Baltimore MD: Williams & Wilkins, 1989.
44. Stewart DE, Robinson GE, Goldbloom DS, Wright C. Infertility and eating disorders. Am J Obstet Gynecol 1990;163(4-1):1196-1199.
45. Svensson L, Westrom L, Ripa KT, Mardh PA. Differences in some clinical and laboratory parameters in acute salpingitis related to culture and serologic findings. Am J Obstet Gynecol 1980;138(7-2):1017-1021.
46. Tanagho EA, Lue TF, McClure RD. Contemporary management of Impotence and infertility. Baltimore MD: Williams & Wilkins, 1988.
47. Toivonen J, Luukkainen T, Allonen H. Protective effect of intrauterine release of levonorgestrel on pelvic infection: three years' comparative experience of levonorgestrel- and copper-releasing intrauterine devices. Obstet Gynecol 1991;77(2):261-264.
48. Trussell J, Kost K. Contraceptive failure in the United States: a critical review of the literature. Stud Fam Plann 1987;18(5):237-283.
49. Washington AE, Gove S, Schachter J, Sweet RL. Oral contraceptives, Chlamydia trachomatis infection, and pelvic inflammatory disease: a word of caution about protection. JAMA 1985;253(15):2246-2250.
50. Whorton MD, Krauss RM, Marshall S, Milby TH. Infertility in male pesticide workers. Lancet 1977;2(8051):1259-1261.
51. World Health Organization. WHO laboratory manual for the examination of human semen and semen-cervical mucus interactions. 2nd ed. Cambridge; New York: Published on behalf of the World Health Organization by Cambridge University Press, 1992.
52. World Health Organization Task Force on the Diagnosis and Treatment of Infertility. Workshop on the investigation of the subfertile couple. Proceedings of the 12th World Congress on Fertility and Sterility, Singapore. In: Ratman S, Teoh E, Anandakumar C (eds). Infertility in the male and female. London: Parthenon Publishing, 1986. (Advances in fertility and sterility series; vol 4).

Education and Counseling

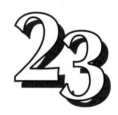

- Successful communication interventions take into account the characteristics of the individual patient and of the specific situation.

- Education conveys knowledge and skill. Counseling elucidates feeling states, and supports and facilitates decision making. Every health care facility needs workers competent in both disciplines.

- Daily choices about personal risk taking exert a powerful influence on health. No care-giver task is more important than helping patients change their personal behavior to reduce risk.

- People change behaviors as a result of new skill more often than new knowledge. Teaching new skills to patients is most helpful when the care-giver keys the intervention to the patient's own readiness for change.

- Informed consent is an educational process, not a piece of paper. The consent form documents the educational process.

FACTORS INFLUENCING EDUCATION AND COUNSELING

The success or failure of our communication effort with patients hinges in large part on our skill at reading the individual patient and the particular situation, and then tailoring an intervention that is compatible with the patient, the place and time, and the issue at hand. Characteristics of the patient influence the issue: age, cultural background, educational attainment, emotional state, and readiness for behavior change. Important characteristics of the situation can include the specific goals of both patient and provider, the time available for the encounter, and the need for a formal informed consent process.

AGE AND DEVELOPMENT

Patients may seek reproductive health care as children, adolescents, or adults, and cognitive and emotional capacities are strongly influenced by age. Developmentally, children move through early, middle, and late adolescence as they approach adulthood,[1] and educational strategies for one stage may be wrong for another. Early adolescents (ages 11-13 or so) are still quite childlike, and late adolescents (age 16 or older) may have many adult characteristics. The care provider may have only moments to ascertain whether a 14-year-old patient is more like a child or like an adult.

A significant portion of patients making their first visit for reproductive care are in midadolescence, about age 14-15. This stage can be distinctly characterized:

- Concrete thinking, oriented to the here and now
- Intense peer involvement around certain issues
- Idealized and romanticized first love relationships

These young people are often beginning sexual and drug and alcohol-using experimentation. Their care providers can help by taking into account their special needs. For example, be respectful of concrete thinking by asking, "Exactly where would you keep your pills? What do you do every day that can remind you to take your pill?" Use the peer involvement issue. Ask, for example, "Do you have any friends who use pills? What do they say about them?" About romance you might say, "I know it's hard to imagine that Mike could have any infections that would hurt you, but it happens sometimes. I'd like to help you stay safe. Love doesn't disinfect anybody!"

Stressful lives can retard cognitive and emotional growth,[1] so assess their developmental status by what patients say and do more than by chronological age.

The ability to plan ahead is a late skill, usually associated with age 16 or older. All methods of birth control call for at least some ability to plan ahead, and are therefore incompatible with the developmental skills of early and middle adolescence. These young people will need your help with intensive skill practice in order to be successful at reducing their risks of pregnancy and STDs.

CULTURE

The cultural values and ideas learned in childhood strongly influence each person. Cultures vary widely in many characteristics that influence reproductive lives. Care providers need to know the cultural values of the patient population, learning, for example:[7]

- What is the ideal family size?
- Who makes sexual decisions?
- What is the typical marriage age?
- How is same-gender sexuality regarded?
- How does this culture understand the causation of illness?
- Who are the powerful healers?
- What is safe to tell the care provider?
- Is the general communication style direct or indirect? Formal or informal?

Balance an understanding of each client's unique personality with an awareness of and respect for influential cultural values and characteristics.

Culturally competent communication skill begins with an awareness of how we ourselves are culture-bound. For example, many clinics use an appointment system (based on Western European cultural values about the importance of punctuality) while serving a patient population that does not share that cultural value, a no-win situation that frustrates everyone.

EDUCATIONAL ATTAINMENT

Successful communication uses communication styles with which patients are comfortable and familiar. Perhaps the most common error is using print materials with patients who do not customarily read. A good screening question might be, "How many newspapers and magazines do you read in a typical week?"[9]

If in your judgment print materials are appropriate, match the readability of materials to the skill in the patient population. College students can usually read almost anything. For other groups, aim for about seventh grade reading level, the U.S. average. Use a tool such as the SMOG formula to determine the reading level of your materials.[3] The SMOG formula is a quick way to get an approximate idea of reading difficulty. Contraceptive consent forms are a good place to start with a reading level assessment.

SMOG Formula for Reading Level

When the text has at least 30 sentences:

1. Count three sets of 10 sentences each, one near the beginning, one in the middle, and one near the end.

2. Circle all words with three or more syllables, including repetitions of the same word. Total all circled words in the 30 sentences.
3. Find the nearest perfect square to your total. (Examples: total is 98, use 100; total is 51, use 49.) Take the square root. (Examples: 100 is 10; 49 is 7.)
4. Add 3 to your square root for the reading grade level. (Examples: 10 plus 3 = thirteenth grade; 7 plus 3 = tenth grade.)

When the text has fewer than 30 sentences:

1. Count all words in text with three or more syllables. Next, count the total number of sentences. Then divide to find the average number of long words per sentence. (Example: 40 circled words divided by 20 sentences = an average of 2 per sentence.)
2. Multiply your average number of long words per sentence by the number of sentences short of 30. (Example: 2 times 10 = 20.)
3. Add your answer to your total number of long words, find the square root, and then add 3. (Example: 20 plus 40 = 60. Nearest perfect square = 64. Square root = 8. 8 plus 3 = eleventh grade.)

The grade level tells you that two-thirds of the U.S. students in that grade could read the sample with 100% comprehension. The standard error of prediction is 1.5 grades in either direction. The two most important strategies for lowering reading levels are to (1) use short words and (2) use short sentences.[2]

EMOTIONAL STATE

Intense feelings of anger, anxiety, fear, disappointment, or even elation must be acknowledged and discussed before effective patient education can begin. "Yes, you are pregnant, and here are your options" is callous as well as ineffective. "Yes, you are pregnant. Can you tell me how this news feels to you?" gets off to a better start. In some situations, it may make sense to defer education until a later visit. People who learn their HIV test is positive often say they remember nothing at all the counselor said after hearing the word "positive." When you and the patient assess the ease and likelihood of a return visit as low or unknown, try to take extra time for processing feelings while you are together.

READINESS FOR BEHAVIOR CHANGE

Not all patients are equally ready to undertake the changes in personal daily life that promote health, such as abstaining from sex or using condoms when there is an STD risk, stopping smoking, or taking birth control pills diligently. Demonstration projects in HIV prevention have based educational interventions on a stages of change model, theorizing that behavior change is incremental, and that interventions must be tailored to the patient's (or target community's) particular position along a continuum of change.[4] Using a model developed in psychotherapy and smoking cessation research,[5,6] scientists have described five steps along the behavior change continuum. These steps, characteristics, and other features are detailed in Table 23-1.

In the individual counseling setting, one or two questions ("What are you doing to protect yourself from accidental pregnancy?" "When would you like to become pregnant?") can help place the patient along the stages of change continuum, so that the limited time available for education can be used effectively.

Table 23-1 Stages of change and educational interventions

Stage	Characteristics	Typical Response to "What do you do to protect yourself from AIDS?"	How to Focus Educational Intervention
Precontemplative	Not aware of risk; denies risk; no plan to change	"Who, me?"	Teach risk awareness facts; show models of desired behavior
Contemplative	Thinking about change; no specific plans	"I've been thinking about that myself."	Assist with priority-setting; teach skills required for change; promote self-efficacy ("You can do this. Think for yourself.")
Ready for Action	Has a plan; some action steps	"I checked out condoms in the drugstore the other day. There must be 30 brands!"	Assist with personal goals; reinforce skills; promote self-efficacy
Action	Change has begun; change is new	"From now on, no sex without condoms! Got them right here in my backpack!"	Reinforce personal goals; promote self-efficacy; show models of desired behavior
Maintenance	Change is in place; change is sustained	"I haven't had sex without condoms in a year now."	Praise success; promote self-efficacy; show models of desired behavior

Sources: O'Reilly and Higgins, 1991.
Prochaska and DiClemente, 1983.
Prochaska and DiClemente, 1984.

Relapse is common with any human behavior change undertaking. Relapsing patients will need extra help with renewed (and perhaps rethought) goal setting, a boost in self-efficacy, and sympathetic understanding.

Patient Goals, Provider Goals, and Time Considerations

Because it is rare to have all the time you need and all the time the patient needs for talking together, it is helpful to use *contracting* in the beginning of an encounter. Contracting makes clear from the outset what your priorities are for the encounter, makes clear approximately how much time is available to talk, and encourages the patient to discuss what is uppermost in her or his mind. For example, contracting with a first visit family planning patient might sound like this: "We have about 20 minutes to talk today, Linda. I want to be sure to tell you about what we have to offer you here, and we always ask health history questions of our new patients. Can you tell me, what do you most want to talk about?"

There are at least five options when education and counseling issues are unfinished and time is not immediately available:

- Schedule a return visit if logistically feasible for the patient.
- Schedule a telephone appointment for more discussion.
- Refer to a hotline for specific issues such as HIV or abuse.
- Offer reading material if appropriate.
- Refer to another care source, such as a prenatal clinic, sex therapist, or substance abuse treatment center.

Need For Formal Informed Consent Procedure

Pill, IUD, and Norplant users, among others, must be given full disclosure about their drugs and procedures in advance. On the basis of this disclosure, the patient must provide an informed and documented consent to care. Help patients view informed consent not as legal paperwork but as a serious process for ensuring safe and effective medical care, beginning with the tone you set as educator. Remember that you do not truly know what the patient has learned until you hear her or him say it back to you in her or his own words. This specialized aspect of patient education is spelled out in detail in the following section.

I NFORMED CONSENT

The importance of informed consent in family planning and reproductive health has three bases: pragmatic, ethical, and legal. Pragmatically, a person who thoroughly understands her or his contraceptive method or device or medical procedure will be more likely to use it safely and effectively. Ethically, every person has a right to thorough information about products or procedures that can affect health. Legally, the clinician must provide adequate information to help the patient reach a reasonable and informed decision about medications, procedures, and devices.

Issues of informed consent are particularly crucial in the field of contraception because of the nontherapeutic nature of these services. Family planning methods and medications are usually initiated at the request of a healthy person and in the absence of traditional medical indications for treatment.

Legal standards for informed consent do not depend on "local community" standards as was formerly the case, but on the "reasonable person" standard. Did the patient receive all the information that a reasonable person would need to make a sound decision and a truly informed consent? It is the responsibility of the clinician to ensure that the patient has sufficient understanding of the proposed medication, device, or procedure and to determine whether the patient is competent to consent on her or his own behalf.

Federal regulations for informed consent to sterilization[8] provide helpful guidance for what types of information constitute informed consent, and this guidance can be applied to the contraceptive field in general. According to these Department of Health and Human Services regulations, informed consent comprises seven basic elements. A simple mnemonic device may prove useful in remembering these seven components. The word to remember is **"BRAIDED"**:

Benefits of the method

Risks of the method (both major risks and all common minor ones), including consequences of method failure

Alternatives to the method (including abstinence and no method)

Inquiries about the method are the patient's right and responsibility

Decision to withdraw from using the method without penalty is the patient's right

Explanation of the method is owed the patient

Documentation that the clinician has covered each of the previous six points, usually by use of a consent form

The importance of a voluntary decision—free from any coercion—is paramount. Documentation is essential, but a written consent form and signature alone are not enough. It may be particularly helpful to document the provision of any print and audiovisual educational aids used to inform the patient.

COMPETENCE TO CONSENT

These are the basic criteria for competence to consent:

- Is the patient capable of understanding the proposed treatment, alternatives, and risks?

- Is the patient capable of rational decision making?

In some situations, the patient's competence is difficult to evaluate. The very young teen, the developmentally disabled person, the intoxicated person, and the mentally ill person are examples of such patients. If you have any doubt regarding competence of the patient, consult with other professionals to determine the appropriate course of action. Be sure to document your consultation in the patient's record.

EDUCATIONAL CONSIDERATIONS FOR CONSENT

Adults and adolescents best learn, and make considered decisions, under the following circumstances:

- In the absence of threat
- When information seems relevant
- When participating actively in the learning process
- When having a chance to ask and receive answers to questions
- With time to digest, and room for insight

Make every effort to provide these elements for the informed consent process. Provide audiotaped or videotaped consent forms (in all appropriate languages) for poor readers, so they can learn by listening. Write consent forms at a manageable reading level, about grade seven or eight. Have the patient repeat what she or he has learned for a clear evaluation of learning and comprehension.

CONSENT FORMS

A number of family planning programs view the consent form as an important piece of patient education literature and provide each patient with a copy to keep.

This practice is entirely consistent with the philosophy of full disclosure, so consider using consent forms that include all the BRAIDED elements and use simple language. Be sure to stress warning signs for serious complications on consent forms, especially for IUDs and hormonal methods.

Remember that all providers of pills, Norplant, and IUDs must give a copy of the FDA-approved and manufacturer-supplied leaflet or pamphlet to each user. Clinic or office consent forms can be written to include a statement such as "I have been given a copy of (title) and have been encouraged to read it carefully."

A sample Norplant consent form follows. It can be adapted or reproduced without permission.

NORPLANT INFORMED CONSENT

Please read this form carefully. You will be asked to sign your name once you **understand** this information **completely.**

Before giving your consent, be sure that you understand both the advantages and the disadvantages of using the Norplant system. This form outlines possible problems that can occur with Norplant, warning signs you should watch for, and side effects that some women experience. If you have any questions as you read, please ask. We will answer any questions you have.

Also, remember that your consent is entirely voluntary. You can change your mind any time before Norplant is inserted. Once Norplant is inserted, you can have it removed any time you want.

As you read, please check (√) each section.

How Norplant Works

The Norplant system consists of six soft, thin rubber (Silastic) capsules that are placed in your upper arm. Each capsule contains 36 milligrams of levonorgestrel, a **hormone** similar to progesterone hormone produced by your ovaries. Levonorgestrel is released through the walls of the capsule to provide a steady flow of low hormone dose.

The Norplant hormone is the same hormone used in several brands of birth control pills; the Norplant dose, however, is much lower.   ❏

Norplant prevents pregnancy by **interfering with ovulation.** It also causes your cervical mucus to be **thick and sticky** so that sperm have trouble reaching your uterus. Because the dose of hormone is steady, the Norplant system provides extremely good birth control protection. No other birth control method for women is as effective except having your tubes tied. **Fewer than 1 woman in 1,000** using Norplant will become pregnant each year. The Norplant system provides steady protection for 5 years. Norplant **does not** protect against sexually transmitted infections. You will need to use condoms or avoid intercourse and other sexual contact if there is any risk of infection from a sex partner.   ❏

Who Should Not Use Norplant

Norplant is **not** a wise choice for women with certain **medical** problems:

- Thrombophlebitis (blood clots in vein) or embolism (clots in lung, eye, brain)
- Abnormal vaginal bleeding that has not been diagnosed
- Pregnancy or suspected pregnancy
- Severe active liver disease or liver tumors
- Breast cancer   ❏

Before having Norplant inserted, be sure to **discuss** with your clinician any serious medical condition you may have. Some examples include: diabetes, high blood pressure, high cholesterol, migraine or other severe headaches, epilepsy, depression, gallbladder, heart, or kidney disease. It is possible that Norplant may not work as well for women taking epilepsy drugs such as Dilantin or Tegretol or the antibiotic Rifampin.   ❏

What to Expect

Almost all women using Norplant have **irregular periods or bleeding,** especially during the first year after it is inserted. You could have many bleeding days, spotting, or irregular periods. Some women skip periods, or have very light periods. Overall, the total amount of blood loss is usually **less** than with normal periods, but the **timing is not as predictable.** These problems tend to decrease after the first year and can sometimes be treated with additional hormone medication.❏

Possible Problems

In the first week after insertion, be alert for itching, pain, pus, or bleeding at the Norplant insertion site. Let your clinician know about any of these problems.

While using Norplant, you will need to watch for **warning signs of serious problems** such as high blood pressure inside your skull, stroke, liver disease, breast cancer, thrombophlebitis, embolism, depression, or accidental pregnancy. If you become pregnant, or develop one of these problems, Norplant may need to be removed. Report any of these warning signs **right away:**

- No period after having a period every month
- Norplant comes out
- Severe depression
- Headache(s), persistent or more frequent or severe than usual
- Blurry or double vision or loss of vision
- Visual sparks or flashes
- Ringing sound in ears
- Feeling dizzy or fainting

- Sudden weakness or numbness on one side
- Shortness of breath
- Coughing blood
- Severe pain in the stomach or abdomen
- Sharp or crushing chest pain
- Unusual swelling or pain in the legs or arms
- Yellowing of the skin or eyes
- Heavy bleeding from the vagina
- Lump in breast ❏

Although pregnancy is very unlikely while using Norplant, you must have a pregnancy test if you have symptoms of pregnancy, or if you go more than 6 weeks with no menstrual bleeding. Tubal (ectopic) pregnancy can occur with Norplant. ❏

These problems with Norplant are **uncommon:**

- Headache
- Ovary enlargement
- Appetite change
- Breast pain or discharge
- Hair loss from scalp
- Difficulty removing implants
- Nervousness

- Nausea or dizziness
- Dermatitis or acne
- Weight gain
- Increased body hair growth
- Skin discoloration over implants
- Numbness in hand or forearm of Norplant arm

If they do occur, these problems usually go away when Norplant is removed. ❏

Inserting and Removing Norplant

The six Norplant capsules, each about $\frac{1}{8}$-inch wide and $1\frac{1}{4}$-inch long, will be inserted just under the skin of your upper arm through a $\frac{1}{8}$-inch incision. Local anesthetic is used before insertion to make the skin temporarily numb. A lot of bruising usually occurs in the insertion area but should disappear within a few weeks. The incision will be protected with a bandage for the first few days. The site will usually heal quickly. No stitches are required, and the scar is small. You will be able to feel the Norplant capsules, and they may be visible under the skin. ❏

After you have used Norplant for **5 years,** or sooner if you choose, the implants will need to be removed because all the hormone may be used up. Removal will require local anesthesia and one or more small incisions. There is usually an additional medical fee for removal. ❏

Your Consent

I have read this Informed Consent summary, and have discussed my questions with my clinician. I also understand the risks and benefits of other methods of birth control including birth control pills, the IUD, the diaphragm, cervical cap, condoms, spermicide, and sterilization surgery. I have thought about all these factors. I **voluntarily choose** to have the Norplant system inserted. I have received a copy of the Norplant system booklet from the manufacturer.

Date _____ Signature _____

Witness _____

REFERENCES

1. Johnson R. Adolescent growth and development. In: Hofmann A, Greydanus D (eds). Adolescent medicine, 2nd ed. Norwalk CT: Appleton & Lange, 1989.
2. Manning D. Writing readable health messages. Public Health Reports 1981; 96(5): 464-465.
3. Office of Cancer Communications. Readability testing in cancer communications. Bethesda MD: National Cancer Institute, 1979.
4. O'Reilly KR, Higgins DL. AIDS community demonstration projects for HIV prevention among hard-to-reach groups. Pub Health Rep 1991;106(6):714-720.
5. Prochaska JO, DiClemente CC. Stages and processes of self-change of smoking: toward an integrative model of change. J Consult and Clini Psychol 1983;51(3):390-395.
6. Prochaska JO, DiClemente CC. The transtheoretical approach: crossing traditional boundaries of therapy. Homewood IL: Dow Jones-Irwin, 1984.
7. Randall-David E. Strategies for working with culturally diverse communities and clients. Washington DC: Association for the Care of Children's Health, 1989.
8. Sterilization of persons in federally assisted family planning projects. Federal Register 1978;43(Nov 8):52146-52175.
9. Wells JA, Sell RL. Learning AIDS: 1991 supplement: a special report on readability, literacy, and the HIV epidemic. New York NY: American Foundation for AIDS Research, 1991.

Adolescent Sexual Behavior, Pregnancy, and Childbearing

24

- One of every eight women aged 15-19 in the United States becomes pregnant each year. This proportion has changed little since the late 1970s.

- This overall constancy masks two offsetting trends: increasing proportions are having sexual intercourse and increasing proportions are using contraception.

- Both pregnancy and birth rates among teens in the United States are very high when compared with those in other developed countries, although rates of sexual activity are similar.

- While everyone agrees that teenage pregnancy is a problem, there is no consensus about a solution.

- Recent research suggests that the consequences of teenage childbearing are not as deleterious as has been claimed.

- That adolescents want to avoid becoming pregnant is sufficient justification for helping them to do so.

- Two-thirds of all STDs occur among persons under 25 years of age.

One in eight women aged 15-19 in the United States becomes pregnant each year. This proportion has changed little since the late 1970s. Consequently, in 1991 about 1.1 million pregnancies occurred among those aged 15-19. Another 57 thousand pregnancies occurred among women aged 14 and younger.[a]

---

a Note that the sum of births, induced abortions and spontaneous abortions among women aged a will not equal pregnancies to women aged a, because women are older when their pregnancies are resolved than when they are conceived. There are more births and induced abortions resulting from pregnancies to women under age 20 than there are births and induced abortions to women under age 20. Estimates of births, abortions and pregnancies for 1991 were obtained by assuming that 1988 rates[28] pertained to 1991 women.[69] The estimated number of intended pregnancies was obtained by assuming that the fraction of pregnancies unintended in 1987[19] pertained to 1991, and the estimated numbers of births by poverty and marital status were obtained in the same manner.[64] The estimated numbers of virgins were obtained by assuming that no ever-married persons in 1991[58] were virgins and that the proportion of virgins among those never married in 1988[61,67] pertained to 1991.

One in 15 men fathers a child while he is a teenager.[41] The sheer magnitude of these statistics has generated widespread public concern: Why do unmarried adolescents become pregnant and what can be done about it?

The overwhelming consensus is that adolescent pregnancy is a serious problem and that public policies and programs should be implemented to reduce its incidence and ameliorate its consequences.

This consensus, however, offers little guidance for formulating public policy because the reasons for concern vary widely.

- Many object to adolescents having sex simply because they are too young.

- Others would draw an important distinction between those who are married and those who are not. Some believe that sex among unmarried persons is unwise or immoral. Approximately 75% of pregnant women aged 15-19 and virtually all those aged 14 and younger are unmarried at the time their pregnancy is resolved. Therefore, in 1991, about 890 thousand women who became pregnant as teenagers resolved their pregnancies outside marriage.

- Others would differentiate pregnancies that are intended from those that are not. Only 222 thousand of the 1.2 million adolescent pregnancies in 1991 were intended.

- Some, including many family planning clinicians, are particularly troubled by the large number of abortions obtained by adolescents: about 384 thousand in 1991 alone.

- Still others view a birth to an adolescent as a tragedy, reasoning that giving birth at an early age not only seriously damages the young woman's life chances and limits her options, but also creates a suboptimal environment for the child. In 1991, about 462 thousand births occurred to women under 20 years of age: about 11 thousand to women less than 15, about 164 thousand to women aged 15-17, and about 287 thousand to women aged 18-19.

While some are concerned about pregnancy or abortion or childbearing among all adolescents, others believe that the problems are particularly acute for the poor or for the very young, although no consensus exists about the definition of the very young. In 1991, about 11 thousand births occurred and 14 thousand abortions were performed among women aged less than 15 and another 164 thousand births occurred and 147 thousand abortions were performed among women aged 15-17. Of the 462 thousand births to women aged less than 20, about 356 thousand (77%) occurred among poor women (those with family incomes ranging from below the poverty level to as much as 50% above). Slightly over half the total (236 thousand or 51%) occurred among women who were both poor and unmarried. Some view the problem primarily as a health issue, others as a moral issue, and yet others as an economic issue.

We have identified three categories of arguments supporting public intervention to "solve" the adolescent pregnancy problem, each suggesting different intervention strategies and target groups. These arguments may be summarized as follows:

1. Unmarried persons, especially young persons, should not engage in sexual intercourse. Our society places far too much emphasis on sex, especially in the media, and public institutions, especially the schools, have abandoned the teaching of traditional values. The solution, therefore, is a vigorous campaign to promote traditional values, particularly chastity among the unmarried. Because other strategies to reduce adolescent pregnancy (*e.g.*, increasing the availability of contraceptive and abortion services) have the undesirable even if unintended effect of "legitimizing" and perhaps even increasing sexual activity, they are unacceptable. The target group is very large. In 1991, 7.9 million women aged 15-19 had never married.[58] Of these, 4.0 million have had intercourse and 3.9 million were still virgins. Likewise, 8.4 million men aged 15-19 had never married,[58] of whom 3.3 million were still virgins.

2. Not many people would seriously promote sex among adolescents. But campaigns with the sole aim of promoting chastity have not proven effective. Because such large proportions of adolescents are sexually active, it seems only prudent to provide accurate information on reproductive biology and contraception starting at an early age. Such information is an essential component of family life education, whose primary goal should be to promote rational and informed decision-making about sexuality. Nevertheless, information will not reduce pregnancy rates unless contraceptive services are also widely available. Preventing pregnancy should reduce the incidence of adolescent childbearing and abortion. The target group here is the sexually active and those about to become sexually active. In 1991, some 4.4 million women and 5.2 million men aged 15-19 had experienced intercourse at least once.

3. While preventing pregnancies is a very important goal, this objective will not be met in the short run. Even if high-quality sex education and contraceptive services were universally available, some adolescents would nevertheless become pregnant. Many of them do not always plan their lives carefully. However, all available contraceptive methods require such planning. Moreover, typical contraceptive failure rates even among more mature women are not low.[65] Therefore, abortion services and/or programs to ameliorate the adverse consequences of

adolescent childbearing must be available, particularly for the poor, who both suffer the consequences to a greater extent and generate more public costs. The target group here is much smaller, consisting in 1991 of abortion services for whatever fraction of the 1.2 million pregnant teenagers who do not wish to carry their pregnancy to term (at least the 411 thousand who actually obtained abortions) and ameliorative programs for the remainder.

These three arguments are not mutually exclusive, and even those persons generally in agreement with one of them may not concur with all the points. Nevertheless, even this simple categorization shows the considerable discrepancies among the solutions advocated by those who view sex, those who view pregnancy, and those who view childbearing (particularly among the poor) as the main aspect of this problem. There is also conflict (by no means limited to adolescents) about the use of abortion as a remedy for an unwanted pregnancy. We return at the end of this chapter for further discussion of intervention strategies. Before doing so, we examine trends and levels of adolescent pregnancy in the United States, contrast the U.S. experience with that in other developed countries, analyze the determinants of adolescent pregnancy, examine the incidence of STDs among adolescents, and analyze the consequences of adolescent childbearing.

L EVELS AND TRENDS IN ABORTION, BIRTH, AND PREGNANCY RATES

Pregnancies can end in births, induced abortions, or spontaneous abortions. Data for the United States are available for only the first two outcomes. Hence, estimates of pregnancies must include estimates of spontaneous abortions. In 1988 (the latest year for which estimates are available), 3% of females aged 14 became pregnant. This proportion rose steadily with age, as can be seen in Figure 24-1, to reach 18% of women aged 18 and 19. The fraction of pregnancies ending in a birth was virtually constant with age (about 51%).

Birth rates among women aged 15-19 declined steadily from 1970 to 1978, rose slightly thereafter, began to decline again in 1983, and rose very sharply in 1988 and 1989 after falling to a record low in 1986.[50] The birth rate among women aged 15-19 was higher in 1989 than in any year since 1973. In contrast, *abortion rates* rose steadily from 1973 (the year abortion was legalized) to 1979, remained relatively constant through 1987, and rose to the highest level yet observed in 1988.[28] As can be seen in Figure 24-2, the increase in abortion rates initially outweighed the decrease in birth rates, however, so that *pregnancy rates* rose slowly but steadily from 1973 to 1981. Pregnancy rates remained relatively constant between 1981 and 1987, before turning sharply upward in 1988.[28] Intentional pregnancies constitute only 19% of all pregnancies among women aged 15-19.[18]

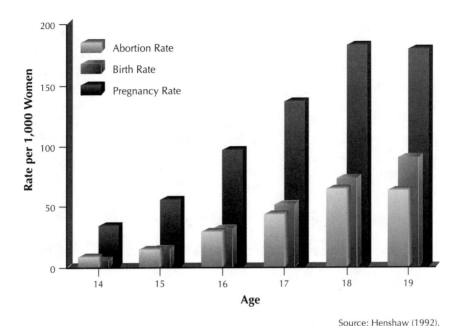

Figure 24-1 Abortions, births, and pregnancies per 1,000 women aged 14-19, by single year of age, United States, 1988

Teenage *pregnancy rates* among blacks are more than twice as high as those among whites (251 per 1,000 black women versus 110 per 1,000 white women aged 15-19 in 1988).[28] Furthermore, because whites and blacks are equally likely to abort a pregnancy, the differential in birth rates is the same: 110 births per 1,000 black women versus 49 per 1,000 white women aged 15-19 in 1989.[50] Comparable data for Hispanics do not exist. Although information on Hispanic origin is collected on birth certificates in almost half the states, it is not gathered in the abortion surveillance systems. The birth rate among 15-19 year old Hispanics (100.8 per 1,000) in 1989 was more than twice that for whites (48.5 per 1,000) and 91% as high as that for blacks (110.4 per 1000).[50] These racial and ethnic differentials are probably due in large part to differences in standards of living and in perceived life chances.

COMPARISON WITH EXPERIENCE IN OTHER COUNTRIES

Pregnancy rates among women under age 20 are considerably higher in the United States than in any other developed country for which data are available, with the exception of Hungary (where the rate is about 5% higher). Even in Hungary the pregnancy rate among women under age 18

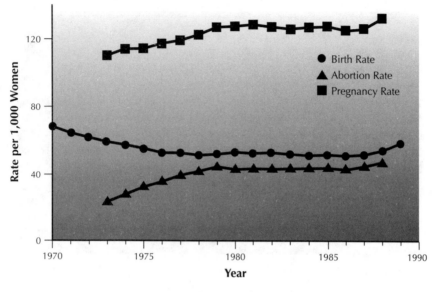

Sources: Birth rates—NCHS (1991).
Abortion and pregnancy rates—Henshaw (1992).

Figure 24-2 Abortions, births, and pregnancies per 1,000 women aged 15-19, United States, 1970-1989

is only three-quarters as high as in the United States. Moreover, *birth rates* among women under age 20 are higher in the United States than in 29 other developed countries. The only developed countries with higher birth rates are Bulgaria, Chile, Cuba, (former) Czechoslovakia, Iceland, Greece, Hungary, Puerto Rico, and Romania. Only Bulgaria, Cuba, Hungary, and Puerto Rico have higher birth rates among women aged 15-17. Both the under-18 and under-20 fertility rates among U.S. blacks are higher than those in any of the other 39 populations (including U.S. whites).[33,72]

Why is the experience in the United States so different? For the six countries (Canada, England and Wales, France, The Netherlands, Sweden, and the United States) examined in a cross-national comparison, the difference in pregnancy rates was not due to cross-national variations in proportions married, since the same qualitative conclusions would be obtained if comparisons were limited to the unmarried.[33] Part of the difference is attributable to the very high teenage pregnancy rates among U.S. blacks, but pregnancy rates for U.S. whites are still much higher than those for women in the other countries. The available evidence indicates that the proportions of teenagers ever having had sexual intercourse are similar in all countries except Sweden, which has much higher proportions at each age, and Canada, where the proportions are lower but the data are less reliable.

Hence, with the possible exception of Canada, higher pregnancy rates in the United States are not caused by more prevalent sexual experience. The contrast between Sweden and the United States is quite extreme: at every age greater proportions of teenagers are virgins in the United States, whereas abortion, birth, and pregnancy rates are far lower in Sweden.

The reason for higher pregnancy rates in the United States is that American teenagers are less likely to use contraceptives, or less likely to use them effectively. Lower proportions of teenage women in the United States use contraceptives regularly than do teenage women in the other five countries. Among users, a smaller fraction relies on the most efficient methods, particularly the pill.

- Contraceptive supplies and services appear to be most widely available, free of charge or at low cost, to adolescents in Sweden, The Netherlands, and England and Wales. In France, the quality of adolescent contraceptive services has steadily improved. Both Canada and the United States lag significantly behind the others.
- Sex education in Sweden is compulsory and is taught in the schools at all grade levels. Information on contraception is provided, and its effectiveness is enhanced by a close link between the schools and adolescent birth control clinics. No other country approaches this level of implementation. In The Netherlands, where teenage pregnancy rates are lowest, sex education in the schools is generally limited to the teaching of reproductive biology. However, sex education has received heavy emphasis in the mass media, and public funding supports educational efforts aimed at adolescents by the private family planning associations.[33]

D ETERMINANTS OF ADOLESCENT PREGNANCY

Although one in eight women aged 15-19 becomes pregnant each year, seven in eight do not. Of those who do, one in two carries the pregnancy to term. A common opinion, expressed in popular books,[12,13] is that many adolescents perceive (however incorrectly) having a child as an attractive alternative to their current situation. They may, for example, be bored in school or have conflicts with parents. Undoubtedly, some do believe that a child is a ticket to independence or to a better life and act accordingly.

However, the vast majority of unmarried adolescents who become pregnant do not intend to do so.[77,79] Intention is seldom adequately characterized by a sharp yes-or-no dichotomy. Therefore, even though only a small minority of teenagers *intend* to become pregnant out-of-wedlock, the strength of the motivation of the rest to *avoid* pregnancy varies considerably.

The motivation to avoid pregnancy is governed by a young woman's perception of the benefits of deferring parenthood. This perception is strongly influenced by both her present circumstances and her belief in her future life chances. For many disadvantaged youth, the benefits of postponed parenthood must seem remote indeed.

Research on black adolescent mothers provides revealing insights about their sexuality and childbearing.[20] Most, if not all, of these findings pertain to all adolescents.

- First, the values adolescents express often differ from their actual behaviors. Their "ideal" sexual code places emphasis on waiting until marriage to have sex and on the practical dangers of becoming pregnant. These values, however, must be "stretched" because of the pressures of everyday life. This ambivalence between the ideal code and actual behavior leads to several real difficulties. To plan to have sex is wrong. Sexual intimacy is excusable only if one is swept away in the heat of passion, without prior thought. Unfortunately, effective contraceptive use requires planning. Once pregnancy has occurred, the young woman tends to deny it exists. As a consequence, adolescents resort to abortion, if at all, later than more mature women.

- Second, many parents (particularly mothers) encourage this charade. While they will warn their daughters not to become pregnant, they offer little guidance for accomplishing this feat. The parents practice denial by pretending that their daughters do not have sex and then express great shock when they become pregnant.

- Third, initial reactions to a pregnancy, even among those who eventually carry it to term, are usually quite negative. Adolescents feel that having a baby would damage their life chances and that they are not mature enough to care for and raise a child. Nevertheless, many feel helpless to alter their fate.

- Finally, as the pregnancy progresses and is accepted (if not welcomed) by parents and friends, the reactions of the expectant mothers become more positive. Their expectations about the future consequences, however, grow unrealistically positive. They underestimate the difficulties of continuing their education and the demands of a child on their time, they overestimate their future economic status, and they underestimate the difficulty of maintaining a quality relationship with the father.

A common misperception is that adolescent fathers have little contact with their children. Roughly half of all adolescent fathers live with their children shortly after birth.[41] Paternal involvement persists for extended periods following the birth, even among those males who do not marry the mothers of their children.[54] Nevertheless, the frequency of contact declines markedly with time.[27]

SEXUAL BEHAVIOR

Why do unmarried adolescents become pregnant? The proximate cause is obviously sexual relations. In 1988, 51% of never-married women aged 15-19 had ever had sexual intercourse, and 39% reported sexual relations during the 3 months preceding the survey. The proportion with some sexual experience rises sharply with age: 1% by age 13, 5% by age 14, 12% by age 15, 26% by age 16, 42% by age 17, 58% by age 18, 76% by age 19, and 82% by age 20. These proportions by race are shown in Figure 24-3. By the time they reach their 18th birthday, well over half of never-married women in the United States have had intercourse. The proportions engaging in regular sexual relations are lower but are nevertheless substantial. For example, among never-married women, 25% of those aged 15-17 and 60% of those aged 18-19 reported sexual intercourse in the 3 months preceding the survey.[67]

The available data suggest a slowdown during the early 1980s in the rapid increase in the proportion of females aged 15-19 who had experienced premarital sexual intercourse (30% in 1971, 41% in 1976, and 43% in 1982).[67,79] However, hopes that this slowdown would continue were dashed by results from the 1988 NSFG. Examination of retrospective reports of age at first

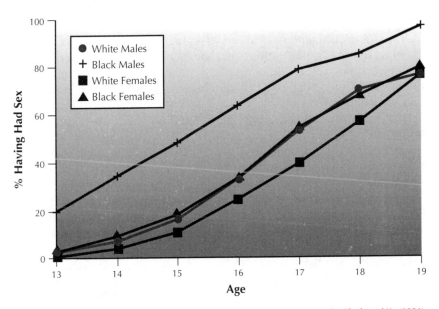

Sources: Males—Sonnenstein, Pleck, and Ku (1991).
Females—Trussell and Vaughan (1991).

Figure 24-3 Percent of never-married men and women who have ever had sex: 1988 NSAM and 1988 NSFG. Life-table tabulations based on retrospective reports of age at first intercourse.

intercourse by women in the 1982 and 1988 NSFGs reveals that the increase between 1982 and 1988 in the fraction of teenagers who have had sexual intercourse was driven almost entirely by increases among whites.

Information on adolescent males is much more limited. The most recent data (shown by race in Figure 24-3) reveal that by their 13th birthday 5% of never-married males have become sexually active. The proportions rise to 11%, 21%, 38%, 58%, 67%, and 79% by the 14th, 15th, 16th, 17th, 18th, and 19th birthdays, respectively.[61]

CONTRACEPTIVE USE

Among teenage women surveyed in 1988, 65% reported use of a contraceptive at first intercourse. Of these, 73% used the condom, 13% relied on withdrawal, and only 13% used the pill.[19] Among teenage women who were currently exposed to the risk of unintended pregnancy, 20% were using no method (down from 30% in 1982) while 47% (up from 44% in 1982) and 27% (up from 15% in 1982) were relying on the pill and condom, respectively.[67]

Why do so many adolescent women fail to use contraceptives? In a 1976 survey, among the never-married sexually active women who did not use a method at the time they last had intercourse even though they did not want to become pregnant, more than half (58%) thought they could not conceive. Of the remainder, one in five stated that they had not expected to have inter- course. Not expecting to have intercourse is an even more important factor in failing to use a contraceptive when adolescents begin sexual activity. For example, among those who did not use a contraceptive even though they thought they could but did not want to become pregnant the only time they had intercourse, 87% did not expect to have sex.[78]

Half of all initial adolescent pregnancies occur within the first 6 months following initiation of intercourse, and 20% in the first month alone. Among adolescents who never practice contraception, 39% become pregnant within 6 months and 66% within 2 years of their initial sexual encounter. Among those who always use a method, the corresponding proportions are 7% and 11%, respectively.[76] Those who do not practice contraception at the time of first intercourse face a high risk of unintentional pregnancy. Who among these become pregnant is largely a matter of chance. Those lucky enough to avoid conception until they initiate use of contraception reduce substantially their risk thereafter.

In focus group sessions, adolescents have revealed an intense desire for pri- vacy concerning their own sexual activity and strong feelings of embarrass- ment when communicating about sexual matters with others: partners, friends, parents, counselors, and physicians. Those who had not attended clin- ics pictured these facilities as dingy places for the poor where they would be treated impersonally and viewed as morally irresponsible.[37] Adolescents are also embarrassed to go to family physicians, who might reveal their secrets, offer unwanted moral advice, or simply not help. Their fears are not ground-less: 22% of physicians in private general or family practice (but only 2% of OB-GYNs) refuse to serve minors, and 19% of GP/FPs (18% of OB-GYNs) pro-vide contraceptive services only with parental consent.[53] These sentiments help to explain the long delay, 23 months on average among women aged 15-24, between initiating sexual relations and the first family planning visit.[49]

SEX EDUCATION

Substantial proportions of teenage women surveyed in 1982 reported that they had discussed specific topics (menstrual cycle, how pregnancy occurs, venereal disease, contraception) with their parents, and even higher pro-portions stated that they had received formal instruction about these top-ics in the schools.[14] For example, among those aged 15, 66% and 52% had discussed how pregnancy occurs and contraception, respectively, with their parents, while 81% and 67% had received instruction on these top-ics in school. At age 18 (when more than half of all never-married women were no longer virgins), the corresponding figures were 67% and 55% with parents and 81% and 74% in the schools.

These figures reveal little about the depth of coverage of the topics. The efficacy of such education is challenged by the fact that only 34% of those who had received both pregnancy and contraceptive instruction in school could correctly identify the time during the menstrual cycle when con-ception is most likely (only 21% with no instruction could do so). A sim-ilarly gloomy conclusion is reached when one examines behavior. Among sexually active teenagers at risk of unintended pregnancy, only 62% of those who had received both pregnancy and contraceptive instruction were cur-rently practicing contraception, compared with 58% of those who had received no instruction.[14]

A 1988 survey of public school teachers in five specialties (biology, health education, home economics, physical education, and school nursing) who taught in grades 7-12 revealed that the overwhelming majority (93%) of their schools offered sex education or AIDS education in some form.[18] In practice, however, only 82%-84% of teachers were in schools that provided instruction in sexual decision-making, abstinence, and birth control methods; 97% of teachers said that sex education classes should include information on where to obtain contraceptives but only 48% were in schools where such information is provided. Most teachers thought that topics related to the prevention of pregnancy and STDs should be covered by grades 7-8 at the latest. However, only about a third of teachers were in schools that by the end of the seventh grade pro-vided information on STDs, sexual decision-making, abstinence, or birth control methods, and only about a sixth were in schools that provided information on birth control sources.

Opposition to teaching about contraceptives and where to obtain them is based on the belief that such information promotes promiscuity. The data, however, do not support this belief. One study found that exposure to contraceptive education had no consistent effect on the probability that a virgin would subsequently begin to have intercourse.[14] A second study found that 15- and 16-year-old adolescents who had ever had a course on sex education were less likely to be sexually experienced than those who had not (17% versus 26%).[21] A third study found that adolescent women who had taken a sex education course had a statistically significant higher probability of initiating intercourse at ages 15 and 16, though they were no more likely to do so at ages 17 and 18.[42] However, the practical importance of the effect at ages 15 and 16 is small. For a typical respondent, having taken a sex education course raised the likelihood of having intercourse by 2-4 percentage points. Church attendance, parental education, and race were much more important determinants.

The studies cited above are all based on retrospective survey data. More rigorous prospective comparisons of actual intervention with control programs confirm that sexuality and contraceptive education does not promote promiscuity. One study evaluated the effects of a school-based program for the primary prevention of pregnancy among inner city adolescents. The program combined sex education, counseling, and contraceptive services. It emphasized the development of personal responsibility, goal-setting, and communication with parents. The results were encouraging. Not only were pregnancy rates reduced substantially when the two schools with the program were compared with two control schools, but among those not sexually active when the program began, the onset of sexual intercourse was postponed.[73,74,75] While this postponement was not large, it was substantial enough to refute the assertion that services such as those provided by that program promote sexual activity. An evaluation of six other school-based programs also found that these interventions did not hasten initiation of intercourse nor increase its frequency among sexually active students.[36] Finally, evaluations of three additional sexuality and contraceptive education programs showed that participants in these programs were less likely to initiate intercourse and that those participants who did start to have intercourse were more likely to use contraception than were nonparticipants.[17,32,35]

S EXUALLY TRANSMITTED DISEASES AMONG ADOLESCENTS

Most public attention to the consequences of teenage sexual behavior focuses on only one outcome: pregnancy. Much less attention is devoted to a second outcome: sexually transmitted diseases (STDs). The incidence of STDs among adolescents increased rapidly during the 1960s and 1970s.

In the 1980s, despite the increase in awareness of STDs caused by HIV prevention messages, rates of genital infections in adolescents have stayed at record high levels.[7] Two-thirds of all STDs occur among persons under 25 years of age.[9]

In the 1980s, gonorrhea infection rates remained nearly constant among teens (with a slight rise among males offset by a decline among females) while they fell among other age groups. Nearly 200 thousand cases were reported among teens in 1989 (about 10 thousand cases among white males, 20 thousand cases among white females, and more than 80 thousand cases among both black males and black females). Unlike gonorrhea, chlamydia infection is not a reportable condition in all 50 states. Nevertheless, most clinical investigations find that rates of chlamydia are at least double those of gonorrhea. The number of visits of teenage women to office-based fee-for-service practices for genital herpes infections increased from 15 thousand in 1966 to 125 thousand in 1989. The number of visits for genital warts caused by the human papillomavirus (HPV) increased from 50 thousand in 1966 to 300 thousand in 1989 among teenage women. Perhaps three times as many women have asymptomatic cervical HPV infection. By the end of the teenage years, about 4% of whites and 17% of blacks have been infected with herpes simplex virus type 2.[7]

By the end of 1992, 378 persons in the United States under the age of 20 with AIDS had been infected with HIV through sexual contact. Given the long latency period from infection with HIV to the development of AIDS, a considerable fraction of the 32,259 persons diagnosed with AIDS at ages 20-29 who had been infected through sexual contact must have been infected while still teenagers.[10]

The epidemiology of STD transmission is the same among adolescents as among adults: unprotected intercourse with multiple partners is very risky. Data from the 1988-1989 General Social Survey of men and women aged 18-44 show that over half of males and 34% of females aged 15-19 who had experienced sexual intercourse in the past year had had two or more partners in that time period.[19] In 1988, 57% of teenage males[60] and 31% of teenage females[67] reported condom use at last intercourse. It is difficult to resolve the discrepancy between these two statistics. The most plausible explanation is that either males overreport use of condoms because they know that it is the socially responsible answer or females underreport condom use when a condom is used as an adjunct to a regular method of contraception. Regardless of the answer, condom use seems to have increased among adolescents. The only plausible explanation for this increase is greater awareness of STDs, primarily HIV. Nevertheless, the disturbing fact remains that a very large fraction of adolescents at risk of acquiring STDs does not use condoms.

CONSEQUENCES OF ADOLESCENT CHILDBEARING

A considerable literature exists on the medical, social, and economic consequences of adolescent childbearing for the mother and for the child. Much is summarized in excellent review articles.[40,63] Unfortunately, many of the studies suffer from analytical flaws or poor experimental design, thereby rendering the conclusions suspect. Many studies report results obtained by analyzing all adolescents as one group, while the evidence suggests that the experiences of younger and older adolescents may differ widely. Many studies are also based on small, selective samples so that results are not easily generalizable.

Perhaps the greatest problem is that the analyst can seldom be sure whether the adverse conditions frequently observed among adolescent mothers are causally related to age at birth. Many studies fail to control for both maternal age and other factors correlated with age at first birth, such as socioeconomic status. Thus the adverse consequences of early childbearing *per se* are frequently overstated. An even more serious analytical problem arises because adolescents are able to select (or at least affect) whether or not they become pregnant or whether or not they will bear a child. Investigators can never study the consequences of adolescent childbearing by conducting a rigorous randomized trial. However, they can try to ensure that adolescent mothers are compared with a control group that is as similar as possible with respect to measurable background variables at an early age, such as achievement, aptitude, motivation, and socioeconomic status. A recent innovative methodological approach controls for a similar family environment by comparing the experiences of pairs of sisters, one of whom gave birth as a teenager and the other of whom did not.[23,24,25,30]

HEALTH CONSEQUENCES

Maternal health. More recent research in the United States has shown that many adverse consequences such as pregnancy-induced hypertension, anemia, toxemia, prematurity, and perinatal and maternal mortality documented in earlier studies were greatly overstated because the controls for socioeconomic status were inadequate or nonexistent.[31,45] The (much reduced) deleterious effects of young maternal age that are still observed when the effect of socioeconomic status is controlled are probably primarily attributable to inadequate prenatal care among adolescents.[44] Adolescents receiving good prenatal care exhibit pregnancy outcomes that are no different from, or better than, those of other women, according to several studies.[1] The problem, of course, is that adolescents, especially the very young, are much less likely to receive any prenatal care or, if they do, are more likely to initiate it later in the pregnancy.[50,59] The reasons for such behavior include not recognizing the pregnancy or desiring to conceal it, not realizing that prenatal care is valuable or available, and not being able to afford it.

When family background characteristics of mothers are controlled by comparing the health of children of sisters who gave birth at different ages, the effects of teen childbearing are mixed and modest.[23] For both blacks and whites, comparisons within sister-pairs (one who had a child as a teenager and one who did not) revealed less adverse effects for infants than did traditional cross-section comparisons. Generally, the differentials for whites were narrowed and for blacks were eliminated or even reversed. Compared with their sisters who first gave birth at older ages, black teen mothers were no more likely to smoke during pregnancy or to have low-birthweight babies and no less likely to breastfeed their infants and to bring them to clinics for well-baby visits. The situation was generally the opposite among whites.

One positive health consequence of teenage childbearing has been identified. The risk of breast cancer increases with the age at which a woman delivers her first full-term child. A woman who bears a child before the age of 18 faces about one-third the risk of a woman whose first birth occurs after the age of 35.[62]

Infant/child health. Comparisons of the children of sisters have also been used to examine the effects of teenage motherhood on the cognitive and socioemotional development of children.[25] For a cross-sectional sample in which the effects of family background are not controlled, the children of women who had first births after age 19 scored consistently better on measures related to child cognitive development than children of teen mothers. But in the sisters comparison, children of teen mothers did no worse than their first cousins whose mothers had first births after age 19. One surprising finding, in light of the racial differences found in infant and maternal health, was that children of white teen mothers did better than their first cousins according to indicators of cognitive development, while children of black teen mothers differed little from their first cousins. British and U.S. studies show that cognitive development of the child is influenced by the age of the mother even after the effects of background variables have been controlled. Children of young mothers fare less well, though the difference is small. In contrast, the results for the social and emotional development of the child are rather inconclusive. In all these studies, however, maternal age proved to have much less influence than did the socioeconomic variables.[1,40,47]

SOCIOECONOMIC CONSEQUENCES

Evidence from the United States suggests that women who have first births at an early age bear subsequent children more rapidly and have more unwanted and out-of-wedlock births, face greater marital instability, are more poorly educated, and have fewer assets and lower incomes later in life.[64] All these conclusions are drawn from studies in which the effects of some important background variables, particularly childhood achievement and motivation, could not be controlled because data were not available. It is plausible, for example, that the lower educational attainment of adolescent mothers is not caused by their having given birth at an early age. They may have left school, even if they had not become pregnant, because they were bored or performing poorly.

One study that does address this issue directly demonstrates that although the adverse outcomes associated with early childbearing are reduced, they are not eliminated when the effects of pre-existing factors are controlled.[6] This study matched each woman who bore a child before age 18 to a woman who did not, on the bases of pre-existing socioeconomic status, academic achievement, aptitude, and educational expectations. The matched sample was used to study differences between groups for selected outcome variables. By age 29, only half of the women in the youngest childbearing group (under age 18) received high school diplomas, whereas nearly all those who postponed childbearing until after age 20 graduated from high school. Similar results hold for college degrees: only 2% of those who bore a child before age 18 obtained a degree before age 29 compared with 22% of those who had not given birth by age 24. Those who bore their first child at an early age also bore subsequent children more rapidly than those who postponed childbearing.

Analysis of data from three national surveys replicates findings from previous studies demonstrating that teenage childbearing leads to substantial long-term socioeconomic disadvantage when those who have births as teens are compared with all those who do not. This finding holds even when the effects of some background characteristics such as mother's and father's education and respondent upbringing in a single-parent family are controlled.[24] These conventional controls, however, may not adequately make the two groups (teen mothers versus others) similar enough that the estimated effect of a teen birth can be interpreted as a causal effect.

When the comparison group is confined to the sisters (who did not have births as teenagers) of the teenage mothers, a different conclusion emerges. In two of the three surveys, standard comparisons seriously overstate the costs of teenage childbearing. In the third survey, the methodology based on sister comparisons leads to the same conclusion as the conventional methodology that controls for several background characteristics.[24,30]

However, even sister comparisons may overstate the deleterious consequences of teen childbearing because they may reflect differences between sisters that are unrelated to the age at first birth. For example, parents may favor, starting at an early age, the daughter they perceive to be the more able. Evidence for this concern arises from the fact that in two of three national surveys, sister comparisons show that a teen birth is associated with a lower probability of graduation from high school. Another study that carefully assessed the timing of the sequence of events (school dropout, pregnancy, and birth) yielded a different conclusion. Models controlling for the effects of several background characteristics show that neither having a birth nor being pregnant (among those who carry the pregnancy to term) while in school increases the risk of subsequently dropping out. Another model reveals that having a birth after dropping out reduces the rate at which women progress to graduation.[68]

Work on (primarily) black adolescents living in Baltimore who became pregnant between 1965 and 1967 has emphasized that the popular belief that early childbearing invariably leads to dropping out of school, many subsequent unwanted births, and welfare dependency is grossly oversimplified. In the period up to 5 years following the birth of their first child, these adolescent mothers did very poorly when compared with their peers who did not bear children. But a follow-up study in 1984 revealed that a substantial majority finished high school, found regular employment, and eventually escaped dependence on welfare.[22] Nevertheless, the authors concluded that the degree of flexibility that teenage mothers have in manipulating their circumstances in later life is definitely limited and that, on average, these women did not fare as well as they would have had they been able to postpone childbearing. Their analysis of which adolescent mothers were more likely to "succeed" later in life is revealing though hardly surprising. Young mothers who had been doing well in school, who had high educational aspirations, and who had more economically secure and better-educated parents were more likely to succeed. Furthermore, those who had no more children in the 5 years following their first birth had fewer constraints in attending school and accruing job experience. The one-quarter of women who remained poor and dependent on welfare were the most likely to experience problems in later life. Hence, identifying this high-risk group is particularly important.

Given these adverse conditions associated with teenage childbearing, one would expect that the children of teenage parents would be relatively disadvantaged. Indeed, such children are more likely to exhibit lower academic achievement and to show a tendency to repeat the early marriage, early childbearing, and high fertility cycle of their parents, even when the effects of other background variables are controlled.[5] The poor educational performance of the children of adolescent mothers is particularly pronounced and debilitating.[22] To what extent the adverse conditions are truly consequences of teenage childbearing as opposed to simply reflecting the pre-existing poorer life chances of women who give birth as teens is still an open question. These adverse conditions are most likely to be found when the mother raises children without the support of the father or her own parents. Fortunately, a finding common to several studies is that those who have children at very young ages are less likely to leave the parental home and are therefore able to achieve a better childrearing environment.[1]

STRATEGIES TO SOLVE THE PROBLEM

The preceding survey of levels and trends in adolescent sexual activity, pregnancy, and childbearing and of the determinants and consequences of such behavior provides insight for evaluating strategies to solve the adolescent pregnancy and STD "problem."

PROMOTING CHASTITY

The most effective way to reduce the incidence of adolescent pregnancy and STDs would be to reduce the proportion of adolescents having sexual intercourse. This is a goal shared by all. However, there is sharp disagreement about whether the best strategy is an abstinence-only approach, an abstinence-based approach that also includes sex and contraceptive education, or an abstinence-based approach that includes not only sex and contraceptive education but also provision of contraceptive services.

The abstinence-only approach is precisely the strategy advocated by social conservatives (particularly organizations such as Right to Life, Concerned Women for America, and American Life League) and embodied in the Adolescent Family Life Act (PL97-75), which has provided millions of dollars per year since 1975 to "promote self-discipline and other prudent approaches to the problem of adolescent premarital sexual relations ... and ... promote adoption as an alternative to adolescent parents." With very few exceptions, rigorous evaluations of the effects on sexual behavior of demonstration projects funded by this act are noticeably lacking. Two evaluations that have been published[11,57] offer no support for the notion that programs that only encourage premarital abstinence can prevent adolescent sexual activity. In contrast, participants in two programs (one a series of parent-daughter workshops designed to delay the onset of intercourse and the other an assertiveness training program designed to help young teenage girls say and mean "No") were only about half as likely to have sexual intercourse for the first time during a 1-year period as were nonparticipants.[26] However, it is far from clear that the differences between the groups are due to program participation because assignment was not random. Instead, those who voluntarily enrolled in the programs constituted the treatment group while those who did not enroll in any program served as the control group. Therefore, it is possible, indeed likely, that participants were self-selected for a higher propensity to remain virgins.

Sex education programs that emphasize personal responsibility among young adolescents and also provide information about sexuality and contraception can postpone the initiation of sexual activity. Such programs move beyond "Just Say No" to help adolescents develop concrete skills for managing interpersonal challenges, such as how to say no to sex when there is no condom or how not to have sex while not losing one's boyfriend.[17,32,35] As discussed below, a more comprehensive strategy that also includes provision of contraceptive services can be effective not only in delaying the onset of first intercourse but also in reducing the incidence of adolescent pregnancy.

PROMOTING CONTRACEPTIVE USE

Given that more than half of unmarried adolescents are sexually active, a practical strategy for reducing adolescent pregnancy would be to promote the effective practice of contraception. Likewise, promoting the use of condoms is a practical strategy for reducing the incidence of STDs, including HIV. This task is formidable. Legitimating the use of currently available contraceptives (including condoms for STD prophylaxis) and making them widely available would require fundamental changes in philosophy on the part of many parents and clinicians; the media; the schools; youth agencies; local, state and federal governments; and the general public. Improving the availability of contraceptives is a difficult enough goal, but it would be much more effective if ways could be found to increase the demand for contraceptives by strengthening the motivation to avoid pregnancy and STDs.

Although the European experience does show that adolescents can use contraceptives very effectively to prevent pregnancy even when the fraction with sexual experience is quite high, three factors that inhibit demand in the United States are largely absent in the United Kingdom, France, The Netherlands, and Sweden: high levels of a fundamentalist, antisex type of religiosity, large pockets of deep poverty, and misunderstanding about the risks and benefits of the pill. The first two factors would be very hard to change because they are such a part of the social fabric.

Antisex fundamentalism. The United States exhibits a sort of religiosity that judges many types of sexual activity, particularly sexual relations among unmarried persons, to be immoral. A belief that protecting "traditional values" is of paramount importance hinders not only the public provision of contraception but also the public discussion about many sexual matters. Concern about the morality of sex, while by no means absent, has less impact on public policy in the other countries. This fundamentalist antisexuality is all the more problematic because messages extolling sexuality are so pervasive in our culture. Unfortunately, as we all recognize, the culture does not promote healthy sexuality (including the use of contraception). Thus, while the "Just Say No" message of the social conservatives is overwhelmed by a permissive sexual culture, any effective countervailing force promoting contraceptive use is absent.

Pockets of deep poverty.   The unequal distribution of income and the existence of a semipermanent underclass in the United States guarantee that many poor adolescents will perceive that they are not sacrificing a bright future by having a child. In the other countries, the state redistributes income to a far greater extent. Moreover, public education, health care delivery, and other social services are more centrally controlled, thereby enabling the establishment of national policies far less subject to the influence of local interest groups.

Myths about the pill.   Reliance on the most effective method of pregnancy prevention, the pill, is much smaller in the United States than in the other countries, among both adolescents and older women. Despite the evidence that the pill is a good pregnancy-prevention method for sexually active adolescents (and almost all women), public perceptions in the United States are heavily influenced by myth (particularly about cancer, future fecundity, and other side effects).[37] Pills in the United States, except in selected clinics, are also much more expensive than in the other countries, where health services in general and contraceptive services in particular are heavily subsidized for all persons.

Increasing the effective practice of contraception is difficult in part because all currently available contraceptives require the type of abstract thinking about the future that many teens have not developed. Hence, a new contraceptive that could be used at the end of cycles during which intercourse occurred (thereby reducing the importance of planning ahead), had few side effects, was relatively inexpensive, and did not require a visit to a physician could reduce adolescent pregnancy significantly. A technological solution is unlikely, however, because (1) such a method would be considered to be an abortifacient and therefore not eligible for federal research and development support and (2) drug companies generally do not believe that developing new contraceptives is profitable.[43] Nevertheless, more effective promotion of currently available "morning after" contraception could significantly reduce unintended pregnancies among teens.[66]

Another problem is that the most effective methods for preventing pregnancy do not reduce the risk of STD transmission. Many health practitioners are concerned that teens will switch from pills to condoms and that the pregnancy rate will consequently rise. Many fear that it will be difficult to convince teens to use both pills and condoms.

INTERVENING THROUGH THE SCHOOLS

The schools are not the cause of adolescent pregnancy, and they cannot be restructured to cure the problem in the absence of other efforts.

Nevertheless, we have little doubt that a combination of providing sex education in the schools, including the provision of contraception information to students at an early age and making contraceptive services widely available, would increase contraceptive utilization rates. Although experience in The Netherlands (where sex education is conducted through a mass media approach) shows that a school-linked approach may not be necessary, we argue that the incidence of teenage pregnancy and STDs could be reduced far more substantially at far less cost if the schools were involved. All adolescents attend school, and broad-based programs seem more likely to foster changes in attitudes and behavior through peer communication.

School-linked interventions can take several forms. One, the first to be evaluated with baseline data and controls, combined sex education, counseling, and contraceptive services in two schools serving predominantly poor inner-city blacks in Baltimore.[73,74,75] The same clinicians who staffed a special off-campus clinic for students in a junior and senior high school also gave lectures, led discussions, and offered individual counseling in the schools during the regular school day. After school hours, the clinic offered additional educational sessions and registered both males and females for individual counseling with a social worker and for contraceptive services. After 28 months of operation, pregnancy rates had decreased more than 30% in the program schools, while they had increased almost 60% in the control schools. Although the success of the program lends strong support to the concept of a school-based model, it is only one of a range of options.[15,16,34] In some situations, the clinic may be categorically oriented to reproductive health. In others, it may provide more general medical and dental services, particularly when it is the only source of care for the targeted population. Comprehensive clinics have the double advantages of (1) not making the reason for a visit immediately obvious to the client's peers or the school administration and (2) teaching adolescents *to use* the system for *all* their health care needs. In some cases the clinic may be located in the school. In other situations, particularly in a politically charged atmosphere, it may be located off campus. Clinics located outside the school can remain open in the evenings, on the weekends, and in the summer when the schools are closed, and they may have more flexibility in serving those who are not currently enrolled.

Several prerequisites for success are necessary.

- First, educational, counseling, and medical (including contraceptive) services must be easily available.

- Second, such services must be provided by, and must be perceived to be provided by, well-trained professionals in a dignified and confidential setting.

- Third, the community must support the program. Without such support, programs have been killed by a tiny minority of opponents.
- Fourth, adequate funding must be available. Separate funding for adolescent family planning invites political controversy but seems necessary because adolescents are not well-served by programs oriented to adults.

The major problem with school-linked programs is that very few can properly be considered interventions *for pregnancy prevention* because they do not offer contraceptive services but instead refer students to other programs, which are aimed primarily at adult women. In practice, there is no real option to make school-linked programs either comprehensive or categorically oriented to reproductive health. Political considerations ensure that programs follow the comprehensive model and that the real decision is whether and to what degree to include family planning services. Ironically, school-linked clinics are *perceived* to be pregnancy prevention centers. Therefore, any global evaluations of school-linked programs will undoubtedly conclude that they are generally ineffective at reducing pregnancy, when in fact the majority are not really designed to do so.

COMMUNITY-WIDE STRATEGIES

Community support is essential for the implementation of pregnancy or STD prevention programs. Community-wide strategies for pregnancy prevention include abstinence education, encouraging contraceptive use when teens do become sexually active, and providing reasons to postpone sexual intercourse or pregnancy by enhancing life options.[3] Joint efforts between diverse community-based agencies (schools, parent groups, health agencies, and youth-serving agencies, community service organizations, churches, media, and businesses) are becoming increasingly important as a means of developing community-wide service delivery programs. Model programs and detailed practical suggestions for successful implementation are described in an excellent guidebook.[2]

Such a strategy was adopted in one community in South Carolina. Before the implementation of a school/community program aimed primarily at reducing adolescent pregnancy by postponing sexual intercourse among virgins and secondarily at promoting contraceptive use among the sexually active, pregnancy rates among women aged 14-17 were among the highest in the state. The program involved the entire community: teachers, religious leaders, social service professionals, community leaders, parents, children, and the media. The goal was to saturate the community with large quantities of pregnancy-prevention educational messages, primarily those promoting the postponement of initial voluntary intercourse. In the 3-year period following introduction of the program, pregnancy rates fell 54% compared with increases in pregnancy rates in three comparison counties.[70]

Originally described as an abstinence plus sex and contraceptive education program, the results seemed to indicate that the active support of the entire community could substitute for actual provision of contraceptive services. A re-evaluation of the program revealed, however, that in fact a school nurse both distributed condoms to males and transported females to family planning clinics run by the health department. The nurse's activities and the community efforts were synergistic. When the active participation of the community waned, pregnancy rates began to rise.[38] Hence, the evidence indicates that a community-wide strategy that includes provision of contraceptive services can effectively reduce rates of adolescent pregnancy.

AMELIORATING THE CONSEQUENCES OF CHILDBEARING

A final strategy commanding wide public support is to ameliorate the negative consequences of adolescent childbearing. Demonstration projects have focused on three priorities for adolescent mothers:

- Ensuring a safe pregnancy and delivery;
- Staying in school (particularly to increase employability); and
- Avoiding additional unintended pregnancies.

Health interventions are very effective. For young women in any socioeconomic category, adequate prenatal and obstetrical care greatly reduces the adverse health consequences to mother and child associated with pregnancy and childbirth at an early age.[4,40]

Some prenatal home-visitation programs for socially disadvantaged women are effective in improving women's health-related behaviors during pregnancy, reducing the incidence of preterm births and low birthweight, and reducing subsequent unintended pregnancies. The more effective programs employ nurses who visit frequently enough during pregnancy and after delivery to establish a therapeutic alliance with the family and who address the material, social, psychological, and behavioral factors associated with maternal and child health. Results of randomized trials of home-visitation programs reveal that attempts to isolate only a few important aspects of such interventions are misguided. Social support during pregnancy is ineffective at improving pregnancy outcomes unless adverse maternal health behaviors are altered. Prenatal home visits alone, without continuing comprehensive postnatal visits, are insufficient to promote well-being past delivery.[51,52]

The next priorities after ensuring a healthy delivery are to keep the mother in school and to prevent further unintended pregnancies. The results of Project Redirection—a comprehensive program whose participants (who were extremely disadvantaged when compared not only with teenagers generally but also with other teen parents) were asked to organize and frequently reorient aspects of their lives while pursuing an education, training for a job, and learning about family planning—are sobering. When compared with those not in the program who served as controls, Redirection participants were more likely to be in school or have graduated, less likely to have become pregnant, and more likely to be practicing contraception at the time of the 1-year follow-up. After 2 years, however, the differentials had vanished.[56] This finding led the investigators to conclude that the impact of the intervention lasted no longer than the participants' stay in the program. Although Project Redirection was based on a research design substantially more rigorous than is typical for teenage parent programs, the comparison group had much wider access to local social service programs than had been anticipated. Thus, comparison of Redirection participants and controls does not reveal the difference in outcomes between "no treatment" and "comprehensive treatment" groups. A supplementary analysis compared four groups: Redirection participants in the program from 1–2 years, Redirection participants in the program for less than 1 year, controls who were ever in a similar program, and controls who were never in any program. The results, which must be interpreted with caution since the outcomes could reflect systematic variation in uncontrolled characteristics such as motivation, suggest that the more services a mother received, the better she performed. Nevertheless, the most reasonable conclusion is that short-term assistance does not have a long-term impact on educational attainment or subsequent pregnancy.

A 5-year follow-up of Project Redirection confirmed this conclusion: the experimental and control groups had equal educational attainment and equal numbers of subsequent pregnancies, on average. The experimental group actually had a greater average number of subsequent births (but fewer abortions) than the control group. In contrast, Redirection participants, when compared with controls, worked more hours and had higher weekly earnings from employment, were less likely to be receiving welfare, and scored higher on a widely used test of parenting ability. Moreover, participants' children showed better cognitive skills and exhibited fewer behavioral problems.[55] These results, though confirming that an intensive short-term program cannot eliminate the long-term disadvantages conferred by poverty, do provide a basis for believing that the prospects for disadvantaged teenage mothers and their children can be improved by such an intervention.

Project Redirection is perhaps the best example of a comprehensive program for pregnant teenagers. Such programs have considerable appeal because they focus on the individual *after* she becomes pregnant, thereby avoiding the controversy surrounding the prevention of adolescent pregnancy and the seemingly insoluble problem of poverty. Moreover, focusing on local communities and the coordination of local programs appears to circumvent the need for additional resources. However, a review of the quality of such comprehensive programs has concluded that the comprehensive model is better suited to political compromise and rhetoric than to effective problem-solving.[71] The authors argue that many comprehensive programs are based on three faulty assumptions: (1) that the requisite services are already locally available and need only be stitched together administratively, (2) that this goal can be accomplished without a further infusion of state and federal financial assistance, and (3) that the adolescent pregnancy problem can be best addressed by targeting services to those already pregnant.

In summary, short-term interventions aimed at ensuring a safe pregnancy and delivery, reducing subsequent fertility, and enhancing educational attainment are expensive, and only those focused on prenatal care appear to be truly effective. The lesson to be learned is that *no band-aid, quick-fix, inexpensive solutions exist for ameliorating the negative outcomes associated with adolescent childbearing.* Given such outcomes—rapid subsequent fertility, low educational attainment, poor marriage prospects, high rates of marital dissolution, and out-of-wedlock childbearing—it is not surprising that a strong association exists between early childbearing and subsequent poverty.[29] Three of four Aid to Families of Dependent Children (AFDC) recipients under age 30 had a first birth as a teenager.[46] A compelling question of public policy, therefore, is the relative effectiveness of fertility prevention versus ameliorative schemes for reducing poverty. Research suggests that preventing adolescent childbearing would be far more effective in reducing the proportion of young women who require public assistance than would increasing education, increasing marriage probabilities, or reducing subsequent fertility among adolescent mothers.[48] Such a finding is reassuring, because the public cost associated with teenage childbearing is substantial. In 1990 over $25 billion was paid through three programs (AFDC, food stamps, and Medicaid) to women who first gave birth as teenagers.[8] The public will pay an average of $18,133 over the next 20 years for each family begun by a first birth to a teenager in 1990. Suppose that this association was truly causal. Then, if all teenage births were delayed until the mother was at least 20 years old, the potential public savings would be $7,253 for each birth delayed and an aggregate $7.15 billion for all births delayed.

However, the revisionist view of the consequences of teenage childbearing warns that the conventional estimates such as those presented above overstate—perhaps substantially—the costs of teenage childbearing and therefore the benefits of reducing its incidence. The subtle danger is that this new work will

> be used to argue that because teen pregnancy is not the linchpin that holds together myriad other social ills, it is not a problem at all. Concern about teen pregnancy has at least directed attention and resources to young, poor, and minority women. It has awakened many Americans to their diminished life chances. If measures aimed at reducing teen pregnancy are not the quick fix for much of what ails American society, there is the powerful temptation to forget these young women altogether and allow them to slip back to their traditional invisible place in American public debate. Teen pregnancy is less about young women and their sex lives than it is about restricted horizons and the boundaries of hope. It is about race and class and how those realities limit opportunities for young people. Most centrally, however, it is typically about being young, female, poor, and non-white and about how having a child seems to be one of the few avenues of satisfaction, fulfillment, and self-esteem. It would be a tragedy to stop worrying about these young women—and their partners—because their behavior is the measure rather than the cause of their blighted hopes.[39]

Perhaps the best argument for supporting programs to reduce the incidence of adolescent pregnancy is not one based on negative consequences or public costs but instead one that simply stresses the fact that the overwhelming majority of pregnant adolescents do not intend to become pregnant. That adolescents want to avoid becoming pregnant is sufficient reason for helping them to do so.

SUGGESTED READING

- Alan Guttmacher Institute (AGI). Teenage pregnancy: the problem that hasn't gone away. New York NY: Alan Guttmacher Institute, 1981.
- Hayes CD (ed). Risking the future: adolescent sexuality, pregnancy and childbearing, Volume I. Washington DC: National Academy Press, 1987.
- Henshaw SK, Kenney AM, Somberg D, van Vort J. Teenage pregnancy in the United States: the scope of the problem and state responses. New York NY: Alan Guttmacher Institute, 1989.
- Hofferth SL, Hayes CD (eds). Risking the future: adolescent sexuality, pregnancy, and childbearing, Volume II. Washington DC: National Academy Press, 1987.

REFERENCES

1. Baldwin W, Cain VS. The children of teenage parents. Fam Plann Perspect 1980;12(1):34-43.

2. Brindis CD. Adolescent pregnancy prevention: a guidebook for communities. Palo Alto CA: Stanford Health Promotion Resource Center, Stanford Center for Research in Disease Prevention, 1991.

3. Brindis C. Reducing adolescent pregnancy: the next steps for program, research, and policy. Fam Life Educator 1990;9(1):3-62.

4. Brown SS. Can low birthweight be prevented? Fam Plann Perspect 1985; 17(3):112-118.

5. Card JJ. Long-term consequences for children of teenage parents. Demography 1981;18(2):137-156.

6. Card JJ, Wise LL. Teenage mothers and teenage fathers: the impact of early childbearing on the parents' personal and professional lives. Fam Plann Perspect 1978;10(4):199-205.

7. Cates W. Teenagers and sexual risk taking: the best of times and the worst of times. J Adolesc Health 1991;12(2):84-94.

8. Center for Population Options. Teenage pregnancy and too-early childbearing: public costs, personal consequences. Washington DC: Center for Population Options, 1992.

9. Centers for Disease Control. Division of STD/HIV prevention annual report, 1991. Atlanta GA: Centers for Disease Control, 1992.

10. Centers for Disease Control and Prevention. HIV/AIDS surveillance: year-end edition. Atlanta GA: Centers for Disease Control and Prevention, 1993.

11. Christopher FS, Roosa MW. An evaluation of an adolescent pregnancy prevention program: is "Just say no" enough. Fam Relat 1990;39(1):68-72.

12. Dash L. When children want children: an inside look at the crisis of teenage parenthood. New York NY: Viking Penguin, 1990.

13. Dash L. When children want children: the urban crisis of teenage childbearing. New York NY: William Morrow, 1989.

14. Dawson DA. The effects of sex education on adolescent behavior. Fam Plann Perspect 1986;18(4):162-170.

15. Dryfoos J. School-based health clinics: a new approach to preventing adolescent pregnancy? Fam Plann Perspect 1985;17(2):70-75.

16. Dryfoos JG. School-based health clinics: three years of experience. Fam Plann Perspect 1988;20(4):193-200.

17. Eisen M, Zellman GL, McAlister AL. Evaluating the impact of a theory-based sexuality and contraceptive education program. Fam Plann Perspect 1990; 22(6):261-271.

18. Forrest JD, Silverman J. What public school teachers teach about preventing pregnancy, AIDS and sexually transmitted diseases. Fam Plann Perspect 1989;21(2):65-72.

19. Forrest JD, Singh S. The sexual and reproductive behavior of American women, 1982-1988. Fam Plann Perspect 1990;22(5):206-214.

20. Furstenberg FF. Unplanned parenthood: the social consequences of teenage childbearing. New York NY: The Free Press, 1976.

21. Furstenberg FF, Moore KA, Peterson JL. Sex education and sexual experience among adolescents. Am J Public Health 1985;75(11):1331-1332.

22. Furstenberg FF, Brooks-Gunn J, Morgan SP. Adolescent mothers and their children in later life. Fam Plann Perspect 1987;19(4):142-151.

23. Geronimus AT, Korenman S. Maternal youth or family background? On the health disadvantages of infants with teenage mothers. Am J Epidemiol 1993;137(2):213-225.

24. Geronimus AT, Korenman S. The socioeconomic consequences of teen child-bearing reconsidered. Q J Econ 1992;107(4):1187-1214.

25. Geronimus AT, Korenman S, Hillemeier MM. Does young maternal age adversely affect child development? Evidence from cousin comparisons. Popul Dev Rev 1994; 20 (in press).

26. Girls Incorporated. Truth, trust and technology: new research on preventing adolescent pregnancy. Indianapolis IN/New York NY: Girls Incorporated, 1991.

27. Hardy JB, Duggan AK, Masnyk K, Pearson C. Fathers of children born to young urban mothers. Fam Plann Perspect 1989;21(4):159-163, 187.

28. Henshaw SK. U.S. teenage pregnancy statistics. New York NY: Alan Guttmacher Institute, 1992.

29. Hofferth SL, Moore KA. Early childbearing and later economic well-being. Am Sociol Rev 1979;44(5):784-815.

30. Hoffman SD, Foster EM, Furstenberg FF. Re-evaluating the costs of teenage childbearing. Demography 1993;30(1):1-13.

31. Hollingsworth DR, Kotchen JM, Felice ME. Impact of gynecologic age on outcome of adolescent pregnancy. In: McAnarney ER (ed). Premature adolescent pregnancy and parenthood. New York NY: Grune and Stratton, 1983:169-190.

32. Howard M, McCabe JB. Helping teenagers postpone sexual involvement. Fam Plann Perspect 1990;22(1):21-26.

33. Jones EF, Forrest JD, Goldman N, Henshaw S, Lincoln R, Rossoff JI, Westoff CF, Wulf D. Teenage pregnancy in industrialized countries. New Haven CT: Yale University Press, 1986. Summarized in Jones EF, Forrest JD, Goldman N, Henshaw S, Lincoln R, Rossoff JI, Westoff CF, Wulf D. Teenage pregnancy in developed countries: determinants and policy implications. Fam Plann Perspect 1985;17(2):53-63.

34. Kenney AM. School-based clinics: a national conference. Fam Plann Perspect 1986;18(1):44-46.

35. Kirby D, Barth RP, Lelend N, Fetro JV. Reducing the risk: impact of a new curriculum on sexual risk taking. Fam Plann Perspect 1991;23(6):253-263.

36. Kirby D, Waszak C, Ziegler J. Six school-based clinics: their reproductive health services and impact on sexual behavior. Fam Plann Perspect 1991;23(1):6-16.

37. Kisker EE. Teenagers talk about sex, pregnancy and contraception. Fam Plann Perspect 1985;17(2):83-90.

38. Koo HP, Dunteman GH, George C, Green Y, Vincent M. Reducing adolescent pregnancy through a school and community-based intervention: Denmark, South Carolina, revisited. Research Triangle Park NC: Research Triangle Institute, 1992

39. Luker K. Dubious conceptions: the controversy over teen pregnancy. Am Prospect 1991;5:73-83.

40. Makinson C. The health consequences of teenage fertility. Fam Plann Perspect 1985;17(3):132-139.

41. Marsiglio W. Adolescent fathers in the United States: their initial living arrangements, marital experience, and educational outcomes. Fam Plann Perspect 1987;19(6):240-251.

42. Marsiglio W, Mott FL. The impact of sex education on sexual activity, contraceptive use, and premarital pregnancy among American teenagers. Fam Plann Perspect 1986;18(4):151-162.

43. Mastroianni L, Donaldson PJ, Kane TT (eds). Developing new contraceptives: obstacles and opportunities. Washington DC: National Academy Press, 1990.

44. McAnarney ER, Thiede HA. Adolescent pregnancy and childbearing: what we learned during the 1970s and what remains to be learned. In: McAnarney ER (ed). Premature adolescent pregnancy and parenthood. New York NY: Grune and Stratton, 1983:375-395.

45. Menken J. The health and demographic consequences of adolescent pregnancy and childbearing. In: Chilman CS (ed). Adolescent pregnancy and childbearing: findings from research. Washington DC: United States Government Printing Office, 1980:157-200.

46. Moore KA, Burt MR. Private crisis, public cost: policy perspectives on teenage childbearing. Washington DC: The Urban Institute Press, 1982.

47. Moore KA, Snyder NO. Cognitive attainment among firstborn children of adolescent mothers. Am Sociol Rev 1991;56(5):612-624.

48. Moore KA, Wertheimer RF. Teenage childbearing and welfare: preventive and ameliorative strategies. Fam Plann Perspect 1984;16(6):285-289.

49. Mosher WD, Horn MC. First family planning visits by young women. Fam Plann Perspect 1988;20(1):33-40.

50. National Center for Health Statistics. Advance report of final natality statistics, 1989. Mon Vital Stat Rep 1991;40(8-Suppl):1-55.

51. Olds DL. Home visitation for pregnant women and parents of young children. Am J Dis Child 1992;146(6):704-708.

52. Olds DL, Kitzman H. Can home visitation improve the health of women and children at environmental risk? Pediatrics 1990;86(1):108-116.

53. Orr MT, Forrest JD. The availability of reproductive health services from U.S. private physicians. Fam Plann Perspect 1985;17(2):63-69.

54. Parke RD, Neville B. Teenage fatherhood. In: Hofferth SL, Hayes CD (eds). Risking the future: adolescent sexuality, pregnancy, and childbearing, Volume II. Washington DC: National Academy Press, 1987:145-173.

55. Polit DF. Effects of a comprehensive program for teenage parents: five years after Project Redirection. Fam Plann Perspect 1989;21(4):164-169, 187.

56. Polit DF, Kahn JR. Project Redirection: evaluation of a comprehensive program for disadvantaged teenage mothers. Fam Plann Perspect 1985;17(4):150-155.

57. Roosa MW, Christopher FS. Evaluation of an abstinence-only adolescent pregnancy prevention program: a replication. Fam Relat 1990;39(4):363-367.

58. Saluter AF. Marital status and living arrangements: March 1991. U.S. Bureau of the Census, Current Population Reports: Population Estimates and Projections, Series P-20, No. 461, 1992.

59. Singh S, Torres A, Forrest JD. The need for prenatal care in the United States: evidence from the 1980 national natality survey. Fam Plann Perspect 1985; 17(3):118-124.

60. Sonenstein FL, Pleck JH, Ku LC. Sexual activity, condom use, and AIDS awareness among adolescent males. Fam Plann Perspect 1989;21(4):152-158.

61. Sonenstein FL, Pleck JH, Ku LC. Levels of sexual activity among adolescent males in the United States. Fam Plann Perspect 1991;23(4):162-167.

62. Speroff L, Glass RH, Kase NG. Clinical gynecologic endocrinology and infertility. Baltimore MD: Williams and Wilkins, 1989.

63. Strobino DM. The health and medical consequences of adolescent sexuality and pregnancy: a review of the literature. In: Hofferth SL, Hayes CD (eds). Risking the future: adolescent sexuality, pregnancy, and childbearing, Vol. II. Washington DC: National Academy Press, 1987:93-122.

64. Trussell J. Teenage pregnancy in the United States. Fam Plann Perspect 1988;20(6):262-272.

65. Trussell J, Kost K. Contraceptive failure in the United States: a critical review of the literature. Stud Fam Plann 1987;18(5):237-283.

66. Trussell J, Stewart F, Guest F, Hatcher RA. Emergency contraceptive pills (ECPs): a simple proposal to reduce unintended pregnancies. Fam Plann Perspect 1992;24(6):269-273.

67. Trussell J, Vaughan B. Selected results concerning sexual behavior and contraceptive use from the 1988 National Survey of Family Growth and the 1988 National Survey of Adolescent Males. Working Paper #91-12. Princeton NJ: Office of Population Research, Princeton University, 1991.

68. Upchurch DM, McCarthy, J. The timing of a first birth and high school completion. Am Sociol Rev 1990;55(2):224-234.

69. U.S. Bureau of the Census. United States population estimates, by age and sex, based on the 1990 census: 1990 and 1991. Suitland MD: U.S. Bureau of the Census, April 16, 1992.

70. Vincent ML, Clearie AF, Schluchter MD. Reducing adolescent pregnancy through school and community-based education. JAMA 1987;257(24):3382-3386.

71. Weatherley RA, Perlman SB, Levine MH, Klerman LV. Comprehensive programs for pregnant teenagers and teenage parents: how successful have they been? Fam Plann Perspect 1986;18(2):73-78.

72. Westoff CF, Calot G, Foster AD. Teenage fertility in developed nations, 1971-1980. Int Fam Plann Perspect 1983;9(2):45-50. Also published in Fam Plann Perspect 1983;15(3):105-110.

73. Zabin LS, Hirsch MB, Smith EA, Streett R, Hardy JB. Evaluation of a pregnancy prevention program for urban teenagers. Fam Plann Perspect 1986; 18(3):119-126.

74. Zabin LS, Hirsch MB, Streett R, Emerson MR, Smith M, Hardy JB, King TM. The Baltimore pregnancy prevention program for urban teenagers. I. How did it work? Fam Plann Perspect 1988a;20(4):182-187.

75. Zabin LS, Hirsch MB, Smith EA, Smith M, Emerson MR, King TM, Streett R, Hardy JB. The Baltimore pregnancy prevention program for urban teenagers. II. What did it cost? Fam Plann Perspect 1988b;20(4):188-192.

76. Zabin LS, Kantner JF, Zelnik M. The risk of adolescent pregnancy in the first months of intercourse. Fam Plann Perspect 1979;11(4):215, 217-222.

77. Zelnik M, Kantner JF. Sexual activity, contraceptive use, and pregnancy among metropolitan-area teenagers: 1971-1979. Fam Plann Perspect 1980;12(5):230-237.

78. Zelnik M, Kantner JF. Reasons for nonuse of contraception by sexually active women aged 15-19. Fam Plann Perspect 1979;11(5):289-296.

79. Zelnik M, Kantner JF, Ford K. Sex and pregnancy in adolescence. Beverly Hills CA: Sage Publications, 1981.

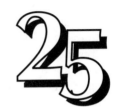

Dynamics of Reproductive Behavior & Population Change

- Contrary to intuition, an abortion does not prevent a birth because the next pregnancy will occur sooner than it otherwise would have.
- Breastfeeding is an important contraceptive for a population even though it may be unreliable for an individual woman or couple.
- Declining fertility inevitably leads to an aging of the population. Caring for an increasing proportion of elderly persons will be a significant problem in many countries.

- Current population growth rates are very high by historical standards and cannot possibly persist indefinitely.
- In developing countries, urbanization occurs primarily because births outnumber deaths, not because of migration from rural to urban areas.
- The impact of AIDS on mortality rates and population growth could be dramatic and devastating in certain areas of the world, particularly in sub-Saharan Africa and Asia.

In the United States, according to current experience, an average woman will bear just under two children in a lifetime that will last about 79 years. In Rwanda, an average woman currently will produce eight children; her life expectancy at birth is around 51 years. We will explore some of the reasons for these differences in the following sections. We will also examine the consequences of rapid population growth, the concepts of population momentum and population aging, and the results of governmental population policy.

Why should these issues be of concern to family planning practitioners? As firm believers in voluntary family planning, the authors of this book stress that we are dedicated to helping individuals achieve their reproductive life goals, whatever they may be. Nevertheless, individual reproductive choices do have aggregate consequences, since they determine the fertility of a population. It is only natural that those involved in family planning and reproductive health would be interested in understanding how the uses of contraception and its effectiveness, the prevalence of abortion, and the duration of lactation affect the aggregate level of fertility in a population. Providing a framework of analysis for this question is one of the goals of this chapter.

Fertility, however, is only one of the determinants of population change. Providing an understanding of the other two components—mortality and migration—is a second goal. A third goal is to acquaint the reader with a few methodological tools for demographic analysis. We emphasize methodology for the sake of neither rigor nor completeness. Instead, we hope to show that such tools are necessary to avoid common pitfalls when thinking about reproductive issues that are of common concern to us all.

DETERMINANTS OF FERTILITY

Why is fertility high in some populations and low in others? First, the childbearing ages have biologic limits. Between menarche and menopause, a woman has about 35 years in which she can produce children. Clearly these limits do constrain fertility, and they do vary somewhat among populations. Second, different populations vary in the proportions of females at each age who are sexually active and therefore exposed to the risk of pregnancy. Third, the spacing between initiation of sexual activity and the first live birth and in the spacing between one live birth and the next vary across populations.

MENARCHE, MENOPAUSE, AND STERILITY

The average age of menarche normally varies only in a narrow range from about age 12 to about age 15.[21] The average age at menopause is much harder to measure; it is easy for a woman to know whether she has had a first period but hard to know if she has had her last. Ordinarily, menopause is assumed to have occurred if a specified period of time (e.g., 1 or 1¹/₂ years) has passed since the last period. Menopause, too, appears to be largely confined to a rather narrow range, from about age 47 to age 51.[21]

These ranges of ages for menarche and menopause imply childbearing spans that could range from about 32 to 39 years. This difference of 7 years, all other factors being equal, could imply a difference in lifetime fertility of as much as 2-3 children, if, during the added 7 years, women experienced the same fertility rates that prevail in the primary childbearing years. For several reasons the difference is likely to be far smaller. First, as previously mentioned, it is not possible to measure directly the age at which menopause occurs, so that 7 years may be an overestimate of the potential difference.

Second, a difference of several years in estimated age at menopause between two populations, even if real, may mean only that in one population women have a longer period of subfecundity (reduced physiological capacity to produce a live birth) before becoming sterile. What we can observe directly is age at last birth, which seems to be near age 41 for several non-contracepting populations for which we have data.[34] Third, differences in age at menarche are unlikely to result in differences in fertility unless entry into a sexual union is tied closely to menarche. In most populations entry into sexual unions takes place considerably after menarche. Therefore, we conclude that though differences in the childbearing span could affect lifetime fertility, in practice the effect is likely to be small, at most a difference of one child over a lifetime and possibly much smaller.

AGE AT MARRIAGE AND PROPORTIONS MARRIED

A major determinant of fertility differences among populations is age at entry into sustained sexual activity.[5] In many populations, sexual intercourse is primarily confined to marriage, so that we can reformulate the statement as follows: Age at marriage, proportions ever marrying, and patterns of marital dissolution and remarriage are powerful determinants of fertility levels. One way to measure the impact of marriage on fertility is to compare the total fertility rates of married women with the total fertility rates of all women. Maximum fertility would be achieved if all women married at menarche and stayed married until menopause. This marriage pattern does not exist in any population. Estimates of the fertility-reducing effects of actual marriage patterns range from lows of 11% in Bangladesh and 14% in Senegal, to highs of 40% in Korea and 43% in Costa Rica.[12]

While proportions of older women currently married do vary across populations, this variation is too small to account for a large portion of observed fertility differentials, particularly because marital fertility rates fall with age. In contrast, the proportion of young women who are married varies considerably. For example, the fraction married among 15- to 19-year-old women varies from lows of 1% in Japan, 2% in South Korea, and 4% in China, to 69% in Bangladesh, 59% in Nepal, and 44% in India.[16] It has been convincingly demonstrated that even if many developing countries adopted modern contraceptive practices, they are not likely to achieve growth rates lower than 1.5% per year without also raising age at marriage.[27] This argument is purely demographic; raising age at marriage lowers total fertility by removing some young women from exposure to risk of childbearing and raises the mean age at childbearing, thereby lengthening the time between generations.[48]

Raising age at marriage is almost certain, moreover, to have effects other than the purely mechanically demographic. The most important is to enhance the status of women, allowing them to stay in school longer to acquire job-related skills, to work outside the home before marriage, and to enter marriage with more physical and emotional maturity and financial security. Such social changes are themselves likely to stimulate a demand for fertility control.[24] Because raising age at marriage does so profoundly alter the social fabric, governments may be unwilling or unable to use this potential instrument of public policy, and in those populations with a high prevalence of consensual unions or premarital childbearing, a change in the legal minimum age at marriage may have little effect on fertility.

BIRTH INTERVAL LENGTH

Populations also differ widely in the length of time between one birth and the next, known as the birth interval. The shorter the average interval between births, the greater the number of births that can be squeezed into the childbearing span, and vice versa. The birth interval can be divided into three parts: waiting time to a conception leading to a live birth, gestation length, and period of postpartum insusceptibility.[32] The second of these parts, the gestation period, does not vary from population to population. There is, however, considerable variation in the other two components.

Waiting time to conceive. The length of time a sexually active woman must wait before conceiving a pregnancy that leads to a live birth is determined by the underlying fecundity (physiological capacity to produce a live birth) of the male and female, the frequency and timing of intercourse, the prevalence and effectiveness of use of contraception, and the frequency of abortion (both spontaneous and induced). Fetal wastage in the absence of induced abortion is certainly not constant across populations, but it is a relatively unimportant cause of differentials in fertility unless the prevalence of syphilis is high (see Effects of STDs). Likewise, fecundity, which declines with age within a given population, does not seem to vary much among populations unless the prevalence of pelvic inflammatory disease is high (see Effects of STDs). Of these four factors, the prevalence and effectiveness of use of contraception and the frequency of induced abortion are the most important sources of fertility differences.

Postpartum insusceptibility. The period of postpartum insusceptibility is primarily governed by the length of lactation. If women do not breastfeed, this period can be as short as 2 months. With prolonged breastfeeding, the period can be up to $1^1/_2$ years on average. For example, urban Nigerian women with primary education breastfeed for an average of 11 months and do not resume menses for an average of 5 months. In rural Senegal, women breastfeed for about 20 months and amenorrhea lasts for 18 months.[37] The contraceptive effect depends on the intensity (frequency and duration) of the infant's sucking, which in turn is heavily influenced by the extent of supplemental feeding, particularly by bottle (see Chapter 17).[11]

Effects of Breastfeeding and Contraception

Consider a typical developing country in which contraceptive practice is minimal and breastfeeding is virtually universal and prolonged. In the absence of contraception, it typically takes young wives about 6 months to become pregnant. Pregnancy lasts an average of 9 months and post-partum insusceptibility lasts 12 months. Then the total birth interval is $6 + 9 + 12 = 27$ months, or 2.25 years; thus, the typical woman has a birth every 2.25 years, so that the average fertility rate per year is $1/2.25 = 444$ per 1,000 sexually active women.[a] A common effect of modernization is to reduce breastfeeding but increase the use of contraception. However, the first change frequently precedes the second.

If breastfeeding is completely abandoned, the duration of postpartum insusceptibility would be reduced to approximately 2 months and the typical birth interval would fall to $6 + 9 + 2 = 17$ months or 1.4 years. Hence, the fertility rate per year among sexually active women would rise to 706 births per 1,000 women ($12/17 \times 1,000$) from 444 per 1,000—a rise of 59%. This simple calculation demonstrates the importance of lactation as a contraceptive to a population, even though no individual woman may rely dependably on it for very long to prevent pregnancy (see Chapter 17). As the use of contraception increases, the waiting time to conception will rise and the birth interval will lengthen accordingly. If all women use effective contraception that reduces the monthly probability of conception by 80% (say from 0.1667 to 0.0333), then the waiting time to conception would rise to about 30 months, since the waiting time can be shown to be the reciprocal ($1/p$) of the monthly probability (p) of conception. This rise would more than compensate for the fall in the postpartum insusceptible period, since the resulting birth interval would become $30 + 9 + 2 = 41$ months. The fertility rate would fall from 706 to 293 per 1,000.

The same reasoning leads us to conclude that breastfeeding has little effect on fertility in the United States. Suppose women use contraception that reduces the monthly probability of conception to 0.01. The typical birth interval would be 111 months in the absence of breastfeeding (100 months to conceive, 9 months of gestation, and 2 months of postpartum insus-ceptibility). Even if breastfeeding produced an average of 8 months of post-partum insusceptibility, then the typical birth interval would increase by only 5%; both the proportion of infants breastfed and the average dura-tion of breastfeeding would have to increase substantially to produce even this effect.

---

[a] We ignore here and in the discussion to follow the effects of spontaneous abortion, which on average would add about 2 months to the average birth interval.

EFFECT OF ABORTION

Many people assume that one abortion will prevent one birth. But we can easily demonstrate that the statement is false. Let's go back to our developing country with a birth interval among young women of 27 months, composed of a waiting time to pregnancy of 6 months, a pregnancy of 9 months, and a period of postpartum insusceptibility of 12 months. Imagine that every other pregnancy is aborted. Thus the waiting time to conception would be composed of the following parts: 6 months to get pregnant the first time; 3 months of gestation until the abortion; 1 month of postpartum insusceptibility; and 6 more months of waiting until the next pregnancy. Thus the total waiting time goes from 6 to 16 months, a rise of 167%. But the birth interval (16 + 9 + 12 months) would increase by only 37%, from 27 to 37 months. Hence, if one aborts every other pregnancy, the fertility rate would decline by only 27%, not 50%. In summary, we know that fertility is inversely related to the length of the total birth interval. Thus, a change in any component will have a less-than-proportional impact on the total, and hence on fertility. But, one might object, an abortion certainly prevents one birth. However, this way of thinking ignores the fact that the next birth will come sooner than it would have. Therefore, while an abortion prevents a particular birth, it reduces the woman's lifetime births by fewer than one if reproductive behavior does not otherwise change.

The same logic reveals that an abortion in a population practicing highly effective contraception will prevent nearly one birth. Suppose that effective contraception reduces the monthly probability of conception to 0.01 and that breastfeeding is minimal. The average birth interval would be 111 months, as described above. If every other pregnancy is aborted, then the birth interval would rise to 215 months, an increase of 94%, and the fertility rate would fall by nearly half (48%). Hence, in the United States, some abortions (those occurring to women who use contraceptives effectively) will prevent nearly one birth while other abortions (those occurring to women who do not use contraceptives effectively) will prevent substantially fewer than one birth.

EFFECTS OF SEXUALLY TRANSMITTED DISEASES

Sexually transmitted diseases have major impacts on fertility in selected populations, though not in the United States.[43] Syphilis is an important cause of fetal loss among women with primary or secondary infections and may be an important factor contributing to low fertility among certain tribal groups in Burkina Faso and the Central African Republic.[21] Untreated pelvic inflammatory disease is a major cause of sterility. The low fertility characteristic of Central Africa (a belt extending from the west coast of Cameroon and Gabon through northern Zaire into southwest Sudan) is thought to be associated with high prevalence of gonorrhea.[1] Mass penicillin campaigns against gonorrhea (New Guinea) and yaws (Martinique) have been followed by pronounced increases in fertility.[21]

EFFECTS OF NUTRITION

A link between nutrition and fertility has been postulated as a relatively simple explanation for variations in marital fertility in populations that do not use birth control.[20] It is suggested that the lower the nutritional status of a population, the lower the fecundity and hence fertility. If nutrition is to have a demographically important impact on fertility, it must affect the waiting time to conception or the duration of postpartum insusceptibility. The evidence suggests that nutritional differences in chronically malnourished populations may be responsible for slight differences in the duration of postpartum insusceptibility. But such differences will not amount to a difference of even one child in completed lifetime fertility. Nutrition does not appear to affect the waiting time to conception in chronically malnourished populations.[6,19,34] Chronic malnutrition probably does result in a delay in menarche, though, as argued above, the impact on fertility is likely to be very small. When food supplies are so short that there is outright famine and starvation, fecundity and hence fertility are reduced. But when malnourishment is chronic and food intake is above starvation levels, there does not appear to be an important nutrition-fertility link.

DETERMINANTS OF MORTALITY

As living conditions in a country improve, the causes of death shift quite dramatically.[40] In developing countries, major causes of death are the infectious diseases. In developed countries, causes of death are concentrated among degenerative diseases such as cancer and cardiovascular disease. This shift occurs primarily because infant and child mortality are much higher in developing countries. Poor nutrition makes children more susceptible to infection and less able to withstand illness that otherwise would not prove fatal. Improvement in living conditions implies better nutrition, sanitation, water supply, and access to public health measures such as vaccination against tetanus, measles, and other common diseases. With such improvements, children survive to older ages, during which degenerative diseases become important.

Among Guatemalan females in 1964, for example, elimination of diarrheal, infectious, and parasitic diseases would have raised expectation of life at birth by 9.1 years, and elimination of cancer and heart disease would have added only 1.7 years. In contrast, elimination of the first three categories of diseases in the United States would have added 0.2 years and the elimination of the two degenerative causes of death 19.6 years.[39] The reason for the contrast between the United States and Guatemala is quite simple. In the United States, virtually nobody died of the infectious diseases, while in Guatemala, only a small fraction of the population lived long enough to die of cancer or heart disease.

An even more interesting contrast occurs in the United States itself. As stated above, elimination of heart disease and cancer would have added 19.6 years to the expectation of life. But the contributions of the two causes are very lopsided. Cancer accounts for only 2.6 years, whereas heart disease accounts for 17.4.

Reproductive and sexual behavior significantly affect mortality in three major ways. First, the total number of children women bear, the ages at which they bear children, and length of intervals between births all affect maternal and infant health. Short intervals between births are associated with higher rates of infant, child, and maternal mortality. Reductions in the number of children women bear would reduce maternal morbidity and mortality. These reductions would be greatest in populations in which fertility is high, health conditions are poor, and reproductive morbidity is common. Parents can minimize the risk of infant and child death by avoiding births at very young and very old ages, by averting high-parity births, and by lengthening the interval between births.[35] Second, breastfeeding significantly lowers the risk of infant and child death.[53] Third, unprotected sexual intercourse entails the risk of transmitting and acquiring STDs, including the human immunodeficiency virus (HIV), the virus that causes AIDS. STDs other than HIV are themselves associated with higher risks of transmitting and acquiring HIV. Pregnant women infected with HIV may transmit the infection to their infants *in utero*, during childbirth, or through breastmilk.

By early 1992, at least 12.9 million people (7.1 million men, 4.7 million women, and 1.1 million children) had been infected with HIV, according to the Global AIDS Policy Coalition (GAPC).[29] Among those infected, about one in five had developed AIDS; among those with AIDS, more than nine in 10 had died. GAPC estimates indicate that in 1990 the United States spent $2.71 and the Europeans spent $1.18 per person for HIV prevention, compared with $0.07 per person in sub-Saharan Africa and $0.03 per person in Latin America. GAPC predicts that as many as 110 million adults will have been infected with HIV before the end of the century. By the year 2000, Asia is projected to account for 42%, sub-Saharan Africa for 31%, Latin America for 8%, North America for 7%, the Caribbean for 6%, and Western Europe for 2% of the cumulative number of HIV infections. Overall, by the end of this century, 90% of all HIV infections will have occurred in developing countries. The impact on infant and child mortality rates and on population growth could be dramatic and devastating in certain areas of the world, particularly in sub-Saharan Africa and Asia.

DETERMINANTS OF MIGRATION

Compared with fertility and mortality, migration is a process that has received relatively less academic attention. It is also the process that is least linked to biology and most linked to economic, social, and political conditions. When assessing the determinants of migration, investigators have traditionally emphasized "push" and "pull" factors. Push factors include extraordinary events such as wars, flood, famines, political/religious persecution, and more ordinary conditions associated with depressed economic conditions: high unemployment, low wages, and little hope. Pull factors are those that attract people to a location. They are often those associated with economic opportunity: good jobs, high wages, and good public services such as education. They may also include attractive environment, religious freedom, and proximity to family or large ethnic groups. These factors help to explain why people in the United States have been moving from the north and east to the south and west, from the frostbelt to the sunbelt. These factors also help explain rural-to-urban migration in developing and developed countries. Urban wages are typically higher and public services are better.

The rapid growth of cities in developing countries is a matter of great concern to policy makers. However, careful examination of available data leads to several conclusions that do not support popular perceptions.[41] First, the rate of out-migration from rural to urban areas is higher in developed than in developing countries. Second, rates of urbanization in currently developing countries are not especially high if compared with currently developed countries when they were in a similar stage of development. Third, the primary determinant of the growth of urban areas in developing countries is the rate of natural increase (birth rate minus death rate) in urban areas. Natural increase accounts for about three-fifths of the growth while net in-migration explains the remaining two-fifths. However, the rate of growth of the absolute size of the urban population, as opposed to the rate of growth of the proportion urban in the total population, is very high by historical standards—precisely because the rate of natural increase is so high. This observation suggests that policies that slow the rate of natural increase, such as provision of family planning services, can have the added benefit of reducing urban growth.

POPULATION GROWTH AND AGE STRUCTURE

The age structure of a population is completely determined by its history of fertility, mortality, and migration. In Figure 25-1, we see two examples of age pyramids, one for the United States and one for Mexico. We notice immediately that the profile for the United States is more nearly vertical (or steeper). Although one might think that the difference is due to mortality, it is, in fact, due almost entirely to fertility. High-fertility populations have age pyramids

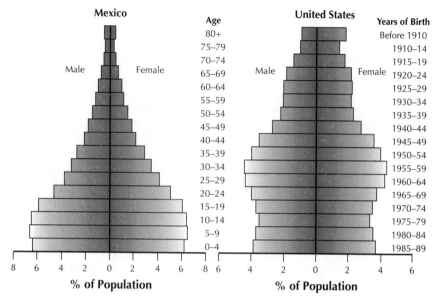

Sources: INEGI (1992); United States Bureau of the Census (1992).

Figure 25-1 Age pyramids for the United States and Mexico, 1990

with bases that are far wider than the middle or the top. This fact can be demonstrated if we consider populations that result from all combinations of three levels of fertility (total fertility rates of 3, 6, and 10 births per typical woman) and two levels of mortality (life expectations of 20 and 65). If the age schedules of fertility and mortality remain constant for a long time, then the age distribution of the population will also become constant. The population itself may grow, shrink, or remain the same size, but the proportion of the population in each age group will remain the same. Such a population is known as a stable population; if its growth rate is zero, it is called stationary. The age distributions of the six stable populations resulting from these combinations of fertility and mortality levels are shown in Figure 25-2. There it can be seen that mortality plays the smaller role in determining the shape of the age profile; moving across a row (changing fertility) causes the age profile to change shape to a far greater extent than moving down a column (changing mortality).

POPULATION MOMENTUM

The current age profile of a population contains momentum, just as a moving locomotive does. This momentum occurs because the number of persons already born implies much about future growth. The easiest way to understand

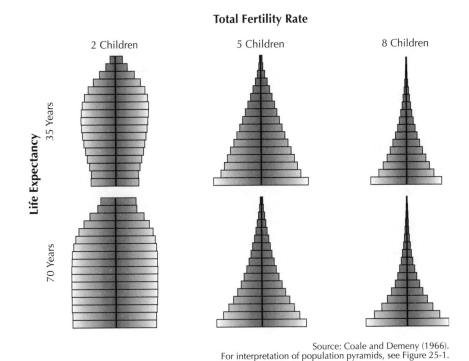

Total Fertility Rate

Figure 25-2 Age pyramids for six stable populations

the power of momentum is to ask how large the population would ultimately be if (1) the number of births in future years remains the same as the number this year, and (2) mortality remains constant. As is demonstrated in the last section of this chapter, a population with the same number of births each year and constant mortality will ultimately have the same age distribution as the underlying life table. The expectation of life (E) is the ratio of total person-years lived to the number of births (B). Then the total person-years lived by the population, or equivalently the total size of the stationary population, is E times B. Consider again the case of the United States and Mexico (see Figure 25-1). The number of births in 1992 in Mexico was 2.5 million and the expectation of life was 69 years.[23] Hence, the ultimate size of the stationary population would be 172.5 million or 97% larger than the 1992 population. In the United States, the number of births was about 4.1 million and the life expectancy about 76 years.[23] Hence, the ultimate size would be 311.6 million, about 22% larger than the 1992 population. We see that the Mexican population currently contains more momentum than does the U.S. population. The larger momentum results from its past high fertility, which has produced an age distribution with a very wide base, as examination of Figures 25-1 and 25-2 reveals.

These calculations are "quick and dirty" estimates. They give a precise answer to the question of what the size of the population would be if the number of births and mortality rates remained constant. But it is very unlikely that the number of births in Mexico will remain the same. From the age distribution shown in Figure 25-1, it is clear that the age-specific fertility rates would have to fall over time for the number of births to remain constant since the number of women of childbearing age will continue to increase for many years. Therefore, the size of the Mexican population is very likely to surpass 172.5 million in the future. In the United States, on the other hand, the number of births would decrease over time since the number of women currently of childbearing age is atypically large (the children of the baby boom). In fact, if the current age-specific mortality and fertility rates continued into the future, the size of the U.S. population (ignoring migration) would shrink to zero in the distant future since the typical woman now bears less than one daughter (see the section on Gross and Net Reproduction Rates at the end of this chapter).

SOCIETAL CONSEQUENCES OF IRREGULAR AGE DISTRIBUTIONS

Age distributions convey more than information about population momentum, however. Often they imply real problems for society. In the United States, the population aged 65 and over rose only from 17% of the working age (18-64) population in 1960 to 20% in 1990. If current trends continue, however, the fraction will rise to 28% by the year 2020 and to 37% by the year 2050.[17,45] Those projections also indicate that the population aged 85 and over will rise only from 2% of the working age population in 1990 to 3% in 2020; however, it will increase rapidly thereafter, reaching 8% in 2050. This rise in the fraction of old persons in the population is mostly the consequence of the rapid decline in fertility levels, from "baby boom" to "baby bust." The increase in population over age 65 has produced a strain on the Social Security system, which relies on the contributions of the current workers to finance benefits for the current retired population. The challenge of caring for the elderly posed by aging of the population is perhaps even more severe in Japan, where changes in the age structure will occur more rapidly than in the United States. For example, the elderly dependency ratio (population aged 65+/population aged 15-64) in Japan will double between 1985 and 2010, from 15.1% to 31.1%, and then rise to 39.1% by 2025.[51] Perhaps of greater importance for social and economic planning is the absolute increase in the number of elderly persons. Between 1990 and 2025, the size of the population aged 65 and over is expected to double in the United States and Japan, to triple in China, and to quadruple in South Korea, Singapore, and Malaysia.[30]

In the United States, fertility fell as a consequence of decisions by millions of couples to limit childbearing. Government policy, especially after the 1973 Supreme Court decision on abortion, did not attempt to limit individual control of reproductive behavior. Two more examples reveal the potential power of government action; they also highlight the value of demographic analysis before action is taken. In 1966 the government of Romania introduced pronatalist policies, including a decree banning virtually all abortions; in addition, importation of oral contraceptives and IUDs was discontinued. The result was as instantaneous as it was stunning.[46,47] Within 8 months the monthly birth rate had doubled; within 11 months it had tripled. The birth cohorts of 1967 and 1968 were twice the size of the cohorts preceding them. What were the economic and social effects? Inadequate hospital care for the babies and their mothers caused infant and maternal mortality to rise sharply. As a consequence of unsafe illegal abortion, maternal mortality increased to a level 10 times that in any other European country. In the 23 years the policy was enforced, more than 10,000 women died from unsafe abortions. Many women who did not resort to unsafe abortion bore unwanted children whom they placed in institutions. Such large-scale warehousing of children overwhelmed these institutions and severely degraded the quality of care. The educational system had to digest a giant bulge of students. Other problems, such as employment and housing, also arose as the large cohorts aged. The government took action because it was worried about low levels of fertility (fertility rates in 1965 implied that the typical woman who lived to age 50 would bear only 1.9 children). Its action certainly had the result of increasing fertility, but obviously the government had not thought clearly about the consequences. The policy was reversed immediately after the Ceaucescu regime was overthrown in December 1989.

Another example illustrates the problems caused by government attempts to lower fertility quickly. From 1979 through 1983, the government of China vigorously promoted the policy of one child per family.[b] What would be the consequences if the one-child policy were strictly adopted? By the year 2035, about a quarter of the population would be aged 65 and over, versus only about 5% today.[15] Only a tiny minority of Chinese are eligible for the state system of social security for the aged, so the state-financed system of old-age security will not be in danger of collapsing. Nevertheless, the traditional family structure would change radically in ways that would jeopardize the family's ability to care for the elderly and reduce its potential as a production unit;

---

[b] Since that time, the government has pursued a more flexible policy by allowing certain categories of couples to have two (but never three) children. Furthermore, clear repudiation from the central government appears to have throttled the excessive zeal with which subordinate officials implemented the policy (mandatory insertion of IUDs for women with one child, abortion for unauthorized pregnancies, and sterilization for couples with two or more children).[2,22]

there would be no brothers, sisters, aunts, or uncles. The one-child policy may have already had the unintended side-effect of inducing female infanticide and female-specific abortion due to a cultural preference for sons.[2,3,59] Results of demographic analysis suggest that the Chinese could meet their aggregate population targets by replacing the one-child policy with a two-child policy having a minimum age at first birth of 27 and a minimum birthspacing interval of 4 years.[7] While the two-child policy would not avoid the adverse age distribution effect, it would offer couples greater choice (they could have one child any time or two children subject to the rules) and reduce the adverse effects on the family.

DEMOGRAPHIC TRANSITION

Students of population long ago observed that the national populations of Western Europe tended historically to undergo first a fall in mortality and only later a fall in fertility. This observation led to a formal description of the process known as the demographic transition, which is shown in Figure 25-3. The paradigm is one of high birth and death rates in the pretransition phase. Birth and death rates were not necessarily equal in every year. Fertility was the more stable. In good years, mortality was low. But the population was subject to chronic food shortage resulting from vagaries of the weather and limited storage and transport capacities, as well as periodic epidemics. Generally, then, mortality fluctuated widely and birth and death rates, on the average, balanced.

At the time of the industrial revolution, improvements in living conditions such as better housing and food distribution networks and public health measures such as the provision of clean water caused mortality to fall. These changes required little or no individual action. Lowering fertility, however, required that individuals make conscious decisions about postponing marriage or controlling fertility within marriage. These personal decisions tended to be induced only after standards of living had improved considerably. Several mechanisms have been suggested. As couples realized that mortality had fallen, they would need to have fewer births in order to attain the same number of surviving children. As the status of women changed, primarily through mass education, high fertility became less desirable to them.[9,10] Moreover, the changing economic value of children would motivate a desire to limit fertility. In traditional societies wealth flows upward, from the young to the old. In modern societies, wealth flows from the old to the young, as parents invest heavily in their children's education.

All developed countries have experienced a demographic transition. For some, however, the lag between the fall in mortality and the fall in fertility was short and for others, long. The strict interpretation of the classical paradigm has been shown to be incorrect. When the countries of Europe are exam-

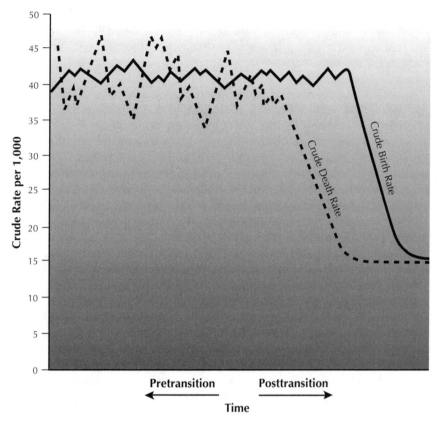

Sources: INEGI (1992); U.S. Bureau of the Census (1992).

Figure 25-3 The demographic transition

ined on a provincial basis, the results indicate that fertility sometimes fell before mortality declined and before education became general.[14] Hence, the demographic transition is a more complicated process than the simple paradigm suggests. Exhaustive analysis of the population history of England reveals that it did not correspond to the prototypical high-pressure regime of high birth and death rates before the transition. Instead, mortality was, on average, moderate and fertility was kept moderate, not through control of marital fertility, but through controls on age at marriage.[58] Other pretransition societies have also been found to have moderate levels of marital fertility.[4,14]

Demographic transition theory is especially relevant if, in addition to telling us why fertility fell historically, it yields predictions about what would cause fertility to fall in currently developing countries. Appeal to the classical statement of the theory would suggest that development is the best contraceptive. Indeed, this was the position taken by many at the World

Population Conference in Bucharest in 1974, a conference split between those who thought that family planning programs were the key to reducing fertility and hence population growth, and those who felt that policy makers should concentrate on development and population would take care of itself.[c]

A careful reading of the historical evidence suggests that (1) declines in marital fertility occurred in a wide variety of social and economic settings, (2) deliberate attempts to limit family size were not only largely absent but also probably unknown prior to the onset of the decline in fertility, even though a substantial fraction of births may have been unwanted, (3) the decline of marital fertility and the adoption of family limitation were essentially irreversible processes once under way, and (4) cultural setting had an important and independent effect on the onset and spread of fertility decline.[26] These considerations lead one to adopt a position midway between the two extremes adopted at Bucharest. The historical record does confirm a relation, albeit loose, between socioeconomic modernization and fertility decline, but historical analysis also reveals an important innovation-diffusion aspect to the practice of fertility control. Hence, emphasis on the right of couples to make and implement an informed decision on the number of children they want to have, and the provision of information and technical assistance to give meaning to this right, particularly when coupled with advances in the status of women, could have a sharp impact on reducing fertility.

Large fractions of women in developing countries desire increased spacing between children or termination of childbearing, according to the considerable evidence from surveys conducted under the auspices of the World Fertility Surveys, the Contraceptive Prevalence Surveys, and the Demographic and Health Surveys.[8,55,56] Hence, as three recent comprehensive reviews of population and development have concluded, voluntary family planning can play an important role in aiding the development process.[31,36,57] While slower population growth would benefit development in most developing countries, it would not automatically make poor countries rich and is no substitute for the elimination of market imperfections.

China illustrates an alternative to voluntary family planning that is clearly effective in reducing fertility and the rate of population growth. However, it is unlikely that many other governments would have the

---

[c] The United States was the leader of the family planning approach in Bucharest but reversed its position at the 1984 World Population Conference held in Mexico City due to intense political pressure from social conservatives, particularly antiabortion groups. The U.S. position that rapid population growth does not hinder and even fosters economic development was supported only by the Vatican. Ironically, those developing countries that had been the most vocal critics of the U.S. position in Bucharest also switched sides in Mexico City.

authority to implement such compulsory policies, even if they had the desire. Recent experience with mass sterilization campaigns in India suggests that coercive or compulsory attempts to bring down the birth rate are more likely to bring down the government instead.

M EASURING FERTILITY, MORTALITY, & POPULATION GROWTH

The population of a state, county, city, or country can change in only three ways: through births, deaths, or migration. New persons can be added by birth or in-migration; persons can exit through death or out-migration. Total world population can change in only two ways: births and deaths.

The question of how to measure these processes immediately arises. For example, how should one compare mortality across populations? In 1992, the United States had an estimated 2.30 million deaths but Rwanda had only 123 thousand deaths.[23] Does the fact that there were almost 19 times as many deaths in the United States as in Rwanda indicate that it is healthier to live in Rwanda? A moment's reflection will convince one that it is not. The United States had a population of 255.6 million people (who were therefore at risk of dying), but Rwanda had a population of only 7.7 million people. If one divides the number of deaths by the population at risk, one obtains the *crude death rate* (CDR). The CDR provides a simple index of mortality conditions. These rates were 9 per 1,000 population (0.009) in the United States and 16 per 1,000 (0.016) in Rwanda.

Many readers will immediately recognize the necessity of controlling for the size of the population at risk of dying when comparing the mortality conditions in different populations. But in other contexts, this same methodological principle is often overlooked. For example, in 1982 the Centers for Disease Control issued a report calling attention to its estimate that for the first time in the United States contraceptive-related deaths outnumbered pregnancy-related deaths.[42] This finding was widely (mis)interpreted by the press to mean that it is just as dangerous to prevent pregnancy as it is to become pregnant. But such reasoning ignores the two different populations at risk in this comparison. Only women who become pregnant can die of pregnancy-related causes. A much larger number of women (more than 5 times as many) is at risk of death from contraception-related causes. Most of the contraceptive-related deaths are estimated to be women who are pill users; even so, nearly twice as many women use the pill as become pregnant. Hence, the risk of death from prevention of pregnancy is far lower than the risk of death from pregnancy.

CRUDE RATES

Rates are defined by demographers to be the number of events divided by the average number of persons exposed to the risk of the event in a year. The denominator of a rate can also be described as the number of *person-years* lived; the concept of person-years is a natural generalization of man-hours or person-hours. Using a rate, such as the CDR, avoids the severe problems in interpretation, as illustrated above, caused by examination of the numerator alone (*e.g.,* deaths), without reference to the population at risk (the denominator). Another example of a rate is the crude birth rate (CBR), the number of births in a year divided by the total midyear population. The difference between the *crude birth rate* and the crude death rate is known as the *crude rate of natural increase* (CRNI). If migration is negligible, the CRNI is also the *crude growth rate* (CGR), usually referred to more simply as the growth rate; otherwise, the CGR is the sum of the crude birth rate and the crude rate of in-migration minus the sum of the crude death rate and the crude rate of out-migration.

The population of the world in mid-1992 was estimated to have been 5.42 billion (see Figure 25-4). It is currently growing at a rate of 1.7% per year.[23] In 1992 approximately 92.1 million people—a number comparable to the total population of Nigeria, the tenth largest country in the world—were added; this growth results in the addition of 252.4 thousand people every day, or 10.5 thousand people every hour. Should this growth of 1.7% continue, in 50 years time the population would be 12.6 billion, and in 100 years would be 29.2 billion. Of course, such growth could not continue indefinitely. Indeed, the growth rate has fallen after having reached a peak of 2.06% per year in the period 1965-1970.[51]

DOUBLING TIME

The growth rate is a simple measure of the rapidity of population growth. It can be used to determine the length of time it would take a population to double, known as the *doubling time*. If a population is growing at a rate of r% per year, then it will double in approximately T = 69.3/r years (see Figure 25-5).[d]

---

[d] This formula is correct for all values of r if r is the continuously compounded (exponential) rate of growth. If r is derived from the formula r = {P(2)/P(1)-1.0} × 100 (*i.e.,* the population this year is r% bigger than the population last year), then the doubling time formula is a very good approximation for values of r up to 10%. The exact formula in this case, used to derive the figures in the text, is T = 1n(2)/1n(1 + r/100), where 1n is the natural logarithm.

The concept of geometric growth or doubling (1, 2, 4, 8, 16 ...) originally led the economist Malthus to the dismal conclusion that population would soon outstrip the food supply.[28] He reached this conclusion by arguing that if population growth continued unchecked, it would increase in a geometric sequence (1, 2, 4, 8, 16, 32, 64, 128 ...), while food supply could grow only in an arithmetic sequence (1, 2, 3, 4, 5, 6, 7, 8 ...). Under such conditions the ratio of food to population would diminish rapidly. Fortunately, as we all know, Malthus' prediction has thus far been incorrect. He failed to foresee improvements in agricultural technology and the widespread acceptance of contraception in many societies.

Nevertheless, geometric growth is still staggering. Many students who are first introduced to the concept are surprised to learn that the world population growth rate is 1.7%. After all, this number is small compared with inflation rates in excess of 10% and interest rates of 15% or more common in many countries. Still, at the current growth rate, the population of the world would double in 41.1 years and quadruple in 82.2 years. To see just how great the current growth rate is, let us compare it with the population growth rate in the past. Imagine that Adam and Eve lived about 100,000 years ago. What average growth rate would result in a population of 2 growing to a population of 5.42 billion in 100,000 years? The answer is a very small number, only 0.0217%. Another way of looking at this issue is to determine what the population of the earth would be if it had grown at 1.7% for 100,000 years. The answer is ridiculously large: approximately the number 249 followed by 730 zeroes! Finally, we might work backwards from the present by asking when Adam and Eve would have lived if the population growth rate had remained constant at 1.7% ever since. A population of two would grow to 5.42 billion in 1,330 years; hence Adam and Eve would have lived in the Garden of Eden in the year 662 A.D., in reality about the time of the great split in Islam between the Shiites and the Sunnis. We see from these three calculations that the current growth rate is very large by historical standards.

PROBLEMS WITH CRUDE RATES

All the rates discussed above are called crude rates because they make no allowance for the age distribution of the population. A simple example will demonstrate that they are indeed crude and that more refined measurement is needed. In 1980, the CDR in Mexico was 6.2 per 1,000 population, while in the United States it was 8.8.[44] One might be tempted to conclude that the United States provided a less healthy environment. In fact, however, the death rates in every age group (0-14, 15-44, 45-64, and 65+) were higher in Mexico. How could this anomaly arise? The answer is quite simple. The crude death rate in the United States was higher because its population was

	Population Estimate, Mid-1992 (millions)	Birth Rate (per 1,000 pop)	Death Rate (per 1,000 pop)	Natural Rate of Increase (annual %)	Population Doubling Time, Years (at current rate)	Population Projection, 2010 (millions)	Infant Mortality Rate (deaths per 1,000 live births)	TFR (avg number of children born to a woman during lifetime)	% Population Under Age 15	% Population Over Age 65	Life Expectancy at Birth, Males	Life Expectancy at Birth, Females	Urban Population (%)	% Married Women Using Contraception (Total)	% Married Women Using Modern Contraception
World	5,420	26	9	1.7	41	7,114	68	3.3	33	6	63	67	43	55	47
More Developed	1,224	14	9	0.5	148	1,333	18	1.9	21	12	71	78	73	72	47
Less Developed	4,196	30	9	2.0	34	5,781	75	3.8	36	4	61	64	34	51	47
Less Developed (Excl. China)	3,031	33	10	2.3	30	4,361	84	4.4	39	4	58	61	37	43	36
Africa	654	43	14	3.0	23	1,085	99	6.1	45	3	52	55	30	—	—
Northern Africa	147	35	8	2.6	26	216	72	4.8	42	4	59	62	43	32	28
Algeria	26.0	35	7	2.8	25	37.9	61	4.9	44	4	65	67	50	36	31
Egypt	55.7	32	7	2.4	28	81.3	73	4.4	41	4	58	61	45	38	35
Libya	4.5	37	7	3.0	23	7.1	64	5.2	50	2	65	70	76	—	—
Morocco	26.2	33	8	2.4	29	36.0	73	4.2	41	4	62	65	46	36	29
Sudan	26.5	45	14	3.1	22	42.2	87	6.5	46	2	52	53	20	9	6
Tunisia	8.4	27	6	2.1	33	11.3	44	3.4	38	5	65	66	53	50	40
Western Africa	182	47	17	3.0	23	312	111	6.7	46	3	48	50	23	7	3
Burkina Faso	9.6	50	17	3.3	21	17.0	121	7.2	48	4	51	52	18	—	—
Côte d'Ivoire	13.0	50	14	3.6	19	25.5	92	7.4	48	3	52	55	43	3	1
Gambia	0.9	46	21	2.6	27	1.6	138	6.3	44	3	42	46	22	—	—
Ghana	16.0	44	13	3.2	22	26.9	86	6.4	45	3	52	56	32	13	5
Guinea	7.8	47	22	2.5	28	11.6	148	6.1	44	3	40	44	22	—	—
Mali	8.5	52	22	3.0	23	14.2	113	7.3	47	4	43	46	22	5	1
Niger	8.3	52	20	3.2	22	15.1	124	7.1	49	3	43	46	15	—	—
Nigeria	90.1	46	16	3.0	23	152.2	114	6.5	45	2	48	49	16	6	4
Senegal	7.9	45	17	2.8	25	13.1	84	6.3	46	3	47	49	37	11	2
Eastern Africa	206	47	15	3.2	22	359	110	7.0	47	3	50	53	19	—	—
Ethiopia	54.3	47	20	2.8	25	94.0	139	7.5	46	3	46	48	12	4	3
Kenya	26.2	45	9	3.7	19	44.8	62	6.7	49	2	59	63	22	27	18
Madagascar	11.9	45	13	3.2	22	21.3	115	6.6	47	3	53	56	23	—	—
Malawi	8.7	53	18	3.5	20	14.9	137	7.7	48	3	48	50	15	7	1
Mozambique	16.6	45	18	2.7	26	26.6	136	6.3	44	3	46	49	23	—	—
Rwanda	7.7	51	16	3.4	20	14.4	117	8.0	48	3	48	51	7	10	1
Somalia	8.3	49	19	2.9	24	13.9	127	6.6	46	3	44	48	24	—	—
Tanzania	27.4	50	15	3.5	20	50.2	105	7.1	48	3	49	54	21	—	—
Uganda	17.5	52	15	3.7	19	32.5	96	7.4	49	2	50	52	10	5	3
Zambia	8.4	51	13	3.8	18	15.5	76	7.2	49	2	51	54	49	—	—
Zimbabwe	10.3	41	10	3.1	22	17.0	61	5.6	45	3	58	61	26	43	36
Middle Africa	72	45	15	3.0	23	122	97	6.1	44	3	49	53	38	—	—
Angola	8.9	47	19	2.8	25	14.9	132	6.4	45	3	42	46	26	—	—
Cameroon	12.7	44	12	3.2	22	23.1	85	6.4	46	3	54	59	42	16	4
Zaire	37.9	46	14	3.1	22	65.6	83	6.1	43	4	50	54	40	—	—
Southern Africa	47	35	8	2.7	26	76	57	4.6	40	4	60	66	52	45	43
South Africa	41.7	34	8	2.6	26	66.0	52	4.5	40	4	61	67	56	48	46
Asia	3,207	26	9	1.8	39	4,207	68	3.2	33	5	63	66	31	56	52
Asia (excl. China)	2,042	30	10	2.0	34	2,787	81	3.9	36	4	60	63	34	47	41
Western Asia	139	36	8	2.8	24	226	63	4.7	41	4	64	68	62	—	—
Iraq	18.2	45	8	3.7	19	34.1	67	7.0	45	3	66	68	73	—	—
Israel	5.2	21	6	1.5	45	6.9	9	2.9	31	9	75	78	91	—	—
Jordan	3.6	39	5	3.4	20	6.4	39	5.6	48	3	69	73	70	35	27
Kuwait	1.4	32	2	3.0	23	3.2	16	4.4	45	1	72	76	—	—	—
Lebanon	3.4	28	7	2.1	33	4.9	46	3.7	40	5	66	70	84	—	—
Saudi Arabia	16.1	42	7	3.5	20	31.1	65	7.1	45	3	63	66	77	—	—
Syria	13.7	45	7	3.8	18	25.6	48	7.1	49	4	64	66	50	—	—
Turkey	59.2	29	7	2.2	32	81.2	59	3.6	35	4	64	69	59	63	31
Yemen	10.4	51	17	3.5	20	19.0	124	7.5	49	3	48	51	25	—	—
Southern Asia	1,231	33	11	2.2	31	1,725	95	4.3	38	4	58	58	26	43	37
Afghanistan	16.9	48	22	2.6	27	34.5	172	6.9	46	4	41	42	18	—	—
Bangladesh	111.4	37	13	2.4	29	165.1	120	4.9	44	3	54	53	14	31	24
India	882.6	30	10	2.0	34	1,172.1	91	3.9	36	4	58	59	26	49	43
Iran	59.7	41	8	3.3	21	105.0	43	6.1	46	3	63	66	54	—	22
Nepal	19.9	42	17	2.5	28	30.2	112	6.1	42	3	50	50	8	14	14
Pakistan	121.7	44	13	3.1	23	195.1	109	6.1	44	4	56	57	28	12	9
Sri Lanka	≈ 17.6	21	6	1.5	46	21.4	19	2.4	35	4	68	73	22	62	40
Southeast Asia	451	28	8	1.9	36	592	61	3.4	37	4	60	64	29	46	43
Cambodia	9.1	38	16	2.2	32	10.5	127	4.5	36	3	47	50	13	—	—
Indonesia	184.5	26	8	1.7	40	238.8	70	3.0	37	4	58	63	31	50	47
Laos	4.4	46	17	2.9	24	7.2	112	6.8	44	4	48	51	16	—	—
Malaysia	18.7	30	5	2.5	27	27.1	29	3.6	37	4	69	73	35	51	30
Myanmar	42.5	30	11	1.9	36	57.7	72	3.9	37	4	56	60	24	5	0
Philippines	63.7	32	7	2.4	28	85.5	54	4.1	39	4	63	66	43	36	22
Thailand	56.3	20	6	1.4	48	69.2	39	2.4	34	4	64	69	18	66	64
Vietnam	69.2	30	8	2.2	31	92.4	45	4.0	39	5	62	66	20	53	38

(continued)

Figure 25-4 1992 World Population Data Sheet of the Population Reference Bureau, Inc.

	Population Estimate, Mid-1992 (millions)	Birth Rate (per 1,000 pop)	Death Rate (per 1,000 pop)	Natural Rate of Increase (annual %)	Population Doubling Time, Years (at current rate)	Population Projection, 2010 (millions)	Infant Mortality Rate (deaths per 1,000 live births)	TFR (avg number of children born to a woman during lifetime)	% Population Under Age 15	% Population Over Age 65	Life Expectancy at Birth, Males	Life Expectancy at Birth, Females	Urban Population (%)	% Married Women Using Contraception (Total)	% Married Women Using Modern Contraception
East Asia	1,386	19	7	1.2	57	1,664	32	2.1	27	6	69	73	34	71	69
China	1,165.8	20	7	1.3	53	1,420.3	34	2.2	28	6	68	71	26	71	70
Hong Kong	5.7	12	5	0.7	99	6.3	7	1.2	21	9	75	80	—	81	75
Japan	124.4	10	7	0.3	217	129.4	5	1.5	18	13	76	82	77	64	60
Korea, North	22.2	24	6	1.9	37	28.5	31	2.5	29	4	66	72	64	—	—
Korea, South	44.3	16	6	1.1	65	51.7	15	1.6	26	5	67	75	74	77	70
Taiwan	20.8	16	5	1.1	62	24.0	6	1.7	27	6	71	76	71	78	62
North America	283	16	8	0.8	89	328	9	2.0	21	12	72	79	75	74	69
Canada	27.4	15	7	0.8	89	32.1	7	1.8	21	11	73	80	78	73	69
United States	255.6	16	9	0.8	89	295.5	9	2.0	22	13	72	79	75	74	69
Latin America	453	28	7	2.1	34	609	54	3.4	36	5	64	70	70	57	48
Central America	118	31	6	2.5	28	166	50	4.1	40	4	65	71	64	49	42
Costa Rica	3.2	27	4	2.4	29	4.5	15	3.3	36	5	75	79	45	70	58
El Salvador	5.6	36	8	2.9	24	7.8	55	4.6	44	4	61	68	48	47	44
Guatemala	9.7	39	7	3.1	22	15.8	61	5.2	45	3	60	65	39	23	19
Honduras	5.5	40	8	3.2	22	8.7	69	5.6	46	3	62	66	44	41	33
Mexico	87.7	29	6	2.3	30	119.5	47	3.8	38	4	66	72	71	53	45
Nicaragua	4.1	38	8	3.1	23	6.4	61	5.0	47	4	59	65	57	27	23
Caribbean	35	26	8	1.8	38	43	54	3.1	33	7	67	71	58	51	48
Cuba	10.8	18	6	1.1	62	12.3	11	1.9	23	9	74	78	73	70	67
Dominican Republic	7.5	30	7	2.3	30	9.9	61	3.6	39	3	66	69	58	50	47
Haiti	6.4	45	16	2.9	24	9.4	106	6.0	45	4	53	56	29	10	10
Puerto Rico	3.7	19	7	1.2	59	3.9	14	2.2	29	10	70	78	72	70	62
South America	300	26	7	1.9	36	399	56	3.2	35	5	64	70	74	62	50
Argentina	33.1	21	8	1.2	56	40.2	26	2.7	30	9	66	73	86	—	—
Bolivia	7.8	36	10	2.7	26	11.3	89	4.9	41	4	58	64	51	30	12
Brazil	150.8	26	7	1.9	37	200.2	69	3.1	35	5	62	68	74	66	57
Chile	13.6	23	6	1.8	39	17.2	17	2.7	31	6	71	76	85	—	—
Colombia	34.3	26	6	2.0	35	45.6	37	2.9	36	4	68	73	68	66	55
Ecuador	10.0	31	7	2.4	29	14.5	57	3.8	41	4	65	69	55	53	41
Peru	22.5	31	9	2.2	32	31.0	76	4.0	39	4	60	63	70	46	23
Venezuela	18.9	30	5	2.5	27	27.3	24	3.6	38	4	67	73	84	—	—
Europe	511	12	10	0.2	338	523	11	1.6	20	14	71	78	75	72	47
Northern Europe	93	14	11	0.3	242	96	9	1.9	19	15	72	79	83	72	66
Denmark	5.2	13	12	0.1	753	5.1	8	1.7	17	16	72	78	85	63	60
Sweden	8.7	14	11	0.3	210	8.9	6	2.1	18	18	75	80	83	78	71
United Kingdom	57.8	14	11	0.3	257	59.9	8	1.8	19	16	73	79	90	72	71
Western Europe	178	12	10	0.2	398	179	7	1.6	18	14	73	79	82	—	—
Belgium	10.0	13	11	0.2	347	9.7	8	1.6	18	15	72	79	95	81	63
France	56.9	13	9	0.4	169	58.8	7	1.8	20	14	73	81	73	81	67
Germany	80.6	11	11	-0.1	—	78.2	8	1.4	16	15	72	78	90	—	—
Netherlands	15.2	13	9	0.5	147	16.6	7	1.6	18	13	74	80	89	76	72
Switzerland	6.9	13	10	0.3	231	6.9	7	1.6	16	15	74	81	60	71	65
Eastern Europe	96	13	11	0.2	369	101	17	1.9	23	11	67	75	63	69	23
Bulgaria	8.9	12	12	0.0	—	8.8	15	1.7	20	13	68	75	68	76	8
Hungary	10.3	12	14	-0.2	—	10.5	15	1.8	20	14	65	74	63	73	62
Poland	38.4	14	11	0.4	187	41.3	16	2.0	25	10	67	76	61	75	26
Romania	23.2	12	11	0.1	578	24.0	26	1.6	23	11	67	73	54	58	5
Southern Europe	144	11	9	0.2	344	146	12	1.5	20	13	72	79	68	70	34
Greece	10.3	10	9	0.1	990	10.4	10	1.5	19	14	73	78	58	—	—
Italy	58.0	10	9	0.1	1,386	56.4	9	1.3	17	14	73	80	72	78	32
Portugal	10.5	11	10	0.1	533	10.8	11	1.4	21	13	71	78	30	66	33
Spain	38.6	10	9	0.2	433	40.1	8	1.3	20	13	73	80	91	59	38
Former USSR	284	17	10	0.7	104	328	39	2.2	26	9	65	74	66	—	19
Belarus	10.3	14	11	0.3	217	11.1	20	1.9	23	10	67	76	67	—	13
Kazakhstan	16.9	22	8	1.4	50	21.9	44	2.7	32	6	64	73	58	—	22
Russia	149.3	14	11	0.2	301	162.3	30	1.9	23	10	64	75	74	—	22
Ukraine	52.1	13	12	0.1	1,155	53.3	22	1.9	22	12	66	75	68	—	15
Uzbekistan	21.3	33	6	2.7	25	32.8	64	4.0	41	4	66	72	40	—	19
Oceania	28	20	8	1.2	57	35	33	2.6	26	9	69	75	71	63	68
Australia	17.8	15	7	0.8	83	21.5	8	1.9	22	11	73	80	85	72	72

Source: 1992 World Population Data Sheet of the Population Reference Bureau Inc., Washington, ©1992 Population Reference Bureau Inc. Used with permission. These pages excerpt several geographic regions of the world from the comprehensive Data Sheet. Limited space has precluded inclusion of other regions or a description of the methodology used to obtain these numbers, though full explanations are given with the printed sheet. For a copy of the complete document, write to the Population Reference Bureau at PO Box 96152, Washington DC 20090–6152. Single copies $3.00, 2–10 copies $2.75 each, 11–50 copies $2.50 each, 51 or more copies $2.25 each. For handling on orders up to $50.00, add $1.00 or 4% of total, whichever is greater. For handling on orders over $50.00, 4% of total will be included on the invoice.

Figure 25-4 1992 World Population Data Sheet of the Population Reference Bureau, Inc.

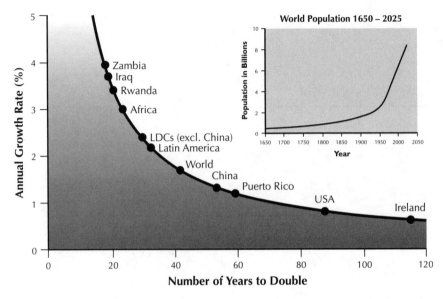

Sources: Haub and Yanagishita (1992); United Nations (1953); United Nations (1991).

Figure 25-5 Doubling time and world population growth curve

older (a much smaller fraction aged 0-14 and a much larger fraction over age 45) than Mexico's. If the United States' age-specific death rates had prevailed in Mexico, the CDR in Mexico would have been only 3.8 instead of 6.2. Similarly, if the Mexican death rates at all ages had prevailed in the United States, the CDR would have been 11.4 instead of 8.8.

Why does the age distribution of a population affect the CDR? It does so because death rates are not the same at every age. A typical example of death rates by age is shown in Figure 25-6. Examination reveals that age-specific death rates after childhood rise with age; the probability of dying at age 60 is much higher than the probability of dying at age 40, which in turn is higher than the probability of dying at age 20. This example helps us to understand why the current CDR in the United States is higher than the CDR in Egypt, Iran, Iraq, Malaysia, Nicaragua, the Philippines, Thailand, and Vietnam, although mortality, when properly measured, is higher in these countries. The crude birth rate is less problematic because childbearing, unlike death, is confined to the middle of the age distribution.

There is a parallel between problems with crude death rates and a crude technique of determining contraceptive effectiveness called the Pearl index, which is calculated as the number of unintended pregnancies divided by the number of women-years of exposure to risk of pregnancy. Each woman contributes to

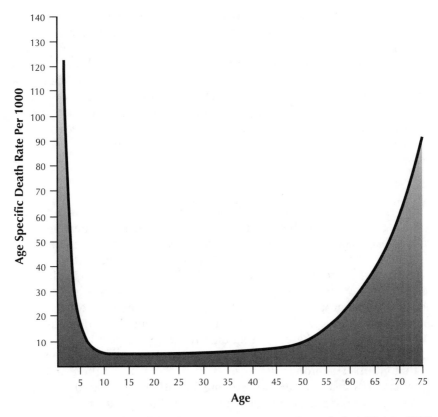

Source: Coale and Demeny (1966).

Figure 25-6 Age-specific mortality rates for a typical population with expectation of life of 50 years

the denominator the number of years of exposure from the beginning of use of a method until the end of the study, until the occurrence of an unintended pregnancy, or until she stops using the method for other reasons. The problem arises because contraceptive failure rates decline with duration of use, just as in the previous mortality example death rates in adulthood rise with age. Failure rates fall with duration of use because those women most prone to fail become pregnant early after starting use, so that over time the group of continuing users becomes increasingly composed of those least likely to fail. As a consequence, the longer the study runs, the more years of exposure each individual woman is allowed to contribute and the lower will be the failure rate.

Hence, two investigators using a data set that was designed to yield estimates of contraceptive failure for the United States as a whole could obtain failure rates of 7.5 and 4.4 per 100 women-years of exposure for the condom.[49] How could the two investigators get such different rates? One (who got 4.4) allowed each woman to contribute a maximum of 5 years of exposure while the other (who got 7.5) allowed each woman to contribute only 1 year. Which investigator is incorrect? Neither. The two rates are simply not comparable. The lesson is that when comparing the effectiveness of different contraceptive methods, one must be careful to ensure that failure is measured in the same way. We suggest, in fact, that the common measure be the probabilities of failure within the first, second, third, fourth, and fifth years of use, calculated by life-table techniques, which are discussed below.

AGE-SPECIFIC RATES

Crude rates can often hide more than they reveal because of the influence of the age structure of the population. Therefore, demographers prefer to calculate age-specific rates. These can be 1-year rates calculated for every single age, but they are more commonly 5-year rates computed for standard 5-year age groups. Age-specific death rates are computed by dividing the number of persons alive in the age group into the number of deaths to persons in that group; they may, of course, be computed for each sex separately. Age-specific birth rates are normally computed in a different way. Only women enter the denominator, since only women bear children. Births to women in each age group are divided by the number of women in that group. The problem with age-specific rates is that there are many numbers. It is inconvenient to compare fertility in the United States and Mexico by looking at 35 single-year age-specific fertility rates, or even seven 5-year rates. Hence, it is desirable to combine age-specific rates into a single fertility or mortality index that is free of any age-distribution effect.

TOTAL FERTILITY RATE

Suppose we simply add all the age-specific fertility rates together. If we do so in the United States, we get 2.0. What does this number mean? Recall that the fertility rate at age 20, for example, is the number of births to women aged 20 divided by the number of women aged 20. Thus, the age-specific fertility rate is the number of babies produced by the typical woman of that age. If we add the fertility rates at ages 20 and 21 together, we get the number of babies produced by the typical woman during the 2-year period from exact age 20 to exact age 22. Therefore, if we add all the age-specific fertility rates together, we get the number of births that the typical woman would have if she experienced the fertility rates prevailing at every age and lived through the end of the childbearing ages. Hence, at current rates, the typical woman would produce 2.0 children by age 50. This index is known as total fertility, or the *total fertility rate* (TFR).

GROSS AND NET REPRODUCTION RATES

If we count just female births (we sum the age-specific female-birth rates), the measure is known as the *gross reproduction rate* (GRR). Because approximately 105 males are born for every 100 females born in all populations (except among blacks, whose sex ratio at birth is about 103 males per 100 females), the fraction of female births is about 0.488. Thus we have the simple relationship that the GRR = 0.488 × TFR. Hence, the GRR in the United States is now about 0.98. This number directly tells us that women are not reproducing themselves; the typical female baby would by age 50 produce only 98% of a daughter. Thus, over the long run (ignoring migration), the population of the United States would shrink if these age-specific birth rates remained constant. Actually, to reach this conclusion, we must also account for the fact that each girl baby does not necessarily live through the childbearing years. If the probability of survival is also factored in, the fertility index is known as the *net reproduction rate* (NRR). It is the number of daughters that the average girl baby will subsequently produce during her lifetime. Because not all girl babies survive to age 50, the NRR is always less than the GRR; the difference increases as mortality becomes higher. If the NRR is greater than 1.0, each female will more than replace herself so that the population will in each succeeding generation grow (ignoring migration); and if the NRR is less than 1.0, it will decline. If the NRR equals 1.0, the population will ultimately neither shrink nor grow—it will become stationary, or constant.

LIFE TABLE AND EXPECTATION OF LIFE

Since each person can die only once, it does not make sense to add the age-specific mortality rates. Instead, we use them to construct a *life table*.[38] A life table can best be imagined as a table showing how many people are still alive at each birthday out of the total number born at a particular time. Suppose that we observe 1,000 births in 1994. Then we simply record the number who have their first birthday in 1995, their second in 1996, and so forth. We can also record how many person-years were lived between birth and age 1, between age 1 and age 2, and so on. If we add up all the years lived and divide by the number who were born, we get the average number of years lived, or the expectation of life at birth. We could also find, for example, the expectation of life at age 40 by dividing the total years lived after age 40 by the number who survived to age 40. While this exercise is revealing, we usually do not want to wait the 100 or so years it would take to find the answer. It is possible, however, to take the current age-specific death rates and convert them into a life table. This life table would not, of course, represent the experience of an actual birth cohort. It tells us at what ages members of a cohort would die if current age-specific mortality rates persisted in the future. Life tables are not mere mathematical games; they affect our everyday lives, for they are used in setting insurance rates and in developing pension plans.

Life-table methodology is not restricted just to deaths. One can use the same techniques to measure contraceptive failure (where initiation of use of a method and accidental pregnancy, respectively, take the place of birth and death in the life table),[54] marital dissolution (marriage replacing birth and divorce or separation replacing death),[33] and other events of interest. In these other applications, the expectation of life is not always the most convenient measure; instead, one may be interested directly in the proportion failing within 12 or 24 months (contraceptive failure) or 5 years (marriage dissolution).

It is also very enlightening to realize that a life table can be thought of as a stationary population.[38] If mortality is constant, and if the number of births remains the same every year, then (ignoring migration) the number of persons at each age will be the same year after year. Furthermore, the number of person-years lived in the life table between ages 6 and 7, for example, will be the same as the number of 6-year-olds in the population.

REFERENCES

1. Adegbola O. New estimates of fertility and child mortality in Africa, south of the Sahara. Popul Stud 1977;31(3):467-486.
2. Aird JS. Coercion in family planning: causes, methods, and consequences. Congressional Record-Senate 1985;S7776-7788.
3. Banister J. China's changing population. Stanford CA: Stanford University Press, 1987.
4. Barclay GW, Coale AJ, Stoto MA, Trussell TJ. A reassessment of the demography of traditional rural China. Popul Index 1976;42(4):606-635.
5. Bongaarts J. A framework for analyzing the proximate determinants of fertility. Popul Dev Rev 1978;4(1):105-132.
6. Bongaarts J. Does malnutrition affect fecundity? A summary of evidence. Science 1980;208(4444):564-569.
7. Bongaarts J, Greenhalgh S. An alternative to the one-child policy in China. Popul Dev Rev 1985;11(4):585-617.
8. Boulier BL. Evaluating unmet need for contraception: estimates for thirty-six developing countries. Working paper 678, Population and Development Series 3. Washington DC: World Bank, 1985.
9. Caldwell JC. A theory of fertility: from high plateau to destabilization. Popul Dev Rev 1978;4(4):553-577.
10. Caldwell JC. Mass education as a determinant of the timing of fertility decline. Popul Dev Rev 1980;6(2):225-255.
11. Campbell OMR, Gray RH. Characteristics and determinants of postpartum ovarian function in women in the United States. Am J Obstet Gynecol 1993;169(1):55-60.
12. Casterline JB, Singh S, Cleland J, Ashurst H. The proximate determinants of fertility. WFS Comparative Studies, Number 39. Voorburg, Netherlands: International Statistical Institute, 1984.

13. Coale AJ, Demeny P. Regional model life tables and stable populations. Princeton NJ: Princeton University Press, 1966.
14. Coale AJ, Watkins SC. The decline of fertility in Europe. Princeton NJ: Princeton University Press, 1986.
15. Coale AJ. Population trends, population policy, and population studies in China. Popul Dev Rev 1981;7(1):85-97.
16. Crews KA, Haub C. Teen mothers: global patterns. Washington DC: Population Reference Bureau, 1989.
17. Day JC. Population projections of the United States, by age, sex, race, and Hispanic origin: 1992 to 2050. Curr Popul Rep [Popul Estim Proj], Series P25-1092. Washington DC: GPO, 1992.
18. Demeny P. Bucharest, Mexico City, and beyond. Popul Dev Rev 1985;11(1): 99-106.
19. Ford K, Huffman SL, Chowdhury AKMA, Becker S, Allen H, Menken J. Birth-interval dynamics in rural Bangladesh and maternal weight. Demography 1989;26(3):425-437.
20. Frisch RE. Demographic implications of the biological determinants of female fecundity. Soc Biol 1975;22(1):17-22.
21. Gray RH. Biological factors other than nutrition and lactation which may influence natural fertility: a review. In: Leridon H, Menken J (eds). Natural fertility. Liege, Belgium: Ordina Editions, 1979:217-251.
22. Greenhalgh S. Shifts in China's population policy, 1984-86: views from the central, provincial, and local levels. Popul Dev Rev 1986;12(3):491-515.
23. Haub C, Yanagishita M. 1992 world population data sheet. Washington DC: Population Reference Bureau, 1992.
24. Henry A, Piotrow PT. Age at marriage and fertility. Popul Rep 1979;7(6), Series M(4).
25. INEGI (Instituto Nacional de Estadistica Geografia e Informatica. Estados Unidos Mexicanos: Perfil Sociodemografico: XI Censo General de Poblacion y Vivienda, 1990. Aguascalientes, Mexico: INEGI, 1992.
26. Knodel J, van de Walle E. Lessons from the past: policy implications of historical fertility studies. Popul Dev Rev 1979;5(2):217-245.
27. Lesthaeghe R. Nuptiality and population growth. Popul Stud 1971;25(3): 415-432.
28. Malthus TR. An essay on the principle of population, as it affects the future improvement of society. London, England: J Johnson, 1798.
29. Mann JM, Tarantola DJM, Netter TW (eds). AIDS in the world. Cambridge MA: Harvard University Press, 1992.
30. Martin LG. Population aging policies in East Asia and the United States. Science 1991;251(4993):527-531.
31. Menken, J (ed). World population and U.S. policy: the choices ahead. New York NY: W.W. Norton, 1986.
32. Menken J, Bongaarts J. Reproductive models in the study of nutrition-fertility interrelationships. In: Mosley WH (ed). Nutrition and human reproduction. New York NY: Plenum Press, 1978:261-311.
33. Menken J, Trussell J, Stempel D, Babakol O. Proportional hazards life table models: an illustrative analysis of socio-demographic influences on marriage dissolution in the United States. Demography 1981;18(2):181-200.
34. Menken J, Trussell J, Watkins S. The nutrition-fertility link: an evaluation of the evidence. J Interdisciplinary History 1981;11(3):425-441.

35. National Research Council. Contraception and reproduction: health consequences for women and children in the developing world. Washington DC: National Academy Press, 1989.
36. National Research Council. Population growth and economic development: policy questions. Washington DC: National Academy Press, 1986.
37. Ndiaye S, Sarr I, Ayad M. Enquête Démographique et de Santé au Sénégal 1986. Columbia MD: Institute for Resource Development, March 1988.
38. Palmore JA, Gardner RW. Measuring mortality, fertility, and natural increase: a self-teaching guide to elementary measures. Honolulu HI: The East-West Center, 1983.
39. Preston SH, Keyfitz N, Schoen R. Causes of death: life tables for national populations. New York NY: Seminar Press, 1972.
40. Preston SH. Mortality patterns in national populations. New York NY: Academic Press, 1976.
41. Preston SH. Urban growth in developing countries: a demographic reappraisal. Popul Dev Rev 1979;5(2):195-215.
42. Sachs BP, Layde PM, Rubin GL, Rochat RW. Reproductive mortality in the United States. JAMA 1982;247(20):2789-2792.
43. Sherris JD, Fox G. Infertility and sexually transmitted disease: a public health challenge. Popul Rep 1983;11(3), Series L(4).
44. Smith DP. Formal demography. New York NY: Plenum Press, 1992: Table 3.3.
45. Spencer G. Projections of the population of the United States, by age, sex, and race: 1988 to 2080. Curr Popul Rep [Popul Estim Proj], Series P25-1018. Washington DC: GPO, 1989.
46. Stephenson P, Wagner M, Badea M, Serbanescu F. Commentary: the public health consequences of restricted induced abortion—lessons from Romania. Am J Public Health 1992;82(10):1328-1331.
47. Teitelbaum MS. Fertility effects of the abolition of legal abortion in Romania. Popul Stud 1972;26(3):405-417.
48. Trussell J. The impact of birthspacing on fertility. Int Fam Plann Perspect 1986;12(3):80-82.
49. Trussell J, Menken J. Life table analysis of contraceptive failure. In: Hermalin AI, Entwisle B (eds). The role of surveys in the analysis of family planning programs. Liege, Belgium: Ordina Editions, 1982:547-571.
50. United Nations. The determinants and consequences of population trends. New York NY: United Nations, 1953: Table 2.
51. United Nations. World population prospects: 1990. New York NY: United Nations, 1991: Table 11.
52. U.S. Bureau of the Census. United States population estimates, by age and sex, based on the 1990 census: 1990 and 1991. Suitland MD: U.S. Bureau of the Census, April 16, 1992.
53. VanLandingham M, Trussell J, Grummer-Strawn L. Contraceptive and health benefits of breastfeeding: a review of the recent evidence. Int Fam Plann Perspect 1991;17(4):131-136.
54. Vaughan B, Trussell J, Menken J, Jones EF. Contraceptive failure among married women in the United States, 1970-1973. Fam Plann Perspect 1977; 9(6):251-258.
55. Westoff CF, Ochoa LH. Unmet need and the demand for family planning. Comparative Studies No. 5. Columbia MD: Institute for Resource Development, July, 1991.

56. Westoff CF, Pebley AR. Alternative measures of unmet need for family planning in developing countries. International Fam Plann Perspect 1981;7(4):126-136.

57. World Bank. World development report, 1984. New York NY: Oxford University Press, 1984.

58. Wrigley EA, Schofield RS. The population history of England 1541-1871. Cambridge MA: Harvard University Press, 1981.

59. Yi Z, Ping T, Baochang G, Yi X, Bohua L, Yongping L. Causes and implications of the recent increase in the reported sex ratio at birth in China. Popul Dev Rev 1993; 19(2):283-302.

Future Methods

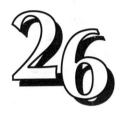

- Renewed emphasis is being placed on developing female-controlled methods that protect against both pregnancy and sexually transmitted infections.
- New IUD designs may reduce side effects such as cramping and excess bleeding.

- In improving continuous hormonal delivery methods such as implants and injectables, goals are to minimize bleeding disruption that occurs with the progestin-only methods and to reduce cost.
- The search for an effective, safe contraceptive vaccine continues. However, none will be available in this century.

A number of contraceptive leads being developed by public and private sector organizations *could* lead to new products before the year 2000. Unfortunately, the always-present uncertainties of scientific progress are confounded to an even greater extent by changing requirements of the Food and Drug Administration and concerns about product liability. Not only have companies dropped their research programs in the face of these obstacles, but more recently other companies have begun refusing to supply raw materials for contraceptive products.

MECHANICAL BARRIER METHODS

In light of the current prevalence of AIDS and other sexually transmitted diseases, researchers and policy makers have placed renewed emphasis on finding methods that are more user friendly and effective. There is great

The authors thank Henry Gabelnick, PhD, Director of the CONRAD Program, for contributing this chapter.

interest in providing methods that are female controlled in order to empower women with a means to protect themselves. Research has focused on enhancing effectiveness and minimizing annoying side effects of barrier methods, which have long provided protection against pregnancy and disease.

Female condom. Available in several European countries, the female condom was recently approved by the FDA. Because of limited supplies, the manufacturer restricted the initial distribution to high-risk populations in public sector clinics. As soon as the larger manufacturing facility is approved, however, general commercial sales will begin in the United States (probably early 1994). Although the clinical studies of this device showed it to be about as effective as other female-controlled barrier methods such as the sponge and cervical cap, analysis of failure under perfect use (used correctly and consistently) indicate a high efficacy.[11] Furthermore, because of its design, the female condom protects all of the vaginal lining, thus providing good protection against pathogens. (See Chapter 9.)

Lea's Shield. Also under development is Lea's Shield, a one-size-fits-all diaphragm-like device with a one-way valve to allow air to escape during placement, thus creating better retention against the cervix. The valve allows uterine and cervical fluids to escape yet prevents sperm from getting into the cervix. The final clinical studies to obtain FDA approval are scheduled to start in early 1994, and approval would be expected in 1998.

Femcap. A cervical cap-like barrier method that has shown promise but is not as far along in testing is the Femcap. Resembling a sailor's cap, it comes in three sizes; the size selection is made based on the user's parity.[9] Femcap should be approved by the end of the decade.

Disposable diaphragm. Clinical studies have yet to begin on a disposable diaphragm that releases the traditional spermicide nonoxynol-9. It is uncertain whether the method will be available before the end of the century.

Polyurethane male condom. Although very effective for fertility and disease prevention when used consistently and properly stored, the latex condom for men all too often goes unused. Some couples complain about its interference with sexual spontaneity and pleasure. Therefore, a search for better materials to improve the feel and durability has been ongoing for some time. A new polyurethane condom with a traditional design will be introduced in the United States in 1994. Alternative designs using polyurethane are also undergoing acceptability and efficacy studies and could be available as early as 1995 or 1996. (See Chapter 7 on Condoms.)

C HEMICAL BARRIERS

Chemical barriers are also being tested to improve spermicidal delivery systems. The new systems would enhance the ease of use and would increase the spreadability and cohesiveness to better protect against HIV and other pathogens as well as sperm. Researchers seek to reduce the amount of vaginal tissue irritation associated with heavy use of nonoxynol-9. Such irritation has been speculated to increase the woman's susceptibility to HIV infection even though nonoxynol-9 kills HIV in the test tube.

Initial clinical studies have begun on new formulations similar to the currently available vaginal contraceptive film (VCF). These new versions are designed to be easier to use and may contain alternative spermicides. Other agents that have an antifertility effect, such as acrosin inhibitors, are in the final stages of preclinical testing. Initial clinical tests will begin in 1994.

In the past couple of years, scientists have placed a priority on developing agents that will provide protection against disease without affecting sperm. Although clinical studies have not begun, the FDA has placed such agents on the fast-track, so it is conceivable that these pathogen-killing chemicals could become available sooner than any new spermicides.

H ORMONAL METHODS

Because hormonal methods have had a good record of safety and efficacy, particularly with the modern formulations, there would appear to be little incentive to drastically change them. However, the introduction of Norplant and Depo-Provera into the United States in recent years has spurred an increased momentum to provide improved versions or competitive products.

Drugs that have little or no oral activity are being evaluated to minimize the possible impact of hormones on nursing babies. The prime candidates are the natural hormone progesterone and a synthetic with the code name ST-1435.[7] Progesterone, which must be delivered at the rate of at least 5 mg per day, has been formulated in vaginal rings, suppositories, and injectable polymeric microspheres. The most likely candidate for approval in the next several years is the vaginal ring. ST-1435, recently named Nestorone, has been incorporated in skin creams, transdermal devices, vaginal rings, and subdermal implants. Although many clinical studies have been conducted, it is too early to say with any certainty which if any of the possible formulations will be available by the year 2000.

Implants

Implanon.   A single implant containing the progestin 3-ketodesogestrel, Implanon should remain effective for 2-3 years. The implant is currently undergoing large-scale clinical trials world-wide and should appear on the market in a few years.[3]

Norplant II.   An improved version of Norplant containing two rods instead of six, Norplant II achieves similar drug levels and duration of action. It may go on the market in the United States as early as 1995 (it is already on sale in Finland).[5]

Biodegradable implants.   To eliminate the need for surgical removal of implants, biodegradable devices are being developed. One system known by the trade name Annuelle consists of pellets the size of grains of rice in which norethindrone is fused with cholesterol.[10] Its duration of action is approximately 2 years and preliminary clinical efficacy studies are near completion. Another biodegradable method called Capronor is made from tubes of polycaprolactone; levonorgestrel permeates through the wall in the same manner as Norplant.[4] It is designed, however, to degrade after the drug has been released over a 2-year period. The availability of either of these methods is 3-5 years away, at the minimum.

Injectables

Levonorgestrel butanoate.   A long-acting ester, levonorgestrel butanoate is an alternative to depot medroxyprogesterone acetate (DMPA). Currently in efficacy trials, it could be available in 5-7 years.

Estrogen-containing injectables.   One of the drawbacks of the implants and injectables that contain only a progestin is the disruption of normal bleeding patterns that often occurs. The World Health Organization (WHO) has tested a number of monthly injectables that contain an estrogen as well as a progestin. One such combination is CycloProvera, which contains 25 mg of DMPA and 5 mg of estradiol cypionate.[6] This combination is being introduced under a licensing arrangement with WHO using the name Cyclofem. Another product called Mesigyna contains 50 mg of norethindrone enanthate and 5 mg of estradiol valerate. Both products are highly effective and minimize bleeding disruptions. The World Health Organization recently endorsed the products. It is quite likely that Cyclofem will be registered in the United States within the next 2 or 3 years.

Vaginal Rings

Vaginal rings provide another method of continuous delivery of progestins. The rings are being evaluated for use with a number of compounds; the most extensively tested ring contains levonorgestrel released at the rate of 20μg/day.[13] Unfortunately, problems associated with possible irritation of the vagina have slowed commercialization. A softer, nonirritating device is being prepared, but it is not clear whether the release rate will be increased to lower the pregnancy rate, which is close to 4 per 100 women-years in clinical studies and would undoubtedly be higher in actual use.

Also being tested are rings that contain both an estrogen and a progestin. These would be used in the same schedule as oral contraceptives: 3 weeks of drug and 1 week without to provide a withdrawal bleed. Several combinations are in various stages of development, but it is unclear when they might be available.

Male Hormonal Methods

Hormonal methods for men are also under investigation. A study using the prototype drug testosterone enanthate (TE) is nearing completion.[14] Although complete suppression of sperm production is not universally achieved, sperm counts in most men may be low enough to provide an acceptable level of protection. The major drawbacks are a long induction period requiring additional contraceptive protection and a weekly injection schedule, which is impractical.

Under study are drug delivery systems that can deliver testosterone for 2-3 months and testosterone-derivative implants that are active for up to a year.[2] Concurrently administered drugs such as peptide hormone analogs or progestins are also being examined in order to improve the efficacy.

INTRAUTERINE DEVICES (IUDS)

Although not a method with universal applicability, the IUD is certainly an excellent method for parous women who are not at risk for STDs.

Frameless IUD. A frameless device eliminates any pressures against the uterus and thus should minimize cramping.[12] A polypropylene thread anchors the copper-releasing sleeves in the myometrium at the fundus. In another version, a biodegradable anchoring cone allows insertion immediately postpartum. Clinical trials of both devices are under way in Europe.

Levonorgestrel IUD. The levonorgestrel IUD, which releases levonorgestrel as the active agent, is extremely effective and should provide 7 years of protection.[8] This IUD is useful for women who have a tendency to bleed excessively. Because of its effect on cervical mucus, it might have a beneficial effect on PID, although more extensive studies would be necessary. The main disadvantage is the cost, which is higher than the copper devices. Although available in Finland, the country of manufacture, its widespread availability remains uncertain. (See Chapter 14 on IUDs.)

VACCINES

The goal of a safe, reversible immunological approach to contraception remains elusive despite the many leads explored over the last two or three decades.

Vaccines for women. The most advanced testing is on hCG-based approaches, either whole molecule or fragments.[1] Both approaches, however, are abortifacients. Thus, even if efficacy, safety, reversibility, and reproducibility could be demonstrated, it is unlikely that any company will pursue hCG-based vaccines. Other antigens that prevent fertilization are more promising from a political point of view but are so early in development that none will be available in this century. They include a variety of sperm and zona pellucida antigens.

Vaccines for men. Potential vaccines for men use either luteinizing hormone releasing hormone (LHRH) or follicle stimulating hormone (FSH). Currently being tested on men with prostate cancer, a vaccine using LHRH linked to tetanus toxoid shuts down the testes to eliminate testosterone as well as sperm production. To maintain libido and potency, the user would need to supplement the vaccine with testosterone. In contrast, the FSH-based vaccine has eliminated sperm while maintaining normal testosterone levels in monkeys.

REFERENCES

1. Aitken RJ, Paterson M, Koothan PT. Contraceptive vaccines. Br Med Bull 1993;49(1):88-99.
2. Bhasin S, Swerdloff RS, Steiner BS, Peterson MA, Meridores T, Galmirini M, Pandian M, Goldberg R, Berman N. A biodegradable testosterone microcapsule formulation provides uniform eugonadal levels of testosterone for 10-11 weeks. J Clin Endocrinol Metab 1992;74:75-83.
3. Davies GC, Li XF, Newton JR. Release characteristics, ovarian activity and menstrual bleeding pattern with a single contraceptive implant releasing 3-ketodesogestrel. Contraception 1993;47(3):251-261.
4. Indian Council of Medical Research Task Force on Hormonal Contraception. Phase II clinical trial with biodegradable subdermal contraceptive implant Capronor. Contraception 1991;44(4):409-417.
5. Indian Council of Medical Research Task Force on Hormonal Contraception. Phase III clinical trial with Norplant II (two covered rods): report on five years of use. Contraception 1993;48(2):120-132.
6. Koetsawang S. The injectable contraceptive: present and future trends. Ann NY Acad Sci 1991;626:30-42.
7. Lahteenmaki PL, Lahteenmaki P. Concentration-dependent mechanisms of ovulation inhibition by the progestin ST-1435. Fertil Steril 1985;44(1): 20-24.
8. Rybo G, Anderson K, Odlind V. Hormonal intrauterine devices. Ann Med 1993;25(2):143-147.
9. Shihata AA, Gollub E. Acceptability of a new intravaginal barrier contraceptive device (Femcap). Contraception 1992;46(6):511-519.
10. Singh M, Saxena BB, Landesman R, Ledger WJ. Contraceptive efficacy of bioabsorbable pellets of norethindrone (NET) as subcutaneous implants: phase II clinical study. Adv Contracept 1985;1(2):31-49.
11. Trussell J, Sturgen K, Strickler J, Dominik R. Contraceptive efficacy of the Reality female condom: comparison with other barrier methods. Fam Plann Perspect (in press).
12. Wildemeersch D, Van der Pas H, Thiery M, Van Kets H, Parewijck W, Delbarge W. The Copper-Fix (Cu-Fix): a new concept in IUD technology. Adv Contracept 1988;4:197-205.
13. World Health Organization Task Force on Long-Acting Systemic Agents for Fertility Regulation. Microdose intravaginal levonorgestrel contraception: a multi-centre clinical trial. I. Contraceptive efficacy and side effects. Contraception 1990;41(2):105-124.
14. World Health Organization Task Force on Methods for the Regulation of Male Fertility. Contraceptive efficacy of testosterone-induced azoospermia in normal men. Lancet 1990;336:955-959.

Contraceptive Failure Rates

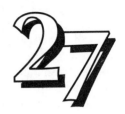

- Failure rates during perfect use reflect how effective methods can be in preventing pregnancy when used consistently and correctly according to instructions.
- Failure rates during typical use reflect how effective methods are as they are actually used and misused.
- Failure rates during typical use generally vary widely for different groups using the same method, primarily due to differences in the propensity to use the method perfectly.
- Empirically based estimates of contraceptive failure rates during perfect use are badly needed, particularly for condoms and for spermicides.

How effective is a given contraceptive method? Although Table 27-1 (reproduced from Table 5-2 on page 113) summarizes our current understanding of the literature, the question cannot be answered with certainty for any given couple. Contraceptive efficacy is a complicated issue. The likelihood that a contraceptive will "fail" to protect the user depends on two major factors:

- Inherent efficacy of the method itself, when used correctly and when used incorrectly
- Characteristics of the user

A general explanation of the sources of evidence and the logic underlying the summary table on contraceptive failure is provided in Chapter 5. In this chapter, we provide a more complete discussion of the derivation of the summary failure rates in Table 27-1 (reproduced from Table 5-2). The chapter also contains tables summarizing the efficacy literature for each method. These are arranged in the order in which they appear in summary Table 27-1. In these tables, all studies were conducted in the United States unless otherwise noted.

Chance

Our estimate of the percentage of women becoming pregnant among those relying on chance is based on populations in which the use of contraception is rare and on couples who report that they stopped using contraceptives because they want to conceive. Based on this evidence, we conclude that 85 of 100 sexually active couples would experience an accidental pregnancy in the first year if they used no contraception. Because this statement could be easily misinterpreted, further clarification is necessary. Available evidence in the United States suggests that only about 40% of married couples who do not use contraception (but who still wish to avoid pregnancy) become pregnant within 1 year.[5] However, such couples are almost certainly selected for low fecundity or low frequency of intercourse. They do not use contraception because, in part, they are aware that they are unlikely to conceive. The probability of pregnancy of 85%, therefore, is our best guess of the fraction of women now using reversible methods of contraception who would become pregnant within 1 year if they were to abandon their current method but not otherwise change their behavior. Couples who have unprotected intercourse for a year without achieving pregnancy are, by definition, infertile (but by no means are they necessarily sterile—see Chapter 20). Table 27-2 summarizes the efficacy studies on women who are neither using contraception nor breastfeeding.

Typical Use of Spermicides, Periodic Abstinence, Diaphragm, Male Condom, and Pill

Our estimates of the probability of failure during the first year of typical use for spermicides, periodic abstinence, the diaphragm, male condom, and pill are the averages of results for married women in the 1976 and 1982 National Surveys of Family Growth (NSFG).[13] They are standardized to reflect the estimated probabilities of failure that would be observed if users of each method had the same characteristics (the same age distribution, the same fraction seeking to prevent further childbearing instead of delaying the next wanted pregnancy, the same parity distribution, and the same fraction living in poverty). For alternative estimates of the efficacy of these methods, see Table 5-3 (on page 115) and the accompanying text.

Withdrawal

Our estimate of the proportion failing during a year of perfect use of withdrawal is purely a guess based on the reasoning that pregnancy resulting from pre-ejaculatory fluid is unlikely.[7,10] The estimate for typical use of withdrawal is the weighted average of the three life-table estimates shown in Table 27-5.

CERVICAL CAP, SPONGE, AND DIAPHRAGM

Our estimates of the probabilities of failure during the first year of perfect use of the cervical cap and sponge correspond with results of a reanalysis of data from clinical trials in which women were randomly assigned to use the diaphragm or sponge or the diaphragm or cervical cap.[15] The results indicate that among parous women who use the sponge perfectly, 19.4%-20.5% will experience a contraceptive failure within the first year. The corresponding range for nulliparous women is 9.0%-9.5%. Among parous women who use the cervical cap perfectly, 25.7%-27.0% will experience a contraceptive failure within the first year. The range for nulliparous women is 7.6%-9.9%. In contrast, parous users of the diaphragm do not appear to have higher failure rates during perfect use than do nulliparous users; 4.3%-8.4% of all women experience an accidental pregnancy during the first year of perfect use of the diaphragm. Our revised estimates in the third column of Table 27-1 (and 5-2) are obtained from the midpoints of these ranges.

We next faced the problem of whether and how to revise the estimates for these methods during typical use (the second column). The proportions failing during the first year of typical use for parous users of the sponge (27.4%) and cervical cap (30.3%) were about twice as high as for nulliparous users of these methods (14.0% and 15.2%, respectively). The evidence for the diaphragm is mixed. In the sponge-diaphragm trial, the proportion failing in the first year of typical use for parous users of the diaphragm (12.4%) was actually lower than that for nulliparous users (12.8%). In the cap-diaphragm trial, the proportion failing among parous users (29.0%) is almost double that among nulliparous users (14.8%).[16] Faced with this information, we set the estimates for nulliparous users of the cervical cap and sponge equal to the estimate for all users of the diaphragm based on the 1976 and 1982 NSFGs (18%). We doubled the estimates for nulliparous users of the cervical cap and sponge to obtain the estimates for parous users.

PERFECT USE OF PERIODIC ABSTINENCE

The perfect-use estimates for periodic abstinence are based on an empirically based estimate of 3.2% for the ovulation method.[12] Common sense dictates that the newer variants of periodic abstinence should be inherently efficacious because they demand abstinence during large portions of each cycle and particularly during times near estimated peak fecundity. They are relatively ineffective in actual use because perfect use is so difficult to achieve, and the consequence of imperfect use is a high risk of pregnancy. The post-ovulation variant of periodic abstinence requires the longest periods of abstinence, followed in order by the sympto-thermal, ovulation, and calendar variants. Consequently, we have assigned probabilities of failure during perfect use that are consistent with that ordering with the realization that we can be confident only about the rate for the ovulation method. Given the dearth of evidence, higher or lower estimates for calendar rhythm would be as plausible and defensible.

PERFECT USE OF SPERMICIDES

Our estimate of the proportion failing during a year of perfect use of spermicides is not empirically based. We reason that spermicides used alone may be less effective and certainly should be no more effective than spermicides used in conjunction with a barrier. However, three studies outside the United States,[1,2,6] in addition to several U.S. studies reviewed earlier,[13] have yielded very low probabilities of spermicide failure during the first year of typical use. Our intuition may lead us to understate the efficacy of spermicides used alone because we ignore the fact that the spermicidal products used alone differ from those used in conjunction with barriers. The modern efficacy literature on spermicides is dominated by studies of suppositories, foams, and film, and high-spermicide efficacy is documented only in these studies. There are few studies of creams and gels used alone, and those with the lowest failure rates are more than 30 years old (Table 27-3). It is plausible that the biophysical properties of foams (and perhaps suppositories and film) result in better dispersion both in the vagina and in cervical secretions. Evidence for this hypothesis can be found in an early randomized trial with a crossover design (so that all subjects used each product); however, even in this study the failure rates for foam are high.[9] We consider it more likely that the spermicide studies suffer from flaws in analysis or design that are not apparent in the brief published descriptions. Therefore, we set the failure rate during perfect use of spermicides equal to the empirically based failure rate during perfect use of the diaphragm.

The first clinical trial of Emko vaginal foam is also one of the few studies to compute separate failure rates for cycles in which the product was used at every act of intercourse and for cycles in which unprotected intercourse occurred.[9] The design of that trial was also quite sophisticated. Women were randomly assigned to six groups. Each group used three different spermicidal products for three cycles each. The six groups represented all possible permutations of orders of use of the three products. If the failure rate for three cycles of consistent use of Emko vaginal foam is extrapolated, then the implied proportion failing in the first year of consistent use is 8.9%.

PERFECT USE OF THE MALE CONDOM

Our estimate of the proportion failing during a year of perfect use of the male condom is based on studies of condom breakage. Under the assumption that

1.5% of condoms break[17,18] and that women have intercourse twice a week, then about 1.5% of women would experience condom breaks during the half-week that they are at risk of pregnancy during each cycle. The per-cycle probability of conception would be reduced by 98.5%, from 0.136 to only 0.002, so that about 2.6% of women would become pregnant each year.[8] If higher percentages of condoms break or slip off the penis during intercourse, then the perfect-use failure rate would be higher. For example, if the condom fails during 3.0% of acts of intercourse, then 5.2% of women would become pregnant each year. If 4.5% of condoms fail, then 7.7% of women would become pregnant each year.

FEMALE CONDOM

The typical-use estimate for the female condom is based on the results of a 6-month clinical trial of the Reality female condom (originally classified as a vaginal pouch); 12.4% of women in the United States experienced a failure during the first 6 months of use.[16] The 12-month probability of failure for users of Reality in the United States was projected from the relation between the failure rates in the first 6 months and the failure rates in the second 6 months for users of the diaphragm, sponge, and cervical cap.[16] The probability of failure during 6 months of perfect use of Reality by U.S. women who met the compliance criteria stipulated in the study protocol was 2.6%. Those who reported fewer than four acts of intercourse during the month prior to any follow-up visit, who did not use Reality at every act of intercourse, who ever reported not following the Reality instructions, or who used another method of contraception were censored at the beginning of the first interval where noncompliance was noted.[3] Under the assumption that the probability of failure in the second 6 months of perfect use would be the same, the probability of failure during a year of perfect use would be 5.1%.

PERFECT USE OF THE PILL

Although the lowest reported failure rate for the combined pill during typical use is 0% (Table 27-11), recent studies offer good evidence that failures do occur, albeit rarely, during perfect use. Hence, we set the perfect-use estimate for the combined pill at the very low level of 0.1%. The combined pill appears to be inherently more effective than the minipill. The lowest reported proportion failing during the first year of use of the minipill is about 1% (Table 27-10), but imperfect use in 15%-20% of cycles probably accounts for half the failures. Consequently, we set the perfect-use estimate for the minipill at 0.5%.

IUD

The estimates for typical use of the Progesterone T and the Copper T 380A are taken directly from the large study for each method shown in Table 27-12. The estimate for LNg 20 is the weighted average of the results from the two studies shown in Table 27-12. The estimate for perfect use of the Copper T 380A was obtained by removing the pregnancies that resulted when the device was not known to be *in situ*,[11] on the perhaps-questionable assumption that these failures should be classified as user failures, and the empirically based assumption that expulsions are so uncommon that the denominator of the perfect-use failure rate is virtually the same as the denominator for the typical-use rate (Table 27-12). The perfect-use estimates for the Progesterone T and LNg 20 were derived analogously. No differences in the typical-use and perfect-use estimates for LNg 20 are apparent due to the fact that only one significant digit is displayed.

NORPLANT AND DEPO-PROVERA

The typical-use estimate for Norplant is taken directly from Table 27-14. Because there is no scope for user error, the typical-use and perfect-use estimates are the same. The typical-use estimate for Depo-Provera is the weighted average of the six studies of the 150-mg dose shown in Table 27-13. While there is scope for imperfect use of injectables because women may miss a scheduled injection, each 150-mg dose provides more than 3 months' protection, perhaps an additional 4–6 weeks. For this reason, and because we have no information concerning pregnancies that may have resulted from late injections, we set the perfect-use estimate equal to the typical-use estimate.

STERILIZATION

The weighted average of the results from the seven vasectomy studies in Table 27-16 analyzed with life-table procedures is 0.02% failing in the year following the procedure. In these studies, pregnancies occurred after the ejaculate had been declared to be sperm-free. This perfect-use estimate of 0.02% is undoubtedly too low, because clinicians are understandably loath to publish articles describing their surgical failures and journals would be reluctant to publish an article documenting poor surgical technique. The difference between typical-use and perfect-use failure rates for vasectomy would depend on the frequency of unprotected intercourse after the procedure had been performed but before the ejaculate had been certified to be sperm-free. We arbitrarily set the typical-use and perfect-use estimates at 0.15% and 0.10%, respectively. For female sterilization, there is no scope for user error. The typical-use and perfect-use estimates are the weighted average

(0.38) of the 12 studies of procedures other than those involving clips (which are clearly less effective) in Table 27-15 analyzed with life-table procedures. We are less concerned about publication bias with female than with male sterilization because the largest studies of female sterilization are based on prospective, multicenter clinical trials, not retrospective reports from one investigator.

CONTINUATION RATES

Contraceptives will be effective at preventing unintended pregnancy only if women or couples continue to use them once they have initiated use. The proportions of women continuing use at the end of the first year for spermicides, periodic abstinence, the diaphragm, the male condom, and the pill were computed in two steps. In the first step, we obtained from the 1988 National Survey of Family Growth the proportions of married women continuing use if (1) change of method and (2) stopped using contraception altogether while still at risk of an unintended pregnancy were the only forms of discontinuation.[4] Other reasons for discontinuing use of a method such as stopped to get pregnant or stopped because not having intercourse are not counted in the discontinuation rate because these reasons are unrelated to the method and do not apply to women seeking to avoid pregnancy and at risk of becoming pregnant. These discontinuation rates are standardized to reflect the estimated probabilities of continuation that would be observed if users of each method had the same characteristics (the same distribution by age, race, and education). In the second step, we multiplied the continuation rates excluding pregnancy (obtained in the first step) by the complement of the probability of becoming pregnant during the first year of typical use (shown in the second column of Table 27-1 and Table 5-2) to obtain the probability of continuing use among those seeking to avoid pregnancy. To obtain the estimate for the cervical cap and sponge, we substituted the probability of continuation (excluding pregnancy) for the diaphragm in the first step. To obtain the estimate for the female condom, we substituted the probability of continuation (excluding pregnancy) for the diaphragm in the first step. The result is the same if one uses instead the probability of continuation for the male condom in the first step.

Proportions continuing use of Depo-Provera at the end of 1 year were calculated from the results of the two WHO trials of the 150-mg dose injected every 90 days shown in Table 27-13. Proportions continuing use of Norplant at the end of 1 year were taken from the results of the Norplant (6 capsule) trial shown in Table 27-14.[11] The estimates for the Progesterone T and the Copper T 380A were taken directly from the large study for each method shown in Table 27-12. The estimate for LNg 20 is the weighted average from the two studies shown in Table 27-12.

TEXT REFERENCES

1. Brehm H, Haase W. Die alternative zur hormonalen kontrazeption? Med Welt 1975;26(36):1610-1617.
2. Dimpfl J, Salomon W, Schicketanz KH. Die spermizide barriere. Sexualmedizin 1984;13(2):95-98.
3. Farr G, Gabelnick H, Sturgen K. The Reality® female condom: efficacy and clinical acceptability of a new barrier contraceptive. Durham NC: Family Health International, 1993.
4. Grady WR, Hayward MD, Florey FA. Contraceptive discontinuation among married women in the United States. Stud Fam Plann 1988;19(4):227-235.
5. Grady WR, Hayward MD, Yagi J. Contraceptive failure in the United States: estimates from the 1982 National Survey of Family Growth. Fam Plann Perspect 1986;18(5):200-209.
6. Iizuka R, Kobayashi T, Kawakami S, Nakamura Y, Ikeuchi M, Chin B, Mochimaru F, Sumi K, Sato H, Yamaguchi J, Ohno T, Shiina M, Maeda N, Tokoro H, Suzuki T, Hayashi K, Takahashi T, Akatsuka M, Kasuga Y, Kurokawa H. Clinical experience with the Vaginal Contraceptive Film containing the spermicide polyoxyethylene nonylphenyl ether (C-Film study group). Jpn J Fertil Steril 1980;25(2):64-68. (In Japanese; translation supplied by Apothecus Inc.)
7. Ilaria G, Jacobs JL, Polsky B, Koll B, Baron P, MacLow C, Armstrong D, Schlegel PN. Detection of HIV-1 DNA sequences in pre-ejaculatory fluid. Lancet 1992;340(8833):1469.
8. Kestelman P, Trussell J. Efficacy of the simultaneous use of condoms and spermicides. Fam Plann Perspect 1991;23(5):226-227, 232.
9. Mears E. Chemical contraceptive trial: II. J Reprod Fertil 1962;4(3):337-343.
10. Pudney J, Oneta M, Mayer K, Seage G, Anderson D. Pre-ejaculatory fluid as potential vector for sexual transmission of HIV-1. Lancet 1992;340(8833):1470.
11. Sivin I. Personal communication to James Trussell, August 13, 1992.
12. Trussell J, Grummer-Strawn L. Contraceptive failure of the ovulation method of periodic abstinence. Fam Plann Perspect 1990; 22(2):65-75.
13. Trussell J, Kost K. Contraceptive failure in the United States: a critical review of the literature. Stud Fam Plann 1987;18(5):237-283.
14. Trussell J, Hatcher RA, Cates W, Stewart FH, Kost K. Contraceptive failure in the United States: an update. Stud Fam Plann 1990;21(1):51-54.
15. Trussell J, Strickler J, Vaughan B. Contraceptive efficacy of the diaphragm, sponge, and cervical cap. Fam Plann Perspect 1993;25(3):100-105,135.
16. Trussell J, Sturgen K, Strickler J, Dominik R. Contraceptive efficacy of the Reality® female condom: comparison with other barrier methods. Fam Plann Perspect 1994;26(2) (in press).
17. Trussell J, Warner DL, Hatcher RA. Condom performance during vaginal intercourse: comparison of Trojan-Enz® and Tactylon™ condoms. Contraception 1992a;45(1):11-19.
18. Trussell J, Warner DL, Hatcher RA. Condom slippage and breakage rates. Fam Plann Perspect 1992b;24(1):20-23.

TABLE REFERENCES

Alderman PM. The lurking sperm: a review of failures in 8879 vasectomies performed by one physician. JAMA 1988;259(21):3142-3144.

Apothecus Pharmaceutical Corporation. VCF®: Vaginal Contraceptive Film™. East Norwich NY: Apothecus Inc, 1992.

Ball M. A prospective field trial of the ovulation method of avoiding conception. Eur J Obstet Gynecol Reprod Biol 1976;6(2):63-66.

Bartzen PJ. Effectiveness of the temperature rhythm system of contraception. Fertil Steril 1967;18(5):694-706.

Belhadj H, Sivin I, Diaz S, Pavez M, Tejada AS, Brache V, Alvarez F, Shoupe D, Breaux H, Mishell DR, McCarthy T, Yo V. Recovery of fertility after use of the levonorgestrel 20 mcg/d or Copper T 380 A intrauterine device. Contraception 1986;34(3):261-267.

Bernstein GS. Clinical effectiveness of an aerosol contraceptive foam. Contraception 1971;3(1):37-43.

Bernstein GS, Clark V, Coulson AH, Frezieres RG, Kilzer L, Moyer D, Nakamura RM, Walsh T. Use effectiveness study of cervical caps. Final report. Washington DC: National Institute of Child Health and Human Development, Contract No. 1-HD-1-2804, July 1986.

Bhiwandiwala PP, Mumford SD, Feldblum PJ. A comparison of different laparoscopic sterilization occlusion techniques in 24,439 procedures. Am J Obstet Gynecol 1982;144(3):319-331.

Board JA. Continuous norethindrone, 0.35 mg, as an oral contraceptive agent. Am J Obstet Gynecol 1971;109(4):531-535.

Boehm D. The cervical cap: effectiveness as a contraceptive. J Nurse Midwifery 1983;28(1):3-6.

Bounds W, Guillebaud J. Randomised comparison of the use-effectiveness and patient acceptability of the Collatex (Today) contraceptive sponge and the diaphragm. Br J Fam Plann 1984;10(3):69-75.

Bounds W, Vessey M, Wiggins P. A randomized double-blind trial of two low dose combined oral contraceptives. Brit J Obstet Gynaecol 1979;86(4):325-329.

Bracher M, Santow G. Premature discontinuation of contraception in Australia. Fam Plann Perspect 1992;24(2):58-65.

Brehm H, Haase W. Die alternative zur hormonalen kontrazeption? Med Welt 1975;26(36):1610-1617.

Brigato G, Pisano G, Bergamasco A, Pasqualini M, Cutugno G, Luppari T. Vaginal topical chemical contraception with C-Film. Ginecol Clinica 1982;3(1):77-80. (In Italian; translation supplied by Apothecus Inc.)

Bushnell LF. Aerosol foam: a practical and effective method of contraception. Pac Med Surg 1965; 73(6):353-355.

Cagen R. The cervical cap as a barrier contraceptive. Contraception 1986;33(5):487-496.

Carpenter G, Martin JB. Clinical evaluation of a vaginal contraceptive foam. Adv Plann Parent 1970;5:170-175.

Chi IC, Laufe LE, Gardner SD, Tolbert MA. An epidemiologic study of risk factors associated with pregnancy following female sterilization. Am J Obstet Gynecol 1980;136(6):768-773.

Chi IC, Mumford SD, Gardner SD. Pregnancy risks following laparoscopic sterilization in nongravid and gravid women. J Reprod Med 1981;26(6):289-294.

Chi IC, Siemens AJ, Champion CB, Gates D, Cilenti D. Pregnancy following minilaparotomy tubal sterilization: an update of an international data set. Contraception 1987;35(2):171-178.

Cliquet RL, Schoenmaeckers R, Klinkenborg L. Effectiveness of contraception in Belgium: results of the second national fertility survey, 1971 (NEGO II). J Biosoc Sci 1977;9(4):403-416.

Debusschere R. Effectiviteit van de anticonceptie in Vlaanderen: resultaten van het NEGO-III-onderzoek 1975-1976. Bevolking en Gezin 1980;1:5-28.

Denniston GC, Putney D. The cavity rim cervical cap. Adv Plann Parent 1981;16(3): 77-80.

Dimpfl J, Salomon W, Schicketanz KH. Die spermizide barriere. Sexualmedizin 1984;13(2):95-98.

Dolack L. Study confirms values of ovulation method. Hospital Progress 1978;59(8): 64-66,72-73.

Dubrow H, Kuder K. Combined postpartum and family-planning clinic. Obstet Gynecol 1958;11(5):586-590.

Edelman DA. Nonprescription vaginal contraception. Int J Gynecol Obstet 1980;18(5):340-344.

Edelman DA, McIntyre SL, Harper J. A comparative trial of the Today contraceptive sponge and diaphragm. Am J Obstet Gynecol 1984;150(7):869-876.

Ellis JW. Multiphasic oral contraceptives: efficacy and metabolic impact. J Reprod Med 1987;32(1):28-36.

Ellsworth HS. Focus on triphasil. J Reprod Med 1986;31(6-Suppl):559-564.

Engel T. Laparoscopic sterilization: electrosurgery or clip application? J Reprod Med 1978;21(2):107-110.

Frank R. Clinical evaluation of a simple jelly-alone method of contraception. Fertil Steril 1962;13(5):458-464.

Frankman O, Raabe N, Ingemansson CA. Clinical evaluation of C-Film, a vaginal contraceptive. J Int Med Res 1975;3(4):292-296.

Gibor Y, Mitchell C. Selected events following insertion of the Progestasert system. Contraception 1980;21(5):491-503.

Glass R, Vessey M, Wiggins P. Use-effectiveness of the condom in a selected family planning clinic population in the United Kingdom. Contraception 1974;10(6):591-598.

Grady WR, Hayward MD, Yagi J. Contraceptive failure in the United States: estimates from the 1982 National Survey of Family Growth. Fam Plann Perspect 1986;18(5):200-209.

Grady WR, Hirsch MB, Keen N, Vaughan B. Contraceptive failure and continuation among married women in the United States, 1970-75. Stud Fam Plann 1983;14(1):9-19.

Hall RE. Continuation and pregnancy rates with four contraceptive methods. Am J Obstet Gynecol 1973;116(5):671-681.

Hawkins DF, Benster B. A comparative study of three low dose progestogens, chlormadinone acetate, megestrol acetate and norethisterone, as oral contraceptives. Br J Obstet Gynaecol 1977;84(9):708-713.

Howard G, Blair M, Chen JK, Fotherby K, Muggeridge J, Elder MG, Bye PG. A clinical trial of norethisterone oenanthate (Norigest) injected every two months. Contraception 1982;25(4):333-343.

Hughes I. An open assessment of a new low dose estrogen combined oral contraceptive. J Int Med Res 1978;6(1):41-45.

Hulka JF, Mercer JP, Fishburne JI, Kumarasamy T, Omran KF, Phillips JM, Lefler HT, Lieberman B, Lean TH, Pai DN, Koetsawang S, Castro VM. Spring clip sterilization: one-year follow-up of 1,079 cases. Am J Obstet Gynecol 1976;125(8):1039-1043.

Iizuka R, Kobayashi T, Kawakami S, Nakamura Y, Ikeuchi M, Chin B, Mochimaru F, Sumi K, Sato H, Yamaguchi J, Ohno T, Shiina M, Maeda N, Tokoro H, Suzuki T, Hayashi K, Takahashi T, Akatsuka M, Kasuga Y, Kurokawa H. Clinical experience with the Vaginal Contraceptive Film containing the spermicide polyoxyethylene nonylphenyl ether (C-Film study group). Jpn J Fertil Steril 1980;25(2):64-68. (In Japanese; translation supplied by Apothecus Inc.)

John APK. Contraception in a practice community. J R Coll Gen Pract 1973; 23(134):665-675.

Johnston JA, Roberts DB, Spencer RB. A survey evaluation of the efficacy and efficiency of natural family planning services and methods in Australia: report of a research project. Sydney, Australia: St. Vincent's Hospital, 1978.

Jones EF, Forrest JD. Contraceptive failure rates based on the 1988 NSFG. Fam Plann Perspect 1992;24(1):12-19.

Jubhari S, Lane ME, Sobrero AJ. Continuous microdose (0.3 mg) quingestanol acetate as an oral contraceptive agent. Contraception 1974;9(3):213-219.

Kambic R, Kambic M, Brixius AM, Miller S. A thirty-month clinical experience in natural family planning. Am J Public Health 1981;71(11):1255-1258. Erratum. Am J Public Health 1982;72(6):538.

Kasabach HY. Clinical evaluation of vaginal jelly alone in the management of fertility. Clin Med 1962;69(4):894-897.

Kase S, Goldfarb M. Office vasectomy review of 500 cases. Urology 1973;1(1):60-62.

Kassell NC, McElroy MP. Emma Goldman Clinic for Women study. In: King L (ed). The cervical cap handbook for users and fitters. Iowa City IA: Emma Goldman Clinic for Women, 1981:11-19.

Keifer W. A clinical evaluation of continuous Norethindrone (0.35 mg). In: Ortho Pharmaceutical Corporation. A clinical symposium on 0.35 mg Norethindrone: continuous regimen low-dose oral contraceptive. Proceedings of a symposium, New York City, February 22, 1971. Raritan NJ: Ortho Pharmaceutical Corporation, 1973:9-14.

Klapproth HJ, Young IS. Vasectomy, vas ligation and vas occlusion. Urology 1973;1(4):292-300.

Klaus H, Goebel JM, Muraski B, Egizio MT, Weitzel D, Taylor, RS, Fagan MU, Ek K, Hobday K. Use-effectiveness and client satisfaction in six centers teaching the Billings ovulation method. Contraception 1979;19(6):613-629.

Kleppinger RK. A vaginal contraceptive foam. Penn Med J 1965;68(4):31-34.

Koch JP. The Prentif contraceptive cervical cap: a contemporary study of its clinical safety and effectiveness. Contraception 1982;25(2):135-159.

Korba VD, Heil CG. Eight years of fertility control with norgestrel-ethinyl estradiol (Ovral): an updated clinical review. Fertil Steril 1975;26(10):973-981.

Korba VD, Paulson SR. Five years of fertility control with microdose norgestrel: an updated clinical review. J Reprod Med 1974;13(2):71-75.

Lane ME, Arceo R, Sobrero AJ. Successful use of the diaphragm and jelly by a young population: report of a clinical study. Fam Plann Perspect 1976;8(2): 81-86.

Ledger WJ. Ortho 1557-O: a new oral contraceptive. Int J Fertil 1970;15(2): 88-92.

Lehfeldt H, Sivin I. Use effectiveness of the Prentif cervical cap in private practice: a prospective study. Contraception 1984;30(4):331-338.

Loffer FD, Pent D. Risks of laparoscopic fulguration and transection of the fallopian tube. Obstet Gynecol 1977;49(2):218-222.

Loudon NB, Barden ME, Hepburn WB, Prescott RJ. A comparative study of the effectiveness and acceptability of the diaphragm used with spermicide in the form of C-film or a cream or jelly. Br J Fam Plann 1991;17(2):41-44.

Luukkainen T, Allonen H, Haukkamaa M, Holma P, Pyörälä T, Terho J, Toivonen J, Batar I, Lampe L, Andersson K, Atterfeldt P, Johansson EDB, Nilsson S, Nygren KG, Odlind V, Olsson SE, Rybo G, Sikström B, Nielsen NC, Buch A, Osler M, Steier A, Ulstein M. Effective contraception with the levonorgestrel-releasing intrauterine device: 12-month report of a European multicenter study. Contraception 1987;36(2):169-179.

Margaret Pyke Centre. One thousand vasectomies. Br Med J 1973;4(886):216-221.

Marshall J. Cervical-mucus and basal body-temperature method of regulating births: field trial. Lancet 1976;2(7980):282-283.

Marshall S, Lyon RP. Variability of sperm disappearance from the ejaculate after vasectomy. J Urol 1972;107(5):815-817.

McIntyre SL, Higgins JE. Parity and use-effectiveness with the contraceptive sponge. Am J Obstet Gynecol 1986;155(4):796-801.

McQuarrie HG, Harris JW, Ellsworth HS, Stone RA, Anderson AE. The clinical evaluation of norethindrone in cyclic and continuous regimens. Adv Plann Parent 1972;7:124-130.

Mears E. Chemical contraceptive trial: II. J Reprod Fertil 1962;4(3):337-343.

Mears E, Please NW. Chemical contraceptive trial. J Reprod Fertil 1962;3(1):138-147.

Morigi EM, Pasquale SA. Clinical experience with a low dose oral contraceptive containing norethisterone and ethinyl oestradiol. Curr Med Res Opin 1978;5(8): 655-662.

Mishell DR, El-Habashy MA, Good RG, Moyer DL. Contraception with an injectable progestin. Am J Obstet Gynecol 1968;101(8):1046-1053.

Moss WM. A comparison of open-end versus closed-end vasectomies: a report on 6220 cases. Contraception 1992;46(6):521-525.

Mumford SD, Bhiwandiwala PP, Chi IC. Laparoscopic and minilaparotomy female sterilisation compared in 15,167 cases. Lancet 1980;2(8203):1066-1070.

Nelson JH. The use of the minipill in private practice. J Reprod Med 1973;10(3): 139-143.

Peel J. The Hull family survey: II. Family planning in the first five years of marriage. J Biosoc Sci 1972; 4(3):333-346.

Postlethwaite DL. Pregnancy rate of a progestogen oral contraceptive. Practitioner 1979;222(1328):272-275.

Potts M, McDevitt J. A use-effectiveness trial of spermicidally lubricated condoms. Contraception 1975;11(6):701-710.

Powell MG, Mears BJ, Deber RB, Ferguson D. Contraception with the cervical cap: effectiveness, safety, continuity of use, and user satisfaction. Contraception 1986;33(3):215-232.

Preston SN. A report of a collaborative dose-response clinical study using decreasing doses of combination oral contraceptives. Contraception 1972;6(1):17-35.

Preston SN. A report of the correlation between the pregnancy rates of low estrogen formulations and pill-taking habits of females studied. J Reprod Med 1974;13(2):75-77.

Rice FJ, Lanctôt CA, Garcia-Devesa C. Effectiveness of the sympto-thermal method of natural family planning: an international study. Int J Fertil 1981;26(3): 222-230.

Richwald GA, Greenland S, Gerber MM, Potik R, Kersey L, Comas MA. Effectiveness of the cavity-rim cervical cap: results of a large clinical study. Obstet Gynecol 1989;74(2):143-148.

Rovinsky JJ. Clinical effectiveness of a contraceptive cream. Obstet Gynecol 1964;23(1):125-131.

Royal College of General Practitioners. Oral contraceptives and health. New York NY: Pitman Publishing Corp., 1974.

Schirm AL, Trussell J, Menken J, Grady WR. Contraceptive failure in the United States: the impact of social, economic, and demographic factors. Fam Plann Perspect 1982;14(2):68-75.

Schmidt SS. Vasectomy. JAMA 1988;259(21):3176.

Schwallie PC, Assenzo JR. Contraceptive use-efficacy study utilizing Depo-Provera administered as an injection once every six months. Contraception 1972;6(4):315-327.

Schwallie PC, Assenzo JR. Contraceptive use-efficacy study utilizing medroxyprogesterone acetate administered as an intramuscular injection once every 90 days. Fertil Steril 1973;24(5):331-339.

Scutchfield FD, Long WN, Corey B, Tyler CW. Medroxyprogesterone acetate as an injectable female contraceptive. Contraception 1971;3(1):21-35.

Sheps MC. An analysis of reproductive patterns in an American isolate. Popul Stud 1965;19(1):65-80.

Sheth A, Jain U, Sharma S, Adatia A, Patankar S, Andolsek L, Pretnar-Darovec A, Belsey MA, Hall PE, Parker RA, Ayeni S, Pinol A, Foo CLH. A randomized, double-blind study of two combined and two progestogen-only oral contraceptives. Contraception 1982;25(3):243-252.

Shroff NE, Pearce MY, Stratford ME, Wilkinson PD. Clinical experience with ethynodiol diacetate 0.5 mg daily as an oral contraceptive. Contraception 1987;35(2):121-134.

Sivin I. International experience with implant contraception. In: Ratnam SS, Teoh ES, Lim SM. Proceedings of the 12th World Congress on Fertility and Sterility, Singapore, October 1986. Vol. 6: Contraception. Park Ridge NJ: Parthenon Publishing Group, 1987:121-126.

Sivin I. Personal communication to James Trussell, August 13, 1992.

Sivin I, El Mahgoub S, McCarthy T, Mishell DR, Shoupe D, Alvarez F, Brache V, Jimenez E, Diaz J, Faundes A, Diaz MM, Coutinho E, Mattos CER, Diaz S, Pavez M, Stern J. Long-term contraception with the Levonorgestrel 20 mcg/day (LNg 20) and the Copper T 380Ag intrauterine devices: a five-year randomized study. Contraception 1990;42(4):361-378.

Sivin I, Shaaban M, Odlind V, Olsson SE, Diaz S, Pavez M, Alvarez F, Brache V, Diaz J. A randomized trial of the Gyne T 380 and Gyne T 380 Slimline intrauterine copper devices. Contraception 1990;42(4):379-389.

Sivin I, Stern J. Long-acting, more effective copper T IUDs: a summary of U.S. experience, 1970-1975. Stud Fam Plann 1979;10(10):263-281.

Smith GG, Lee RJ. The use of cervical caps at the University of California, Berkeley: a survey. Contraception 1984;30(2):115-123.

Smith M, Vessey MP, Bounds W, Warren J. C-Film as a contraceptive. Br Med J 1974;4(5939):291.

Squire JJ, Berger GS, Keith L. A retrospective clinical study of a vaginal contraceptive suppository. J Reprod Med 1979;22(6):319-323.

Tatum HJ. Comparative experience with newer models of the copper T in the United States. In: Hefnawi F, Segal SJ (eds). Analysis of intrauterine contraception. Amsterdam, The Netherlands: North Holland, 1975:155-163.

Tietze C, Lewit S. Comparison of three contraceptive methods: diaphragm with jelly or cream, vaginal foam, and jelly/cream alone. J Sex Res 1967;3(4):295-311.

Tietze C, Lewit S. Evaluation of intrauterine devices: ninth progress report of the cooperative statistical program. Stud Fam Plann 1970;1(55):1-40.

Tietze C, Poliakoff SR, Rock J. The clinical effectiveness of the rhythm method of contraception. Fertil Steril 1951;2(5):444-450.

Trussell J, Grummer-Strawn L. Contraceptive failure of the ovulation method of periodic abstinence. Fam Plann Perspect 1990;22(2):65-75.

Trussell J, Hatcher RA, Cates W, Stewart FH, Kost K. Contraceptive failure in the United States: an update. Stud Fam Plann 1990;21(1):51-54.

Trussell J, Kost K. Contraceptive failure in the United States: a critical review of the literature. Stud Fam Plann 1987;18(5):237-283.

Tyler ET. Current developments in systemic contraception. Pac Med Surg 1965;93(1A):79-85.

Valle RF, Battifora HA. A new approach to tubal sterilization by laparoscopy. Fertil Steril 1978;30(4):415-422.

Vaughan B, Trussell J, Menken J, Jones EF. Contraceptive failure among married women in the United States, 1970-1973. Fam Plann Perspect 1977;9(6):251-258.

Vessey M, Huggins G, Lawless M, McPherson K, Yeates D. Tubal sterilization: findings in a large prospective study. Br J Obstet Gynaecol 1983;90(3):203-209.

Vessey M, Lawless M, Yeates D. Efficacy of different contraceptive methods. Lancet 1982;1(8276):841-842.

Vessey MP, Lawless M, Yeates D, McPherson K. Progestogen-only oral contraception. Findings in a large prospective study with special reference to effectiveness. Br J Fam Plann 1985;10(4):117-121.

Vessey MP, Villard-Mackintosh L, McPherson K, Yeates D. Factors influencing use-effectiveness of the condom. Br J Fam Plann 1988;14(2):40-43.

Vessey M, Wiggins P. Use-effectiveness of the diaphragm in a selected family planning clinic population in the United Kingdom. Contraception 1974;9(1):15-21.

Vessey MP, Wright NH, McPherson K, Wiggins P. Fertility after stopping different methods of contraception. Br Med J 1978;1(6108):265-267.

Wade ME, McCarthy P, Braunstein GD, Abernathy JR, Suchindran CM, Harris GS, Danzer HC, Uricchio WA. A randomized prospective study of the use-effectiveness of two methods of natural family planning. Am J Obstet Gynecol 1981; 141(4):368-376.

Westoff CF, Potter RG, Sagi PC, Mishler EG. Family growth in metropolitan America. Princeton NJ: Princeton University Press, 1961.

Wolf L, Olson HJ, Tyler ET. Observations on the clinical use of cream-alone and gel-alone methods of contraception. Obstet Gynecol 1957;10(3):316-321.

World Health Organization. A multicentered phase III comparative clinical trial of depot-medroxyprogesterone acetate given three-monthly at doses of 100 mg or 150 mg: I. Contraceptive efficacy and side effects. Contraception 1986;34(3): 223-235.

World Health Organization. A multicentered phase III comparative study of two hormonal contraceptive preparations given once-a-month by intramuscular injection: I. Contraceptive efficacy and side effects. Contraception 1988;37(1):1-20.

World Health Organization. A prospective multicentre trial of the ovulation method of natural family planning. II. The effectiveness phase. Fertil Steril 1981;36(5):591-598.

World Health Organization. Multinational comparative clinical evaluation of two long-acting injectable contraceptive steroids: norethisterone oenanthate and medroxyprogesterone acetate. Contraception 1977;15(5):513-533.

World Health Organization. Multinational comparative clinical trial of long-acting injectable contraceptives: norethisterone enanthate given in two dosage regimens and depot-medroxyprogesterone acetate. Final report. Contraception 1983;28(1):1-20.

Woutersz TB. A low-dose combination oral contraceptive: experience with 1,700 women treated for 22,489 cycles. J Reprod Med 1981;26(12):615-620.

Woutersz TB. A new ultra-low-dose combination oral contraceptive. J Reprod Med 1983;28(1-Suppl):81-84.

Wyeth Laboratories. NORPLANT® SYSTEM prescribing information. Philadelphia PA: Wyeth Laboratories, December 10, 1990.

Yoon IB, King TM, Parmley TH. A two-year experience with the Falope ring sterilization procedure. Am J Obstet Gynecol 1977;127(2):109-112.

Table 27-1 Percentage of women experiencing a contraceptive failure during the first year of typical use and the first year of perfect use and the percentage continuing use at the end of the first year, United States

Method (1)	% of Women Experiencing an Accidental Pregnancy within the First Year of Use		% of Women Continuing Use at One Year[3] (4)
	Typical Use[1] (2)	Perfect Use[2] (3)	
Chance[4]	85	85	
Spermicides[5]	21	6	43
Periodic Abstinence	20		67
Calendar		9	
Ovulation Method		3	
Sympto-Thermal[6]		2	
Post-Ovulation		1	
Withdrawal	19	4	
Cap[7]			
Parous Women	36	26	45
Nulliparous Women	18	9	58
Sponge			
Parous Women	36	20	45
Nulliparous Women	18	9	58
Diaphragm[7]	18	6	58
Condom[8]			
Female (Reality)	21	5	56
Male	12	3	63
Pill	3		72
Progestin Only		0.5	
Combined		0.1	
IUD			
Progesterone T	2.0	1.5	81
Copper T 380A	0.8	0.6	78
LNg 20	0.1	0.1	81
Depo-Provera	0.3	0.3	70
Norplant (6 Capsules)	0.09	0.09	85
Female Sterilization	0.4	0.4	100
Male Sterilization	0.15	0.10	100

Emergency Contraceptive Pills: Treatment initiated within 72 hours after unprotected intercourse reduces the risk of pregnancy by at least 75%.[9]

Lactational Amenorrhea Method: LAM is a highly effective, *temporary* method of contraception.[10]

Source: Updated from Trussell et al. (1990). See text.

1   Among *typical* couples who initiate use of a method (not necessarily for the first time), the percentage who experience an accidental pregnancy during the first year if they do not stop use for any other reason.

2   Among couples who initiate use of a method (not necessarily for the first time) and who use it *perfectly* (both consistently and correctly), the percentage who experience an accidental pregnancy during the first year if they do not stop use for any other reason.

3   Among couples attempting to avoid pregnancy, the percentage who continue to use a method for one year.

4   The percents failing in columns (2) and (3) are based on data from populations where contraception is not used and from women who cease using contraception in order to become pregnant. Among such populations, about 89% become pregnant within one year. This estimate was lowered slightly (to 85%) to represent the percent who would become pregnant within one year among women now relying on reversible methods of contraception if they abandoned contraception altogether.

5   Foams, creams, gels, vaginal suppositories, and vaginal film.

6   Cervical mucus (ovulation) method supplemented by calendar in the pre-ovulatory and basal body temperature in the post-ovulatory phases.

7   With spermicidal cream or jelly.

8   Without spermicides.

9   The treatment schedule is one dose as soon as possible (but no more than 72 hours) after uprotected intercourse, and a second dose 12 hours after the first dose. The hormones that have been studied in the clinical trials of postcoital hormonal contraception are found in Nordette, Levlen, Lo/Ovral (1 dose is 4 pills), Triphasil, Tri-Levlen (1 dose is 4 yellow pills), and Ovral (1 dose is 2 pills).

10   However, to maintain effective protection against pregnancy, another method of contraception must be used as soon as menstruation resumes, the frequency or duration of breastfeeds is reduced, bottle feeds are introduced, or the baby reaches 6 months of age.

Table 27-2 Summary of studies of pregnancy rates among women neither contracepting nor breastfeeding[a]

Reference	N for Analysis	Life-Table 12-Month Failure Rate	Characteristics of the Sample	LFU[g]	Comments
Grady et al., 1986	1,028	43.1	All married	20.6[r]	1982 NSFG; estimate far too low; see text
Sivin and Stern, 1979	420	78.1	48% nulliparous	?	Following removal of copper-medicated IUD for planned pregnancy
Vessey et al., 1978	779	82	All nulligravid	?	Oxford/FPA study following cessation of method use for planned pregnancy; conceptions leading to a live birth
Tatum, 1975	553	84.6		17.2	Following removal of copper-medicated IUD for planned pregnancy
Sivin, 1987	96	87	All parous	?	Chile, Dominican Republic, Finland, Sweden, United States; following removal of Norplant for planned pregnancy
Tietze and Lewit, 1970	378	88.2	89% aged 15–29	19.0	Following removal of nonmedicated IUD for planned pregnancy
Sheps, 1965	397	88.8	All married Hutterites	?	Conceptions leading to the first live birth following marriage among women reporting no fetal losses before the first conception
Vessey et al., 1978	1,343	89	All parous	?	Oxford/FPA study following cessation of method use for planned pregnancy; conceptions leading to a live birth
Belhadj et al., 1986	110	94.0[c]	All parous; aged 18–36	9.1	Brazil, Chile, Dominican Republic, Singapore, United States; following removal of medicated IUD for planned pregnancy

Notes:
a Updated from Trussell and Kost (1987), Table 1.
c Calculated by James Trussell from data in the article.
g Most of these studies incorrectly report the loss to follow-up rate as the number of women lost at any time during the study divided by the total number of women entering the study. Thus, these are the rates presented in the table. However, the correct measure of LFU would be a gross life-table rate. When available, 12-month rates are denoted by the letter "g."
r Nonresponse rate for entire survey.
For table references, see reference section.

Table 27-3 Summary of studies of contraceptive failure: spermicides[a]

Reference	Method Brand	N for Analysis	Life-Table 12-Month Failure Rate	Pearl Index Index	Pearl Index Total Exposure	Pearl Index Maximum Exposure	Characteristics of the Sample	LFU[g]	Comments
Edelman, 1980	S'positive	200		0.0	2,682 Mo.	?		?	Study conducted by Jordan-Simmer, Inc., as reported by Edelman
Squire et al., 1979	Semicid Suppository	326	0.3				69% aged 20–34; 55% married; "well educated", "highly motivated"; 24% prior use of oral contraceptives	0.0[c]	89% reported exclusive use of foam
Iizuka et al., 1980	Vaginal Contraceptive Film (C-Film)	168		0.6	2,161 Mo.	?	All women had been pregnant before; 20% aged < 25, 64% aged 25–34, 17% aged 35+	?	Japan
Brehm and Haase, 1975	Patentex Oval	10017		0.9[c]	63,759 Cy.	?	18% aged < 21, 20% aged > 35; 46% parity 0	?	Germany
Dimpfl et al., 1984	Patentex Oval	482	1.5				22% aged < 21, 25% aged > 31; 44% parity 0; 60% married	?	Denmark, Germany, Poland, Switzerland
Bushnell, 1965	Emko Vaginal Foam	130		1.8	2,737 Mo.	57 Mo.	Aged 17–51; 76% aged 20–35	?	
Carpenter and Martin, 1970	Emko Pre-fil Vaginal Foam	1778		3.4[c]	17,200 Cy.	18 Cy.	69% aged 21–35; 24% ≥ 12 years education; 44% no previous contraceptive experience	14.2[c]	All women agreed to exclusive use of foam
Brigato et al., 1982	Vaginal Contraceptive Film (C-Film)	37		3.9[c]	924 Mo.	?		?	Italy
Wolf et al., 1957	Preceptin Vaginal Gel	112		4.2[c]	1,145 Mo.	29 Mo.	All aged 13–40; mean aged = 25[t]; all married	8.9[c]	

(continued)

Table 27-3 Summary of studies of contraceptive failure: spermicides[a] *(cont.)*

Reference	Method Brand	N for Analysis	Life-Table 12 Month Failure Rate	Pearl Index Index	Pearl Index Total Exposure	Pearl Index Maximum Exposure	Characteristics of the Sample	LFU[g]	Comments
Bernstein, 1971	Emko Pre-fil Vaginal Foam	2,932		4.3[c]	28,332 Cy.	20 Cy.	70% aged 21–35; 39% ≥12 years education	16.1[c]	All women agreed to exclusive use of foam
Tyler, 1965	Delfen Vaginal Foam	672		6.0	9,486 Cy.	>16 Mo.	Rates for full applicator doses and half doses combined	?	
Kleppinger, 1965	Delfen Vaginal Foam	138		7.5	1,116 Mo.	19 Mo.	53% aged 21–30; 27% postpartum	0.0[c,g]	
Dubrow and Kuder, 1958	Delfen Vaginal Cream	338		7.6	633 Mo.	12 Mo.	Mean age = 25; 93% ≤12 years education; 39% black; 45% Puerto Rican[t]	59.5[c]	
Apothecus, 1992	Vaginal Contraceptive Film (C-Film)	824[c]		7.9[c]	6,695[c] Mo.	?		?	Belgium, Netherlands, Britain, Germany, Switzerland, Denmark, Sweden, Israel, Egypt; results never published; quality of study unknown
Dubrow and Kuder, 1958	Preceptin Vaginal Gel	835		8.1	3,728 Mo.	23 Mo.	Mean age = 25; 93% ≤12 years education; 39% black; 45% Puerto Rican[t]	45.1[c]	
Wolf et al., 1957	Delfen Vaginal Cream	875		8.9[c]	5,232 Mo.	30 Mo.	All aged 13–40; mean age = 25[t]; all married	13.0[c]	
Frankman et al., 1975	Vaginal Contraceptive Film (C-Film)	237		9.0	1,866 Mo.	23 Mo.		?	Sweden; data included in Apothecus (1992)
Rovinsky, 1964	Delfen Vaginal Cream	251		9.1	2,915 Mo.	67 Mo.	70% aged 20–34; 55% Puerto Rican; 10% ≥ 13 years education	28.0[c]	

(continued)

Table 27-3 Summary of studies of contraceptive failure: spermicides[a] *(cont.)*

Reference	Method Brand	N for Analysis	Life-Table 12-Month Failure Rate	Pearl Index Index	Pearl Index Total Exposure	Pearl Index Maximum Exposure	Characteristics of the Sample	LFU[g]	Comments
Vessey et al., 1982		?		11.9	303 Yr.	?	All white; at recruitment aged 25–39 and married; at enrollment, all women had been using the diaphragm, IUD, or the pill successfully for at least 5 months	0.3[t,v]	Oxford/FPA study
Jones and Forrest, 1992		267	13.4				Aged 15–44[t]	21[r]	NSFG 1988; failure rate when standardized and corrected for estimated underreporting of abortion = 30.2[s]
Vaughan et al., 1977		596	14.9[s]				Aged 15–44; all married[t]	19.0[r]	NSFG 1973
Grady et al., 1983		1,106	17.5[s,c]				Aged 15–44; all married[t]	18.2[r]	NSFG 1973 and 1976
Schirm et al., 1982		1,106	17.9[s]				Aged 15–44; all married[t]	18.2[r]	NSFG 1973 and 1976
Mears, 1962	Emko Vaginal Foam	425		18.0[c]	722 Cy.	3 Cy.	Pearl index of 9.3 among consistent and 48.4 among inconsistent users	> 20[c,t]	Britain; postal trial
Kasabach, 1962	Koromex A Jelly	242		21.0[c]	2,058 Mo.	24 Mo.	36% aged 25–35; all married; 68% "had a high school education"; all parous	19.3[c]	
Bracher and Santow, 1992		89	21.5				27% aged < 20, 56% aged 20–29, 17% aged 30+; 49% parity 0; 87% married or cohabiting[t]	25[r]	Australian Family Survey; first use of method
Grady et al., 1986		284	21.8[s]				Aged 15–44; all married[t]	20.6[r]	NSFG 1982

(continued)

Table 27-3 Summary of studies of contraceptive failure: spermicides[a] (cont.)

Reference	Method Brand	N for Analysis	Failure Rate				Characteristics of the Sample	LFU[g]	Comments
			Life-Table 12-Month Failure Rate	Pearl Index					
				Index	Total Exposure	Maximum Exposure			
Frank, 1962	Koromex A Jelly	824		24.8[c]	5,767 Mo.	12 Mo.	72% aged 21–35	17.0[c]	
Tietze and Lewit, 1967	Emko Vaginal Foam	779	28.3				86% < age 30; all married; 47% ≥ high school completion; 75% nonwhite	6.9[g]	
Tietze and Lewit, 1967	Cooper Creme and Creme Jel, Koromex A, Lactikol Creme and Jelly, Lanesta Gel	806	36.8				79% < age 30; all married; 53% ≥ high school completion; 75% nonwhite	3.4[g]	
Mears, 1962	Volpar Foaming Tablets	425		48.2[c]	728 Cy.	3 Cy.	Pearl index of 44.4 among consistent and 64.1 among inconsistent users	>20[c,t]	Britain; postal trial
Mears and Please, 1962	Vaginal Cream	678		49.6[c]	707 Cy.	3 Cy.	Pearl index of 31.4 among consistent and 132.0 among inconsistent users	>41[c,t]	Britain; postal trial
Smith et al., 1974	Vaginal Contraceptive Film (C-Film)	63[c]		55.7[c]	194[c] Mo.	<15[c] Mo.	Aged 16–35	9.5[c]	Britain; data included in Apothecus (1992); trial terminated for ethical reasons

(continued)

Table 27-3 Summary of studies of contraceptive failure: spermicides[a] *(cont.)*

Reference	Method Brand	N for Analysis	Failure Rate				Characteristics of the Sample	LFU[g]	Comments
			Life-Table 12-Month Failure Rate	Pearl Index					
				Index	Total Exposure	Maximum Exposure			
Mears and Please, 1962	Volpar Foaming Tablets	678	59.0[c]		705 Cy.	3 Cy.	Pearl index of 47.8 among consistent and 106.7 among inconsistent users	>41 [c,t]	Britain; postal trial

Notes:

a Updated from Trussell and Kost (1987), Table 2.

c Calculated by James Trussell from data in the article.

g Most of these studies incorrectly report the loss to follow-up rate (LFU) as the number of women lost at any time during the study divided by the total number of women entering the study. Thus, these are the rates presented in the table. However, the correct measure of LFU would be a gross life-table rate. When available, 12-month rates are denoted by the letter "g."

r Nonresponse rate for entire survey.

s Standardized: Vaughan et al., (1977) (1973 NSFG)—intention (the average of rates for preventers and delayers); Grady et al., (1983) (1973 and 1976 NSFG)—intention. Our calculation (the average of rates for preventers and delayers); Schirm et al., (1982) (1973 and 1976 NSFG)—intention, age, and income; Grady et al., (1986) (1982 NSFG)—intention, age, poverty status, and parity; Jones and Forrest (1992) (1988 NSFG)—duration, age, marital status, and poverty status.

t Total for all methods in the study.

v The authors report that LFU for "relevant reasons (withdrawal of cooperation or loss of contact)" was 0.3% per year in the 1982 study. In the 1982 study, women had on average been followed for 9.5 years; if 0.3% are LFU per year, then 2.8% would be LFU in 9.5 years. LFU including death and emigration is about twice as high as LFU for "relevant reasons."

Mo. = months.

Cy. = cycles.

For table references, see reference section.

Table 27-4 Summary of studies of contraceptive failure: periodic abstinence[a]

Reference	Method	N for Analysis	Life-Table 12-Month Failure Rate	Pearl Index — Index	Pearl Index — Total Exposure	Pearl Index — Maximum Exposure	Characteristics of the Sample	LFU[g]	Comments
Trussell and Grummer-Strawn, 1990	Ovulation	725	3.2				Mean age = 30; proven fertility; agreed to use OM alone; cohabiting; 765 of 869 learned OM to satisfaction of teachers; 725 entered effectiveness study	?	Reanalysis of W.H.O. (1981) trial: failure rate based on 13 cycles of *perfect use*
Rice et al., 1981	Calendar + BBT	723	8.2				Aged 19–44; 9% aged 19–24, 54% aged 25–34, 37% aged 35–44; all parity 1+	3.4[c]	United States, France, Colombia, Canada, Mauritius
Dolack, 1978	Ovulation	329		10.5[c]	3,354 Cy.	?	Aged 19–48; mean age = 28; 40% had used oral contraceptives prior to study	18.0[c]	
Johnston et al., 1978	Cervical Mucus + BBT + Other Signs	268	13.3[c]				73% aged 22–32; all married or de facto married; 48% ≥ 12 years education (n = 460)	33.9[c,t]	Australia; failure rate based on 13 cycles
Wade et al., 1981	Cervical Mucus + BBT + Calendar	239	13.9[c]				Aged 20–39; 78% married	11.4[c,g]	Random assignment to OM or CM + BBT + Cal
Johnston et al., 1978	Calendar + BBT + Other Signs	192	14.3				73% aged 22–32; all married or de facto married; 48% ≥ 12 years education (n = 460)	33.9[c,t]	Australia; failure rate based on 13 cycles
Tietze et al., 1951	Calendar	409		14.4	7,267 Mo.	>60 Mo.	57% aged 25–34	13.4[c,t]	

(continued)

Table 27-4 Summary of studies of contraceptive failure: periodic abstinence[a] *(cont.)*

Reference	Method	N for Analysis	Failure Rate Life-Table 12-Month Failure Rate	Pearl Index Index	Pearl Index Total Exposure	Pearl Index Maximum Exposure	Characteristics of the Sample	LFU[g]	Comments
Vessey et al., 1982	Rhythm	?		15.5	161 Yr.	?	All white; at recruitment aged 25–39 and married; at enrollment, all women had been using the diaphragm, IUD, or the pill successfully for at least 5 months	0.3	Oxford/FPA study
Klaus et al., 1979	Ovulation	?	15.8[n]				67% aged 18–34; 52% ≥ 13 years education; some use of concurrent methods	2.9[n]	Failure rate based on only 12 cycles
Johnston et al., 1978	Cervical Mucus + BBT + Other Signs + Other Methods	94	16.0				78% aged 22–32; all married or de facto married; 53% ≥ 12 years education ("other" not limited to rhythm)	33.9[c,t]	Australia; failure rate based on 13 cycles
Grady et al., 1986	Rhythm	167	16.1[s]				Aged 15–44; all married[t]	20.6[r]	NSFG 1982
Bracher and Santow, 1992	Rhythm	137	17.9				14% aged <20, 75% aged 20–29, 11% aged 30+; 46% parity 0; 92% married or cohabiting	25[r]	Australian Family Survey; first use of method
Kambic et al., 1981, 1982	Ovulation or Cervical Mucus + BBT	235	18.2[n]				81% aged 20–34; 83% married; approx. 30% used barrier methods concurrently[t]	6.5[n]	
Ball, 1976	Ovulation	124		16.8[c]	1626 Cy.	22 Cy.	Aged 20–39	1.6[c]	Australia
Grady et al., 1983	Rhythm	412	18.3[s,c]				Aged 15–44; all married[t]	18.2[r]	NSFG 1973 and 1976

(continued)

Table 27-4 Summary of studies of contraceptive failure: periodic abstinence[a] *(cont.)*

			Failure Rate						
			Life-Table	Pearl Index					
Reference	Method	N for Analysis	12-Month Failure Rate	Index	Total Exposure	Maximum Exposure	Characteristics of the Sample	LFU[g]	Comments
Johnston et al., 1978	Ovulation + Other Methods	71	18.8				80% aged 22–32; all married or de facto married; 49% ≥ 12 years education ("other" not limited to rhythm)	33.9[c,t]	Australia; failure rate based on 13 cycles
Vaughan et al., 1977	Rhythm	220	19.1[s]				Aged 15–44; all married[t]	19.0[r]	NSFG 1973
W.H.O., 1981	Ovulation	725	19.6				Mean age about 30; proven fertility; agreed to use OM alone; 54% desired no more children; 765 of 869 learned OM to satisfaction of teachers; 725 entered effectiveness study	?	New Zealand, India, Ireland, Philippines, El Salvador; rate based on 13 cycles
Jones and Forrest, 1992	Rhythm	289	20.9				Aged 15–44[t]	21[r]	NSFG 1988; failure rate when standardized and corrected for estimated under-reporting of abortion = 31.4[s]
Bartzen, 1967	BBT	335		21.3[c]	4,824 Cy.	58 Mo.	Aged 19–45; mean age = 28	11.6[c]	
Schirm et al., 1982	Rhythm	412	23.7[s]				Aged 15–44; all married[t]	18.2[r]	NSFG 1973 and 1976

(continued)

Table 27-4 Summary of studies of contraceptive failure: periodic abstinence[a] (cont.)

Reference	Method	N for Analysis	Failure Rate Life-Table 12-Month Failure Rate	Pearl Index Index	Pearl Index Total Exposure	Pearl Index Maximum Exposure	Characteristics of the Sample	LFU[g]	Comments
Marshall, 1976	Ovulation + BBT	84		23.9[c]	1,195 Cy.	32 Mo.	67% aged 20–34	1.2[c]	Britain
Johnston et al., 1978	Ovulation	586	26.4				69% aged 22–32; all married or de facto married; 44% ≥12 years education	33.9[c,t]	Australia; failure rate based on 13 cycles
Wade et al., 1981	Ovulation	191	37.2[c]				Aged 20–39; 74% married	13.8[c,g]	Random assignment to OM or CM + BBT + Cal

Notes:
a Updated from Trussell and Kost (1987), Table 3.
c Calculated by James Trussell from data in the article.
g Most of these studies incorrectly report the loss to follow-up rate (LFU) as the number of women lost at any time during the study divided by the total number of women entering the study. Thus, these are the rates presented in the table. However, the correct measure of LFU would be a gross life-table rate. When available, 12-month rates are denoted by the letter "g."
n Only net rates available for this study.
r Nonresponse rate for entire survey.
s Standardized: Vaughan et al., (1977) (1973 NSFG)—intention (the average of rates for preventers and delayers); Grady et al., (1983) (1973 and 1976 NSFG)—intention. Our calculation (the average of rates for preventers and delayers); Schirm et al., (1982) (1973 and 1976 NSFG)—intention, age, and income; Grady et al., (1986) (1982 NSFG)—intention, age, poverty status, and parity; Jones and Forrest (1992) (1988 NSFG)—duration, age, marital status, and poverty status.
t Total for all methods in the study.
v The authors report that LFU for "relevant reasons (withdrawal of cooperation or loss of contact)" was 0.3% per year in the 1982 study. In the 1982 study, women had on average been followed for 9.5 years; if 0.3% are LFU per year, then 2.8% would be LFU in 9.5 years. LFU including death and emigration is about twice as high as LFU for "relevant reasons."
For table references, see reference section.

Table 27-4 **663**

Table 27-5 Summary of studies of contraceptive failure: withdrawal[a]

Reference	N for Analysis	Failure Rate				Characteristics of the Sample[w]	LFU[g]	Comments
		Life-Table 12-Month Failure Rate	Pearl Index					
			Index	Total Exposure	Maximum Exposure			
Vessey et al., 1982	?		6.7	674 Yr.	?	All white; at recruitment aged 25–39 and married; at enrollment, all women had been using the diaphragm, IUD, or the pill successfully for at least 5 months	0.3[t,v]	Oxford/FPA study
Bracher and Santow, 1992	94	14.2				25% aged <20, 66% aged 20–29, 9% aged 30+; 57% parity 0, 92% married or cohabiting	25[r]	Australian Family Survey; first use of method
Westoff et al., 1961	~74		16.7	1,287 Mo.	?	All married; all white	5.7[r]	FGMA study
Cliquet et al., 1977	2,316	17.3				All aged 30–34 living in Belgium; 93% living as married[t]	22[r]	Belgium; 1971 National Survey on Family Development (NEGO II)
Debusschere, 1980	3,561	20.8				Aged 16–44 living in Flanders; 85% married[t]	40[r]	Belgium; 1975–1976 National Survey on Family Development (NEGO III)
Peel, 1972	62		21.9	1,640 Mo.	60 Mo.	All married	2.9[t]	Britain; Hull Family Survey

Notes:
a Updated from Trussell and Kost (1987), Table 1.
c Calculated by James Trussell from data in the article.
g Most of these studies incorrectly report the loss to follow-up rate (LFU) as the number of women lost at any time during the study divided by the total number of women entering the study. Thus, these are the rates presented in the table. However, the correct measure of LFU would be a gross life-table rate. When available, 12-month rates are denoted by the letter "g."
r Nonresponse rate for entire survey.
t Total for all methods in the study.
v The authors report that LFU for "relevant reasons (withdrawal of cooperation or loss of contact)" was 0.3% per year in the 1982 study. In the 1982 study, women had on average been followed for 9.5 years; if 0.3% are LFU per year, then 2.8% would be LFU in 9.5 years. LFU including death and emigration is about twice as high as LFU for "relevant reasons."
w Unless otherwise noted, characteristics refer to females.
For table references, see reference section.

Table 27-6 Summary of studies of contraceptive failure: cervical cap[a, b]

		Failure Rate					
		Life-Table	Pearl Index				
Reference	N for Analysis	12-Month Failure Rate	Index	Total Exposure	Maximum Exposure	Characteristics of the Sample	LFU[g]	Comments
Denniston and Putney, 1981	110	8.0[d,n]				98% aged 20–35; 70% nulliparous	20.9[c]	
Cagen, 1986	620	8.1[n]				87% aged 20–34; 80% always used spermicide and 14% never did	38.5[c]	LFU = "no response"
Koch, 1982	372	8.4				76% aged 20–29; 65% college graduates	8.0[c]	Women advised also to use condom for the first several cap uses
Richwald et al., 1989	3,433	11.3				Mean age 29.0; 91% white non-Hispanic; 80% unmarried; almost 60% college graduates; 64% one or more previous pregnancies; 6.1% failure rate among perfect users, 11.9% among imperfect users	18[g]	Women advised to use extra spermicide or use condoms during first 2 months of use; 15 sites; 14 in Los Angeles, 1 in Santa Fe
Powell et al., 1986	477	16.6				67% aged 25–34 "about half" unmarried; 97% high school graduates; 17% using the pill when fitted for cap	43.8[c]	Canada; back-up methods encouraged (including the "morning after pill," used by 23 women in cases of cap dislodgement)

(continued)

Table 27-6   **665**

Table 27-6 Summary of studies of contraceptive failure: cervical cap[a,b] (cont.)

Reference	N for Analysis	Failure Rate				Characteristics of the Sample	LFU[g]	Comments
		Life-Table 12-Month Failure Rate	Pearl Index					
			Index	Total Exposure	Maximum Exposure			
Bernstein et al., 1986	687[c]	17.4				95% aged ≤ 35, 16% married, 96% ≥ high school completion	26.3[c,g]	Random assignment to the diaphragm or cervical cap
Kassell and McElroy, 1981	90		18.1[c]	731 Mo.	12 Mo.	Mean age = 23.6; mean education = 14.7 years	10.0[c]	
Boehm, 1983	47		18.1[c]	397 Mo.	12 Mo.		31.6	All women reported exclusive use of cap
Lehfeldt and Sivin, 1984	130	19.1				37% aged 16–25; 72% college graduates; 91% nulliparous	7.2[c]	All women agreed to exclusive use of cap
Smith and Lee, 1984	33	27.0				80% aged 20–29; clients at university student health service	1.5–4.6[c]	Regular users for whom the cap (with spermicide) was the sole method used "during the fertile portion of the cycle"

Notes:
a Updated from Trussell and Kost (1987), Table 4.
b All entries pertain to the Prentif Cavity-rim cap except for Smith and Lee (1984) and Powell et al., (1986), which included both Cavity-rim and Vimule caps.
c Calculated by James Trussell from data in the article.
d 6-month net rate; 12-month rate not available.
g Most of these studies incorrectly report the loss to follow-up (LFU) rate as the number of women lost at any time during the study divided by the total number of women entering the study. Thus, these are the rates presented in the table. However, the correct measure of LFU would be a gross life-table rate. When available, 12-month rates are denoted by the letter "g."
n Only net rates are available for this study.
For table references, see reference section.

Table 27-7 Summary of studies of contraceptive failure: sponge[a]

Reference	N for Analysis	Life-Table 12-Month Failure Rate	Characteristics of the Sample	LFU[g]	Comments
Jones and Forrest, 1992	227	14.5	Aged 15–44[t]	21[r]	NSFG 1988
Edelman et al., 1984	722	17.0	89% aged 20–34; 28% married; 77% ≥ 13 years education; 94% white, 49% never-married; 38% used oral contraceptives prior to entering study	33.2[c,g]	Random assignment to the diaphragm or sponge
McIntyre and Higgins, 1986	723	17.4	89% aged 20–34; 28% married; 77% ≥ 13 years education; 94% white, 49% never-married; 38% used oral contraceptives prior to entering study	33.2[c,g]	A reanalysis of data used by Edelman et al. (1984); random assignment to the diaphragm or sponge; much higher rate for parous women
Bounds and Guillebaud, 1984	126	24.5	92% aged 20–34; all married/consensual union; "most" ≥ 13 years education; 99% white	1.7[g]	Britain; random assignment to the diaphragm or sponge

Notes:
[a] Updated from Trussell and Kost (1987), Table 4.
[c] Calculated by James Trussell from data in the article.
[g] Most of these studies incorrectly report the loss to follow-up (LFU) rate as the number of women lost at any time during the study divided by the total number of women entering the study. Thus, these are the rates presented in the table. However, the correct measure of LFU would be a gross life-table rate. When available, 12-month rates are denoted by the letter "g."
[r] Nonresponse rate for entire survey.
[t] Total for all methods in the study.
For table references, see reference section.

Table 27-8 Summary of studies of contraceptive failure: diaphragm[a]

		Failure Rate						
		Life-Table	Pearl Index					
Reference	N for Analysis	12-Month Failure Rate	Index	Total Exposure	Maximum Exposure	Characteristics of the Sample	LFU[g]	Comments
Lane et al., 1976	2,168	2.1[c]				61% aged 21–34; 71% unmarried; 92% white	1.1[c,g]	Failure rate downward biased due to improper exposure allocated to women LFU
Vessey and Wiggins, 1974	4,052		2.4	5,909 Mo.	>60 Mo.	All white; at recruitment aged 25–39 and married; all had been using the diaphragm for at least 5 months at enrollment; no previous pill use	1.0[v]	Oxford/FPA study
Vessey et al., 1982	?		5.5	2,582 Yr.	24 Mo.	All white and aged 25–34; all married at recruitment; at enrollment, all women had been using the diaphragm, IUD, or the pill successfully for at least 5 months	0.3[t,v]	Oxford/FPA study
Loudon et al., 1991	269		8.7	2,350 Mo.	12 Mo.	Mean age = 28.6; 57% gravidity 0; 68% married or cohabiting; 54% already using the diaphragm at start of trial	>3.7	Britain; random assignment of spermicide: either C-Film or jelly
Dubrow and Kuder, 1958	873		9.3	5,814 Mo.	48 Mo.	Mean age = 25; 39% black; 45% Puerto Rican; 93% ≤ 12 years education[t]	38.0[c]	
Jones and Forrest, 1992	472	10.4				Aged 15–44[t]	21[r]	NSFG 1988; failure rate when standardized and corrected for estimated underreporting of abortion = 22.0[s]
Hall, 1973	347	10.6				Approximately 75% aged 20–24; 47% black; 38% Hispanic; all postpartum	16.0	

(continued)

Table 27-8 Summary of studies of contraceptive failure: diaphragm[a] *(cont.)*

		Failure Rate						
			Pearl Index					
Reference	**N for Analysis**	**Life-Table 12-Month Failure Rate**	**Index**	**Total Exposure**	**Maximum Exposure**	**Characteristics of the Sample**	**LFU[g]**	**Comments**
Bounds and Guillebaud, 1984	123	10.9				90% aged 20–34; all married/ consensual union; "most" ≥ 13 years education; 96% white	0.0	Britain; random assignment to the diaphragm or sponge
Edelman et al., 1984	717	12.5				88% aged 20–34; 55% never married; 76% ≥13 years education; 94% white; 39% used oral contra- ceptives prior to entering study	37.8[c,g]	Random assignment to the diaphragm or sponge
McIntyre and Higgins, 1986	717	12.9				88% aged 20–34; 55% never married; 76% ≥ 13 years education; 94% white; 39% used oral contra- ceptives prior to entering study	37.8[c,g]	A reanalysis of data used by Edelman et al. (1984); random assignment to the diaphragm or sponge
Vaughan et al., 1977	166	13.1[s]				Aged 15–44; all married[t]	19.0[r]	NSFG 1973
Grady et al., 1983	349	14.3[c,s]				Aged 15–44; all married[t]	18.2[r]	NSFG 1973 and 1976
Bernstein et al., 1986	707[c]	16.7				96% aged ≤ 35; 17% married; 97% ≥ high school completion	33.5[c,g]	Random assignment to the diaphragm or cervical cap
Grady et al., 1986	257	17.0[s]				Aged 15–44; all married[t]	20.6[r]	NSFG 1982
Tietze and Lewit, 1967	1,197	17.9				86% aged < 30; all married; 60% ≥ high school completion; 50% white	7.2[g]	

(continued)

Table 27-8 Summary of studies of contraceptive failure: diaphragm[a] *(cont.)*

		Failure Rate						
		Life-Table 12-Month Failure Rate	Pearl Index			Characteristics of the Sample	LFU[g]	Comments
Reference	N for Analysis		Index	Total Exposure	Maximum Exposure			
Schirm et al., 1982	349	18.6 [s]				Aged 15–44; all married[t]	18.2 [r]	NSFG 1973 and 1976
Bracher and Santow, 1992	219	21.0				12% aged < 20; 77% aged 20–29, 11% aged 30+; 56% parity 0; 87% married or cohabiting	25 [r]	Australian Family Survey; first use of method

Notes:

a Updated from Trussell and Kost (1987), Table 5.

c Calculated by James Trussell from data in the article.

g Most of these studies incorrectly report the loss to follow-up (LFU) rate as the number of women lost at any time during the study divided by the total number of women entering the study. Thus, these are the rates presented in the table. However, the correct measure of LFU would be a gross life-table rate. When available, 12-month rates are denoted by the letter "g."

r Nonresponse rate for entire survey.

s Standardized: Vaughan et al., (1977) (1973 NSFG)—intention (the average of rates for preventers and delayers); Grady et al., (1983) (1973 and 1976 NSFG)—intention. Our calculation (the average of rates for preventers and delayers); Schirm et al., (1982) (1973 and 1976 NSFG)—intention, age, and income; Grady et al., (1986) (1982 NSFG)—intention, age, poverty status, and parity; Jones and Forrest (1992) (1988 NSFG)—duration, age, marital status, and poverty status.

t Total for all methods in the study.

v The authors report that LFU for "relevant reasons (withdrawal of cooperation or loss of contact)" was 0.3% per year in the 1982 study and "about 10 per 1,000" per year in the 1974 study. In the 1982 study, women had on average been followed for 9.5 years; if 0.3% are LFU per year, then 2.8% would be LFU for 9.5 years. LFU including death and emigration is about twice as high as LFU for "relevant reasons."

For table references, see reference section.

Table 27-9 Summary of studies of contraceptive failure: condom[a]

Reference	N for Analysis	Failure Rate				Characteristics of the Sample [w]	LFU [g]	Comments
		Life-Table 12-Month Failure Rate	Pearl Index					
			Index	Total Exposure	Maximum Exposure			
Potts and McDevitt, 1975	397	2.1[b]				77% males ≥ age 40; all married	4.8[c]	Britain; postal trial of spermicidally lubricated condom
Peel, 1972	96					All married	2.9[t]	Britain; Hull Family Survey
Glass et al., 1974	2,057	4.2	3.9	3,698 Mo.	60 Mo.	All white; at recruitment aged 25–39 and married; at enrollment, all women had been using the diaphragm, IUD, or the pill successfully for at least 5 months	<1.0[v]	Oxford/FPA study
Vessey et al., 1988	?		4.4	10,000[c] Yr.	24 Mo.	All white; at recruitment aged 25–39 and married; at enrollment, all women had been using the diaphragm, IUD, or the pill successfully for at least 5 months	?	Oxford/FPA study
John, 1973	85		5.7[c]	261 Yr.	> 7 Yr.	?	?	Britain; retrospective survey
Vessey et al., 1982	?		6.0	4,317 Yr.	24 Mo.	All white and aged 25–34; all married at recruitment; at enrollment, all women were using the diaphragm, IUD, or the pill successfully for at least 5 months	0.3[t,v]	Oxford/FPA study
Jones and Forrest, 1992	1,728	7.2				Aged 15–44[t]	21[r]	NSFG 1988; failure rate when standardized and corrected for estimated underreporting of abortion = 15.8[s]
Bracher and Santow, 1992	262	8.1				16% aged < 20, 65% aged 20–29, 19% aged 30+; 48% parity 0; 83% married or cohabiting	25[r]	Australian Family Survey; first use of method

(continued)

Table 27-9 Summary of studies of contraceptive failure: condom[a] *(cont.)*

Reference	N for Analysis	Failure Rate — Life-Table 12-Month Failure Rate	Failure Rate — Pearl Index — Index	Failure Rate — Pearl Index — Total Exposure	Failure Rate — Pearl Index — Maximum Exposure	Characteristics of the Sample[w]	LFU[g]	Comments
Schirm et al., 1982	1,223	9.6[s]				Aged 15–44; all married[t]	18.2[r]	NSFG 1973 and 1976
Grady et al., 1983	1,223	9.7[sc]				Aged 15–44; all married[t]	18.2[r]	NSFG 1973 and 1976
Vaughan et al., 1977	696	10.1[s]				Aged 15–44; all married[t]	19.0[r]	NSFG 1973
Grady et al., 1986	526	13.8[s]				Aged 15–44; all married[t]	20.6[r]	NSFG 1982
Westoff et al., 1961	~212		13.8[c]	10,062 Mo.	?	All married	5.7[r]	FGMA study

Notes:
a Updated from Trussell and Kost (1987), Table 6.
b 24-month rate; 12-month rate not published.
c Calculated by James Trussell from data in the article.
g Most of these studies incorrectly report the loss to follow-up rate (LFU) as the number of women lost at any time during the study divided by the total number of women entering the study. Thus, these are the rates presented in the table. However, the correct measure of LFU would be a gross life-table rate. When available, 12-month rates are denoted by the letter "g."
r Nonresponse rate for entire survey.
s Standardized: Vaughan et al., (1977) (1973 NSFG)—intention (the average of rates for preventers and delayers); Grady et al., (1983) (1973 and 1976 NSFG)—intention. Our calculation (the average of rates for preventers and delayers); Schirm et al., (1982) (1973 and 1976 NSFG)—intention, age, and income; Grady et al., (1986) (1982 NSFG)—intention, age, poverty status, and parity; Jones and Forrest (1992) (1988 NSFG)—duration, age, marital status, and poverty status.
t Total for all methods in the study.
v The authors report that LFU for "relevant reasons (withdrawal of cooperation or loss of contact)" was 0.3% per year in the 1982 study. In the 1982 study, women had on average been followed for 9.5 years; if 0.3% are LFU per year, then 2.8% would be LFU in 9.5 years. LFU including death and emigration is about twice as high as LFU for "relevant reasons."
w Unless otherwise noted, characteristics refer to females.
For table references, see reference section.

Table 27-10 Summary of studies of contraceptive failure: minipill[a]

Reference	Method Brand	N for Analysis	Failure Rate — Life-Table 12-Month Failure Rate	Pearl Index — Index	Pearl Index — Total Exposure	Pearl Index — Maximum Exposure	Characteristics of the Sample	LFU[g]	Comments
Postlethwaite, 1979	Femulen (Ethynodiol diacetate 0.5 mg)	309	1.1[c]				Aged 17–48	21.0[c]	Britain
Shroff et al., 1987	Femulen (Ethynodiol diacetate 0.5 mg)	425	1.1[n]				72% aged 16–34; 25% nulligravid	12.7[c]	Britain; authors employed by manufacturer
Board, 1971	Micronor (Norethindrone 0.35 mg)	154		1.3	1,882 Mo.	19 Mo.		?	
Keifer, 1973	Micronor (Norethindrone 0.35 mg)	151		1.68	2,141 Mo.	26 Mo.	Aged 18–45; 84% aged 21–35; 74% previous oral contraceptive users; at least 32% current users at start	4.6[c]	
Vessey et al., 1985		?		1.98[c]	404 Yr.	12 Mo.	All white and aged 25–34; all married at recruitment; at enrollment, all women had been using the diaphragm, IUD, or the pill successfully for at least 5 months	.3[t,v]	Oxford/FPA study
Korba and Paulson, 1974	Ovrette (Norgestrel 0.075 mg)	2202		2.19[c]	29,006 Mo.	67 Mo.		?	Authors employed by manufacturer
McQuarrie et al., 1972	Micronor (Norethindrone 0.35 mg)	318		2.64[c]	3,453 Cy.	27 Mo.	Aged 16–42; mean age = 26; all white	2.2[c]	
Nelson, 1973	Megestrol acetate (0.5 mg)	342		2.7	3,552 Mo.	41 Mo.		14.6[c]	

(continued)

Table 27-10 Summary of studies of contraceptive failure: minipill[a] *(cont.)*

Reference	Method Brand	N for Analysis	Failure Rate Life-Table 12-Month Failure Rate	Pearl Index Index	Pearl Index Total Exposure	Pearl Index Maximum Exposure	Characteristics of the Sample	LFU[g]	Comments
Jubhari et al., 1974	Quingestanol acetate (0.3 mg)	382	2.9[n]				Mean age = 23; "predominately white, single and nulliparous"	14.0	
Hawkins and Benster, 1977	Norethisterone (0.35 mg)	200	6.8				Mean age = 25; postpartum women, 71% within 3 months of delivery[t]	5.2[c]	Britain
Hawkins and Benster, 1977	Megestrol acetate (0.5 mg)	174	8.7				Mean age = 25; postpartum women, 71% within 3 months of delivery[t]	8.4[c]	Britain
Sheth et al., 1982	Levonorgestrel (0.30 mg)	128	9.5[n]				Mean age = 25.7	2.1[t]	Yugoslavia and India
Hawkins and Benster, 1977	Chlormadinone acetate (0.5 mg)	182	9.6				Mean age = 26; postpartum women, 71% within 3 months of delivery[t]	3.3[c]	Britain
Sheth et al., 1982	Norethisterone (0.35 mg)	130	13.2[n]				Mean age = 25.6	2.1[t]	Yugoslavia and India

Notes:
a Updated from Trussell and Kost (1987), Table 8.
c Calculated by James Trussell from data in the article.
g Most of these studies incorrectly report the loss to follow-up (LFU) rate as the number of women lost at any time during the study divided by the total number of women entering the study. Thus, these are the rates presented in the table. However, the correct measure of LFU would be a gross life-table rate. When available, 12-month rates are denoted by the letter "g."
n Only net rates available for this study.
t Total for all methods in the study.
v The authors report that LFU for "relevant reasons (withdrawal of cooperation or loss of contact)" was 0.3% per year in the 1982 study. In the 1985 study, women had on average probably been followed for 12.5 years; if 0.3% are LFU per year, then 3.7% would be LFU in 12.5 years. LFU including death and emigration is about twice as high as LFU for "relevant reasons."
For table references, see reference section.

Table 27-11 Summary of studies of contraceptive failure: combined oral contraceptives[a]

Reference	Method Brand	N for Analysis	Failure Rate				Characteristics of the Sample	LFU[g]	Comments
			Life-Table 12-Month Failure Rate	Pearl Index					
				Index	Total Exposure	Maximum Exposure			
Preston, 1972	Norlestrin 2.5 (80%)	378	0.0[c]				Aged 15–46; 46% aged 25–34; 36% white; 64% on pill at start	9.5	Author employed by manufacturer; pill not marketed
Ledger, 1970	Ortho-Novum 1/80	144	0.0[c]				All aged 14–43; mean age = 24; mostly graduate students or wives of students	14.0[c]	
Woutersz, 1981	Lo/Ovral	1,700		0.12	22,489 Cy.	53 Cy.	65% aged 20–29; 55% on pill at start	23.8	Author employed by manufacturer
Korba and Heil, 1975	Ovral	6,806		0.19	127,872 Cy.	110 Cy.	Mean age = 25; 26% white; approximately 80% had not used other oral contraceptives within 3 months	?	Mexico, Puerto Rico and United States; author employed by manufacturer
Ellis, 1987	Ortho-Novum 7/7/7	619		0.22	909[c]Yr.	?	Mean age = 24.5; 40.5% nulligravid	?	United States, Canada, France
Morigi and Pasquale, 1978	Modicon	1,168		0.24[c]	16,345 Cy.	53 Cy.	Aged 13–54; 85% aged 19–36; 61% previous use of oral contraceptives	?	Mexico, Puerto Rico, Canada, and United States; author employed by manufacturer
Hughes, 1978	Ovamin	453	0.24[c]				Aged 16–40; % new users not stated	11.9[c]	Britain
Vessey et al., 1982	50 µg estrogen	?		0.25	10,400 Yr.	24 Mo.	All white and aged 25–34; all married at recruitment; at enrollment, all women had been using the diaphragm, IUD, or the pill successfully for at least 5 months	0.3[t,v]	Oxford/FPA study

(continued)

Table 27-11 Summary of studies of contraceptive failure: combined oral contraceptives[a] *(cont.)*

Reference	Method Brand	N for Analysis	Failure Rate — Life-Table 12-Month Failure Rate	Failure Rate — Pearl Index — Index	Failure Rate — Pearl Index — Total Exposure	Failure Rate — Pearl Index — Maximum Exposure	Characteristics of the Sample	LFU[g]	Comments
Royal College, 1974		23,611		0.34	?	48 Mo.	75% aged 20–34; all married/ living as married; 62% on pill at start (20% new users)	32.0[c]	Britain
Woutersz, 1983	Nordette	1,130		0.35	11,064 Cy.	31 Cy.	71% aged 20–30; 48% no use of hormones and not pregnant within 60 days of start	8.1[c]	Author employed by manufacturer
Vessey et al., 1982	< 50 µg estrogen	?		0.38	3,158 Yr.	24 Mo.	All white and aged 25–34; all married at recruitment; at enroll-ment, all women had been using the diaphragm, IUD, or the pill successfully for at least 5 months	0.3[t,v]	Oxford/FPA study
Preston, 1974 and 1972	Norlestrin 2.5 (60%)	1,192		0.63[c]	14,536 Cy.	>18 Cy.	Aged 14–47; 35% aged 25–34; 47% white; 56% on pill at start	13.7	Author employed by manufacturer; pill not marketed
Preston, 1974 and 1972	Norlestrin 2.5 (40%)	1,393		0.94[c]	15,265 Cy.	> 18 Cy.	Aged 13–42; 27% aged 25–34; 39% white; 49% on pill at start	16.3	Author employed by manufacturer; pill not marketed
Ellsworth, 1986	Triphasil	1,264		1.09	8,349 Cy.	34 Cy.	All < age 38	?	17 U.S. Centers
Preston, 1974 and 1972	Norlestrin 1.0 (60%)	1,872		1.47[c]	20,341 Cy.	> 18 Cy.	Aged 14–44; 30% aged 25–34; 42% white; 55% on pill at start	13.1	Author employed by manufacturer; pill not marketed
Preston, 1974	Norlestrin 1.0 (20%)	276		1.59[c]	2,449 Cy.	?		?	Author employed by manufacturer; pill not marketed
Vaughan et al., 1977		2,434	2.0[s]				Aged 15–44; all married[t]	19.0[r]	NSFG 1973

(continued)

Table 27-11 Summary of studies of contraceptive failure: combined oral contraceptives[a] *(cont.)*

			Failure Rate					
			Life-Table	Pearl Index				
Reference	Method Brand	N for Analysis	12-Month Failure Rate	Index	Total Exposure	Maximum Exposure	Characteristics of the Sample	LFU[g]	Comments
Bracher and Santow, 1992		1,830	2.2				42% aged < 20, 49% aged 20–29, 9% aged 30+; 67% parity 0; 45% married or cohabiting	25[r]	Australian Family Survey; first use of method
Schirm et al., 1982		4,487	2.4[s]				Aged 15–44; all married[t]	18.2[r]	NSFG 1973 and 1976
Grady et al., 1983		4,487	2.5[c,s]				Aged 15–44; all married[t]	18.2[r]	NSFG 1973 and 1976
Bounds et al., 1979	Microgynon-30	55	2.6[c]				Aged 16–39; mean age = 26; 62% used oral contraceptives as last contraceptive before study	5.5[c]	Britain; failure rate based on only 12 cycles
Grady et al., 1986		856	2.9[s]				Aged 15–44; all married[t]	20.6[r]	NSFG 1982
Jones and Forrest, 1992		3,041	5.1				Aged 15–44; all married[t]	21[r]	NSFG 1988; failure rate when standardized and corrected for estimated underreporting of abortion = 7.3[s]
Preston, 1974	Norlestrin 1.0 (40%)	313		5.80[c]	1,570 Cy.	?		?	Author employed by manufacturer; pill not marketed

(continued)

Table 27-11   **677**

Table 27-11 Summary of studies of contraceptive failure: combined oral contraceptives[a] *(cont.)*

Reference	Method Brand	N for Analysis	Failure Rate				Characteristics of the Sample	LFU[g]	Comments
			Life-Table 12-Month Failure Rate	Pearl Index					
				Index	Total Exposure	Maximum Exposure			
Bounds et al., 1979	Loestrin-20	55	5.9 [c]				Aged 16–39; mean age = 26; 65% used oral contraceptives as last contraceptive before study	5.5 [c]	Britain; failure rate based on only 12 cycles
Preston, 1974	Norlestrin 2.5 (20%)	178		10.45 [c]	871 Cy.	?		?	Author employed by manufacturer; pill not marketed

Notes:

a Updated from Trussell and Kost (1987), Table 8.

c Calculated by James Trussell from data in the article.

g Most of these studies incorrectly report the loss to follow-up (LFU) rate as the number of women lost at any time during the study divided by the total number of women entering the study. Thus, these are the rates presented in the table. However, the correct measure of LFU would be a gross life-table rate. When available, 12-month rates are denoted by the letter "g."

r Nonresponse rate for entire survey.

s Standardized: Vaughan et al., (1977) (1973 NSFG)—intention (the average of rates for preventers and delayers); Grady et al., (1983) (1973 and 1976 NSFG)—intention. Our calculation (the average of rates for preventers and delayers); Schirm et al., (1982) (1973 and 1976 NSFG)—intention, age, and income; Grady et al., (1986) (1982 NSFG)—intention, age, poverty status, and parity; Jones and Forrest (1992) (1988 NSFG)—duration, age, marital status, and poverty status.

t Total for all methods in the study.

v The authors report that LFU for "relevant reasons (withdrawal of cooperation or loss of contact)" was 0.3% per year in the 1982 study. In the 1982 study, women had on average been followed for 9.5 years; if 0.3% are LFU per year, then 2.8% would be LFU in 9.5 years. LFU including death and emigration is about twice as high as LFU for "relevant reasons."

For table references, see reference section.

Table 27-12 Summary of studies of contraceptive failure: IUD[a]

Reference	Method Brand	N for Analysis	Life-Table 12-Month Failure Rate	Characteristics of the Sample	LFU[g]	Comments
Luukkainen et al., 1987	LNg20	1,821	0.1	15% aged 17–25, 60% aged 26–35, 25% aged 36–40; 7% parity 0, 27% parity 1, 50% parity 2, 16% parity 3+	5.7[c]	Denmark, Finland, Hungary, Norway, Sweden
Sivin et al., 1990	LNg20	1,124	0.2	Mean age = 26.6; mean parity = 2.4	5.7[g,x]	Brazil, Chile, Dominican Republic, Egypt, Singapore, United States
Sivin et al., 1990	TCu380A Slimline	698	0.3	Mean age = 28.5; mean parity = 2.7; 47.4% prior IUD use	6.0	Randomized trial of TCu380A and TCu380A Slimline. Egypt, Chile, Sweden, Dominican Republic, Brazil
Sivin et al., 1990	TCu380A	298	0.4	Mean age = 28.1; mean parity = 2.6; 49.0% prior IUD use	9.7	Randomized trial of TCu380A and TCu380A Slimline. Egypt, Chile, Sweden, Dominican Republic, Brazil
Sivin and Stern, 1979	TCu380A	3,536	0.8	72% age 20–29; 64% nulliparous	18.3[n]	
Gibor and Mitchell, 1980	Progestasert	6,261	2.0[n]	United States (51%), Canada (5%), and at least 11 other countries	?	Authors employed by manufacturer; multi-country study
Bracher and Santow, 1992		408	3.9	10% aged < 20, 68% aged 20–29, 22% aged 30+; 25% parity 0; 87% married or cohabiting	25[r]	Australian Family Survey; first use of method
Vaughan et al., 1977		576	4.2[s]	Aged 15–44; all married[t]	19.0[r]	NSFG 1973

(continued)

Table 27-12 Summary of studies of contraceptive failure: IUD[a] (cont.)

Reference	Method Brand	N for Analysis	Life-Table 12-Month Failure Rate	Characteristics of the Sample	LFU[g]	Comments
Schirm et al., 1982		1,070	4.6[s]	Aged 15–44; all married[t]	18.2[r]	NSFG 1973 and 1976
Grady et al., 1983		1,070	4.8[c,s]	Aged 15–44; all married[t]	18.2[r]	NSFG 1973 and 1976
Grady et al., 1986		235	5.9[s]	Aged 15–44; all married[t]	20.6[r]	NSFG 1982

Notes:

a Updated from Trussell and Kost (1987), Table 7.

c Calculated by James Trussell from data in the article.

g Most of these studies incorrectly report the loss to follow-up (LFU) rate as the number of women lost at any time during the study divided by the total number of women entering the study. Thus, these are the rates presented in the table. However, the correct measure of LFU would be a gross life-table rate. When available, 12-month rates are denoted by the letter "g."

n Only net rates available for this study.

r Nonresponse rate for entire survey.

s Standardized: Vaughan et al., (1977) (1973 NSFG)—intention (the average of rates for preventers and delayers); Grady et al., (1983) (1973 and 1976 NSFG)—intention. Our calculation (the average of rates for preventers and delayers); Schirm et al., (1982) (1973 and 1976 NSFG)—intention, age, and income; Grady et al., (1986) (1982 NSFG)—intention, age, poverty status, and parity.

t Total for all methods in the study.

x Irving Sivin, personal communication to James Trussell, August 13, 1992.

For table references, see reference section.

Table 27-13 Summary of studies of contraceptive failure: injectables[a]

Reference	Method Brand	N for Analysis	Life-Table 12-Month Failure Rate	Characteristics of the Sample	LFU[g]	Comments
W.H.O., 1988	Depo-Provera 25 mg + Estradiol Cypionate 5 mg (30-Day)	1,168	0.0	Aged 18–35; mean age = 26; proven fertility	11.4[g]	Egypt, Thailand, Mexico, Guatemala, Cuba, Indonesia, Pakistan, U.S.S.R., Philippines, Italy, Hungary, Chile
W.H.O., 1986	Depo-Provera 150 mg (90-Day)	607	0.0	Mean age = 27.7[t]	8.6[g]	7 developing countries
Mishell et al., 1968	Depo-Provera 150 mg (90-Day)	100	0.0[c]	59% aged 21–30	24.0[c]	Injection immediately postpartum
Howard et al., 1982	Norigest 200 mg (56-Day)	383	0.0[c]		6.5[n]	Britain
W.H.O., 1983	Depo-Provera 150 mg (90-Day)	1,587	0.1	Mean age = 27.4[t]	8.1	87% of women from 9 developing countries
W.H.O., 1988	Norigest 50 mg + Estradiol Valerate 5 mg (30-Day)	1,152	0.18	Aged 18–35; mean age = 26.7; proven fertility	10.5[g]	Egypt, Thailand, Mexico, Guatemala, Cuba, Indonesia, Pakistan, U.S.S.R., Philippines, Italy, Hungary, Chile
Scutchfield et al., 1971	Depo-Provera 150 mg (90-Day)	650	0.2[c]	66% aged 20–34; 50% married;	6.8[n]	
Schwallie and Assenzo, 1973	Depo-Provera 150 mg (90-Day)	3,857	0.3	86% aged 20–39	18.6	Primarily United States; also Chile, Jamaica, Mexico; authors employed by manufacturer
W.H.O., 1983	Norigest 200 mg (60-Day)	789	0.4	Mean age = 27.4[t]	7.1	87% of women from 9 developing countries
W.H.O., 1986	Depo-Provera 100 mg (90-Day)	609	0.4	Mean age = 27.7[t]	8.2[g]	7 developing countries
W.H.O., 1983	Norigest 200 mg (84-Day)	796	0.6	Mean age = 27.4[t]	7.4	87% of women from 9 developing countries

(continued)

Table 27-13 Summary of studies of contraceptive failure: injectables[a] (cont.)

Reference	Method Brand	N for Analysis	Life-Table 12-Month Failure Rate	Characteristics of the Sample	LFU [g]	Comments
W.H.O., 1977	Depo-Provera 150 mg (84-Day)	846	0.7	87% aged 20–34	6.2	10 developing countries
Schwallie and Assenzo, 1972	Depo-Provera 300 mg (180-Day)	991	2.3[n]	88% aged 20–39	28.9	United States, Chile; authors employed by manufacturer
W.H.O., 1977	Norigest 200 mg (84-Day)	832	3.6	84% aged 20–34	5.8	10 developing countries

Notes:
a Updated from Trussell and Kost (1987), Table 9.
c Calculated by James Trussell from data in the article.
g Most of these studies incorrectly report the loss to follow-up (LFU) rate as the number of women lost at any time during the study divided by the total number of women entering the study. Thus, these are the rates presented in the table. However, the correct measure of LFU would be a gross life-table rate. When available, 12-month rates are denoted by the letter "g."
n Only net rates available for this study.
t Total for all methods in the study.
For table references, see reference section.

Table 27-14 Summary of studies of contraceptive failure: Norplant[a]

Reference	Method Brand	N for Analysis	Life-Table 12-Month Failure Rate	LFU[g]	Comments
Sivin, 1992	Norplant-2 (2 Rods)	1,389	0.09[y]	1.1	Chile, Dominican Republic, Finland, Sweden, United States
Sivin, 1992	Norplant (6 Capsules)	2,470	0.09[cz]	2.1	Brazil, Chile, Denmark, Dominican Republic, Finland, Jamaica, Sweden, United States

Notes:
a Updated from Trussell and Kost (1987), Table 9.
c Calculated by James Trussell from data provided by Sivin (1992).
g Gross 12-month life-table calculation.
y Proportions failing in the second and third years are 0.37% and 0.35%, respectively.
z Three pregnancies removed because conception preceded implant; if these are included, proportion failing is 0.21%. Proportions failing in the second, third, fourth, and fifth years are 0.5%, 1.2%, 1.6%, and 0.4%, respectively (Wyeth Laboratories 1990).
For table references, see reference section.

Table 27-15 Summary of studies of contraceptive failure: female sterilization[a]

Reference	Procedure	N for Analysis	Failure Rate				Characteristics of the Sample	LFU[g]	Comments
			Life-Table 12-Month Failure Rate	Pearl Index					
				Index	Total Exposure	Maximum Exposure			
Engel, 1978	Laparoscopy	182	0.0[c]				"No failures" presumably some women followed for at least 12 months	?	
Valle and Battifora, 1978	Laparoscopy	165	0.0[c]				"Failure rate after 2 years follow-up is zero" all aged 22-38; 80% had at least 12 months follow-up	?	
Vessey et al., 1983	Procedures other than laparotomy and laparoscopy	345		0.0	331 Yr.	12 Mo.	All white; at recruitment aged 25-39 and married; at enrollment, all women had been using the diaphragm, IUD, or the pill successfully for at least 5 months	0.3[v]	Oxford/FPA study
Chi et al., 1980	Culdoscopy: Pomeroy	392	0.0				Mean age = 32[t]	?	IFRP (19 countries)
Loffer and Pent, 1977	Laparoscopy	1,717	0.0[c]	0.0[c]		≥ 6 Mo.	Duration of follow-up not reported	?	
Chi et al., 1987	Minilaparotomy: Pomeroy	445	0.0[c]				Median age = 32	31.6	IFRP (19 countries)
Bhiwandiwala et al., 1982	Rocket Clip	630	0.18[u]					42.1[c,t]	IFRP (27 countries)
Chi et al., 1980	Minilaparotomy	3,988	0.24				Mean age = 32[t]	?	IFRP (19 countries)
Bhiwandiwala et al., 1982	Electrocoagulation	6,542	0.26[u]				Mean age = 32[t]	42.1[c,t]	IFRP (27 countries)

(continued)

Table 27-15 Summary of studies of contraceptive failure: female sterilization[a] *(cont.)*

Reference	Procedure	N for Analysis	Failure Rate				Characteristics of the Sample	LFU[g]	Comments
			Life-Table 12-Month Failure Rate	Pearl Index					
				Index	Total Exposure	Maximum Exposure			
Vessey et al., 1983	Laparotomy: all procedures	743		0.28	716 Yr.	12 Mo.	All white; at recruitment aged 25–39 and married; at enrollment, all women had been using the diaphragm, IUD, or the pill successfully for at least 5 months	0.3[t,v]	Oxford/FPA study
Mumford et al., 1980	Minilaparoscopy: Pomeroy	2,022	0.3[u]					?	IFRP (23 countries)
Chi et al., 1981	Electrocoagulation	3,594	0.32[c]					?	IFRP (19 countries)
Bhiwandiwala et al., 1982	Tubal Ring	5,046	0.47[u]					42.1[c,t]	IFRP (27 countries)
Mumford et al., 1980	Minilaparoscopy: Ring	1,324	0.51[u]					?	IFRP (23 countries)
Vessey et al., 1983	Laparoscopy: Tubal Diathermy	776		0.53	755 Yr.	12 Mo.	All white; at recruitment aged 25–39 and married; at enrollment, all women had been using the diaphragm, IUD, or the pill successfully for at least 5 months	0.3[t,v]	Oxford/FPA study
Chi et al., 1981	Tubal Ring	4,106	0.54[c]					?	IFRP (19 countries)
Chi et al., 1980	Laparoscopy: Rocket Clip	457	0.59				Mean age = 32[t]	?	IFRP (19 countries)
Mumford et al., 1980	Laparoscopy: Rings	4,262	0.60[u]					?	IFRP (23 countries)

(continued)

Table 27-15 Summary of studies of contraceptive failure: female sterilization[a] *(cont.)*

Reference	Procedure	N for Analysis	Failure Rate				Characteristics of the Sample	LFU[g]	Comments
			Life-Table 12-Month Failure Rate	Pearl Index					
				Index	Total Exposure	Maximum Exposure			
Vessey et al., 1983	Laparoscopy: Rings, Clips, etc.	379		0.60	334 Yr.	12 Mo.	All white; at recruitment aged 25–39 and married; at enrollment, all women had been using the diaphragm, IUD, or the pill successfully for at least 5 months	0.3[t,v]	Oxford/FPA study
Chi et al., 1987	Minilaparotomy: Rings and Clips	1,416		0.79	1,143 Yr.	12 Mo.	Median age = 32 years	13.5	IFRP (19 countries)
Yoon et al., 1977	Falope Ring	902		1.33[c]	3,617[c] Mo.	12 Mo.		21.0[c]	
Hulka et al., 1976	Spring Clip	1,079	2.3[c]					9.5[c]	United States, UK, Jamaica, Thailand, Singapore, El Salvador (defective clips)
Chi et al., 1981	Spring Clip	1,699	4.19[c]					?	IFRP (19 countries) (defective clips)
Chi et al., 1980	Culdoscopy: Tantalum Clip	498	8.19				Mean age = 32[t]	?	IFRP (19 countries)

Notes:

[a] Updated from Trussell and Kost (1987), Table 10.

[c] Calculated by James Trussell from data in the article.

[g] Most of these studies incorrectly report the loss to follow-up (LFU) rate as the number of women lost at any time during the study divided by the total number of women entering the study. Thus, these are the rates presented in the table. However, the correct measure of LFU would be a gross life-table rate. When available, 12-month rates are denoted by the letter "g."

[t] Total for all methods in the study.

[u] Study did not report whether the cumulative life-table failure rate was net or gross.

[v] The authors report that LFU for "relevant reasons (withdrawal of cooperation or loss of contact)" was 0.3% per year in the 1983 study. In the 1983 study, women had on average probably been followed for 10 years; if 0.3% are LFU per year, then 3.0% would be LFU in 10 years. LFU including death and emigration is about twice as high as LFU for "relevant reasons."

For table references, see reference section.

Table 27-16 Summary of studies of contraceptive failure: vasectomy[a]

Reference	N for Analysis	Failure Rate				Characteristics of the Sample	LFU[g]	Comments
		Life-Table 12-Month Failure Rate	Pearl Index					
			Index	Total Exposure	Maximum Exposure			
Moss, 1992	6,220	0.0[c]					?	1 pregnancy 10 years after vasectomy
Schmidt, 1988	5,000	0.0[c]					?	Presumably 0 pregnancies
Alderman, 1988	5,331	0.0[c]				5,331 of 8,879 had at least 2 post-op semen tests	?	Canada; 4 pregnancies, 4.5–8.6 years after vasectomy
Kase and Goldfarb, 1973	500	0.0[c]				2% ≥ age 41	?	1 pregnancy 15 months after vasectomy
Vessey et al., 1982	?		0.08	2,500 Yr.	24 Mo.	Females aged 25–34; all married at recruitment	0.3[t,v]	Oxford/FPA study
Margaret Pyke Center, 1973	1,000	0.1[c]				24% ≥ age 41	?	Britain; 1 pregnancy in first year
Klapproth and Young, 1973	1,000	0.2[c]				35% ≥ age 41	10.0?	2 pregnancies, 3 and 4 months after vasectomy
Marshall and Lyon, 1972	200	0.5[c]				Aged 25–60; "majority" aged 35–39	?	1 pregnancy 3 months after vasectomy

Notes:
a Updated from Trussell and Kost (1987), Table 10.
c Calculated by James Trussell from data in the article.
g Most of these studies incorrectly report the loss to follow-up (LFU) rate as the number of women lost at any time during the study divided by the total number of women entering the study. Thus, these are the rates presented in the table. However, the correct measure of LFU would be a gross life-table rate. When available, 12-month rates are denoted by the letter "g."
t Total for all methods in the study.
v The authors report that LFU for "relevant reasons (withdrawal of cooperation or loss of contact)" was 0.3% per year in the 1982 study. In the 1982 study, women had on average been followed for 9.5 years; if 0.3% are LFU per year, then 2.8% would be LFU in 9.5 years. LFU including death and emigration is about twice as high as LFU for "relevant reasons."
For table references, see reference section.

Selected Family Planning Resources

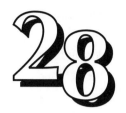

Many resources are available to family planning practitioners and clients. Although it is beyond the scope of this chapter to include the many excellent materials, the authors hope it is nonetheless helpful to provide a partial listing of educational aids.[a]

A number of organizations and associations offer an array of family planning resources such as pamphlets and fact sheets:

American College Health Association	(1-301-963-1100)
American Social Health Association	(1-800-227-8922)
Association of Reproductive Health Professionals	(1-202-466-3825)
Center for Population Options	(1-202-347-5700)
Education Training Research Associates (ETR)	(1-800-321-4407)
National Association of Nurse Practitioners in Reproductive Health	(1-202-466-4825)
Planned Parenthood Federation of America	(1-212-875-3351)
Sex Education and Information Council of the U.S. (SEICUS)	(1-212-819-9770)

---

[a] This list of resources will be maintained and updated by Bridging The Gap Communications, Inc. Call (1-800-721-6990) to request an updated list or to suggest that a resource be added.

CLIENT EDUCATION

RESOURCES BY THE AUTHORS OF THIS BOOK

Some of the authors of *Contraceptive Technology* have created resources that can be used by clients.

- "Listen carefully." This audiotape by Dr. Robert Hatcher describes how to take birth control pills, encourages condom use if needed, and describes proper condom use. Available in large numbers for your office through a local Parke Davis representative.
- "Emergency contraceptive kit." Conceived by Dr. Felicia Stewart, this kit provides instructions for how to use emergency hormonal contraceptives (postcoital pills), background information on postcoital pills, and three condoms to avert the need for postcoital pills in the future. Available in large numbers through Bridging the Gap Communications, Inc. (1-800-721-6990).
- *Understanding Your Body: Every Woman's Guide to Gynecology and Health.* Written by Stewart F, Guest F, Stewart G, Hatcher R, this reference book was published in 1987 by Bantam Books (1-800-223-5780).
- *Safely Sexual.* Written by Kowal D, Hatcher R, Trussell J, et al., this handbook will be published by Irvington Publishers, Inc. (1-800-282-5413).

Teenagers and University Students

Young clients respond best to materials tailored specifically to them. The following list contains print and video resources created by the authors of this book or their institutions to help educate and counsel teens and college students:

- "Planning for the future: Norplant, a contraceptive option for young women." In this videotape, predominantly inner-city teenagers discuss Norplant. Available through Bridging the Gap Communications, Inc. (1-800-721-6990).
- "Postponing sexual involvement: an educational series for young teens and one for pre-teens." The series contains a leader's guide and a videotape for each age group. There is also a parent series for each age group. Available through Emory/Grady Teen Services Program (1-404-616-3513).
- *Doctor, am I a Virgin Again? Cases and Counsel for a Healthy Sexuality.* This book, written by Hatcher, Dammann, and Convisser, presents anecdotes and instructions. Available through Bridging the Gap Communications, Inc. (1-800-721-6990).

- *The Quest for Excellence: From AIDS and Alcohol to Self-esteem and Healthy Sexuality.* This minibook was written by Dr. Robert Hatcher for teens. Available through Bridging the Gap Communications, Inc. (1-800-721-6990).
- *Sexual Etiquette 101.* Aimed at older teens and college students, this minibook was written by Dr. Robert Hatcher. Available through Bridging the Gap Communications, Inc. (1-800-721-6990).

PHARMACEUTICAL HOUSE RESOURCES

Do not overlook or disregard the materials offered by pharmaceutical houses. Some promote a product in addition to providing useful information. Here are just a few examples:

Written Materials

- Package inserts. Almost every contraceptive has a patient package insert. Some provide excellent information. Some are easier to read than others. All are free.
- "Today's Copper IUD." This written brochure describes the copper IUD. Contact your local GynoPharma representative, or call 1-800-322-4966. Consent forms are available in Spanish, English, and Chinese.
- "Insertion and removal and care of the diaphragm." Each pad of 50 tear-off sheets contains a fairly generic set of instructions for the diaphragm. Although produced by Koromex and Koroflex, the material could be used for other diaphragms.
- "Time to talk." This pamphlet for parents encourages dialogue between parents and children about sex. Call Organon (1-800-631-1253).

Videotapes

- "Health guide for the woman over 35 who uses oral contraception." This videotape features Dr. Art Ulene. It is produced and available from Syntex Laboratories through local representatives.
- "Menopause: modern expectations." Clients placed on Estrace may call Mead Johnson at 1-800-321-1335 for both videotape and a series of 12 monthly newsletters on ERT.
- "Norplant system." This counseling film for clients is available through Wyeth Laboratories.

RESOURCES FOR PROFESSIONALS

A great many resources are available for clinicians, counselors, and demographers. The limited lists that follow represent the array of educational materials and sources.

PERIODICALS

- "Contraceptive Technology Update," monthly newsletter (1-800-688-2421).
- "AIDS Clinical Care," monthly journal (1-800-843-6356).
- "American Journal of Public Health," monthly journal (1-202-789-5600).
- "American Journal of College Health," bimonthly journal (1-800-365-9753).
- "Clinical Proceedings," a publication of the Association of Reproductive Health Professionals (1-202-466-3825).
- "Contraception Report," free quarterly publication sponsored by a grant from Wyeth-Ayerst Laboratories (1-908-647-8080).
- "Contraception," monthly journal (1-617-438-8464).
- "Family Planning Perspectives," bimonthly journal (1-800-825-0061).
- "World Population Data Sheet," annual wall chart (1-800-877-9881).

VIDEOTAPES

- "The Emory method for rapid Norplant removal." An instructional videotape that shows how to remove Norplant implants in only a few minutes. Available through Bridging the Gap Communications, Inc. (1-800-721-6990).
- "Norplant: counseling film for clinicians, counselors and staff." Available at no cost from Wyeth Laboratories (1-800-777-6180).
- "Norplant system: insertion and removal techniques." Available from Wyeth Laboratories (1-800-777-6180).
- "Hormonal needs for the perimenopausal woman." Available through Parke Davis (1-800-722-4783).
- "Copper T 380 A ... ParaGard." This videotape is for both clients and clinicians. Available through GynoPharma (1-800-322-4966) or your GynoPharma representative.

MATERIALS IN THE PUBLIC DOMAIN

Material in the public domain clearly state that you may use them as is or adapt them for your local use. Some include excellent tables, figures, or photographs. Use of these materials may save you extensive work and financial resources. They may be copied without permission.

- Angle M, Murphy C. *Guidelines for Clinical Procedures in Family Planning. A Reference for Trainers,* 1993. Program for International Training in Health (INTRAH), University of North Carolina, 208 North Columbia, Chapel Hill, NC 27514 (1-919-966-5636).

- Centers for Disease Control and Prevention. *STD Treatment Guidelines, 1993.* Write CDC, Division of STD/HIV Prevention, 1600 Clifton Rd., NE, Atlanta 30333 (1-404-639-1819).
- Centers for Disease Control and Prevention. "Mortality and Morbidity Weekly Report." This weekly periodical covers wide range of topics from AIDS, condom use, and HPV to cancer and steroid hormones, smoking, and maternal mortality and contraceptive use by teenagers (1-202-783-3238).
- Center for Population Options. "Fact Sheets." Set of 20 updated fact sheets on subjects ranging from adolescent pregnancy, sex, and HIV to school-based health centers, condom use, and substance abuse (1-202-347-5700).
- McIntosh N, Kinzie B, Blouse A. *IUD Guidelines for Family Planning Service Programs.* A problem-solving reference manual, 1992. JHPIEGO, 550 N. Broadway St., Baltimore, MD, 21205 (1-410-955-8558).
- Population Information Program at Johns Hopkins. *Population Reports.* Monographs cover condoms, pills, Norplant, injectable contraceptives including Depo-Provera, sterilization, and STDs. Population Information Program, Johns Hopkins University, 527 St. Paul Place, Baltimore, MD 21202 (1-410-659-6300).
- American Health Consultants. Information inserts for patients in "Contraceptive Technology Update." Topics range from instructions on specific contraceptives to headaches, STDs, and menopause (1-800-688-2421 or 404-262-7436).

Reference Books

Barbach LG. *For Yourself: The Fulfillment of Female Sexuality.* Garden City NY: Anchor Press, 1976.

The Boston Women's Health Collective. *The New Our Bodies, Ourselves.* New York NY: Simon & Schuster, 1993.

Harlap S, Kost K, Forrest JD. *Preventing Pregnancy, Protecting Health: A New Look at Birth Control Choices in the United States.* New York and Washington, DC: The Alan Guttmacher Institute, 1991.

Hatcher RA, Trussell J, Stewart F, Stewart GK, Kowal D, Guest F, Cates W, Policar M. *Contraceptive Technology.* New York NY: Irvington Publishers, 1993.

Hatcher RA, Wysocki S, Kowal D, Guest FJ, Trussell J, Stewart F, Stewart GK, Cates W. *Family Planning at Your Fingertips.* Durant OK: Essential Medical Information Systems; New York NY: Irvington Publishers, 1993.

Holmes KK, Mardh PA, Sparling FP, Wiesner PJ, Cates W Jr, Lemon SM, Stamm WE (eds). *Sexually Transmitted Diseases*, 2nd ed. New York NY: McGraw-Hill, 1990.

Speroff L, Glass R, Kase NG. *Clinical Gynecologic Endocrinology and Infertility*, 3rd ed. Baltimore MD: Williams & Wilkins, 1989.

Speroff L, Darney PD. *A Clinical Guide for Contraception*. Baltimore MD: Williams & Williams, 1992.

Stamm WE, Kaetz SM, Beirne MB, Ashman JA. *The Practitioner's Handbook for the Management of STDs*. Seattle WA: Health Sciences Center for Educational Resources, 1988.

Stewart F, Guest F, Stewart GK, Hatcher, RA. *Understanding Your Body: Every Woman's Guide to Gynecology and Health*. New York NY: Bantam Books, 1987.

CONFERENCES

The authors of *Contraceptive Technology* present annual conferences based on updated information from the book:

- "Contraceptive Technology." These annual conferences are held on the East and the West coasts in March or April. Co-sponsored by Contemporary Forums and Association for Reproductive Health Professionals. All the authors of *Contraceptive Technology* will be in attendance (1-510-828-7100).

- "Quest For Excellence In Reproductive Health." This annual conference sponsored by the Department of Gynecology and Obstetrics and the Regional Training Center for Family Planning, Emory University School of Medicine, is held in Atlanta, Georgia, in the fall of each year (1-404-727-5695).

A number of other organizations also host annual conferences for family planning providers:

AIDS Training Centers. AIDS training from a nationwide system of AIDS Education Training Centers (1-301-443-6364).

ARHP. The Association of Reproductive Health Professionals hosts a range of conferences each year on subjects ranging from adolescent pregnancy and STDs to contraceptive technology and contraceptives for high-risk women (1-202-466-3825).

Planned Parenthood. National, regional, and local Planned Parenthood affiliates hold annual conferences throughout the year on an array of family planning topics (1-212-541-7800).

NFPRHS. The National Family Planning and Reproductive Health Association also holds early spring meetings in Washington, DC, for all public sector programs (1-202-628-3535).

Summer Internships

For more than 25 years, Emory University has sponsored a 10-week fellowship for the leaders of tomorrow to "sign up for life" and become involved in reproductive health issues. Applicants may be students in college, medical, or nursing school, or may be practicing nurse practitioners, physicians, health educators, or counselors. Applications must be postmarked March 1 or earlier for the next summer program. Call Maxine Keel (1-404-616-3709).

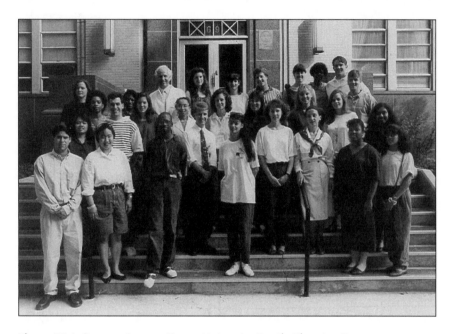

Figure 28.1 Summer interns, Emory University Family Planning Program

Left to right, Front Row: Joel Goldsmith (University of Pennsylvania '95); Maureen Park (Cornell University '94); Terrance Wade (Avondale High School '94); Brian Sullivan (Mary Washington College '93); Elizabeth Flores (Georgia State '96); Rachel Ferencik (University of North Carolina–Chapel Hill '93); Dr. Ani Shakarishvili (Tbilissi, Georgia); Felicia Brown (Longwood College '95); Priti Bhansali (University of Pennsylvania '96); Lily Wong (Cornell University '94); Elliot Austin (Cornell University '92); Eleanor Hatcher (Davidson College '95); Rashida West (Oxford of Emory University '97); Amy Lowery (University of North Carolina); Erica Shoemaker (Cornell University '94); Staci Martin (Florida State University '93); Meredith Talbot (Oberlin College '93); Arefa Mossajee (Emory University '94); Chandra Harrell (Harvard/Radcliffe '95); Malika Levy (University of Pennsylvania '95); Gwen Jackson (Crim High School '94); Dr. Robert A. Hatcher (Program Director); Anne Zweifel (University of Virginia '94); Michelle Simmons (University of Florida School of Medicine '96); Todd Warner (University of Florida School of Medicine '96); Shelley Golden (Yale University '94); Maxine Keel (Program Coordinator); Jay Marque (US Air Force Academy '94); Chad Hamilton (US Air Force Academy '94).

Table 28-1   Hotlines and "800" phone numbers

AIDS Information Hotline (CDC)	1-800-342-2437
AIDS Hotline (CDC)	1-800-227-8922
Alza Corporation	1-800-634-8977
American Health Consultants (AIDS/health newsletters)	1-800-688-2421
Ansell Laboratories NJ; institutional sales	1-800-524-1377
Apothecus: VCF film	1-800-227-2393
Bantam Books: sales	1-800-223-5780
Berlex Laboratories (pills)	1-800-237-5391
Bridging the Gap Communications, Inc.	1-800-721-6990
Burroughs Wellcome (AZT, antibiotics)	1-800-722-9292
Carter Wallace Laboratories (condoms)	1-800-833-9532
Churchill Films	1-800-334-7830
Contraceptive Technology Update	1-800-688-2421
Education Training Research Associates	1-800-321-4407
GynoPharma Inc. (Copper T 380-A)	1-800-322-4966
HIV Tel Service for Clinicians; San Fran General Hospital	1-800-933-3413
Irvington Publishers, Inc.	1-800-282-5413
Mayer Laboratories (condoms)	1-800-426-6366
Mead Johnson Drug Information (pills/ERT)	1-800-321-1335
Medical World Conferences	1-800-825-2900
Okamoto (condoms)	1-800-283-7546
Organon (pills/Time to Talk program for parents)	1-800-631-1253
Parke Davis	1-800-722-4783
Physician's World: Contraception in the '90s	1-800-223-8978
Population Reference Bureau (Population Data Sheet)	1-800-877-9881
Safetex Laboratories (condoms)	1-800-426-2092
Schmid Laboratories (condoms)	1-800-827-0987
Smart Practice (non-allergenic condoms/gloves)	1-800-522-0800
Tambrands	1-800-523-0014
Upjohn Laboratories	1-800-253-8600
Wisconsin Pharmacal (Reality Female Condom)	1-800-274-6601
Wyeth Laboratories	1-800-777-6180
Norplant Foundation for Free Norplant Implants	1-703-706-5933

Glossary

A

Abortion The expulsion or extraction of the products of conception from the uterus before the embryo or fetus is capable of independent life. Abortions may be spontaneous or induced. Spontaneous abortions are commonly called miscarriages. Induced abortions are voluntary interruptions of pregnancy or therapeutic abortions. Incomplete abortion occurs when some products of conception, usually the placenta, remain inside the uterus. Missed abortion is when the fetus has died in utero and some or all of the nonliving products of conception remain in the uterus.

Abortion rate The number of abortions per 1000 women aged 14 to 44 in a given year.

Abortion ratio The number of abortions per 1000 live births.

Abscess A localized collection of pus.

Abstinence Refraining from sexual intercourse.

Acquired immunodeficiency syndrome (AIDS) A disease defined by a set of signs and symptoms, caused by the human immunodeficiency virus (HIV), transmitted through body fluids (e.g., semen, blood) and characterized by compromised immune response.

Adenopathy Any disease of the lymph nodes or glands; swelling.

Adhesion Abnormal sticking together of body tissues, usually by bands of scar tissue which form between two tissues following inflammation.

Adolescence The transition years between puberty and adulthood; the teenage years.

Adnexa Refers to the appendages and accessory organs of the uterus, including the ligaments, ovaries, fallopian tubes, abdominal cavity.

Afterbirth The placenta and associated membranes which are expelled after delivery of an infant.

AIDS See Acquired immunodeficiency syndrome.

Age-specific fertility rate Births in a single year to 1000 women of a specific age.

Amenorrhea The absence or suppression of menstruation. This state is normal before puberty, after menopause, and during pregnancy and lactation.

Amniocentesis Removal of amniotic fluid from the uterus. This procedure may be done to determine fetal chromosomal and biochemical abnormalities, fetal maturity, or fetal sex.

Amnion The inner membrane which forms a fluid-filled sac surrounding and protecting the embryo or fetus. The amnion and the chorion together are called the fetal membranes or the bag of waters.

Ampulla The wide upper end of the vas deferens where spermatozoa are stored. Also refers to the widening of the fallopian tubes.

Androgen A natural steroid hormone found in males and females. It is responsible for producing masculine characteristics (e.g., deep voice, facial hair) by stimulating the sex organs of the male. Androgens are produced chiefly by the testes but also by the adrenal cortex and the ovary.

Anemia A reduction in the quantity of red blood cells per unit volume of blood to below normal levels.

Anorgasmia Inability to have an orgasm. Also called preorgasmia.

Anovulation Temporary or permanent cessation of ovulation.

Anteverted Tipped or tilted forward, as an anteverted uterus.

Areola Pigmented area surrounding the nipple of the breast.

Artificial insemination Introduction of semen into the uterus or oviduct by other than natural means.

Aspiration Removal of contents from a body cavity by suction.

Azoospermia Absence of living sperm in semen.

B

Bacterial vaginosis (BV) Disease of the vagina caused by infection with certain bacteria.

Band-aid surgery A tubal ligation procedure done through an incision small enough to be covered with a band-aid.

Barrier method A contraceptive method that establishes a physical barrier between the sperm and ovum, e.g., condom, diaphragm, foam, sponge, cervical cap. Some of the barrier contraceptives are used in conjunction with a spermicidal agent.

Bartholin's glands Small glands found on either side of the vaginal entrance which secrete small amounts of lubricating fluid. Also called vestibular glands.

Basal body temperature method (BBT) A method of contraception that uses daily temperature readings taken immediately after waking to identify the time of ovulation; approximately 24 hours after ovulation the BBT increases.

Biopsy Removal of tissue from a living body for diagnostic purposes.

Billings method See Periodic abstinence methods.

Bimanual examination Two-handed examination of the pelvic structures performed by inserting gloved finger(s) of one hand into the vagina and/or rectum, while pressing with the other hand on the lower abdominal wall.

Biphasic Two different phases, as in biphasic basal body temperature which shows a rise in temperature in the second half of the cycle suggesting ovulation has occurred.

Birth rate (or Crude birth rate) The number of live births per 1000 of the mid-year population in a given year. Compare with Growth rate and Death rate.

Breakthrough bleeding Bleeding at a time in the cycle other than the menstrual period. Also see Menorrhagia and Metrorrhagia.

C

Caesarean section (also Cesarean) Surgical delivery of a baby through an abdominal and uterine incision. Also called C-section.

Candida A genus of yeast-like fungi. Candida is part of the normal flora of the skin, mouth, intestinal tract, and vagina but may cause disease when it grows to outnumber the other normal flora.

Cannula A hollow tube for insertion into a body cavity.

Capacitation The process by which sperm become capable of penetrating an egg, which occurs in the female reproductive tract.

Carcinoma A new cancerous growth originating in any of the epithelial tissues of the body and characterized by invasive growth and rapid spread to other parts of the body.

Castration Removal of the gonads (testes or ovaries).

Cautery Use of heat, electricity, or chemicals to destroy abnormal or excessive tissue.

Cervical cap Small latex cap that covers the cervix. Users of this barrier method of birth control must spread spermicidal cream or jelly inside the cap.

Cervical crypts Small indentations which line the length of the cervical canal and contain mucus; may serve as a reservoir for sperm.

Cervical intraepithelial neoplasia (CIN) A sexually transmitted disease exhibiting early cancerous or precancerous changes of cervical epithelial cells.

Cervicitis Inflammation of the cervix most commonly due to infection, exposure to chemicals (e.g., spermicidal agents), foreign bodies (e.g., cervical caps, tampons), or partially expelled intrauterine devices.

Chancre The primary lesion of syphilis, which appears as a hard, painless sore or ulcer often on the penis or vaginal tissue.

Chancroid A sexually transmitted disease caused by the *Hemophilus ducreyi* bacterium and characterized by a soft sore on the genitals which becomes painful and discharges pus.

Childbearing years The reproductive age span of women, assumed for statistical purposes to be 15 to 44 years in the United States. In other countries, the range is often set at 15 to 49 years.

Chlamydia trachomatis A microorganism that can cause vaginitis, urethritis, cervicitis, pelvic inflammatory disease, and lymphogranuloma venereum (LGV). Women with positive chlamydia cultures are more likely to have the following: cervical discharge (yellow or green), erythema, ectopy, friability, and white blood cells on microscopic evaluation of cervical secretions. Also called chlamydia, mucopurulent cervicitis, and nongonococcal urethritis (in men).

Chloasma Splotchy, brownish skin discoloration associated with high estrogen levels. May affect pregnant women and oral contraceptive users. Also called mask of pregnancy.

Circumcision In males, surgical removal of the loose skin (foreskin) covering the end of the penis. Often performed shortly after birth. In females, surgical removal of part or all of the clitoris and/or labia minora.

Climacteric A prolonged period of time during which there is a decrease in estrogen production, characterized by a decrease in the frequency of ovulatory cycles and partial atrophy of secondary sexual characteristics. Within that time span, the woman stops menstruating; this event is called the menopause.

Clitoris A small, pea-sized, hooded, erectile body located on the vulva above the vagina. It is situated between the labia minora in front of the urethra. It is the anatomical homologue of the penis in the male and is highly responsive to sexual stimulation.

Cohort A group of people experiencing an event (births, marriages, etc.) at the same time who are observed through time.

Coitus Entry or penetration of the penis into the vagina. Also called intercourse or copulation.

Coitus interruptus Removing the penis from the vagina just prior to ejaculation. Also called withdrawal or pulling out.

Colposcopy Technique of visualizing the cervix and vaginal mucosa magnified 10 to 20 times normal size, making it possible to see structures invisible to the naked eye.

Colpotomy Incision through the lateral fornices or posterior fornix of the vagina into the cavity surrounding the uterus and adnexal structures.

Conception Generally the beginning of pregnancy. Conception is usually equated with the fertilization of the ovum by the sperm, but is sometimes equated with the implantation of the fertilized ovum in the uterine lining.

Condom A cylindrical sheath of latex or sheep intestine worn over the penis during intercourse as a barrier method of contraception and as a prophylactic against sexually transmitted disease. Some condoms contain a spermicide to kill sperm to decrease the risk of pregnancy should a condom break or should semen leak over the outer rim of the condom. Also called a rubber.

Condyloma Wart-like skin growth which may appear on the internal and external sex organs or anus caused by the *Condylomata acuminata,* a sexually transmitted condition caused by the human papillomavirus. *Condyloma acuminata* infections may lead to cervical, vulvar, and penile cancer. Also called venereal warts, flat condylomata, HPV warts, and papillomavirus warts.

Congenital   Existing at, or before, birth.

Contraceptive prevalence rate   A measure of the extent of contraceptive practice among a defined population group at a point in time. The numerator and denominator generally come from household surveys with the numerator consisting of the number of defined women estimated to be practicing contraception, including male-oriented methods.

Contraindication   A medical condition that renders a course of treatment (that might otherwise be recommended) inadvisable or unsafe.

Corpus luteum   Hormone-producing cells which develop from the ovarian follicle once a ripened ovum has been expelled. It produces progesterone to prepare the endometrium for implantation. During the second half of the cycle, if conception does not occur, the corpus luteum degenerates, leaving visible scars called the corpora albicans. If pregnancy does occur, the corpus luteum persists and functions through the first half of pregnancy. During pregnancy it is stimulated by human chorionic gonadotrophin (HCG).

Cowper's glands   Small glands at the base of the penis which secrete lubricating fluids into the urethra. Also called bulbourethral glands.

Crude birth rate   See Birth rate.

Cryosurgery   An operation which employs extremely decreased temperatures, achieved through liquid nitrogen or carbon dioxide, to destroy diseased tissue such as precancerous abnormalities of the cervix or vaginal walls, or warts on the vaginal walls, vulva, or cervix.

Cul-de-sac   The closed pouch located between the anterior surface of the rectum and the posterior surface of the uterus.

Culdocentesis   Aspiration of fluid from the space behind the uterus by puncture of the posterior vaginal wall or cul-de-sac.

Cunnilingus   Erotic stimulation of the female external genitalia with the tongue, lips, and mouth.

Curettage   Removal of tissue by scraping with a spoon-shaped instrument called a curette. Used to remove the endometrial lining of the uterus. (The C in D&C.)

Cyst   A walled sac containing gas, liquid, or semi-solid material.

Cystocele   Bulging of the bladder into the vagina.

Cytology   Study of cells.

Cytomegalovirus   A virus related to the herpes virus, capable of producing a sexually transmitted disease which is usually asymptomatic but may result in non-specific febrile illness, pneumonitis, hepatitis, or mononucleosis.

D

D&C   Dilation and curettage; dilation of the cervix with use of a sound or laminaria, and scraping of the uterine lining. This procedure is often used during abortion.

D&E   Dilation and evacuation; dilation of the cervix and evacuation of the uterine contents using vacuum techniques.

Death rate   See Birth rate for analogous definition.

Demographic transition   The historical shift of birth and death rates from high to low levels in a population. The decline in mortality usually precedes the decline in fertility, resulting in rapid population growth during the transition period.

Demography   The scientific study of human populations, including size and age/sex composition. Includes a study of influencing factors such as fertility, mortality, migration, nuptuality, etc.

Dependency ratio   The ratio of the economically dependent part of the population to the productive part; arbitrarily defined as the ratio of the elderly (65+ years) plus the young (15 years and younger), to the population in the working ages (15-64 years).

Depo-Provera Injectable form of medroxyprogesterone acetate; see Injectable contraceptives.

DES See Diethylstilbestrol.

Diaphragm The soft, rubber, dome-shaped device worn over the cervix and used with spermicidal jelly or cream for contraception. Diaphragms are circular, shallow, rubber domes with a firm but flexible outer rim. They fit between the posterior vaginal wall (posterior fornix) and the recess behind the pubic arch. Sizes vary from 50 to 105 mm in diameter.

Diathermy Heating of body tissues due to their resistance to the passage of high-frequency electromagnetic radiation, electric currents, or ultrasonic waves. In medical diathermy, tissues are warmed but not damaged; in surgical diathermy (electrocoagulation), tissues are destroyed.

Diethylstilbestrol (DES) A nonsteroidal synthetic estrogen provided extensively in the 1940s and 1950s to prevent miscarriages. It is not clear that DES is of any benefit in the prevention of miscarriages, and its uses for this purpose has been discontinued. Women exposed in utero to DES are at an increased risk of developing a clear cell adenocarcinoma of the vagina, miscarrying, having an ectopic pregnancy, or delivering a premature baby.

Dilation (Dilatation) To stretch beyond normal dimensions, usually in the context of the cervix. The instruments most commonly used to dilate the cervical canal are called Hegar dilators. Laminaria are also used to dilate the cervix. (The D in D&C.)

Doubling time The number of years required for a population of an area to double its present size, given the current rate of population growth. Also used to describe the rate of growth of a tumor.

Douche Cleansing the vaginal canal with a liquid; not an effective means of birth control or STD prevention.

Dysmenorrhea Painful menstruation. Usually cramping midline lower abdominal pain. May be associated with low back pain, nausea, diarrhea, or upper thigh pain.

Dyspareunia Difficult or painful sexual intercourse.

Dysplasia Abnormal development of cells or tissues. Dysplasia, as a Pap smear diagnosis, corresponds to Class III or cervical intraepithelial neoplasia (CIN).

Dysuria Painful or difficult urination.

E

Eclampsia Generalized seizure related to pregnancy occurring after the 24th week of gestation. Eclampsia is usually accompanied by high blood pressure, edema, and protein in the urine.

Ectopic Out of place; an ectopic pregnancy occurs when the embryo implants outside the uterus, usually in the fallopian tube. Much less commonly, implantation may occur in the endocervical canal, on the ovary, or within the abdominal cavity.

Edema Excessive fluid retention, swelling.

Egg An ovum; a female gamete; an oocyte; a female reproductive cell at any stage before fertilization.

Ejaculation Expulsion of semen from the penis.

Embryo The developing conceptus through the first 7 to 8 weeks of gestation, after which it is called a fetus.

Endocrine glands Ductless glands which secrete hormones into the blood stream.

Endometriosis A condition in which endometrial glands are present outside the uterus in abnormal locations such as the tubes, ovaries, peritoneal cavity and bowel; produces abnormal vaginal bleeding and dysmenorrhea. It may also produce abdominal, pelvic, or rectal pain.

Endometritis Inflammation of the endometrium or uterine lining.

Endometrium The mucous inner lining of the uterus.

Enteric infections A group of sexually transmitted diseases caused by the bacteria, viruses, protozoa, and organisms that produce intestinal disease.

Epidemic Increase in the number of cases of a disease over the expected rate of occurrence for a given population.

Epididymis A coiled tubular structure where sperm cells mature and are nourished, and which connects the testes to the vas deferens.

Episiotomy An incision in the perineum to facilitate passage of the baby's head during childbirth while minimizing injury to the woman.

Erection Hardening of the clitoris or penis caused by a rush of blood during sexual excitement.

Estrogen The primary female hormones; any natural or artificial substance that induces estrogenic activity, more specifically, the hormones estradiol and estrone produced by the ovary. Estrogens are produced chiefly by the ovary but also by the adrenal cortex and the testis.

Exocrine glands Glands which secrete substances, such as tears or saliva, through ducts to surfaces and organs. Also see Endocrine glands.

F

FDA Food and Drug Administration in the United States.

Fecundity The physiological capacity of a woman, man, or couple to produce a live child. Compare with Fertility.

Fellatio Erotic stimulation of the penis with the lips, tongue, and mouth.

Fertility The actual output of births, as opposed to the potential output.

Fertility awareness A method of birth control in which a couple charts cyclic signs of the woman's fertility and ovulation, using basal body temperature, mucus changes, and other signs to determine fertile periods.

Fetus The developing conceptus after 7 to 8 weeks postfertilization (the end of the embryonic period) until birth.

Fibroadenoma Benign breast tumor(s) consisting of proliferative ductal epithelium and fibrous stroma. Probably associated with estrogen stimulation as it occurs in young women. Increases in size are noted in pregnancy. Black women are more likely to develop this tumor and are more likely to develop it at an early age.

Fibrocystic breast disease Benign breast tumor(s) involving multiple cysts in the terminal ducts and acini of the breast. Believed to be estrogen dependent. Breast cancer is twice as common in women with some types of fibrocystic breast disease. Also known as cystic mastitis, chronic cystic breast disease, cystic hyperplasia, and cystic adenosis.

Fibroids Tumors of the muscle and connective tissues of the uterus that usually remain benign. Also called myomas (or myomata) and leiomyomas (or leiomyomata).

Fibromyoma A tumor composed of both fibrous and muscular tissue.

First trimester The first 12 weeks of pregnancy.

Follicle A small secretory sac or cavity. One type of follicle is an ovarian follicle which is a very small sac in the ovary in which an ovum matures and from which the egg is released.

Follicle stimulating hormone (FSH) Anterior pituitary hormone which stimulates the ovary to ripen egg follicles. FSH stimulates sperm production in the male testes.

Forceps Grasping instrument used to facilitate delivery or rotation of the baby's head; other forceps are used to grasp other tissues, cotton balls, intrauterine devices, etc.

Foreskin A retractable fold of skin over the head of the penis. It is removed during circumcision.

FSH See Follicle stimulating hormone.

Fundus The part of a hollow organ farthest from its opening. The fundus of the uterus is farthest from the cervix.

G

Gardnerella vaginalis See Bacterial vaginosis.

General fertility rate   The number of live births per 1000 women aged 15 to 44 years in a given year.

Gonadotropin   A substance having an affinity for, or a stimulating effect on, the gonads. There are three varieties: anterior pituitary, chorionic (from pregnant women's urine), and equine (from the serum of pregnant horses).

Gonadotropin releasing hormone (GnRH)   A hormone released from the hypothalamus that signals the pituitary gland to release the gonadotropin's luteinizing hormone (LH) and follicle stimulating hormone (FSH).

Gonads   An organ that produces sex cells (e.g., the testis and ovary).

Gonorrhea   A common sexually transmitted disease characterized by a pus-like discharge from urethra or cervix and caused by the bacterium *Neisseria gonorrhoeae*, a gram negative diplococcus. This infection has also been called GC, clap, the drip, and gonococcus.

Gossypol   A derivative of the cottonseed plant believed to induce infertility in males; being used experimentally as a male contraceptive in China. Also known to have spermicidal properties when employed as a vaginal contraceptive.

Granuloma   A growth or chronically inflamed area; usually firm, nodular, and containing macrophages.

Granuloma inguinale   A sexually transmitted disease that is characterized by single or multiple subcutaneous nodules that erode to form ulcers, caused by the bacterium *Calymmatobacterium granulomatis* (formerly called Donovania granulomatis).

Gravid   Pregnant.

Gravidity   The number of pregnancies.

Gross reproduction rate   The number of daughters that will be born to the average female who survives to age 50.

Growth rate   The rate at which a population is increasing or decreasing in a given year due to natural increase (births minus deaths) and net migration, expressed as a percentage of the base population.

H

Hematocrit   The volume percentage of red blood cells in whole blood.

Herpes   A group of contagious viral diseases which can cause sores on the mouth or the genitals.

Huhner's test   Examination of the secretions obtained from the vaginal fornix and endocervical canal after coitus to determine the number and condition of spermatozoa and the extent to which they have penetrated the cervical mucus.

Human chorionic gonadotropin (HCG)   A glycoproteinaceous hormone produced by the placenta which maintains the corpus luteum and causes it to secrete estrogen and progesterone. Measured in urine and blood to detect pregnancy.

Human immunodeficiency virus (HIV)   The virus that causes AIDS. It causes a defect in the body's immune system by invading and then multiplying within white blood cells.

Human papillomavirus (HPV)   A genus of viruses which include those causing papillomas (small nipple-like protrusions of the skin or mucous membrane) and warts in humans.

Hydrocele   Swelling of the scrotum due to fluid build-up in the sac of the membrane covering the testicle.

Hymen   A membrane that partially covers the entrance to the vagina.

Hypothalamus   Part of the brain just above the pituitary which helps to regulate basic functions such as sleep, appetite, body temperature, fertility. The hypothalamus is influenced by higher cortical levels of the brain and controls hormone production by the pituitary.

Hysterectomy   Surgical removal of the uterus.

Hysterogram   An X-ray of the uterus or record of the strength of uterine contractions.

I

Implantation   The process whereby an ovum 6 or 7 days after fertilization burrows into the lining of the uterus and attaches itself firmly. Successful implantation is essential to the development of the embryo.

Impotence   Inability to have or sustain an erection.

Infant mortality rate   The number of deaths among infants under 1 year of age in a given year per 1000 live births in that year.

Infertility   Failure, voluntary or involuntary, to produce offspring. Primary infertility: The woman has never conceived despite cohabitation, exposure to the possibility of pregnancy, and the wish to become pregnant for at least 12 months (World Health Organization definition). Secondary infertility: The woman has previously conceived but is subsequently unable to conceive despite cohabitation, exposure to the possibility of pregnancy, and the wish to become pregnant for at least 12 months (WHO).

Informed consent   Explanation to a patient of a diagnosticor therapeutic approach so that he or she may make a rational decision about it. Components of informed consent include explanation of the benefits, risks, and alternatives of an approach; the opportunity of the patient to ask questions and decide whether to proceed with the approach; detailed instructions; and documentation that those steps have been carried out.

Injectable contraceptives   Hormonal contraceptives given by injection. Two examples of injectable progestins are Depo-Provera (DMPA or medroxyprogesterone acetate), and norethindrone enanthate.

In situ   Confined to place of origin with no spread to other tissues, e.g., carcinoma in situ.

Intrauterine device (IUD)   A flexible, usually plastic device inserted into the uterus to prevent pregnancy. May contain metal (generally copper) or hormones for added effectiveness. It produces a local sterile inflammatory response caused by the presence of a foreign body in the uterus which causes lysis of the blastocyst and sperm, and/or the prevention of implantation. IUDs may also prevent fertilization due to deleterious effects on spermatozoa as they pass through the uterus.

Introitus   The opening of the vagina to the outside.

In vitro   Outside the living organism and in an artificial environment.

In vitro fertilization   A procedure in which an egg is removed from a ripe follicle and fertilized by a sperm cell outside the human body. The fertilized egg is allowed to divide in a protected environment for about 2 days and then is inserted back into the uterus of the woman.

Involution   The return of the uterus to a normal, nonpregnant size after parturition.

IUD   See Intrauterine device.

K

Kegel's exercises   Exercises designed to tighten the muscles at the opening of the vagina, usually recommended for postpartum women or treatment of urinary incontinence.

Keratinization   The formation of keratin or a horny layer.

L

Labia   A lip or lip-like structure. The labia majora are folds of skin on either side of the entrance to the vagina and are covered with hair in most adult women. The labia minora are the smaller hairless folds of tissue just within the labia majora.

Lactation   The secretion of milk. The ideal means for most women to feed their newborn infant. Breast milk transfers immunoglobulins, albumin, vitamin B^{12} binding globulin, lactobacilli, lactoferin, macrophages, neutrophils, complement, lactoglobulin, and certain medications and drugs from mother to infant. Lactation can produce anovulation.

Laminaria   A plug of sterile dried kelp (seaweed) which expands when in contact with water and can thus be placed in the cervical canal to dilate the cervix.

Laparoscopy   Surgical inspection of the abdominal cavity and pelvic structures through a narrow lighted tube.

Laparotomy   A surgical incision into the abdomen.

LH   See Luteinizing hormone.

Libido   Sexual drive.

Life expectancy   The average number of additional years a person would live if current mortality trends were to continue. Most commonly cited as life expectancy at birth.

Life table   A table showing the fraction of survivors at each age of an original birth cohort.

LMP   Last menstrual period. Often used to calculate length of pregnancy.

LRF analogs   Numerous synthetic chemical substances similar to naturally produced luteinizing hormone releasing factor (LRF), a hypothalamus-controlled secretion from the anterior pituitary gland. They are under study as contraceptives and agents to treat infertility.

Luteinizing hormone (LH)   Anterior pituitary hormone which causes a follicle to release a ripened ovum and become a corpus luteum. In the male it stimulates testosterone production and the production of sperm cells.

M

Mammary glands   Glands from which milk comes during breastfeeding.

Mammography   X-rays of the breast to detect abnormal tissue.

Marital fertility rate   Number of live births per 1000 married women aged 15 to 44 years in a given year (usually reported as rates withing specific age groups).

Mastalgia   Breast discomfort or pain; there may be accompanying breast fullness or enlargement.

Mastectomy   Surgical removal of the breast; simple mastectomy removes only breast tissue while radical mastectomy includes removal of lymph nodes and chest muscles.

Masturbation   Stimulating one's own sex organs for pleasure.

Maternal mortality ratio   The number of deaths to women due to pregnancy or childbirth complications per 100,000 live births in a given year.

Menarche   The beginning of menstruation; i.e., the first menstrual period. This occurs during puberty but may not signify the beginning of full adult fecundity because ovulation may be irregular or absent for some time. Early cycles tend to be anovulatory; however, there are reports of pregnancy prior to menarche.

Menorrhagia   Increased amount of menstrual flow, but not greater than 7 days in duration.

Menopause   Cessation of menstruation; i.e., the last episode of physiologic uterine bleeding. After the menopause a woman is permanently sterile. Surgical menopause refers to the removal of a woman's ovaries before natural menopause occurs.

Menses   Menstrual flow.

Metrorrhagia   1. Increased duration of menstrual flow beyond 7 days, or bleeding between periods. 2. Postpartum uterine hemorrhage due to insufficient contraction of the uterine muscles.

Minilaparotomy   Female sterilization procedure in which the fallopian tubes are ligated or cauterized through a small abdominal incision.

Minipill   Oral contraceptive containing no estrogen and generally less than 1 mg of a progestational agent per pill.

Miscarriage   Spontaneous abortion before the fetus is viable. Also see Abortion.

Mittelschmerz   Lower abdominal pain associated with ovulation; this pain occurs in the middle of the cycle. In a high percentage of women experiencing this symptom, it occurs just before ovulation, resulting from the LH peak-induced rise in prostaglandins which cause contractions of the fallopian tube, uterus, and/or gastrointestinal tract. The pain of mittelschmerz may also be due to a chemical peritoneal irritation caused by bleeding from the ovulation site, or it may be due to pressure as the follicle expands just prior to ovulation.

Moniliasis   Infection caused by yeast-like organisms, usually in the vagina and the vulva or under folds of skin in other areas. Usually, the organism is *Candida albicans.* Also called candidiasis, monilia, *Candida albicans,* fungus infection, and yeast. Yeast infection causes a thick, white discharge; itching, redness, or swelling around the labia; and sometimes itching and redness on the upper thighs. Some women have no symptoms at all. Men may be symptom-free or may develop urethritis, sores on the penis, or inflammation of the tip of the penis.

Monophasic   A one-level basal body temperature (BBT) curve demonstrating no rise in temperature during the menstrual cycle. Indicative of anovulation.

Morning-after birth control   A method of birth control to be used following unprotected sexual intercourse; e.g., hormones, IUDs, and prostaglandin suppositories.

Morning-after pill   A hormonal drug that temporarily disrupts the uterine environment to prevent implantation of the fertilized egg if taken within 72 hours after unprotected intercourse. Morning-after pills may also prevent ovulation.

Morning sickness   Nausea of pregnancy.

Mucus method   A method of birth control in which a couple charts the cyclic changes in cervical mucus patterns and abstains from intercourse during fertile days. Also called ovulation method or Billings method. Also see Periodic abstinence.

Multipara   A woman who has had two or more pregnancies resulting in viable fetuses.

Mycoplasma   Mycoplasma are the smallest free-living organisms, somewhere between viruses and bacteria in size. In adults most illnesses caused by mycoplasma are thought to be sexually transmitted. The two genital mycoplasmas found in the reproductive tracts of about half of all sexually active men and women, *Mycoplasma hominis* and *Ureaplasma urealyticum,* are poorly understood at present. In women, mycoplasma have been associated with vaginitis, PID, fever following abortion, fever following delivery, spontaneous abortion, low birthweight infants, infertility, pyelonephritis, and ectopic pregnancy.

Mycoses   Infections caused by fungi.

Myometrium   The muscle layer of the uterus.

N

Natural increase   The surplus or deficit of births over deaths in a population in a given time period.

Neonatal   Pertaining to the first 4 weeks after birth. Early neonatal: pertaining to the first week after birth.

Net migration rate   The number of immigrants minus the number of emigrants per 1000 base population in a given area in a given year. May be positive (net in-migration) or negative (net out-migration).

Net reproduction rate   The number of daughters who will be born to the average female in her lifetime.

Node   A small, circumscribed swelling or knot of cells.

Nongonococcal urethritis (NGU) Bacterial infection other than a gonorrheal infection, often associated with chlamydia, with manifesting symptoms of discharge, dysuria, and itching.

Nullipara   A woman who has never delivered a live infant; also written Para 0.

O

Obstetrics   That specialty of medicine caring for the management of pregnancy and its complications.

OC   See Oral contraceptive.

Oligomenorrhea Infrequent menstrual flow, with intervals between menses longer than 37 days and shorter than 90 days. Also scanty menstrual flow and irregular intervals are common.

Oophorectomy Surgical removal of one or both ovaries.

Oral contraceptives (OC) Various progestin/estrogen or progestin compounds in tablet form taken sequentially by mouth; the pill. Estrogenic and progestational agents have contraceptive effects by influencing normal patterns of ovulation, sperm or ovum transport, cervical mucus, implantation, or placental attachment.

Orgasm A series of muscular contractions in the genital and pelvic areas that occurs at the peak of sexual excitement, resulting in a release of sexual tension.

Osteoporosis An abnormal softening, porousness, or reduction in the quantity of bone, resulting in structural fragility. Causes appear to include estrogen deficiency, thyroid imbalance, calcium deficiency, prolonged immobilization, and adrenal hyperfunction, which result in more bone resorption than formation.

Ovaries The female gonads; glands where ova are formed; also the primary source of female hormones, estrogen and progesterone.

Ovulation The release of an ovum from the ovarian follicle in the ovary during the female menstrual cycle.

Ovulation method See Periodic abstinence methods.

Ovum The egg cell.

Oxytocin A hormone produced by the pituitary gland. As the baby suckles, impulses are sent to the posterior pituitary. The hormone oxytocin is released causing the milk let-down reflex. Oxytocin also causes the uterine muscles to contract.

P

Palpation Feeling with the hands to determine information about the condition of the body.

Panhysterectomy The surgical removal of the uterus, ovaries, and fallopian tubes.

Papanicolaou smear (Pap smear) A screening test for cervical cancer in which cells scraped from the surface of the cervix are placed onto a slide and examined under a microscope. The Pap test may also detect cancer of the uterus, ovary, or vagina; infections; or the level of estrogenic stimulation of the cervix.

Parity The number of live births a woman has had; a woman of zero parity has had no live births, a woman of parity one has had one live birth, etc.

Parturition The act of giving birth.

Pearl index The number of pregnancies per 100 woman-years exposure, usually used as a measure of contraceptive failure.

Pediculosis pubis Infestation of the pubic area with pubic lice. Pubic lice are parasites, small blood-sucking insects much like head lice. They are usually transmitted by sexual intimacy but may be spread by sharing clothing or a bed with an infected person. Also called crabs, papillons d'amour, and *Phthirus pubis*.

Pelvic inflammatory disease (PID) Inflammation of the pelvic structures, especially the uterus and tubes, whose precipitating or contributing cause quite often is a sexually transmitted disease, *e.g.*, gonorrhea, chlamydia, or both. Also called pelvic infection, polymicrobial pelvic infection, tubal infection, and salpingitis.

Perinatal The time period from the 28th week of pregnancy to 4 weeks after birth. May be defined as the time period from the 28th week of pregnancy to 1 week after birth.

Periodic abstinence methods Contraceptive methods that rely on timing of intercourse to avoid the ovulatory phase of a woman's menstrual cycle; also called fertility awareness or natural family planning. 1. The basal body temperature (BBT) method uses daily temperature readings to identify the time of ovulation. 2. In the ovulation or Billings method, women identify the relationships of changes in cervical mucus to fertile and infertile days. 3. The sympto-thermal method charts changes in temperature, cervical mucus, and other symptoms of ovulation (*e.g.,* intermenstrual pain).

Peritoneum   The strong, smooth membrane which surrounds and contains the abdominal organs. Often is punctured in illegal abortion procedures, resulting in infection and often death.

Pessary   A device placed in the vagina or the uterus to support pelvic structures or prevent pregnancy. The diaphragm is a modern form of a pessary. Also a medicated vaginal suppository.

Phimosis   Abnormal tightness of the foreskin, so that it can not be drawn back over the glans of the penis; also the analogous condition in the clitoris.

Pituitary gland   A small gland located at the base of the brain beneath the hypothalamus; serves as one of the chief regulators of body functions, including fertility. Most endocrine glands in the body are controlled by the pituitary. Also known as the hypophysis.

Placenta   The circular, flat, vascular structure within the pregnant uterus which provides nourishment and eliminates wastes for the developing embryo and fetus and is passed as afterbirth after the baby is born.

PMS   See Premenstrual syndrome.

POC   Progestin-only contraceptive.

Population pyramid   A special type of bar chart that shows the distribution of a population by age and sex. Most countries fall into one of three general types of pyramids: (1) Expansive: a broad base relative to the middle, indicating a high proportion of children and a rapid rate of population growth; (2) Constrictive: a base that is narrower than the middle of the pyramid, usually the result of a recent rapid decline in fertility; (3) Stationary: a pyramid with gradually declining numbers in each age group, tapering off more rapidly at the older ages, indicating a moderate propor-

tion of children and a slow or zero rate of growth.

Postpartum   After childbirth.

PPNG   Penicillinase-producing *Neisseria gonorrhoeae;* a penicillin-resistant strain of gonorrhea.

Preeclampsia   See Toxemia.

Pregnancy interval   Length of time that has elapsed between the end of one pregnancy and the end of the next, or between marriage and the end of the first pregnancy or between the end of the most recent pregnancy and the time of inquiry; normally measured in months.

Pregnancy wastage   Occurs when the woman is able to conceive but unable to produce a live birth. Pregnancy wastage occurs when pregnancy ends in miscarriage, stillbirth, or a nonsurviving premature infant.

Premature   Occurring before the proper time. A premature infant is one born before 37 weeks of gestation, or sometimes arbitrarily defined as an infant weighing 1000 to 2499 grams (2.2 to 5.5 pounds) at birth. In some countries where adults are smaller than in the United States, the upper limit is 2250 grams. Other criteria such as crown-heel length (less than 11.5 cm) have been used.

Premature ejaculation   Ejaculation which occurs too rapidly relative to a standard set by a man or his partner.

Premenstrual syndrome (PMS)   A set of physical and emotional experiences which may occur during the period prior to menses. Symptoms may include the following: breast fullness and tenderness, headache, weight gain, bloatedness, thirst, increased appetite, acne, lower back pain, cramping, lower abdominal pain, clumsiness, fear of losing control, violence, irritability, outbursts of anger, anxiety, crying, fatigue, depression, suicidal ideas, confusion, increased sexual desire, forgetfulness, mood swings, hyperactivity, and a craving for sweets, salt, and alcohol.

Prenatal   Existing or occurring before birth.

Preterm An infant born at any time before 37 to 38 weeks of gestation.

Primagravida A woman who is pregnant for the first time.

Progesterone A steroid hormone produced by the corpus luteum, adrenals, or placenta. It is responsible for changes in the uterine endometrium in the second half of the menstrual cycle which are preparatory for implantation of the fertilized ovum, development of maternal placenta after implantation, and development of mammary glands.

Progestins A large group of synthetic drugs that have a progesterone-like effect on the uterus.

Prolactin A hormone produced by the anterior lobe of the pituitary gland that stimulates milk secretion. As a baby sucks the breast, impulses are sent from the areola of the nipple to the vagus nerve and then to the anterior pituitary. The anterior pituitary secretes the hormone prolactin, which stimulates glands in the breast to produce milk. The anterior pituitary and prolactin are thought to be important in the long-term maintenance of milk secretion.

Prostaglandin Refers to a group of naturally occurring, chemically related long-chain fatty acids that have certain physiological effects (stimulate contraction of uterine and other smooth muscles, lower blood pressure, affect action of certain hormones). When prostaglandins are produced as the endometrial lining degenerates, they may cause mild to severe menstrual cramps, diarrhea, nausea, and vomiting. Oral contraceptives diminish the prostaglandins released by the endometrial lining, decreasing menstrual cramps in users.

Pruritus Itching.

Puberty The age when sex organs become functionally operative and secondary sex characteristics develop. Puberty is defined as the state or quality of being first capable of bearing offspring or the period at which sexual maturity is reached. The dictionary says the age of puberty is commonly designated legally as 14 years for boys and 12 years for girls. For a girl, puberty means producing an ovum, and for a boy it is manufacturing spermatozoa. Secondary sexual characteristics in girls include breast development, enlargement of the hips, and development of axillary and pubic hair. In boys they include appearance of pubic, facial, and axillary hair; growth of the penis, testicles and scrotum; and deepening of the voice.

Pubic lice See Pediculosis pubis.

Puerperium The 6 weeks after childbirth. Also called postpartum period.

Purulent Containing or producing pus.

R

Replacement level fertility The level of fertility at which a cohort of women on the average are having only enough daughters to replace themselves in the population. By definition, replacement level is equal to a net reproduction rate of 1.00: one daughter per woman.

Retroversion Bent backward on its vertical axis, i.e., retroverted uterus; also called tipped uterus. This is a normal variant occurring in approximately one-fifth of women.

Rhythm See Periodic abstinence.

S

Salpingectomy Surgical removal of the fallopian tubes.

Salpingitis Inflammation of one or both fallopian tubes causing lower abdominal pain, tenderness, and cervical discharge.

Scabies Contagious skin disease due to a mite which burrows beneath the skin causing intense itching. Also called mites and *Sarcoptes scabiei*.

Scrotum The external pouch containing testicles in men.

Semen The thick, whitish fluid which normally contains sperm and seminal secretions and is ejected during ejaculation.

Seminal vesicles Two glandular structures located behind the prostate gland which secrete a component of semen.

Seminiferous tubules Convoluted tubules in the testicles that produce sperm.

Sepsis (also Septicemia) The presence of various pathogenic bacteria or their toxins in the blood or tissues, resulting in chills and fever. See Toxic shock syndrome.

Sexually transmitted disease (STD) Any disease that is communicated primarily or exclusively through intimate sexual contact. Sexually transmitted diseases have been estimated to cause from 20% to 40% of infertility in the U.S. STDs can adversely affect fertility by three primary mechanisms: pregnancy wastage, prenatal deaths, and damage to male or female reproductive capacity. Also called venereal disease or VD, sexually transmitted infections, or STIs.

Sign Any objective evidence of a disease, as opposed to the subjective sensations (symptoms) perceived by the patient.

Sonogram Sound echo images of soft internal structures. Also called ultrasonography, can be used to determine size and position of the fetus, the placenta, a developing follicle, or a tumor.

Sounding Introducing an elongated probe called a sound into the uterine cavity to measure its dimensions.

Speculum An instrument for viewing the inside of the vagina and the cervix, or any other canal or cavity.

Sperm Male reproductive cell.

Spermatocele A swelling in the scrotum that occurs when the epididymis becomes cystic.

Spermatogenesis The formation of spermatozoa.

Spermicide A chemical substance that kills sperm, particularly foam, creams, jellies, and suppositories used for contraception. The spermicides used in almost all currently marketed spermicides are surfactants, surface-active compounds that destroy sperm cell membranes.

Spinnbarkeit A test to determine cervical mucus viscosity. A thread of cervical mucus is stretched between two glass slides and its length is measured. The time at which it can be drawn to maximum length (lowest viscosity) usually precedes or coincides with the time of ovulation.

Sponge The light fibrous skeleton of certain aquatic animals used as an absorbent. Natural sea sponges have been used for centuries as contraceptives. In 1983 the U.S. Food and Drug Administration approved a vaginal contraceptive sponge, the Today™ sponge, a polyurethane sponge that contains 1 gram of the spermicide nonoxynol-9. It comes in one size which is available without a prescription.

Spotting A small amount of bleeding at a time in the cycle other than menses; light irregular flow, often prolonged; the term metrorrhagia could also be used.

STD See Sexually transmitted disease.

Stable population A closed (no migration) population with an unchanging age distribution caused by unchanging age-specific fertility and mortality rates, and consequently an unchanging rate of growth.

Stationary population A stable population with a rate of growth of 0%.

Sterilization (Tubal ligation, Vasectomy) A surgical procedure which leaves the male or female incapable of reproduction. Sterilization is the most commonly employed method of birth control in the world.

Steroidogenesis The natural production of steroids. The usual progression of hormones is from progesterone and other progestins to androgens to estrogens.

Stricture Tightening or narrowing of a duct or hollow organ.

Subcutaneous Beneath the skin.

Suppository A medicine placed in a body orifice to dissolve and sometimes to be absorbed. Birth control suppositories contain spermicidal chemicals. They melt inside the vagina leaving spermicide to kill sperm.

Symptom Subjective evidence of disease or the condition of the patient.

Sympto-thermal method See Periodic abstinence methods.

Syndrome A set of symptoms which together characterize a condition or disease.

Syphilis A sexually transmitted disease caused by *Treponema pallidum*, a spirochete with 6-14 regular spirals and characteristic motility.

T

Teratogenic Tending to produce anomalies in formation, as in physical defects of the fetus in utero.

Testosterone Male sex hormone produced in the testes. Testosterone is the most potent male sex hormone.

Term An infant born any time from the beginning of the 38th week (260 days) to the end of the 41st week (287 days) of gestation.

Thyroid releasing hormone (TRH) Hypothalamic hormone which causes release of TSH, thyroid stimulating hormone, by the anterior pituitary. TRH also causes the release of prolactin.

Thyroid stimulating hormone (TSH) Anterior pituitary hormone which stimulates the thyroid gland.

Thyroid function tests Tests done to assess the function of the thyroid. Modern assessment of thyroid function is relatively easy utilizing radioimmunoassay of free T_4 (thyroxin), TSH (thyroid-stimulating hormone), and T_3 (triiodothyronine).

Total fertility rate (TFR) The average number of children that would be born alive to a woman (or group of women) during her lifetime if she were to pass through her childbearing years conforming to the age-specific fertility rates of a given year.

Toxemia A term applied to hypertension, albuminuria, and edema when found in pregnancy. The condition usually develops after the 20th week of gestation or early in the presence of trophoblastic disease. It can lead to convulsions. Also known as preeclampsia.

Toxic shock syndrome (TSS) A severe illness characterized by a sudden high fever, vomiting, diarrhea, aches, and a sunburn-like rash. The disease usually occurs in menstruating women using tampons; thought to be caused by a vaginal infection with *Staphylococcus aureus*.

Trichomoniasis Infestation of the vagina with microscopic protozoan organisms called trichomonads resulting in irritation, itching, redness, an objectionable odor, pain, frequency of urination and/or a yellow-green or a whitish-gray, foul-smelling, watery or frothy discharge.

TSS See Toxic shock syndrome.

Tubal ligation A surgical procedure in which the fallopian tubes are cut, tied, or burned to prevent the passage of ova. It does not interfere with menstruation or sexual capability but should be regarded as a permanent form of sterilization. Also called TL.

Tubal patency Unobstructed fallopian tubes.

Tubal reanastomosis A surgical procedure in which the cut ends of the fallopian tube are brought together.

U

Ureter Tube that transports urine from the kidneys to the bladder.

Urethra The tube which drains urine from the bladder to the outside of the body. In women, the opening of the urethra is between the clitoris and the vagina. In men, the urethra travels the length of the penis transporting both urine and semen.

Urinary tract infection (UTI) Infections of the urethra, bladder, ureters, or kidneys; often associated with trauma from diaphragm use, other barrier methods, and frequent intercourse. Symptoms include lower back pain and painful urination.

Uterus The hollow, pear-shaped, muscular, elastic reproductive organ where the fetus develops during pregnancy.

V

Vacuum aspiration   Removal of tissue by the creation of negative pressure through the removal of air.

Vagina   The 3- to 5-inch long muscular tube leading from the external genitals of the female to the uterus. The external opening, called the introitus, may be diminished by a membrane called the hymen. Sometimes called the birth canal, the vagina is the passageway through which babies are born and menstrual fluid flows. The vagina widens and lengthens during sexual arousal.

Vaginal hysterectomy   Surgical removal of the uterus through the vagina.

Vaginismus   Painful, spastic, usually involuntary contraction leading to constriction of the female pelvic muscles which can occur during intercourse or during a pelvic examination. It tends to occur when a woman senses that something is about to penetrate the opening of the vagina.

Vaginitis   Inflammation of the vagina. Often caused by a change in the vaginal environment by factors such as foreign bodies (tampons, cervical caps), trauma, broad spectrum antibiotics, extensive douching, IUD expulsion, certain systemic diseases, obesity, excessive moisture, tight clothing, and a number of infectious agents.

Vaginosis   See Bacterial vaginosis.

Varicocele   Dilated varicose veins in the spermatic cord. This condition usually presents as a baggy swelling of the scrotum. It may be a cause of infertility.

Vas deferens   The tube through which sperm pass from the testes to the ejacula-tory duct and then into the urethra. It is this tube which is cut in the male sterilization procedure called a vasectomy. Also called ductus deferens.

Vasectomy   A surgical procedure in which segments of the vas deferens are removed and the ends tied to prevent passage of sperm. Vasectomy should be regarded as a permanent form of sterilization although reversal is possible.

Venereal disease (VD)   See Sexually transmitted disease.

Venereal warts   See Condyloma.

Vulvovaginitis   Inflammation of both vulva and vagina.

W

Wassermann test   The original blood test for syphilis. Since the Wassermann test is not syphilis specific (other diseases can cause a positive test), newer tests for syphilis (specific for the agent *T. pallidum*) such as VDRL, FTA, and RPA, have been developed.

Withdrawal   See Coitus interruptus.

Withdrawal bleeding   Menstrual bleeding which occurs when the level of hormonal support to the endometrial lining decreases.

Y

Yeast   See Candida and Moniliasis.

Z

Zero growth   A population neither growing nor shrinking.

Zygote   The fertilized egg before it starts to divide.

Index

Adolescents, 571-600
    contraception and, 580-581, 589-
        590
    sexual behavior, 579-580
    childbearing, 584-588
    condom use, 580, 583
    intercourse, premarital, 588
    pregnancy, 574-579
Adoption, 555
Age
    contraceptive use by, 109
Age distribution, consequences of, 612-
    614, see also Population
Alcohol
    and pregnancy, 469
    and infertility, 541
Allergies, 204-206, 313
Amenorrhea (missed periods), 258-259,
    494-498
    estrogen and progestin challenge,
        496
    evaluating, 495-497
    pituitary function studies, 496-497
    postpartum
    with oral contraception, 258
    treatment, 488-490
Amniocentesis, 480
Amnio-infusion, 480
Androgens, G, see Oral contraceptives
    (OCs); and Menstrual cycle
Anemia, 365-367
Anorgasmia, G
    female, 20-22
Anovulation, G
Antibiotics
    and abortion, 482
    oral contraception and, 270-271
    prophylactic with IUDs, 361-362
Antiprostaglandin drugs, 490-491
Arcing spring diaphragm, 210
Asherman's syndrome, 351
Arthritis, 490

BRAIDED mnemonic (for informed con-
    sent counseling), 565
Bacterial vaginosis, 87-88, 206
    and Pap smears, 523
Barrier methods, 191-221, see also
    Cervical caps; Contraceptive
    sponges; Diaphragms; and Vaginal
    spermicides

advantages, 191, 201-204
cervical cap, 196, 211-204
checking supplies, 214-215
choosing method, 200-201
and CIN risk, 204
clinician's role in efficacy, 200-201
condom, 17-18, 147-177, 192-194
contraceptive sponge, 194
contraindications, 204-205
cost, 201
counseling and education, 208-212
diaphragm, 195, 209-211
differences in, 196
disadvantages, 204-207
effectiveness, 198
efficacy, 198-201, see also Failure
    rates, contraceptives
fitting, 209-212
HIV infection, 206
history, 191-192
instructions for use, 213-218
mechanism of action, 192
noncontraceptive benefit, 202
oil-based products and medications,
    209
options, 192-196
and Pap smear abnormalities, 207
and pregnancy, 207
postpartum use, 441
rules for use, 197-198
STDs, 197, 203-204
spermicides, see Vaginal spermicides
and toxic shock syndrome, 207
and urinary tract infections, 206
Basal body temperature method, 332,
    336-337, see also Menstrual cycle,
    charting
Bethesda Classification System (TBS), 518,
    520-521
Billings method, 332-333, see also
    Menstrual cycle, charting
Birth control pills, see Oral contraceptives
    (OCs)
Birth defects
    and Accutane, 256
    late fertilization, 331
    oral contraceptives, 267, 275
    spermicides, 186, 207
Bladder infections, see Cystitis; and
    Urinary tract infections
Bleeding, 259-260

Chastity, adolescent, 588-589, *see also*
    Pregnancy, adolescent
Children
    STDs in, 86
    sexual abuse, 86
Chlamydia, 90, 234, 539, *see also*
    Chlamydia trachomatis;
    Lymphogranuloma venereum;
    Mucopurulent cervicitis;
    Nongonococcal urethritis; *and* PID
Chlamydial infections
    barrier methods and, 203-204
    and infertility, 539
    oral contraception and, 234
    spermicides and, 183-185
Chlamydia trachomatis, 90, *see also*
    Chlamydia; *and* Chlamydial infec-
    tions
Chloasma, 262
    oral contraception and, 262
CIN, *see* Cervical intraepithelial neoplasia
Climacteric, *see* Menopause
Clinical problems, *see* Oral contraceptives
    (OCs)
Coil spring diaphragm, 210
Coitus interruptus (withdrawal), 18, 341-
    344
    advantages and disadvantages, 342-
    343
    effectiveness, 341-342, *see also*
    Failure rates, contraceptive
    history of, 341
    and HIV infection, 341
    instructions for use, 344
    mechanism of action, 341
Colon cancer
    and oral contraception, 277
Combination pill, 223-284, *see also* Oral
    contraceptives (OCs)
    mechanism of action, 233-234
Combined oral contraceptives, *see* Oral
    contraceptives (OCs)
Compliance, *see* specific methods
Complications, *see* specific methods
Conception, *see* Pregnancy; *and*
    Menstrual cycle, charting
Condoms, 9-10, 110-111, 145-177
    adolescents and, 583
    advantages, 161-167
    breakage, 156-159
    counseling issues, 169-180
    disadvantages, 167-168

effectiveness, 154-160
failures, 154-155, *see also* Failure
    rates, contraceptives
female, 192-194
and HIV infection, 56, 161
history of, 145
instructions for users, 171-174
and latex sensitivity, 153, 167-168
lubricants and, 158
lubricated, 152
manufacturers of, 147-148
mechanism of action, 146
natural skin, 152
noncontraceptive benefits, 160-167
and oral contraceptives, 250
postpartum use, 171
programs, 168-171
and STDs, 153, 161-167
spermicidal, 146, 181
storing, 174
synthetic, 153, 167
and teenagers, 169
testing of, 159-160
trends in use, 145
types of, 147-152, 632
use with second method, 155-156
with spermicides, 155
women and, 167, 171-172
Condyloma acuminata, *see* Warts, genital
Confidentiality, 61-64
Consent forms, 566, *see also* Chapter 23
Contraception, 107-143, 515-432, *see also*
    Contraceptives; Family planning;
    and specific methods
    after abortion, 485
    cost, 133
    efficacy, 113-123, *see also* Chapter
    27
    emergency, 415-432, *see also*
    Contraception, postcoital
    failure, 114, 117-118
    family planning and, 107
    future methods, 631-636
    in HIV-infected women, 67
    imperfect use, 119
    major health risks, 124
    male, 635, 636
    and menopause, 499
    noncontraceptive benefits of, 128-
    129
    personal considerations, 130, 133,
    134-135

sexual dysfunctions, 33-35
Cramping, *see also* Dysmenorrhea
   and IUDs, 367-368
   menstrual, 488-490
Cream, contraceptive, 180, 188, *see also*
   Vaginal spermicides
Cryosurgery, 540
Cystitis, 204, 211, 235, *see also* Urinary
   tract infection; *and* Acute urethral
   syndrome
Cysts, breast, *see* Breasts
Cysts, ovarian, 257, 506-507, *see also*
   Adnexal masses
   and minipills, 300, 316
   and Norplant, 299
   and oral contraceptives, 230
Cytopathology, *see* Cervical cytological
   screening
D&E (Dilation and evacuation), 478, *see*
   also Abortion
DES, *see* Diethylstilbestrol
Danazol, 416-417, 422
Danger (warning) signs
   Depo-Provera, 321
   in early pregnancy, 464-469
   female sterilization, 408
   IUDs, 375
   Norplant, 320
   oral contraceptives, 276
   postcoital contraception, 427
   progestin-only pills, 332
   toxic shock syndrome, 214
   vasectomy, 410
Demographic transition theory, 614-617,
   see also Population
Depo-Provera (DMPA), 285-287, 290-293,
   299, 310-314, 320-321
   age of woman, 295-296
   advantages, 294
   amenorrhea and, 293
   breastfeeding and, 294-295, 314
   bone loss, 298
   breast cancer, 310, 312
   breast tenderness, 298
   and cancer risk, 321
   continuation rates, 290
   contraindications, 311
   cost, 291
   danger signs, 321
   disadvantages, 299
   dose, 319
   and drug interactions, 313

   effect on future fertility, 311
   effectiveness, 290
   efficacy, *see* Failure rates, contracep-
     tives
   history of, 285, 310
   indications for use, 313-314
   instructions for users, 320
   lipoprotein profile, 299
   mastalgia, 298
   mechanism of action, 286
   menstrual effects, 296-297, 313
   postpartum use, 295
   problems with, 312-313
   side effects and complications, 313
   vs. Norplant, 313-314
   weight gain, 311
Depression
   oral contraception and, 234, 262-
     263, 267
Desogestrel, 225, 257
Diabetes 245, 247
   diabetes mellitus, 245
   and oral contraception, 245
   gestational, 245
Diaphragms, 209-211 *see also* Barrier
   methods
   choice of, 209
   cystitis and, 204, 211
   disinfecting fitting samples, 212
   disposable, 632
   effectiveness, 198
   efficacy of, 198-201, *see also* Failure
   rates, contraceptives
   fitting, 209-211, 213
   and HIV infection, 203-206
   history of, 191-192
   insertion of, 216
      checking position, 211, 216
   instructions for use, 213-218
   removal of, 217-218
   toxic shock syndrome and, 213
Diet
   during early pregnancy, 470
   and lactation, 446
   and PMS, 493
Diethylstilbestrol (DES), 418
Dilantin (phenytoin)
   oral contraception and, 255
Dilation and evacuation (D&E), 478 *see*
   also Abortion
Dilators, 480-481
Douching, 182, 214, 508

and PID, 508
Drug use, 52-54, *see also* Chapter 4
Drugs, interacting with oral contraception, 269, 271-272
Drugs, affecting efficacy of oral contraception, 270-271
Dysfunctions, sexual, *see* Sexual dysfunctions
Dysmenorrhea (painful menstruation), 488-490
  primary, 488
  secondary, 488
  effect of contraception, 488
  treatment, 488-490
Dyspareunia (painful intercourse), 22-24
Dysplasia, 518, *see also* Cervical cytological screening; and Abnormal Pap smears
Dysuria-pyuria syndrome, *see* Acute urethral syndrome

ELISA (enzyme linked immunosorbent assay), 58, 459
Ectopic pregnancy, *see* Pregnancy, ectopic
Education, *see* Counseling and Education
Effectiveness, of contraceptives, *see* specific methods
Efficacy, of contraceptives, 111-123, *see also* Failure rates, contraceptive
  counseling goals, 122-123
  factors influencing efficacy
    influence of investigator, 120-121
    inherent efficacy, 119
    methodological pitfalls, 121-122
    user characteristics, 119-120
  failures in a lifetime, 117
  over time, 117
  perfect use, 112-114
  typical use, 112-114
Ejaculation, 14, 25, 28-29
  delayed, 28-29
  female, 14
  premature, 25
Emergency contraception, *see also* Contraception, postcoital
  advantages, 429
  contraindications, 422
  cost, 420
  disadvantages, 422-423
  indications for use, 420-422
  instructions for use, 426-427

legal issues, 428-429
mechanism of action, 416-419
problems and follow-up, 425-426
provision of, 423-425
public policy issues, 429
side effects, 422-423
treatment methods, *see* Contraception, postcoital
Endometrial cancer, 231, 240, 292
  hormone treatment and, *see* Menopause
  and oral contraception, 240
Endometriosis, 232
  oral contraception and, 255
Epilepsy, *see* Seizure disorders
Erective difficulty, 26-28
Escherichia coli, 206
Estrogen, 224, 252-253, 255
  in combined OCs, 224, 252-253
  deficiency, and OCs, 255
  determining safety of use, 252-253
  and menopause, 499-500
  in menstrual cycle, 43
Estrogens, 224-226, 243
  actions associated with, 224
  arthrogenesis and, 237-238
  estrogen-induced thrombosis, 243
  ethinyl estradiol, 224-226
  mestranol, 224
Ethinyl estradiol, 224-226, 241
  metabolism, 224
  potency versus mestranol, 225
Ethynodiol diacetate, 225

FSH (follicle stimulating hormone), 43-44
Failure rates, contraceptive, 637-687, *see also* Chapter 27
  cervical cap, 639, 665-666
  chance, 638, 654
  combined OCs (perfect use) 641, 675-678
  continuation rates, 643, 652-653
  Depo-Provera, 642, 681-682
  diaphragm, 639, 688-670
  female condom, 641
  female sterilization, 684-686
  IUD, 642, 679-680
  male condom (perfect use), 640-641, 671-672
  minipill (progestin-only pill), 673-674
  Norplant, 642, 683

periodic abstinence (perfect use), 639, 660-663

spermicides (perfect use), 640, 655-659

sponge, 639, 667

vasectomy, 687

withdrawal, 638, 664

Family planning, *see also* Chapter 28; *and* specific subjects

and AIDS, 54-55

and contraception, 107-108

counseling and education, 559-569

current goals, 29

and infertility, 543-556

and informed consent, 564-566

and legal considerations, 564

resources, 689-696

and STDs, 80-81

and sexuality, 1

Fecundity, G, *see* Infertility

Female condoms, 632, *see also* Reality female condom; *and* Barrier methods

insertion of, 215-216

removal of, 217

Fertility, *see also* Fertility awareness; Infertility; *and* Pregnancy

demographic transition, 614-617

determinants of, 602-607

future fertility, *see* specific methods

measuring, 617-626

normal cyclic span in individual, 602

nutrition, effect on, 607

STDs, effect on, 606-606

Fertility after discontinuing contraception, *see* specific methods

Fertility awareness, 327-340, *see also* Menstrual cycle, charting

Flat spring diaphragm, 210

Fibroids, *see* Leiomyomata

Film, contraceptive, 180, 188 *see also* Vaginal spermicides

Foam, contraceptive, 180, 188 *see also* Vaginal spermicides

Follicle stimulating hormone, *see* FSH

Galactorrhea

oral contraception and, 263-264

Gallbladder disease

and oral contraception, 247

Gel, contraceptive, 180, 188 *see also* Vaginal spermicides

General Social Survey (GSS), 8

Genital ulcers, *see* Ulcers, genital

Genital warts, *see* Warts, genital

Gestodene, 225, 257

Gilbert's disease, 247

Goldman, Emma, 191

Gonadotropin releasing hormone (GNRH), 394

Gonorrhea, 92-93, 539

barrier methods and, 203-204

and infertility, 539

Granuloma inguinale, 93-94

Gross reproduction rate (GRR), 625

HCG (human chorionic gonadotropin), 46, 454-455

HDL

protective nature of

HIV infection, 51-75, *see also* AIDS; and Chapter 3

and abstinence, *see* Safer sex

adolescents, 52, 59

anal intercourse, 162

antibody testing, 59-64

charting, 63-64

clinical course, 64-65

and condoms, 56, 161-167

confidentiality and, 61-64

counseling and education, 54-59

and contraception, 56-58, 66-67

epidemic trends, 51-53

global impact, 51

infection control, 70

and injecting drug users, 52-54

and IUDs, 347, 352

medical care, 64-69

menstrual cycle, 68

minorities, 52

and oral contraceptives, 57

perinatal transmission, 68

and population growth, 68

and pregnancy, 63, 68-69

prevention, 54-59

risk assessment, 30-33, 54

safer sex options, 55

and spermicide, 56-57, 183-185

symptoms, 65

transmission, 56

and workplace safety, 69-71

HPV, *see* Human papillomavirus

HSV, *see* Herpes simplex virus

Headache

and oral contraceptives, 245

and Norplant, 302, 308
Heart disease, *see also* Cardiovascular
    disease
    and oral contraceptive use, 235-236
    and IUDs, 356
Hemophilus ducreyi, 89
Hepatic disease
    oral contraception and, 240-241,
    244
Hepatitis
    oral contraception and, 94-95
Hepatocellular adenomas (HCA), 239,
    277
Hepatocellular carcinoma (HCC), 240,
    277
    and STDs, 77
Herpes genitalis, 95-96, *see also* Herpes
    simplex virus
Herpes simplex virus (HSV), 95, 524
    and HIV infection, 68
Hirsutism
    oral contraception and, 229
History-taking, 29-35, 249, 257-268
    menstrual, *see* Menstrual problems
    and oral contraceptives, 249, 257-
    268
    sexual, 29-33
Home pregnancy tests, *see* Pregnancy,
    testing
Homosexuality, *see* Same-gender sexual
    behavior
Hormone treatment
    and amenorrhea, 497-498
    postmenopausal, 501-503
Hormones, 43-50
    levels and pregnancy, 455
    in menstrual cycle, 43-50
Human chorionic gonadotropin, *see* HCG
Human immunodeficiency virus, *see* HIV
    infection; and AIDS
Human papillomavirus (HPV), 96, 515,
    520, 540, see also Warts, genital; *and*
    Cervical intraepithelial neoplasia
    barrier methods and, 204
    and infertility, 540
Hypertension
    and oral contraception, 236, 245
Hypothalamus, 39, 47
Hypothyroidism, 496
Hysterectomy, 540

IUDs (Intrauterine devices), 347-377
    advantages, 351
    and bleeding, 365-367
    contraindications, 354-356
    cost, 350-351
    counseling and education, 364-365
    and cramping, 367-368
    danger signs, 375
    disadvantages, 351-352
    and ectopic pregnancy, 353, 356
    effectiveness, 349-350
    efficacy of, *see* Failure rates, contra-
    ceptive
    emergency contraception with, 417-
    418
    expulsion of, 352, 368-369
    finding a displaced, 371-373
    and HIV infection, 347, 352
    history of, 348
    indications for use, 351
    infections with, 374
    insertion, 353-364
        prophylactic antibiotics, 361-
        362
        technique, 358-360
        timing, 353, 356-357
    instructions for use, 374-375
    intrauterine pregnancy, 352-353
    and lactation, 362
    life span of, 348-349
    mechanism of action, 347-348
    and menstruation, 352
    noncontraceptive benefits
    nulliparous women, 361
    options, 348
    and Pap smears, 525
    and PID, 352, 373-374
    and perforation, 371-373
    and postcoital contraception, 417
    postpartum insertion, 362-363
    postplacental insertion, 362-363
    and pregnancy, 352-353, 370-371
    progestin-releasing IUD, 349, *see also*
    Progestin-only contraceptives
    removal, 364
    side effects and complications, 365-
    374
    string problems, 369-370
    termination rates, 357
    types of, 348-349
        LNG-20, 349
        ParaGard (TCu-380A), 348

Luteinizing hormone, see LH
Lymphogranuloma venereum (LGV),
   96-97

Malaria, 540
Malthus, 619
Mammography, 262
Mastalgia, 261-262, *see also* Breasts
Masturbation, 19
Mechanism of action, *see* specific
   methods
Medroxyprogesterone acetate, *see*
   Depo-Provera
Melanoma, 277
Menarche, 602
Menopause, 498-506
   abnormal bleeding, 505
   age of onset, 498
   breast cancer risk, 500
   contraception, 499
   estrogen treatment, 499-500
      alternatives to, 504
   hormone treatment
      contraindications, 501
      products and regimens, 501-503
      side effects, 501
   medical management issues, 499,
      504-505
   osteoporosis, 500
   uterine cancer risk, 500
Menstrual cycle, 39-50
   fertilization and early pregnancy,
      46-47
   follicular phase, 43-44
   and HIV infection, 68
   luteal phase, 45-46
   nonreproductive hormonal roles,
      49-50
   ovulation, 44-45
   regulation, 49
Menstrual cycle, charting, 327-340, *see*
   also Fertility awareness
   advantages, 329
   basal body temperature charting,
      332, 336-337
   and birth defects, 331
   calendar charting, 332, 335-336
   cervical mucus charting, 332-334.
      337-338
   for conception, 330, 336, 337, 339
   for contraception, 330, 336, 337,
      339

contraindications, 330
cost, 320
disadvantages, 330-331
effectiveness, 328-329, *see also*
   Failure rates, contraceptive
indications for use, 330-339
instructions, 334
mechanism of action, 328
and PMS, 330
and pregnancy, 331
sympto-thermal charting, 330-334
Menstrual effects, *see also* Menstrual
   problems; Amenorrhea;
   Dysmenorrhea; PMS; *and* specific
   methods
   of combination OCs, 229-230, 234
   of Depo-Provera, 296-297, 313
   of IUDs, 352
   of Norplant, 296-299
   of progestin-only contraceptives,
      296
   of progestin-only pills, 315-319
Menstrual problems, 487-512, *see also*
   Amenorrhea; Dysmenorrhea;
   Menstrual effects; *and* PMS
Menstruation, *see* Menstrual cycle;
   Menstrual effects; *and* Menstrual
   problems
Metabolic effects, of contraceptives, *see*
   Oral contraceptives (OCs); *and*
   Progestin-only contraceptives
Methods, *see* Contraceptives; Abortion;
   and Menstrual cycle, charting
Mifepristone, *see* RU486
Migraine headaches
   oral contraception and, 264-265
Minilaparotomy, *see* Sterilization, female
Minipills, *see* Progestin-only pills
Missed pills, impact on contraception,
   see Oral contraceptives (OCs); *and*
   Progestin-only pills
Mittelschmerz, 229, 333
Molluscum contagiosum, 97-98
Monogamy, *see* Safer sex options
Morning after contraception, *see*
   Emergency contraception; *and*
   Contraception, postcoital
Mortality, G, 607-608, *see also* Population
Morbidity, G, *see* Population
Mucopurulent cervicitis, 98
Mucus method, *see* Cervical mucus chart-
   ing; *and* Menstrual cycle, charting

and condoms, 250
continuation rates, 227
contraindications, 242-248
convenience of, 234
cost, 228, 234, 251
counseling and education, 248
danger signs, 276
and depression, 234, 262-263, 267
and diabetes, 235, 245
and diarrhea, 274
disadvantages of, 234-242
and drug interactions, 269-272
and dysmenorrhea, 488
effectiveness, 227-228, 273
efficacy, *see* Failure rates, contracep--
    tive
and endometriosis, 255
estrogen in, 224, 252
estrogenic effects of, 224, 241-242,
    254
and galactorrhea, 263-264
and gallbladder disease, 239
and HIV infection, 234
and hirsutism, 239
and headache, 234, 235, 264-265
health benefits, 232-233
and heart attack, 243
and hepatocellular adenomas, 239,
    244
and hypertension, 236, 245
indications for use, 232
infections and, 230-231, 272
and infertility, 544
instructions for users, 272-276
interactions, 268-272
and iron, 239
and lab tests, 278-279
and lactation, 246, 250
and lipids, 255-268
low-dose, 238, 251-253
and mastalgia, 261-262
mechanism of action, 223-224
medical problems, 232
and menstrual problems, 229-230
metabolic effects, 238-239, 244,
    269
    carbohydrate metabolism, 239
    glucose intolerance, 238
    liver function, 244, 269
missed pills, 274
and nausea and vomiting, 234, 266,
    274

noncontraceptive benefits, 251-254,
    272
and osteoporosis, 232
and ovarian cysts, 230
and PID, 230-231
and PMS, 230
potency, 225-227
and postcoital contraception, 232,
    416
postpartum, 250
postpill fertility, 230
potency of hormones, 255-256
and pregnancy, 266-267, 275
prescribing, 251-257
progestin in, 225
progestational effects of, 224, 242
protection against PID, 230-231
reversibility, 229-230
and STDs, 250-251
safety, 228-229
and sexual intercourse, 272
and sickle cell disease, 246
side effects, 241-242
and skin conditions, 257-258
and smoking, 248, 249-250, 276
and spotting, 254, 259-260
starting, 249
and stroke, 236
and teenagers, 250
thrombosis, 254
triphasic, 230
and vision, 263
and vomiting, 234, 274
and weight gain, 267-268
Orgasm, 13, *see also* Anorgasmia
Osteoporosis, 232
Ovarian cancer
    oral contraception and, 231
Ovarian cysts, *see* Cysts, ovarian
Ovulation, *see also* Menstrual cycle
    in-home detection tests, 334
    and menstrual cycle charting, 332-
        333
    pain at, 299
    progestin-only minipills and, 316-
        317
Ovum, viability of, *see* Infertility
Oxytocin, 481

PID (Pelvic inflammatory disease), 99-
    101, 203-204
    and diaphragms, 204

and IUDs, 352, 373-374
and oral contraceptives, 230-231
and STDs, 203-204
treatment, 100
PLISSIT model of therapy, 33-35
PMS (Premenstrual syndrome), 490-494
diagnosis, 492
effect of contraception, 494
management of, 493-494
symptoms, 492
Pap smears, 207, 249, *see also* Cervical
cytological screening
abnormalities, 207, 521-527
atypical, 525
and barrier methods, 207
false negative rate, 518
IUDs, 525
inadequate, 522
infection, 523-524
oral contraception and, 249
reporting, 518-521
specimen problems, 522
screening intervals, 517-520
Papillomavirus, G
Papovavirus, G
Paracervical block, 363-364
ParaGard IUD, 348
Partner notification, 81
Pearl index, G, 121
Pelvic inflammatory disease, *see* PID
Penile glans sensitivity, 14-15
and condoms 167
Periodic abstinence, see Menstrual cycle,
charting; and Fertility awareness
Pessary, G
Phenytoin, *see* Dilantin
Pill, the, *see* Oral contraceptives (OCs)
Pituitary gland, 39, 48, 496-497
Pomeroy technique, 388
Population, 601-629
and abortion, 606
age-specific rates, 624
and age structure, 209-614
and birth interval length, 604
breastfeeding and contraception,
effects of, 605
consequences of irregular age distribution, 612-614
crude birth rate (CBR), 618
crude death rate (CDR), 617
crude growth rate (CGR), 618
crude rate of natural increase (CRNI)

crude rates, 618, 619-624
and demographic transition, 614-617
determinants of fertility, 602-607
doubling time, 618-619
government policy, 613-614
gross reproduction rate (GRR), 625
and HIV infection, 608
life tables, 625-626
and marriage, 603-605
measuring, 617-626
migration, determinants of, 609
momentum, 610-612
mortality, determinants of, 607-698
net reproduction rate (NRR), 625
and nutrition, 607
and STDs, 606-607
total fertility rate (TFR), 624-625
Population growth, 609-614
fertility, determinants of, 602-607
migration, determinants of, 609
mortality, determinants of, 607-608
rate of, 617-626
Population, world, 620-621
Postcoital contraception, *see*
Contraception, postcoital
Postpartum contraception, *see*
Contraception, postpartum
Poxvirus, 97
Pre-ejaculate, 17
Pre-ejaculatory fluid, 17
Pregnancy, 46-47, 230, 453-471
and alcohol, 469
and cat fecal matter, 470
clinical evaluation for client, 454
counseling, 468-469
diagnosing, 454
and diet, 470
and drug use, 470
and exercise, 470
fear of, 15
and HIV infection, 68-69
hormone levels and, 455
and IUDs, 352-353, 370-371
management of early, 464-469
and oral contraceptives, 230
planning for optimal, 469-470
and STDs, 84-85, 470
and smoking, 469
and spermicides
unintended, 2, *see also* Pregnancy,
adolescent
testing, 454-464

Pregnancy, adolescent, 571-600, *see also* Pregnancy
arguments for public intervention, 573-574
and chastity, 588-589
consequences, 584-588
and contraceptive use, 580-581, 589-590
determinants, 577-578
and HIV infection, 583
and public policy, 593-596
and schools, 590-591
and sex education, 581-582
and sexual behavior, 579-580
solutions, 588-596
trends and levels in U.S., 574-575
U.S. compared with other countries, 575-577
Pregnancy, ectopic, 465-467, *see also* PID; *and* specific methods
and cramping, 465-467
Depo-Provera and, 293
diagnosis, see Pregnancy
IUD and, 353, 355
Norplant and, 293
and oral contraceptives, 231
progestin-only contraceptives, 299
progestin-only pills and, 300
and pregnancy testing, 465
and STDs, 77
and sterilization, 403
Pregnancy, testing
agglutination inhibition, 461
beta subunit radio immunoassay (RIA), 459, 461
ectopic pregnancy, 465-467
enzyme immunoassay (ELISA), 459
home pregnancy tests, 462
and hormone levels, 455-459
immunometric, 459
interpretation of tests, 562-464
types of tests, 460
Premature ejaculation, *see* Ejaculation; and Rapid ejaculation
Premenstrual syndrome, *see* PMS
Prentif cervical cap, 196, *see also* Cervical cap; *and* Barrier methods
Pritchard technique, 386
Progestasert IUD, 348, 359, *see also* IUDs; *and* Progestin-only contraceptives
Progesterone, 45-46, 633
in menstrual cycle, 45-46

Progestin, 225, *see also* Progestin-only contraceptives
in combined OCs, 225
Progestin-only contraceptives, 285-326, *see also* Depo-Provera; Norethindrone enanthate; Norplant; Progestin-only pills; *and* Vaginal rings
Progestin-only pills, 285-286, 288, 290-292, 300, 315-317, 321-322, see also Progestin-only contraceptives
advantages, 292-294
and age of woman, 295-296
and amenorrhea, 293
and back-up methods, 321
and breastfeeding, 291, 294-295, 443
choices, 315
contraindications, 316
cost, 291
danger signs, 322
delivery systems, 287
disadvantages, 285, 296-298, 300
effectiveness, 288, *see also* Failure rates, contraceptive
history of, 286
indications, 294-296
instructions for users, 321-322
mechanism of action, 286
and menstrual cycle disturbances, 296, 315-319
missed pills, 317
noncontraceptive benefits, 292-293
postpartum use, 295
reversibility, 293
and vomiting and diarrhea, 322
and weight gain, 297
Progestin-releasing IUDs, *see* Progestasert; *and* Progestin-only contraceptives
Progestins, 225-226, 256-257
new, 256-257
potency of, 225-226
Project Hope, 5, 8
Prolactin, G, 261
Prolactin secretion, 261, 264
Prostaglandin E2, 479-480
Prostaglandin inhibitors, 490-491, 494

Rh screening, 464
RU 486, 418, 479
Rape, *see* Sexual assault
Reality female condom, 192-194

insertion, 215-216
  instructions for use, 214-218
  removal, 217
Reproductive life plan, 543
Reproductive life span, 131-132
Reversibility, *see* specific methods
Rhythm method, *see* Calendar charting;
  Menstrual cycle, charting; *and*
  Fertility awareness
Rifampin, 255, 269, 271
  oral contraception and 255

SIL (squamous intraepithelial lesion),
  520, 525-528, *see also* Cervical cytological screening
STDs (Sexually transmitted diseases), *see*
  also specific diseases
  and adolescents, 582-583
  and barrier methods, 197, 203-204
  catalog of, 86-103
  and condoms, 81, 161-167
  consequences of, 77
  and contraception, 81-82
  counseling, 80, 83
  defined, 86-103
  diagnosis and treatment, 82-84
  and diaphragms, 81
  and ectopic pregnancy, 77
  and family planning, 80-81
  and infertility, 531, 535, 539-540
  IUDs and, 352, 373-374
  long-term sequelae, 77
  and oral contraceptives, 230-231,
    272
  and pregnancy, 84-85
  prevention, 79-80
  neoplastic sequelae of, 77
  Norplant and
  reporting, 82
  resources, 86
  and sexual assault and abuse, 85-86
  and spermicides, 183-185
  and tubal occlusion, 77
Safer sex
  and abstinence, 140-143
  counseling, 53-59
  monogamy, 55
  options, 55
Saline, hypertonic, 479
Same-gender sexual behavior, 8-9
Sanger, Margaret, 191

Schistosomiasis, 540
Seizure disorders
  and Depo-Provera, 294, 313
  oral contraception and, 255
Sex behaviors, 2-11, 579
Sex surveys, 3-10
Sex, *see* Sexuality; *and* Sexual intercourse
Sexual abuse, 86
Sexual assault, 85-86
Sexual dysfunctions, 19-29
  counseling and education, 33-35
  and fatigue, 20
  female, 20-25
  and history taking, 29, 20, 33
  and illness, 20, 26-27
  loss of desire, 19-20
  male, 25-29
  therapy, 33-35
Sexual expression, range of, 12, 140-141
Sexual intercourse
  age at first, 4
  anal, 3, 5, 8, 159, 162
  nonvoluntary, 10
  oral, 162
  painful, *see* Dyspareunia
  physiology, 12-19
  vaginal, 156
Sexual history taking, 29-35
Sexual risk taking, 2, 10
Sexuality, *see* also Sexual expression,
  range of; and Sexual dysfunctions
  and behavior patterns, 2-11
  female response, 13-14
  history taking, 29-35
  male response, 14-15
  physiology, 12-19
  same-gender sexual behavior, 8-9
  stages of sexual response, 13-14
  PLISSIT model of therapy, 33-35
  safer sex, 12-19
Sexually transmitted diseases, *see* STDs
Sickle cell disease, 246
Side effects, *see* specific methods
  of oral contraception, 234-242
SMOG Formula for Reading Levels, 561-
  562
Smoking
  and infertility, 541
  and oral contraceptives, 248-250,
    276
  and pregnancy, 469

Sperm, *see also* Infertility
  antibodies, and vasectomy, 384-385
Spermicidal condoms, *see* Condoms
Spermicide, *see* Vaginal spermicides
Spinnbarkeit, G
Sponge, contraceptive, *see* Contraceptive sponges; and Barrier methods
Spontaneous abortion, 331, *see also* Pregnancy
Staphylococcus aureas, 213
Sterility, 602
Sterilization, 379-414, *see also* Sterilization, female; *and* Vasectomy
  and age of client, 398
  BRAIDED mnemonic, 400
  counseling for, 398-400
  cost, 382
  effectiveness, 380-382, *see also* Failure rates, contraceptive
  and informed consent, 401
  and infertility, 545-546
  mechanism of action, 380
  permanency of, 405-407
  policy/legal issues, 400-401
  reversal of, 405-407
  vasectomy, 395-398
Sterilization, female (tubal ligation), *see also* Sterilization
  advantages, 382-383
  and anesthesia, 394-395, 402
  and cesarean section, 393
  complications, 401-404
  danger signs, 408
  disadvantages, 384
  and ectopic pregnancy, 403
  effectiveness, 380-381
  hysterectomy, 391-392, 404
  indications for use, 383
  instructions for clients, 407-409
  laparoscopy, 389-390, 402-403
  and menstruation, 404
  minilaparotomy
    subumbilical, 392
    suprapubic, 386-387
  postabortion, 392-395
  postpartum, 392-395
  and pregnancy, 403
  reversal of, 406-407
  transcervical approach, 391
  vaginal approach, 391
Sterilization, male, *see* Vasectomy

Stroke, 236, *see also* Oral contraceptives (OC)
Suppositories, spermicidal, 180, 188 *see also* Vaginal spermicides
Sympto-thermal charting (method), 333, *see also* Menstrual cycle, charting; *and* Fertility awareness
Syphilis, 101-102

TCu-380A IUD, *see* ParaGard; *and* IUDs
T-Mycoplasma, 540
Tactylon condom, 153
Teenage pregnancy rates, *see* Pregnancy, adolescent
Testosterone, 635
Thrombosis, 235-238, 243, 254
  oral contraception and, 254
  estrogen-induced thrombosis, 254
"TODAY" sponge, 194
Total contraceptive failure rate (TCFR), see Chapter 27
Total fertility rate (TFR), 62-625
Toxic shock syndrome (TSS), 207, 213-214, 507-509
  and barrier methods, 207. 508
  danger signs, 214
  and menstrual hygiene, 509
Toxoplasmosis, 540
Treponema pallidum, G, 191
Trichomonas vaginalis, G, 102
Trichomonas vaginitis, 102
Trichomoniasis, 102-103
  and barrier methods, 203-204
Triphasic pills, 251
Triphasil, 251
Tubal infertility, *see* Infertility; PID; *and* STDs
Tubal ligation, *see* Sterilization, female
Tuberculosis, 540
Tumors, breast, *see* Breasts
Tumors, liver, *see* Hepatocellular adenomas
Tumors, ovarian, *see* Cysts, ovarian; *and* Adnexal masses

Uchida technique, 386
Ulcers, genital, 206
Urea, hypertonic, 480
Urinary tract infection, 204, 206, *see also* Cystitis; and Acute urethral syndrome
  and diaphragms, 204, 211

Vaginal Contraceptive Film (VCF), 180,
188, *see also* Film, contraceptive; *and*
Vaginal rings, 634, *see also*
Progestin-only contraceptives
Vaginal spermicides, 179, 181-192, *see
also* Nonoxynol-9; *and* Barrier methods
advantages of, 179, 183-184
and birth defects, 186
common usage errors, 187-188
condoms with, 187
cost, 182
diaphragm with, 195, 216
disadvantages of, 185-186
effectiveness of, 186
failure rates, 181
and family planning, 186
and HIV infection, 183-185
inserting, 188
instructions for use, 187-188
mechanism of action, 179
and pregnancy, 186
side effects, 185-186
types of, 180-181
Vaginismus, 24-25
Vaginitis, *see* Bacterial vaginosis
Vasectomy, *see also* Sterilization
advantages of, 383
complications, 404-405
danger signs, 410
disadvantages, 384
effectiveness, 382, *see also* Failure
rates, contraceptive

instructions for clients, 409-410
long-term effects, 384-385
no-scalpel, 397-398
and pregnancy, 384
procedure, 394-397
reversal of, 407
Venereal disease (VD), *see* STDs
Venereal warts, *see* Warts, genital
Vitamin B$_6$, 262
Voluntary surgical contraception (VSC),
see Sterilization
Vulvovaginitis, *see* Bacterial vaginosis

Warts, genital, 90-92
Weight change
Depo-Provera and, 311-312
Norplant and, 297
oral contraception and, 267-268
progestin-only pills and, 297
Western blot test, 63
Wide-seal diaphragm, 210
Withdrawal method, *see* Coitus interruptus
World population, *see* Population; *and*
Population growth

Yeast infection, 184, *see also* Candidiasis;
and Candida albicans
"Yuzpe" regimen, 416, *see also*
Contraception, postcoital

IRVINGTON PUBLISHERS, INC.
522 E. 82nd Street, Suite 1
New York, New York 10028

Order Form

Description		Unit Price	Quantity	Total
Contraceptive Technology **New 16th Edition** AIDS and Abnormal Pap Smears	paper cloth	$22.95 $39.50		
Contraceptive Technology 1990-1992 15th Edition AIDS and Condoms	paper	$9.95		
Contraceptive Technology 1988-1989 14th Edition AIDS and Family Planning	paper cloth	$7.48 $17.25		
Contraceptive Technology 1986-1987 13th Edition Sexually Transmitted Diseases	paper	$7.48		
Contraceptive Technology 1984-1985 12th Edition Population and Family Planning	paper cloth	$6.47 $11.50		
Contraceptive Technology 1982-1983 11th Edition Infertility	paper cloth	$3.47 $8.47		
Contraceptive Technology 1979-1981 10th Edition Teenage Contraception	paper cloth	$2.47 $6.47		
Contraceptive Technology 1978-1979 9th Edition	paper	$2.47		
Safely Sexual *	paper cloth	$12.95 $24.95		
Family Planning At Your Fingertips	paper	$19.95		

* For **Safely Sexual**, order by MasterCard, Visa, or Purchase Order <u>only</u>.

Name

Address

City _____ State _____ Zip _____

Telephone

Method of Payment: □ Check □ Money Order
□ Purchase Order (Institutions Only) □ MasterCard □ Visa

Credit Card #:

Expiration Date____/____

Signature

Prices are subject to change without notice. All sales final. No returns.**
Contact Irvington Publishers for discount information on quantity orders.
(25 copies or more)

** Our standard returns policy applies for bookstores.

Subtotal

Add 10% for postage and handling

NY residents add sales tax (NYC 8.25%)

TOTAL DUE (US funds only)

Credit card or institutional purchase orders may be faxed 24 hours a day to (603) 669-7945, or may be placed by phone between 9:30am and 7:30pm EST at (603) 669-5933 or between 9:00am and 5:00pm EST at (800) 282-5413.

This 16th edition of Contraceptive Technology is current until publication of the 17th edition, which is scheduled for release in January 1997. Please write to Irvington Publishers to be notified of the publication of the 17th edition.

Note to Book Sellers:
Book returns require written permission from the publisher. Write to:

Irvington Publishers, Inc.
Warehouse
195 McGregor St.
Manchester, NH 03102.

Please photocopy or clip the order form on the opposite side and mail with your check, credit card information, or purchase order to:

IRVINGTON PUBLISHERS, INC.
522 E. 82nd Street, Suite 1
New York, NY 10028

Network

Organizations involved in family planning, reproductive health, and population activities

**AIDS Clinical Trials
Information Service**
P.O. Box 6421
Rockville, MD 20849-6421
800-TRIALSA [874-2572]
301-738-6616 FAX

Alan Guttmacher Institute
120 Wall Street
New York, NY 10005
212-248-1111
212-248-1951 FAX

**American Association of
Sex Educators, Counselors,
and Therapists**
435 North Michigan Avenue
Suite 1717
Chicago, IL 60611
312-644-0828
312-644-8557 FAX

**American College Health
Association**
P.O. Box 28937
Baltimore, MD 21240-8937
410-859-1500
410-859-1510 FAX

**American College of
Obstetricians and
Gynecologists**
409 12th Street, S.W.
Washington, D.C. 20024-2588
202-638-5577
202-484-5107 FAX

**American Social Health
Association**
P.O. Box 13827
Research Triangle Park,
NC 27709
919-361-8400
919-361-8425 FAX

**Association of
Reproductive Health
Professionals**
2401 Pennsylvania Avenue,
N.W., Suite 350
Washington, D.C. 20037-1718
202-466-3825
202-466-3826 FAX

**Association for Voluntary
Surgical Contraception
(AVSC)**
79 Madison Avenue
New York, NY 10016
212-561-8000
212-779-9439 FAX

Catholics for a Free Choice
1436 U Street, N.W.
Suite 301
Washington, D.C. 20009-3997
202-986-6093
202-332-7995 FAX

**CDC National AIDS
Information
Clearinghouse (CDC NAC)**
P.O.Box 6003
Rockville, MD 20849-6003
800-458-5231
TTY/TDD 800-243-7012
301-738-6616 FAX

**Center for Communications
Programs**
The Johns Hopkins University
527 St. Paul Place
Baltimore, MD 21202
301-659-6300
410-659-6300 FAX

**Centre for Development
and Population
Activities (CEDPA)**
1717 Massachusetts Avenue,
N.W., Suite 202
Washington, D.C. 20036
202-667-1142
202-332-4496 FAX

**Centers for Disease
Control and Prevention
(CDC)**
1600 Clifton Road, N.E.
Atlanta, GA 30333
404-639-3311 (Information)

**Center for Population
Options (CPO)**
1025 Vermont Avenue, N.W.
Suite 210
Washington, D.C. 20005
202-347-5700
202-347-2263 FAX

**Columbia University
Center for Population
and Family Health**
60 Haven Avenue, B-3
New York, NY 10032
212-305-6960
212-305-7024 FAX

**Committee on Population
National Research Council**
2101 Constitution Avenue
Washington, D.C. 20418
202-334-3167
202-334-3768 FAX

**Contraceptive Research
and Development
(CONRAD) Program**
1611 North Kent St., Suite 806
Arlington, VA 22209
703-524-4744
703-542-4770 FAX

**Demographic Health
Surveys Macro
International Inc.**
8850 Stanford Blvd., Suite 4000
Columbia, MD 21045
410-290-2800
410-290-2999 FAX

**East-West Program
on Population**
1777 East-West Road
Honolulu, HI 96848
808-944-7444
808-944-7490 FAX

**Education Programs
Associates (EPA)**
1 West Campbell Avenue
Building D, Room 40
Campbell, CA 95008
408-374-3720
408-374-7385 FAX

**Emory University Family
Planning Program**
Department of Gynecology
and Obstetrics
69 Butler Street, N.E.
Atlanta, GA 30303
404-616-3680
404-223-3071

**ETR (Education,Training,
Research)**
4 Carbonero Way
Scotts Valley, CA 95066
408-438-4060
408-438-4284 FAX

**Family Health
International (FHI)**
P.O.Box 13950
Research Triangle Park Branch
Research Triangle Park, NC
27709
919-544-7040

Ford Foundation
320 E. 43rd Street
New York, NY 10017
212-573-5000
212-599-4584 FAX

**Hewlett Foundation
(William and Flora)**
525 Middlefield Road
Suite 200
Menlo Park, CA 94025-3495
415-329-1070
415-329-9342 FAX

**International Planned
Parenthood Federation**
902 Broadway, 10th Floor
New York, NY 10010
212-995-8800
212-995-8853 FAX

IPAS
P.O. Box 100
Carrboro, NC 27510
919-967-7052
919-929-0258 FAX

**International Union for
the Scientific Study of
Population (IUSSP)**
Rue des Augustins, 34
4000 Liege
Belgium
32-41-22-40-80

John Snow, Inc. (JSI)
210 Lincoln Street
Boston, MA 02111
617-482-9485
617-482-0617 FAX

Johns Hopkins University
Department of Population
Dynamics
School of Hygiene and
Public Health
605 North Wolfe Street
Baltimore, MD 21205
301-995-3260
301-995-0792 FAX

**Los Angeles Regional
Family Planning Council**
3600 Wilshire Boulevard
Suite 600
Los Angeles, CA 90010
213-386-5614
213-383-4069 FAX

**National Abortion
Federation (NAF)**
1436 U Street, N.W.,
Suite 103
Washington, D.C. 20009
202-667-5881
510-642-4006 FAX

**National Association of
Nurse Practitioners
in Reproductive Health**
2401 Pennsylvania Avenue,
N.W. #350
Washington, D.C. 20037-1718
202-466-4825
202-466-3826 FAX

**National Family Planning
and Reproductive Health
Association, Inc. (NFPRHA)**
122 C Street, N.W., Suite 380
Washington, D.C. 20001-2109
202-628-3535
202-737-2690 FAX

**National Institute of
Child Health and Human
Development**
Center for Population
Research
6130 Executive Blvd.
Executive Plaza North,
Room 611
Bethesda, MD 20892
301-496-1101
301-496-0962 FAX

Northwestern University
Program for Applied Research
on Fertility Regulation
680 North Lake Shore Drive
Suite 1225
Chicago, IL 60611
312-908-6558
312-908-0014 FAX

Pathfinder Fund
9 Galen Street, Suite 217
Watertown, MA 02171-4501
617-924-7200
617-924-3833 FAX

**Planned Parenthood
of Atlanta**
100 Edgewood Avenue
Suite 1604
Atlanta, GA 30303
404-688-9300
404-688-0621 FAX

**Planned Parenthood of
Maryland**
610 N. Howard Street
Baltimore, MD 21201
301-576-1400
301-385-2762 FAX

**Planned Parenthood of
Minnesota**
1965 Ford Parkway
St. Paul, MN 55116
612-698-2401
612-698-2405 FAX

**Planned Parenthood of
the Rocky Mountains**
1537 Alton Street
Aurora, CO 80010-1712
303-360-0006
303-360-7462 FAX

**Planned Parenthood of
Sacramento Valley**
2415 "K" Street
Sacramento, CA 95816
916-446-5037
916-446-2994 FAX

**Planned Parenthood of
San Francisco-
Alameda Counties**
815 Eddy Street, Suite 300
San Francisco, CA 94109
415-441-7858
415-776-1449 FAX

**Planned Parenthood of
Seattle-King County**
2211 E. Madison
206-328-7734
206-328-7522 FAX

**Population Association
of America (PAA)**
1722 "N" Street, N.W.
Washington, D.C. 20036
202-429-0891
202-785-0146 FAX

**Population
Communication Services**
Johns Hopkins University
527 St. Paul Place
Baltimore, MD 21202
301-659-6300
410-659-6266 FAX

Population Council
1 Dag Hammarskjold Plaza,
9th Floor
New York, NY 10017
212-339-0500
212-755-6052 FAX

**Population Action
International**
1120 19th Street, N.W.
Washington, D.C. 20036-
36787
202-659-1833
202-293-1795 FAX

**Population Information
Program**
Johns Hopkins University
527 St. Paul Place
Baltimore, MD 21902
301-659-6300
410-659-6266 FAX

Population Institute
107 2nd Street, N.E.
Washington, D.C. 20002
202-544-3300
202-544-0068 FAX

**Population Reference
Bureau**
1875 Connecticut Ave, N.W.
Suite 520
Washington, D.C. 20009
202-483-1100
202-328-3837 FAX

Princeton University
Office of Population Research
21 Prospect Avenue
Princeton, NJ 08544
609-258-4870
609-258-1039 FAX